Plastic and Reconstructive Breast Surgery

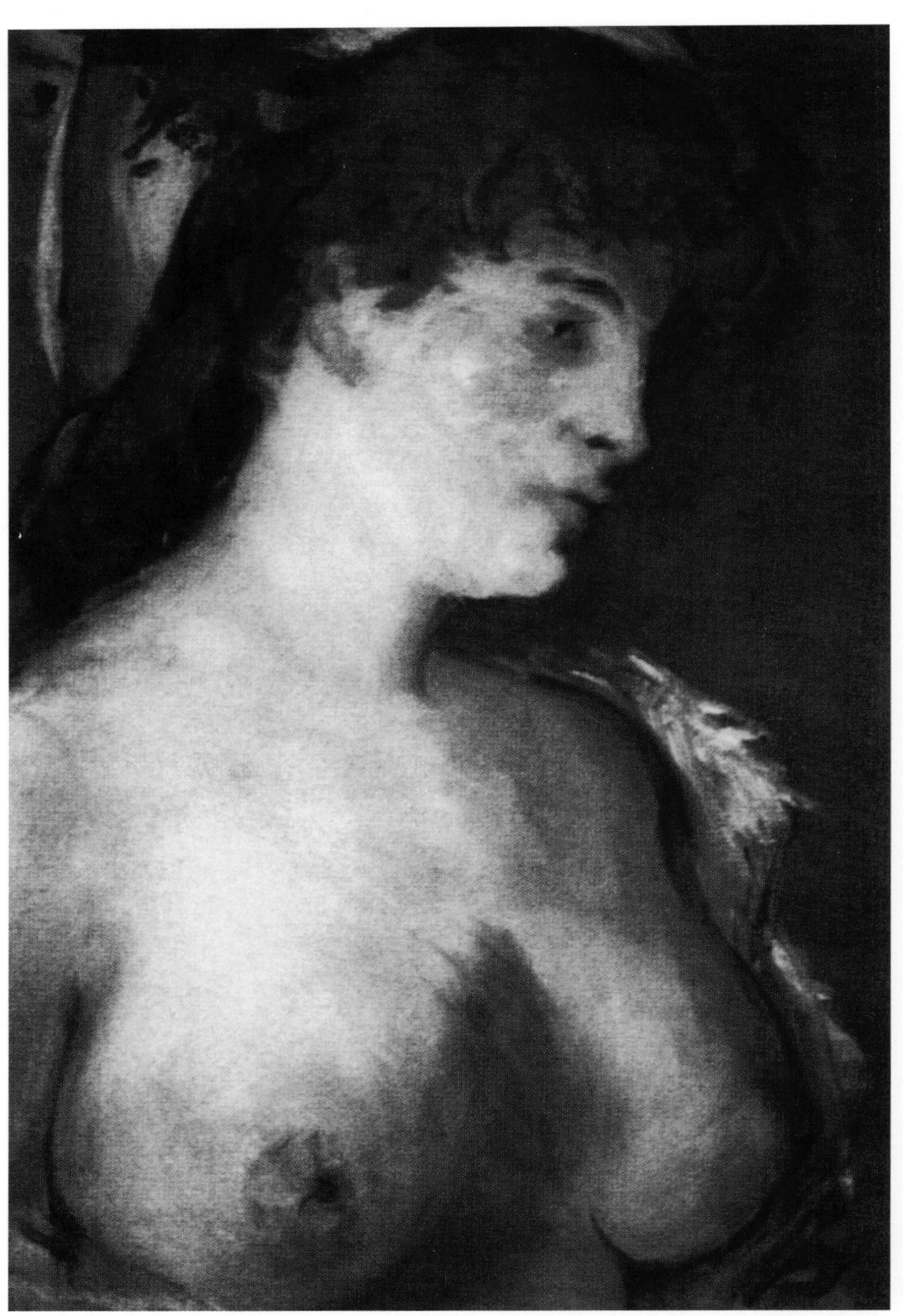

Volume I

Plastic and Reconstructive Breast Surgery

Second Edition

JOHN BOSTWICK III, M.D.

Professor and Chairman, Division of Plastic, Reconstructive, and Maxillofacial Surgery, Emory University School of Medicine, Atlanta, Georgia

ILLUSTRATORS

Alexandra W. Baker, M.S.M.I.

David L. Baker, M.A.

Kip Carter, M.S., C.M.I.

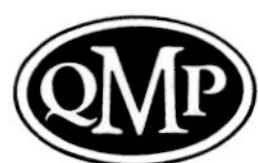

Quality Medical Publishing, Inc.

ST. LOUIS, MISSOURI

2000

Cover art: Henri Matisse, Nu bleu IV, 1952, gouache découpée. Musée Matisse, Ville de Nice. © 1999 Sucession H. Matisse, Paris/ Artists Rights Society (ARS), New York. Photograph, Maurice Bérard.

Part opener art: Henri Matisse, Nu bleu I, 1952, gouache découpée. Fondation Beyeler, Riehen/Basel. © 1999 Sucession H. Matisse, Paris/Artists Rights Society (ARS), New York.

Printed in China.

This book presents current scientific information and opinion pertinent to medical professionals. It does not provide advice concerning specific diagnosis and treatment of individual cases and is not intended for use by the layperson. The author and publisher will not be responsible or liable for actions taken as a result of the opinions expressed in this book.

PUBLISHER *Karen Berger*

PROJECT MANAGER *Carolita Deter*

PRODUCTION *Susan Trail, Carolyn Reich*

DESIGN *Diane M. Beasley, Susan Trail, David Berger*

Quality Medical Publishing, Inc.
11970 Borman Drive, Suite 222
St. Louis, Missouri 63146
Telephone: 1-800-348-7808
Web site: http://www.qmp.com

LIBRARY OF CONGRESS CATALOGING-IN-PUBLICATION DATA

Library of Congress catalog card number 99046503.

ISBN 1-57626-104-2

VT/EB/EB
5 4 3 2

To my mother

Dorothy Bostwick

who has always been there for me

Preface to the Second Edition

The marathon continues. Over the span of nine years with hundreds of miles and manuscripts completed, I am once again committed to the daunting task of translating my craft to the written word. Although the terrain is now more familiar, the challenges are still formidable and exhilarating. As in running, fresh experiences are found at every bend in the road as I encounter each new patient and as medical and scientific advances open up new horizons.

Like its predecessor, this book was born on the roads, the product of early morning musings and late night inspiration. Although totally revised and updated, this edition builds on the foundation established previously. I have attempted to retain what is still viable and valuable, replace methods outdated and abandoned, and incorporate the latest proven techniques and technology. The approach remains personal and clinical throughout.

Ultimately, the first edition of any book must be viewed as a rough draft. Despite the tremendous investment of time and energy that is requisite for any writing project, it suffers from a lack of perspective that can only be gained with time. A revision, however, gives the author a chance to step back and view his work with greater objectivity and to redefine previous practice in light of current understanding. This has been my experience in working on this new edition.

At a casual glance, the table of contents may seem all too familiar. Only one new chapter has been added; that is the one on endoscopic breast surgery. A closer look at the chapters themselves, however, will reveal both subtle and dramatic alterations. The structure remains basically the same, but the content has been refined and expanded to reflect the dynamic nature of the specialty and the natural evolution that is to be expected in a practice after nine years have elapsed.

As with the first edition, the book consists of two volumes comprising four parts. The first volume focuses on aesthetic breast surgery and the second on reconstructive surgery. Despite this arbitrary division, these topics cannot be viewed as discrete subjects. The lessons learned from one operative approach are readily applied to the other. Consequently, some topics are dealt with in several chapters. This overlap is intentional to allow the reader to explore each topic in depth without the inconvenience of paging back and forth between chapters. The preface from the first edition has also been retained to provide a sense of continuity and to remind the reader of the evolutionary process that shapes an author's task at hand.

Obviously, since breast surgery is predominantly a feminine issue, the female patient remains the focus of the book. The surgeon who operates on a woman's breasts must be sensitive to her unique psychological, social, and emotional concerns and be prepared to address her compelling demand for information. I noted in the previous edition that patients are becoming more informed and involved in their own health care; this trend has gained momentum. Today's more knowledgeable and demanding patient is often frustrated by managed health care and the new economics that has pervaded the practice of medicine. Accordingly, the surgeon operating in this milieu and treating these women must be more responsive to their needs in the face of mounting restrictions. To help the surgeon respond to the patient's desire for communication, additional information has been added throughout on patient consultation and evaluation and on frequently asked questions and answers.

Ultimately surgical judgment is the measure of the success of any operation or treatment. Thus clinical problem solving has become an even greater component of this book. Additional algorithms have been provided to guide the surgeon in assessing the various treatment options available and to determine the treatments of choice. For this reason also, the patient evaluations have been reworked to provide better insight into the factors that shape the decision-making process.

The book has grown exponentially over time as our knowledge has evolved. Many new patient examples and operative sequences have been included as have new drawings depicting the procedural steps. Patient descriptions have been more fully developed and long-term results depicted to permit readers to critically evaluate how the results of these operations endure over time and to assess problems and shortfalls. Additional features enhance the educational experience for the reader and provide direction for selecting the best operative approach for the individual patient. Surgical plans have been added for operative sequences and key points and clinical caveats have been highlighted.

Volume I on aesthetic surgery has been extensively revised to include many recent advances. The chapter on implants has been totally rewritten, expanded, and updated in light of FDA restrictions, currently available options, and patient concerns. A new chapter has been added to cover the basics of endoscopic breast surgery and specific endoscopic applications have been included in each of the clinical chapters. The chapters on reduction mammaplasty and mastopexy have grown considerably; they now include comprehensive sections on vertical incision techniques to reflect my increasing reliance on these procedures. Information on standard and ultrasound-assisted liposuction applications and limited incision techniques has been added as well as a more complete discussion of aesthetic problems, such as those related to gynecomastia and treatment of axillary and lateral fullness.

In Volume II on reconstructive surgery the increasing popularity of immediate breast reconstruction has dictated a major expansion of this chapter and of the improved options and natural results now available for women having skin-sparing mastectomy and immediate reconstruction with autologous tissue. Additionally, the chapters on latissimus dorsi, TRAM, and microsurgical flaps have been rewritten and updated to reflect new advances that promote the safety, reliability, and aesthetic potential of these flaps. Information has been added on the Rubens flap, on TRAM flap delay, on autologous and endoscopic latissimus dorsi flaps, and on nipple reconstruction techniques such as the C-V flap.

Breast cancer therapy is undergoing a transformation, as is health care in general. Today the goal of breast cancer treatment is to avoid permanent breast loss while at the same time providing optimal cancer treatment. In accordance with this widely accepted philosophy, lumpectomy with irradiation has become a viable option for most women diagnosed with early breast cancer. The plastic surgeon performing breast reconstruction has a valuable role to play in treating women with breast cancer, but this role has changed over the years. As a member of the breast cancer team, the plastic surgeon must work even more closely with oncologic surgeons and other members of the team to provide input on a range of issues that influence patient care. The best placement of incisions, the need for additional tissue to fill partial mastectomy defects, and the best reconstructive approach to follow skin-sparing or standard modified radical mastectomy surgery are all issues that must be addressed. With the increasing emphasis on immediate breast reconstruction after mastectomy and quadrantectomy, the reconstructive surgeon is often involved earlier in the process and must be able to knowledgeably address patient questions about not only reconstructive issues but also their oncologic concerns. With this in mind, the breast cancer chapter has been totally rewritten and substantially expanded to include additional information on breast cancer research, advances in genetic research and therapy, and recent developments in cancer therapy. Information is also provided in this chapter and others on reconstructive techniques that may be necessary when breast-conserving surgery is chosen, such as endoscopic harvest of latissimus muscle to supplement tissue requirements after partial mastectomy.

"In Retrospect," the final chapter of the book, reviews the many options for aesthetic and reconstructive breast surgery that have evolved over the years and assesses those that have withstood the test of time. This personal and reflective account summarizes my experience as a breast surgeon.

• • •

After 29 years, neither my passion for breast surgery nor my passion for running has diminished; if anything they have increased. Despite the forces propelling health care today, I remain encouraged by the major advances that continue to shape surgical practice and contribute to improved patient care. It is a privilege to play a small part in this process. This book remains a personal record of my ongoing fascination with the art and science of breast surgery, which is built on the contributions of my predecessors and colleagues. I hope my successors will find it a source of inspiration and innovation as they approach new challenges and seek to build their own legacy.

John Bostwick III

Preface to the First Edition

The Marathon

To the committed runner, practically nothing compares to the satisfaction derived from a long, invigorating run. Writing a book is much like running a marathon. Training, practice, and patience must be invested before entering the race; determination and endurance propel the runner across the finish line. After a hard run the marathoner checks his time to evaluate his performance. A personal record is the goal, much as it is for the breast surgeon, who must carefully assess the results of his surgery to refine and improve them.

In a marathon the runner must maintain his pace despite numerous obstacles. The writing process presents similar hurdles, highs and lows, false starts. The publisher prods and I am brought back to the realities of all too pressing deadlines. Sufficient time is never available yet excellence demands the time to focus and concentrate. The effort brings its own rewards. The ultimate "high" stems from seeing your ideas and the craft that you practice each day taking concrete shape in the form of the emerging book.

The Book

The role of author did not come easily. The ideas and concept for this book evolved during long runs on quiet roads as I reflected on the day's activities, sorted through the problems I had seen, and assessed the techniques available to correct them. A desire to share insights gleaned and lessons learned from clinical experience, building on the cumulative examples of others, was my motivation.

This book encompasses the anatomic and aesthetic principles, inherent complexities, and technical developments that shape and influence the clinical practice of plastic surgery of the breast. The casual reader may view its separate volumes as two distinct works: one aesthetic and one reconstructive. That is not my intention. Training, experience, and proficiency in both are essential to produce the best clinical results. Applications and relationships are finely drawn throughout these pages, beginning with the initial chapters in which the anatomic, aesthetic, and technical foundations of breast surgery are established, and concluding with the final chapter's retrospective review of past results in light of current knowledge. The approach reflects a personal philosophy with a strong clinical focus.

The female patient dominates this discussion, although the male surfaces briefly in the chapters on aesthetic and reconstructive problems. She is, after all, the patient at greatest risk for breast cancer and, for her, breasts have always had far greater societal and symbolic significance than their anatomy and physiology would suggest. She is also the patient who is seen most often for breast surgery. Today's patient is better informed and is often determined to play an active role in her own health care. The breast surgeon operating in this milieu must be sensitive and responsive to these issues. The key to excellent operative results lies in understanding and communicating with the patient, carefully analyzing her physical and psychological situation, identifying her expectations, and finding the means to meet them.

Personal observations based on clinical experience precede each chapter. These brief introductions highlight insights found within the chapters. Another recurring feature is "Concerns of Patient and Surgeon," which focuses on specific patient inquiries and hidden concerns about the operations under discussion. In my experience it is always better to address these concerns immediately. If the communication process is established early, many future misunderstandings and disappointments can be avoided.

Although I have attempted to eliminate unnecessary repetition, some information warrants repeating. At times topics have been reexamined for the reader's convenience to permit concentration on a particular technique or discussion without the need to frequently refer to other sections of the book. This repetition underscores the significance of these issues to the practice of breast surgery. Versatility is another recurrent theme. To individualize care we need to be well versed in and experienced with different operations. This does not mean that the newest techniques or devices should be immediately embraced and the old discarded. It is important, however, despite personal preferences, to be conversant with the possibilities and limitations of all the available options.

Because plastic surgeons and our patients judge the success of an operation visually, results and the steps taken to reach them are liberally illustrated throughout this book. Multiple patient examples demonstrate the range of problems and possibilities for surgical correction. Short- and long-term results, complications, and surgical shortcomings are also depicted.

In consideration of the patient's central role in this book, the first chapter is devoted to the dynamic interaction between the patient and surgeon. Beginning with the first patient contact, it takes the reader through the entire process from initial consultation to the development of a treatment plan. Along the way it weaves together all of the different elements—patient concerns and expectations, history-taking and physical examination, documentation, informed consent, clinical decision making, and surgical techniques—to show how they interrelate. Effective doctor-patient communication cements the process to facilitate patient satisfaction. The concerns and psychological issues addressed in the first chapter are thematic throughout the book.

Next, fundamental chapters on surgical anatomy and applied aesthetics lay the groundwork for future technique-oriented chapters. An aesthetic construct is presented and then applied to patient examples to show how these ideals can be realistically approximated.

A book about breast surgery cannot ignore the topic of breast implants and expanders; these are integral components of many aesthetic and reconstructive surgical procedures. Smooth-surface and rough-surface implants and expanders are referred to throughout this book. Correct selection and use of these devices may have a substantial impact on the patient's result and possible postoperative problems. Rod Hester has contributed his considerable expertise in this area, resulting in a chapter on implants and expanders that includes the scientific and clinical aspects of this topic, evaluates the different options available, and presents state-of-the-art applications. Not everyone will want to use polyurethane-covered implants. Discussion of these options does not imply advocacy, but represents personal clinical experience and current applications. The traditional, standard implants and expanders will continue to fill a role as promising new devices are developed.

In Part II: Aesthetic Breast Surgery the emphasis changes from fundamentals to clinical decision making and operative technique. Surgical options, planning decisions, step-by-step operative sequences, patient examples, and management of postoperative complications are considered as well as implant and expander selection, oncologic factors, preservation of function, and scar length and placement. Special aesthetic problems necessitating secondary corrections and specific deformities not easily categorized are included in the final chapter in this volume.

Part III: Reconstructive Breast Surgery focuses on the restorative aspects of breast surgery for rehabilitation after mastectomy. It presents the spectrum of operations available for breast reconstruction and the information needed to safely select and perform these procedures. It is clinical, comprehensive, and replete with specific case examples. It begins with a chapter on breast cancer written by Jack Coleman, who provides an overview of this topic. Breast cancer is a serious threat to all women, and as such it factors into the planning of any breast operation. Conscientious patient care demands knowledge of the specifics of breast cancer, avoidance of procedures that might compromise detection or treatment, and coordination with other specialists to effectively manage the breast cancer patient.

The following chapter, entitled "Decisions in Breast Reconstruction," reviews the choices facing the reconstructive breast surgeon. Flow charts trace the thought process involved in making specific technical decisions. The specifics of available tissue and tissue expansion reconstruction are discussed, as are the flap operations and the touches that artistically refine and complete the breast reconstruction. Chapters on immediate reconstruction, prophylactic mastectomy and reconstruction, and reconstruction after radiation are also included. Prophylactic mastectomy remains controversial; however, increasing patient awareness of breast cancer risks continues to make it an important component of plastic surgery of the breast and one that warrants reappraisal. The effects of radiation on reconstruction will have a growing importance as more women are selecting conservative surgery and radiation to treat their breast cancer. Similarly, immediate breast reconstruction is gaining growing acceptance among patients and surgeons; requests for this approach have increased dramatically.

Not all of the operations discussed will be embraced by each reader. All surgeons do not have a team to perform microsurgery or some of the complex flap procedures described. Others are comfortable with surgical approaches such as the latissimus dorsi flap that have proved safe and predictable over time. Knowledge of these newer techniques is nevertheless important for optimal patient counseling and individualization of care. A chapter on TRAM reconstruction includes basic operative steps as well as many of the refinements that enhance its safety and predictability. Microsurgical techniques are also detailed; they offer expanding possibilities for access to donor tissues for breast reconstruction. Foad Nahai, a master microsurgeon, has contributed a chapter on this topic. It defines the role of microsurgery in breast surgery with attention to available donor sites. "Finishing Touches" brings together a number of techniques for refining and enhancing the final breast reconstruction. Nipple-areola reconstruction, including new procedures using nonspecific tissues and medical tattoo, figures prominently.

Past experience and present knowledge meld into one in Part IV: In Retrospect. It is neither aesthetic nor reconstructive in content, yet it is both. Lessons learned in reconstructive surgery can then be applied to improve aesthetic results, and conversely aesthetic techniques can be combined with reconstructive procedures to provide superior surgical results.

• • •

The surgeon like the marathoner must constantly reassess his record and in so doing set new goals. Science is not static and the art of breast surgery is never completely mastered. This book documents but one point in the continuum. It is my personal record tracing my compelling, ongoing fascination with the craft that I practice. My goal is to add to the body of knowledge that has served us so well and to provide a vehicle for future growth and creativity.

John Bostwick III

Acknowledgments

The environment at Emory University School of Medicine has been an especially favorable milieu for plastic surgery. I have been fortunate to witness and participate in many significant developments during my residency and tenure. The Division of Plastic Surgery, established under the leadership of Dr. M.J. Jurkiewicz with the support of the late Dr. W. Dean Warren as Chairman of the Department of Surgery, was built on a firm foundation of basic surgical principles. Dr. William C. Wood carries on this tradition of strict adherence to the highest scientific standards. His expertise in surgical oncology of the breast has contributed to the outstanding patient care and breast cancer research for which this institution is known. Early investigations involving the microcirculation and experience with musculocutaneous flaps led to the first latissimus dorsi musculocutaneous island flap breast reconstruction by Dr. William Schneider, Dr. Louis Hill, and Dr. Robert Brown. Shortly thereafter Dr. Carl Hartrampf, Dr. Michael Scheflan, and Dr. Paul Black introduced the TRAM flap. The pioneering work of Dr. Foad Nahai established the inferior gluteus maximus musculocutaneous flap for free flap breast reconstruction. Dr. Jack Coleman III extended the applications of autologous tissue transfer for chest reconstruction. In more recent years, Dr. Grant Carlson has further delineated the efficacy and safety of skin-sparing mastectomy while Dr. Glyn E. Jones, Dr. Felmont F. Eaves III, and Dr. Carl Price have been at the forefront of endoscopic applications in aesthetic and reconstructive breast surgery. Dr. Jones, Dr. Nahai, Dr. Eaves, and Dr. Coleman have graciously contributed to this book and deserve special tribute for their efforts.

The surgical oncology team at Emory is unparalleled in my estimation. Dr. Waldo Powell was my mentor in this area for a number of years, providing ongoing guidance and support. He along with Dr. William C. Wood, Dr. Douglas Murray, Dr. Toncred Styblo, Dr. Roger Foster, and Dr. Grant Carlson provides the highest level of care to breast cancer patients.

The faculty of the Division of Plastic Surgery continues to maintain that the plastic surgery residents are its greatest resource, for their unique perspective will continue to push the boundaries of current practice and pave the way for new developments in plastic and reconstructive surgery.

Several have generously given their time and assistance to enable me to write this book. My associates, Dr. Jack Culbertson and Dr. Glyn Jones, have been particularly supportive and have assumed additional clinical responsibilities to allow me to devote hours to the preparation of the manuscript that I would not otherwise have had available. Mrs. Cathy McCrary and Mrs. Royce Trotman, despite their already sometimes overwhelming tasks scheduling clinical and academic activities, have cheerfully accepted the added burden that my authorship has placed on them.

The role of the medical artist is crucial to this project, as demonstrated by Kip Carter's illustrations retained from the first edition. In this edition, Alexandra W. Baker and David L. Baker have contributed their unique talents to vividly illustrate new and current techniques. Their sensibility to this subject matter greatly enhances the concepts presented here. With anatomic preciseness, these gifted artists were able to capture the essence of aesthetic and reconstructive breast surgery.

When it became apparent that this book needed a major revision, I once again looked to Karen Berger, President of Quality Medical Publishing, for guidance and support. Her expertise in medical publishing has served me well over the years, and my respect for her abilities has continued to grow. Our collaboration on *A Woman's Decision: Breast Care, Treatment, and Reconstruction* has underscored her unique and comprehensive understanding of the myriad aspects of breast cancer management and breast reconstruction, which have such an impact on the quality of life of many women. Her encouragement, advice, and input were critical to the organization, writing, and development of the current revision. She and her staff deserve my sincere appreciation for the care, attention, and unparalleled skill that have become their trademark in medical publishing.

Contents

VOLUME I

VOLUME II

Plastic and Reconstructive Breast Surgery

PART I
Fundamentals

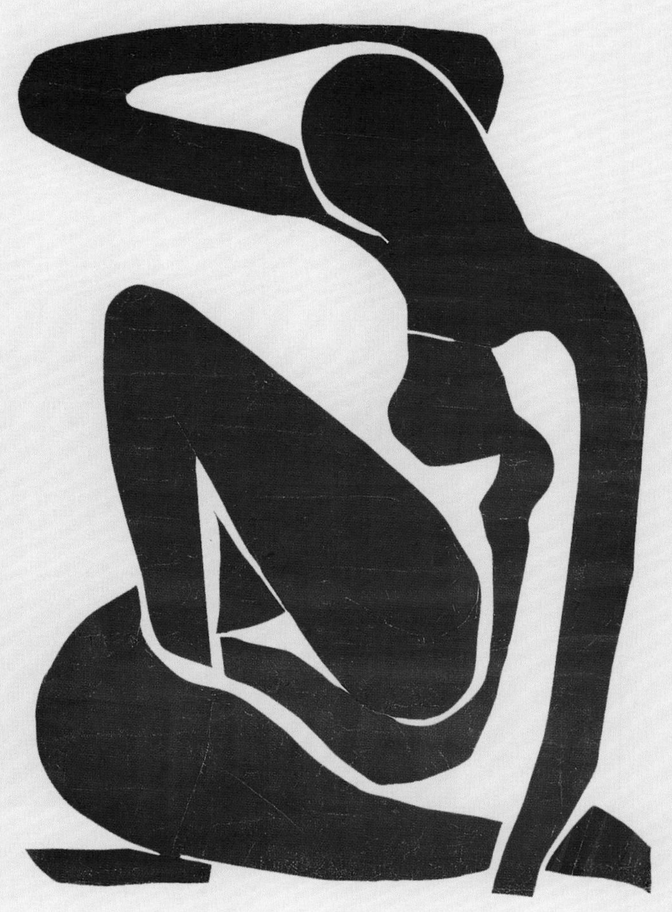

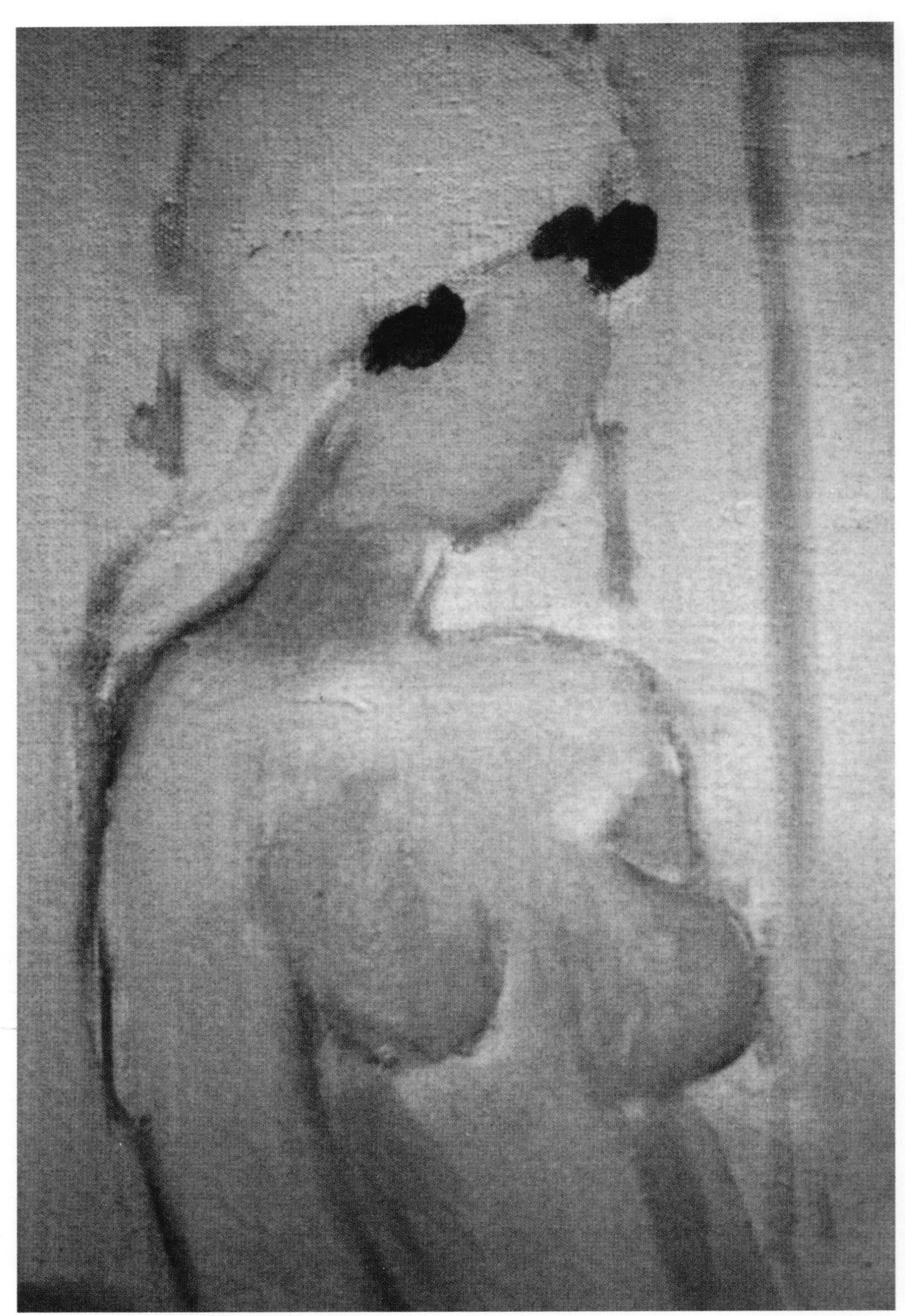

1 The Patient and Surgeon

Key Topics

Preliminary Impressions

Medical History

Physical Examination

Oncologic Evaluation

Photographic Documentation

Digital Imaging

Communication

Discussing the Options

Developing a Treatment Plan

Timing

Patient Education

Postoperative Recovery

Medical-Legal Considerations

Patient Evaluation and Treatment: Case Examples

Observations

By altering a woman's breasts, we as surgeons are tampering with a delicate anatomic balance and subtle psychological complexities. Our obligations to our patients demand that we prepare ourselves to meet this challenge. For surgery to be successful it is crucial that we be sensitive to the powerful emotional forces breast surgery unleashes. We must both elicit and intuit patient expectations, carefully weighing psychological, physical, and oncologic factors before selecting the appropriate surgical approach. Individualization of care becomes a treatment priority.

For me, the greatest satisfaction in breast surgery derives from the interactions with patients. Each patient presents a problem that invites solution. Assembling the clues to individual motivations and expectations is a skill that demands practice and finesse. The surgeon's ability to gather these clues is key to patient satisfaction and excellent results. He must know what to look for and what to expect. An investment of time and a willingness to listen, probe, and decipher contribute to patient understanding. To acquire this skill the surgeon must develop a particular mind-set. This chapter offers the reader insight into that mind-set; it traces the developing doctor-patient relationship, analyzing the process from the initial contact with the patient, through patient assessment and selection, to the decision to operate and formulation of an individualized surgical plan. Along the way it explores the different levels of thinking that are required of the surgeon if he is to succeed in the goal of treating the whole patient.

Preliminary Impressions

I begin forming preliminary impressions about a patient even before our first meeting. I do this by conferring with the people who have referred her to me, whether other doctors or former patients. From her referring physicians or friends I gather medical, psychological, and social background data on this patient to help me understand her particular problems and expectations, identify any preconceived ideas she may have, and determine whether I can provide assistance. In the case of the breast reconstruction patient I confer with other members of the breast management team to gain insights from their assessment of this patient. I also consult with my office staff who talked with the patient on the phone and set up the initial appointment. It helps to know how many times she called the office, if she asked specific questions, and what her psychological state appeared to be. If a woman has called numerous times before her first appointment, perhaps rescheduling with each call, I am forewarned of potential problems. Any behavioral eccentricities are noted: if she was impatient, rude, or attracted attention by some bizarre apparel or behavior. Valuable insight can be gained in this way. It also helps to know what area of the country the woman is from. Over the years I have observed definite differences in regional and national preferences for breast size and shape. For instance, women from the Sun Belt often desire larger breasts than their counterparts in the Midwest and Northeast. Many American women are primarily focused on breast shape, volume, and symmetry and will accept some scars as a trade-off; European, South American, and Asian women, however, are less accepting of scarring. These women expect smaller breasts with inconspicuous scars; techniques that produce shorter scars are indicated. Reviewing all of this preliminary data gives me some insight into the patient before our first meeting.

The initial consultation sets the tone for the doctor-patient relationship. Ideally, it should take place in a quiet, relaxed, unpressured environment. The focus of this meeting is on establishing an atmosphere of caring and concern and an effective line of communication. I try to put the patient at ease and let her know that I have a genuine interest in helping her. This is best accomplished in my office with the patient fully dressed and more comfortable in expressing her thoughts. It is very difficult for a woman to share her deepest emotional concerns when she is undressed, embarrassed, and preoccupied with covering herself with an examining gown or a flimsy drape.

It is essential to understand the motivations that have prompted this woman to seek a surgeon's advice. Her social history and significant influences in her life should be investigated. Who has recommended that she come for consultation? Did another member of the breast team or a colleague refer her? Has she seen or been operated on by several other surgeons? Did an article about a specific procedure prompt her to make the appointment? Did one of my other breast surgery patients refer her? Is a boyfriend, husband, mother or other relative, or friend dictating the decision or exerting too much influence on her? When an operation is done to please another person, there is a great likelihood that the results will be unsatisfactory to both. A family's support for breast surgery, however, is important and significantly influences a woman's satisfaction with the outcome. A husband is not always supportive of his wife's decision to have an elective operation. He is also hesitant to be too encouraging lest he give the impression that he is dissatisfied with her appearance as it is. He usually goes along with her desire because it is important to her and he recognizes and accepts her need. The cooperation of the husband, family, and friends should be solicited to help the patient through the customary postoperative pain, frequent psychological letdown, and possible situational depression.

I provide the direction for this interview and for subsequent consultations by asking open-ended questions that allow the patient to explain her motivations and concerns and relate her story. Questions as simple as, Why are you here? Can you tell me about your problem? What do you want me to do for you? Why do you want to have this operation? What do you want this surgery to accomplish? and Do you have any specific preferences for a particular surgical procedure? may elicit valuable insights into the patient's self-image and expectations for change. If a patient has already decided that she wants a specific augmentation incision, a particular type of implant, or a "tummy-tuck" breast reconstruction and is in my office for that reason, I need to find this out early during the first interview. I must first understand her expectations and perceptions before expressing my opinions. Many patients come to me because they desire a certain procedure, and they know that I perform it. If I can identify particular patient preferences at the outset, and if these preferences are within the realm of realistic possibility, then, after we have reviewed the other options, I can save myself and the patient valuable time initially and can focus with the patient on an individualized surgical plan.

The goal of each question is to evaluate the patient on a number of different levels: psychological, oncologic, aesthetic, and surgical. All aspects of patient care are considered, not just what a particular operation will accomplish. I am seeking clues to the woman. How does she feel about her breasts, and how does her breast size dictate her feelings about her self-worth? Is she depressed? Have other situations or life events contributed to her psychological state? Does she appear to be extremely anxious about the prospect of surgery, the possibility of scars, or the use of implants? Is her conversation agitated? Is eye contact established? Does she say, "Doctor, it is up to you. You are the artist; now just make me pretty"? Patients with this seemingly laudatory and all-accepting approach can be problematic. This is often a setup for later disappointment when the result does not measure up to previously unexpressed, idealized expectations and discontent prevails. Her concept of her deformity and expectations for surgical improvement must be carefully explored and defined before I decide that I can help her.

Some women reject their breasts and femininity, desiring a masculine appearance. They are seen in the group of patients requesting reduction mammaplasty and prophylactic mastectomy. It is a wise investment of time to analyze these individuals further and perhaps counsel them not to have the operation or certainly not before referring them for psychiatric consultation before an operation is scheduled. Other women may have such diminished, distorted, or unrealistic body images that any reasonably sized and even oversized breasts will not be sufficient to boost their feelings of femininity and sense of self-worth to an acceptable level. Still others, while appearing disheveled and overweight, may actually see themselves as svelte and attractive or view the operation as a panacea that will magically transform them both physically and emotionally. Obviously their appearance is incompatible with their unrealistic expectations for change.

While many motivations are appropriate and reasonable, the surgeon must be alert to the possibility of deep-seated insecurities and actual psychopathology that cannot possibly be resolved with breast surgery. A woman may have a conscious or subliminal agenda for her life tied to the expected change to be initiated by the operation. When this operation does not begin this anticipated series of events, she will be seriously disappointed. It is always helpful to inquire why the patient is coming for surgery at this time. What is going on in her life? I am always wary of the patient who requests aesthetic breast surgery "as soon as possible," especially "emergency" augmentation mammaplasty. She may be experiencing an emotional crisis that must be resolved in other ways. Perhaps there are unusual pressures precipitated by marital problems, death in the family, or a recent divorce. The patient might be requesting this operation for secondary gain, that is, salvaging a relationship or attracting a suitor. ***Whatever the reason, emergency aesthetic breast surgery is never a good idea for the surgeon or for the patient.*** The motivation for breast surgery should come from within the patient and usually should have been a recognized need for some time before she actually requests the surgical change.

The breast cancer patient's motivation and sense of urgency when requesting breast reconstruction cannot be considered in the same category as the woman seeking cosmetic changes. Although the fear of breast cancer is shared by all women, it is understandable for the breast cancer patient to feel particularly apprehensive, insecure, and diminished by her cancer, its local and systemic treatment, and the mastectomy experience. After breast cancer treatment many women experience feelings of loss, disfigurement, and defeminization; they fear rejection by significant individuals and inability to sustain intimate relationships. Now that immediate breast reconstruction is common, many of these feelings can be obviated. Frequently a woman's request for an immediate reconstructive procedure is inspired by her desire to "put her cancer experience behind her and get on with her life." For her it is a positive move toward rehabilitation, a "return to wholeness."

Time spent learning about the patient's motivations and expectations can prevent future problems and help the patient and surgeon develop a basic level of understanding and trust. ***Good listening skills are crucially important and key to conducting an effective patient interview.*** Silence, a tool that is often underutilized, can be applied to real advantage. A surgeon who establishes good eye contact with the patient and listens quietly and attentively, smiling and nodding at the appropriate moments, can simultaneously reassure the patient and allow her to open up and express herself freely.

A thorough patient evaluation with a detailed medical history and physical examination that focuses on prior breast or other aesthetic operations completes these preliminary observations. When all of these pieces come together and the surgeon and patient have a clear idea of realistic expectations for surgery, a treatment plan evolves.

Medical History

Information gathered from the medical history influences the decision to operate and the particular treatment approach selected; this information should be detailed. For the sake of convenience, the history and examination are divided into two categories, listing all general medical and physical considerations in one section, such as medications, allergies, previous operations, and history of psychiatric problems, and all oncologic and breast monitoring considerations in another. With this type of organization I get a quick overall impression of the patient's health and can immediately identify those patients with a high-risk status.

The patient's weight should be stable and within the normal range for her size and body frame before she has breast surgery. ***When the woman is more than 30 pounds above her ideal weight, the risks of local as well as general complications are increased.*** Significant weight changes that have taken place within the past year and plans for weight reduction should be noted; these changes will affect the surgical plan. Weight loss after breast reduction can cause a decrease in breast size, possibly resulting in patient distress over breasts that are now perceived as "too small." For example, an overweight teenager with mammary hypertrophy may consider her breasts too small a few years later when weight loss or involutional atrophy have further diminished breast size.

A detailed family history with particular attention to any history of breast problems, breast cancer, other cancers, or anesthetic risks such as malignant hyperthermia is essential; it will identify increased patient risks. Specific questions should probe for any breast problems the patient has experienced previously. She should be asked whether she has had and been treated for breast abnormalities, tumors, infections, fibrocystic change, mastitis, or breast cancer and if she has had radiation of the breast and chest region even as an infant or child. Such data alert the breast surgeon to potential problems and the need to monitor the patient who has had previous breast cancer for possible recurrence. Previous histopathologic diagnoses are noted and considered. Results of recent mammograms and other breast images are assessed.

A patient's history of previous medical or psychological treatment also warrants attention. If possible, her other doctors should be consulted. If a potential psychological or health problem is uncovered during the history or physical examination, the problem should be analyzed and worked through with the patient's other doctors before surgery is planned. This is essential when systemic disease or a condition that might contraindicate general anesthesia or impair the proposed procedure is suspected. It is always a good policy to check with the internist, family physician, or gynecologist to confirm her health status and ensure that a timely history and physical examination are available prior to any procedure as well as to discuss if there are any physician's recommendations that need to be considered.

Prior bleeding conditions are documented and all medications that can affect coagulation are discontinued before an operation. ***Heparin and warfarin (Coumadin) are major anticoagulants. Patients requiring these medications because of life-threatening thromboembolic risks should not have elective aesthetic breast surgery because of the high risk of bleeding.*** If an operation is deemed essential for breast reconstruction or specific wound problems, selection of these patients and their preoperative management should be closely coordinated with their internists. ***Salicylates, other drugs affecting platelet function, nonsteroidal analgesics such as ibuprofen, and anti-inflammatory drugs contribute to intraoperative and postoperative bleeding, thereby increasing the probability of transfusions and hematoma; these, too, should be discontinued when possible several weeks before the operation or accommodated in the surgical plan.*** Autologous whole blood should be available if excess blood loss is anticipated. Patients are asked to donate 2 units of their own blood prior to surgery. Chronic steroid use for collagen vascular, pulmonary, and hematologic diseases poses special problems and may be a contraindication to an operation or to the use of breast implants. Steroids should be discontinued during the perioperative period and the patient's internist should be consulted to determine the indications for steroid use and to agree on the proper course of action. Birth control pills should also be discontinued before the operation because they affect breast size, cause vascular engorgement, and increase blood coagulability. Some diet medications can cause cardiac problems and should be avoided prior to an operation. The patient should be asked if she is taking any herbal or homeopathic remedies. These may adversely affect the outcome of surgery and as a caution should be discontinued. For example, St. John's wort contains a monoamine oxidase inhibitor and can lead to unstable blood pressure during anesthesia. If possible, the operation should be scheduled 1 to 2 weeks after menses to minimize vascular engorgement of the breasts and reduce blood loss.

Drugs To Avoid Before Surgery

For the 3- to 4-week period prior to the scheduled date of your surgery, do not take any medication that contains aspirin. Aspirin affects the blood's ability to clot and could increase your tendency to bleed during surgery and during the postoperative period. If you need minor pain medication, take Tylenol. If you are allergic to Tylenol or unable to take it for some other reason, notify us so that we may arrange for a suitable substitute. The following drugs have undesirable side effects that may cause abnormal bleeding or bruising.

A.P.C.
Achromycin
Acoda
Acuprin
Advil
Aleve
Alka-Seltzer
Alka-Seltzer Plus
Amitriptyline
Amoxapine
Anacin
Anadynos
Anaprox
Anexsia with codeine
Ansaid
Aphrodyne
Argesic-SA
Arthritis Pain Formula
Arthritis Strength
Arthropan
A.S.A.
Ascriptin
Ascriptin A/D
Ascriptin Extra
Ascriptin with codeine
Aspergum
Atromid-S
Axotal
Azdone tablets
Azolid
B-A-C
Bayer
B.C. tablets & powder
Bexophene
Buf-Tabs
Buff-A Comp
Buff-A Comp No. 3
Buffaprin
Bufferin Arthritis Strength
Bufferin Extra Strength
Bufferin with codeine No. 3
Buffets II
Buffinol
Butazolidin
Cama arthritis pain reliever
Carbamazepine
Carisoprodol
Cheracol capsules
Chlor-Trimeton
Clinoril
Co-Tylenol
ColBenemid
Colchicine
Comtrex
Congesprin Chewable
Cope tablets
Coricidin
Cosprin tablets
CP-2 tablets
Damason-P tablets
Darvon Compound
Darvon Compound-65
Darvon N with A.S.A.
Dasin
Desipramine
Dia-Gesic
Disalcid
Dolobid
Dolprn
Donnatal
Doxepin
Dristan
Durasal tablets
Easprin
Ecotrin
Efficin
Elavil
Emagrin
Empirin
Emprazil
Encaprin
Endep
Equagesic
Equazine M
Etrafon
Eutron
Eutronyl
Excedrin
Fastin
Feldene
Fenfluramine
Fiogesic
Fiorgen PF
Fioricet
Fiorinal
Fish oil
Flagyl
Flexeril
Four Way cold tablets
Furazolidone
Furoxone
Gaysal-S
Gelpirin
Gemnisin
Goody's extra strength headache powders
Haltran
Heparin
Ibuprofen
Imipramine
Indocin
Indomethacin
Isocarboxazid
Liquiprin
Limbitrol DS
Lodine
Lortab
Ludiomil
Magnaprin
Magsal
Maprotiline
Marnal
Marplan
Matulane
Measurin
Meprobamate
Meclomen
Medipren
Methcarbamol with aspirin
Micrainin
Midol
Mobidin
Mobigesic
Monoamine oxidase inhibitors
Motrin
Mysteclin F
Nalfon
Naprosyn
Naproxen
Nardil
Nicobid (gum or patch)
Norgesic
Norgesic Forte
Norpramin
Nortriptyline
Norwich
Novahistine
Nuprin

Drugs To Avoid Before Surgery—cont'd

Oraflex	Phenylbutazone	Sinequan	Tolectin
Ornade	Pondimin	Sinutab	Tolmetin
Orphenesic	Ponstel	SK-65 Compound	Toradol
Orudis	Presalin	Soma Compound	Tranylcypromine
Oxycodone	Procarbazine	St. John's wort	Triaminicin
Pabalate	Propoxyphene Compound 65	St. Joseph's aspirin	Triavil
PAC	Protriptyline	St. Joseph's cold tablets	Trigesic
Pamelor	Prozac	Stanback	Trilisate
Panasal	Pyrroxate caplets	Stendin	Trimipramine maleate
Pargyline	Redux	Sulindac	Uracel
Parnate	Relefen	Sumycin	Vanquish
Pedia-profen	Robaxisal	Supac	Verin
Pepto-Bismol	Roxiprin tablets	Surmontil	Vibramycin
Percodan tablets	Ru-Tuss	Synalgos-DC capsules	Vitamin E
Percodan-Demi tablets	Rufen	Tagamet	Vivactil
Perphenazine	S-A-C	Talwin Compound caplets	Voltaren
Persantine	Saleto	Tegretol	Warfarin (Coumadin)
Phenaphen with codeine	Salocol	Tenuate Dospan	Zomax
Phenelzine	Sine-Aid	Tetracycline	ZORprin
Phenergan	Sine-Off sinus medicine	Tofranil	Zyloprim
Phentermine			

The surgeon needs to know how many other surgical procedures the patient has had and which of these were elective. Multiple previous aesthetic procedures can indicate an insatiable cosmetic surgery patient whose body image is poor, who has unobtainable expectations, and who may actually be harmed by further operations. Prior operations should be discussed with the patient and if possible with the surgeon or surgeons who performed them. Her opinion of her other doctors should be elicited. In my experience, when a patient denigrates another surgeon, noting how poorly he functioned and related to her, and then tells me how highly I have been recommended and of her conviction that I will right all of the previous perceived wrongs, I know that it is only a matter of time until I am entered on her growing list of those "other surgeons who haven't measured up." If the woman is particularly critical of previous surgeons or has a history of changing doctors after each procedure or seeking repeated consultations and elective surgical procedures, then caution is in order. ***It is much easier to say "no" at the outset than to have to deal with a problem patient later, possibly after a procedure proves to be a disappointment to her.***

Previous radiation treatment and operations, systemic diseases such as hypertension, diabetes, and autoimmune and collagen diseases such as lupus, rheumatoid arthritis, and scleroderma all affect tissue vascularity and wound healing; they must be considered when deciding which operation is best for the patient and accommodated in the preoperative plan. These conditions and the medications to treat them affect macrocirculation and microcirculation and can cause flap and tissue loss and contribute to delayed wound healing and infections. ***I am extremely reluctant to place breast implants in women with a history of autoimmune disease, scleroderma, or symptoms of polyarthritis.*** Radiation oncologists have found that patients with autoimmune disease also respond poorly to radiation therapy. The extent of systemic disease must be evaluated and the potential risks explained to the patient to determine if an operation should be planned for this individual. Developmental, menstrual, and obstetric histories, the amount of breast fullness during pregnancy and lactation, the degree of postpartum breast involution and response to hormones, especially birth control pills, and future plans for pregnancy and breast-feeding all influence the surgical decision-making process and are detailed in the history.

A history of cigarette smoking is also elicited and recorded. Tobacco smoking should be discontinued in the perioperative period to reduce the acute vasoconstrictive effects of nicotine as well as more general complications such as heart or lung problems, hypercoagulability, and poor circulation. ***Cigarette smoking can contribute to loss of the nipple-areola, delayed healing of incisions, flap loss, wide scars, infections, and fat necrosis.*** A growing body of evidence suggests a possible cumulative effect of cigarette smoking that can amplify these problems, especially if the patient has the equivalent of 40 pack-years or more. A pack-year is the equivalent of smoking one package or 20 cigarettes per day for 1 year. Therefore a patient who smokes two packages of cigarettes per day for 20 years has a 40 pack-year consumption of cigarettes. The long-term effect of this habit will not be reversed with a few hours or days of cigarette abstinence. Environmental tobacco smoke can also affect microcirculation and should be avoided in the perioperative period.

Physical Examination

A thorough physical examination adds to the patient profile. Before the patient undresses, a visual assessment of her general appearance will provide additional clues. An overemphasis on grooming, dressing, and cosmetics may indicate the patient is a perfectionist who may have unobtainable expectations for the correction of a perceived problem. The opposite, a disheveled appearance, inattention to personal hygiene or grooming, or exhibitionist dressing or behavior, may also indicate underlying psychopathology, overmedication, or even signs of early Alzheimer's disease.

GENERAL

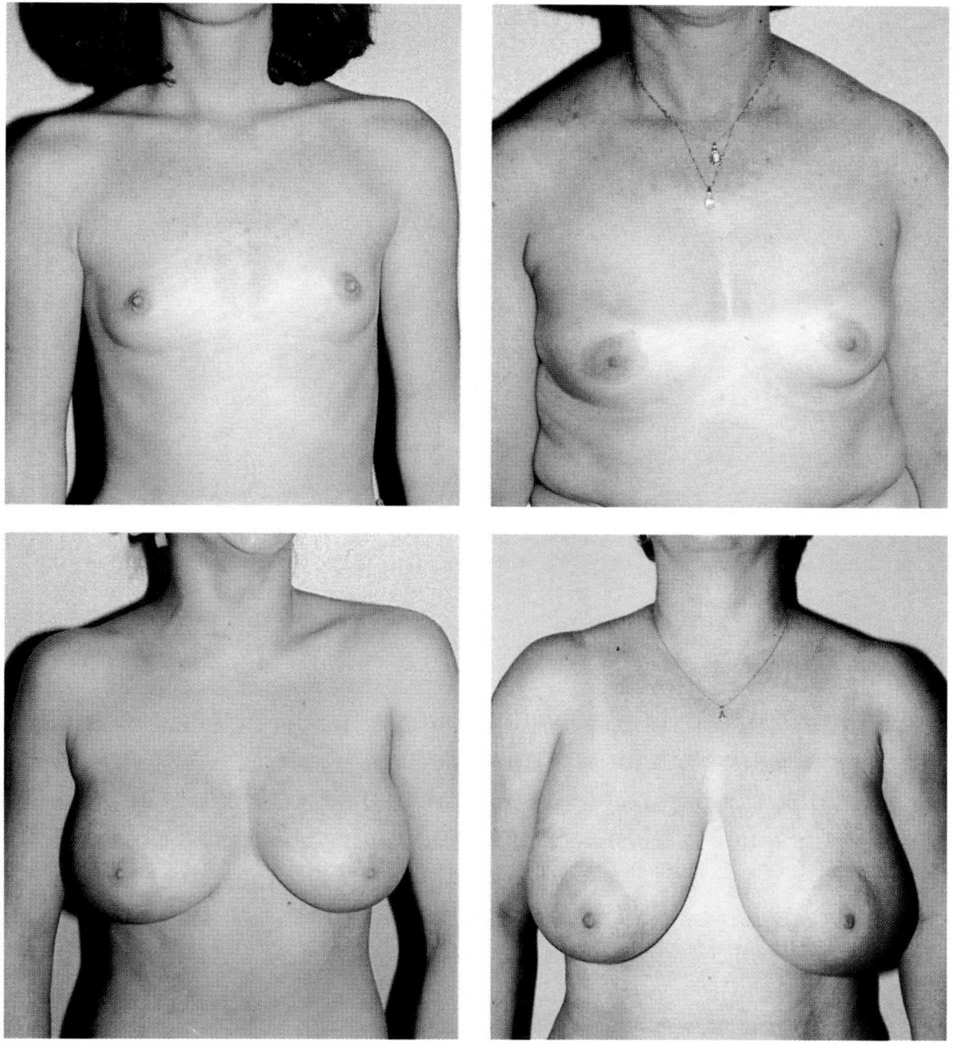

The patient's general body shape and the proportions of her torso are observed to get an idea of ideal breast size in relation to total body form. Unnaturally thin or obese patients may have other related psychological and nutritional problems such as an eating disorder or a medical condition that should be fully investigated before surgery is planned. Thoracic cage shape and contour significantly determine symmetric breast appearance; therefore patients with scoliosis and an asymmetric chest may appear to have unequal breasts. All individuals exhibit some degree of asymmetry. These asymmetries are identified, particularly frontally and circumferentially, pointed out to the patient, photographed, and documented in the record. ***If the plastic surgeon fails to note and tell the patient about asymmetries preoperatively, the patient will certainly point them out postoperatively.***

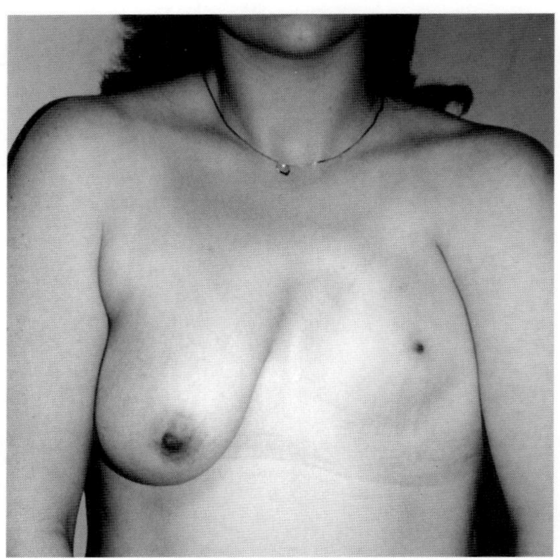

Chest wall musculature is also evaluated; absence of the pectoral muscle and sometimes the latissimus dorsi muscle seen in patients with Poland's syndrome is frequently associated with unilateral breast hypoplasia as well as other anomalies of the chest wall, its musculature, and the upper extremity and hand. Bulky musculature such as that seen in patients who are bodybuilders should also be considered in planning breast surgery. This has implications for implant placement as well as the use of musculocutaneous flaps and incision placement.

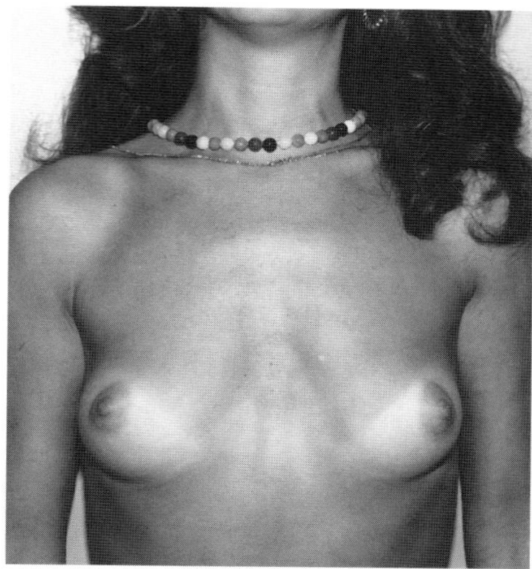

The location of the breasts on the chest wall and the size of the breasts are noted. Patients with pectus excavatum deformities often have breasts that point medially toward the central chest concavity, whereas those with pectus carinatum have breasts that point more laterally.

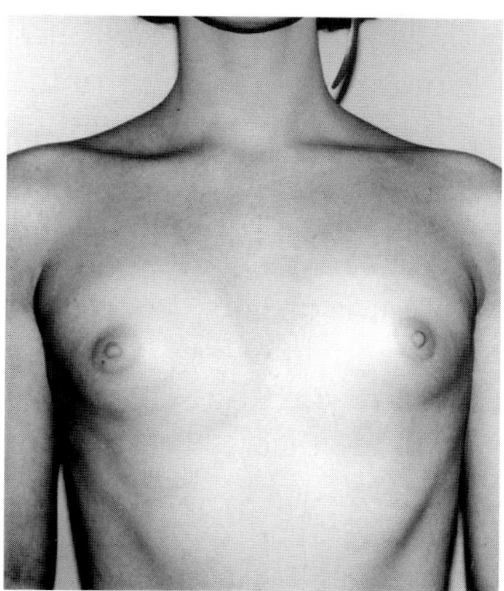

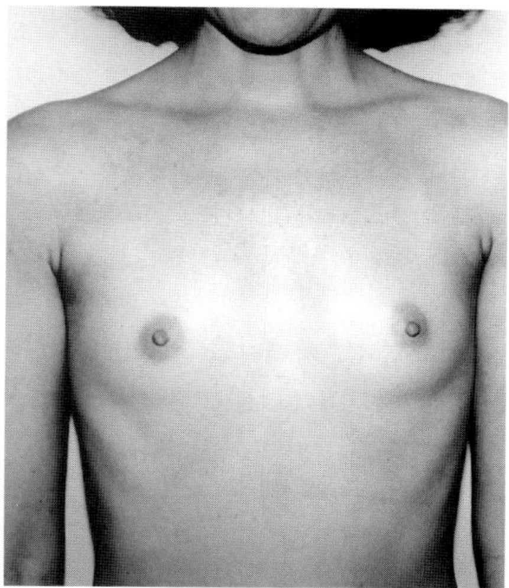

Breast width is compared to chest wall width. Women with wide or normal chests sometimes have disproportionately narrow, constricted, or tubular breasts; the surgical plan must accommodate these variations, particularly for augmentation or reduction, in which case the breast base will have to be widened using breast implants or narrowed by vertical resection. Similarly, patients with narrow chests need surgical procedures that will produce breasts with narrower base proportions. Abnormal growth of certain breast quadrants can lead to subtle or marked nipple malposition. Constricted breasts should also be identified; their management requires additional corrective measures.

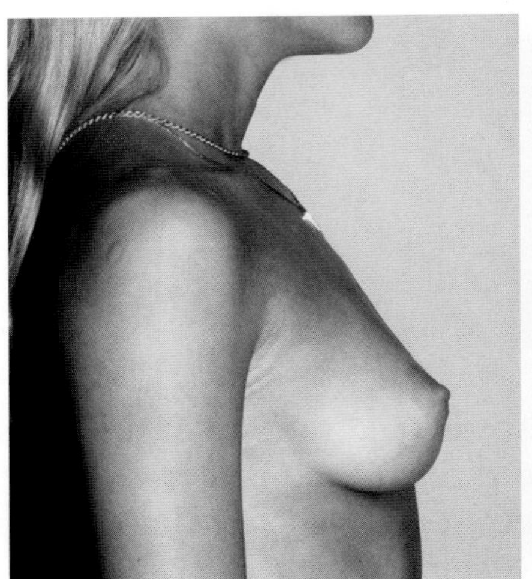
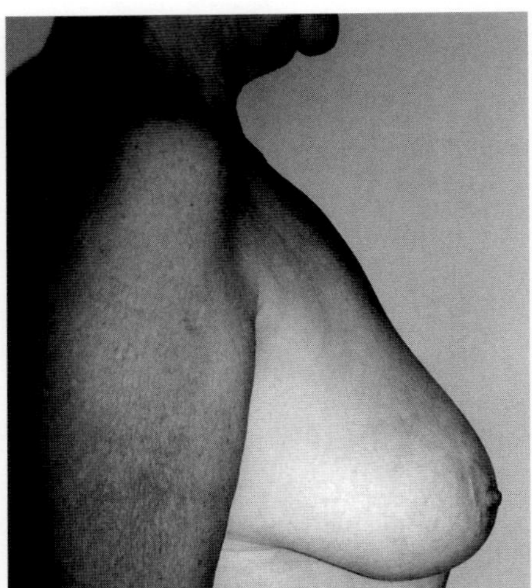

The presence of axillary fullness and medial and lateral breast folds related to the patient's weight must be pointed out to the patient and addressed in the surgical plan. Specifically, the surgeon needs to determine if there is good lateral, medial, and lower breast definition. Does the flow of the breast disappear laterally onto the side and back? I generally explain to the patient that although this lateral fat is not breast tissue, it must be incorporated in the breast operation to achieve the most aesthetic appearance and so that they will not appear more full and prominent laterally after surgery. Such excess lateral fullness in the overweight patient is usually the reason the result of breast surgery is disappointing to the patient as well as the surgeon. Techniques using standard liposuction or ultrasound-assisted liposuction have facilitated treatment of these areas of tissue excess. These tools enable the plastic surgeon to extend the modification of the breast to the surrounding area, thereby improving the overall appearance.

BREAST

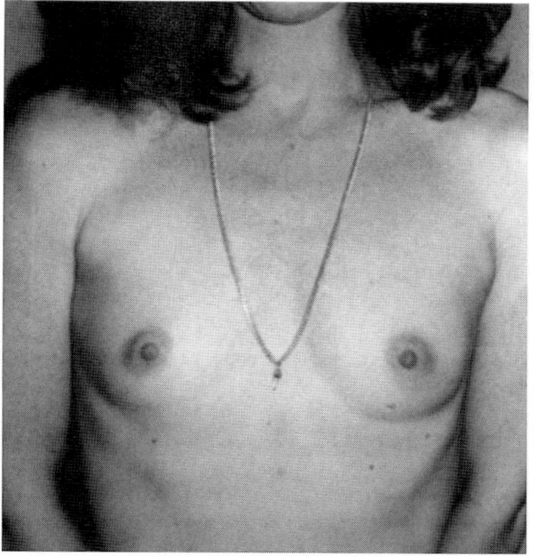
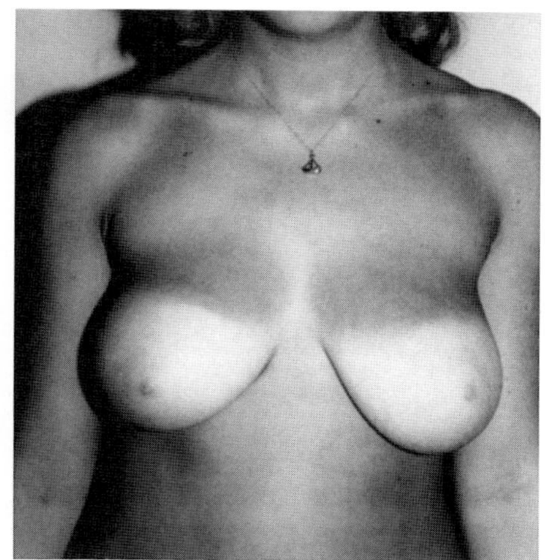
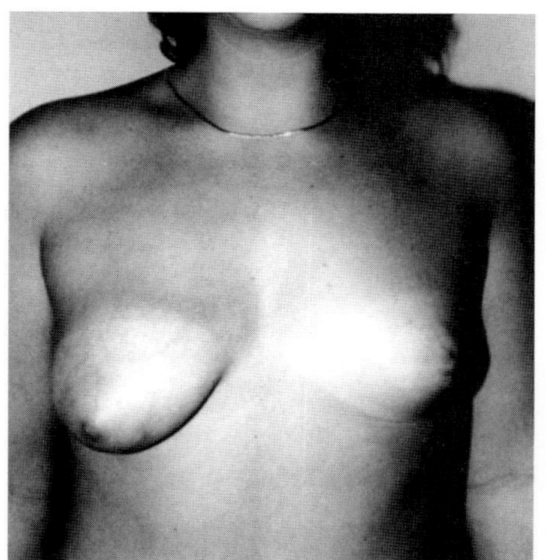
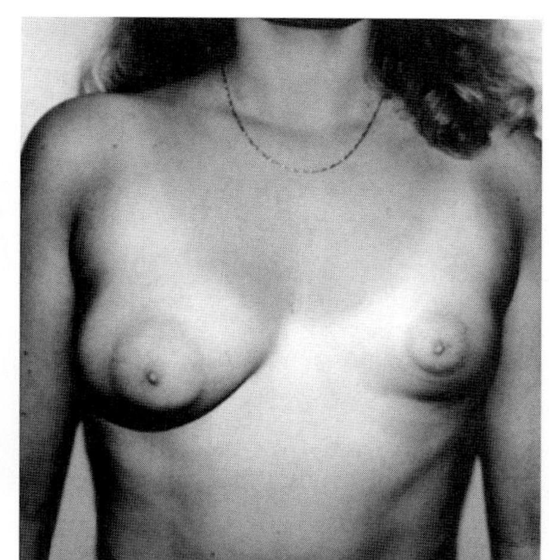
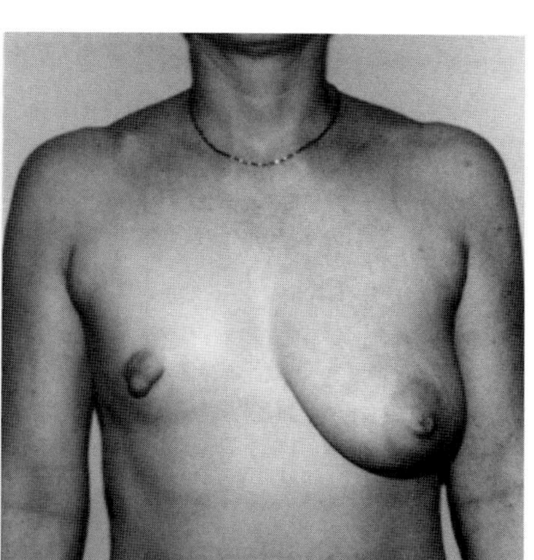

Breast size, shape, proportion, consistency, and symmetry are assessed. Because no two women have the same configuration of physical characteristics, the surgeon will be evaluating and treating patients who demonstrate a range of conditions. That is why it is so important to have a thorough knowledge of breast morphology and to be well versed in a variety of surgical techniques so that the diagnosis and treatment plan can be individualized for each patient and for each specific breast problem.

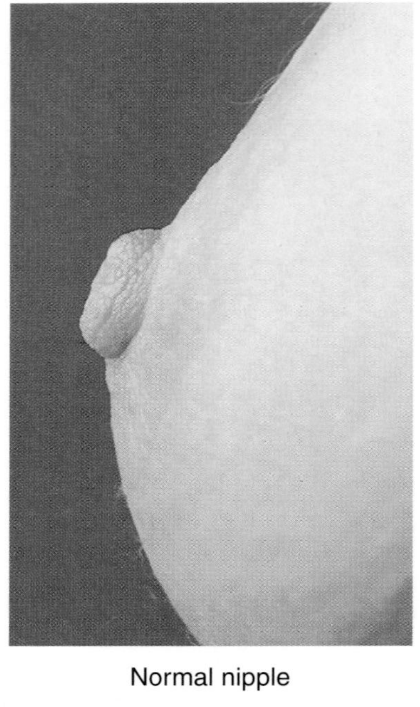

Normal nipple

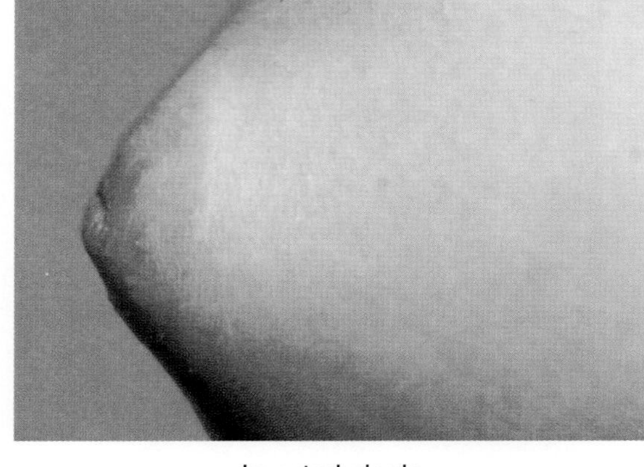

Inverted nipple

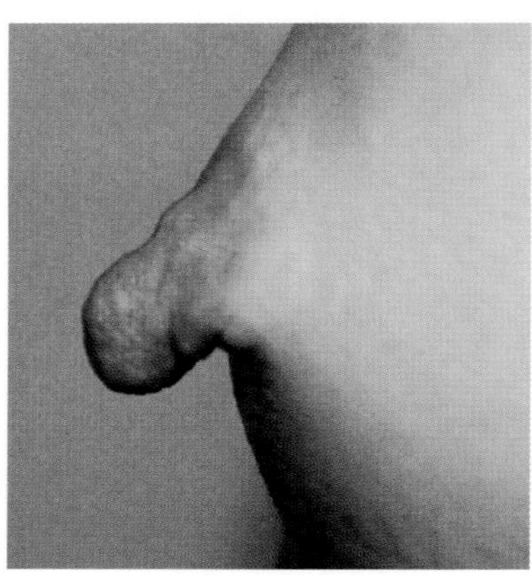

Nipple hyperplasia

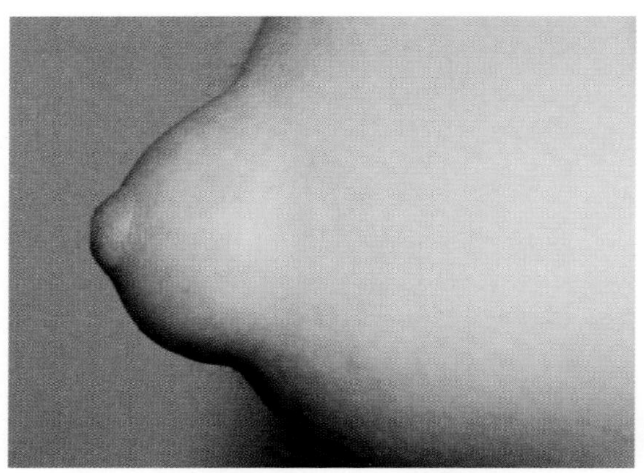

Tubular nipple-areola

The position, size, projection, diameter, symmetry, inclination, and mobility of the nipple-areolae on the glandular tissue are also checked. Again, the possible variations in nipple development should be considered and addressed during a breast procedure. Measurement of the nipple-areolar position as related to the midbreast line and the inframammary breast crease will influence the selection of technique for reduction, mastopexy, and augmentation mammaplasty and to match an opposite breast during reconstruction. The mobility of the breast over the musculofascial layer is an important predictor of the postoperative response of the breast to aesthetic corrections. Breast flow, mobility, and position with the patient in the supine and oblique positions are carefully observed; the goal is to preserve a natural appearance and mobility postoperatively.

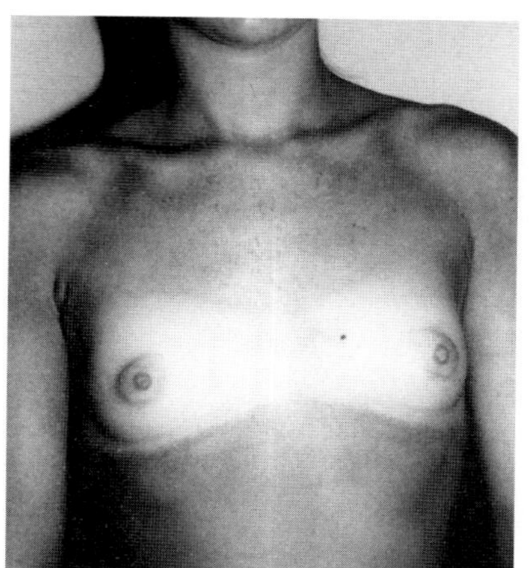
Teenager with normal tight breast skin without striae, atrophy, or ptosis

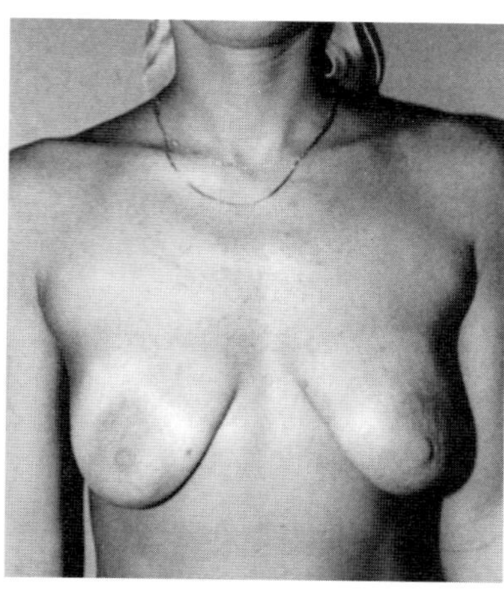
22-year-old patient whose breasts have striae, ptosis, and involutional atrophy

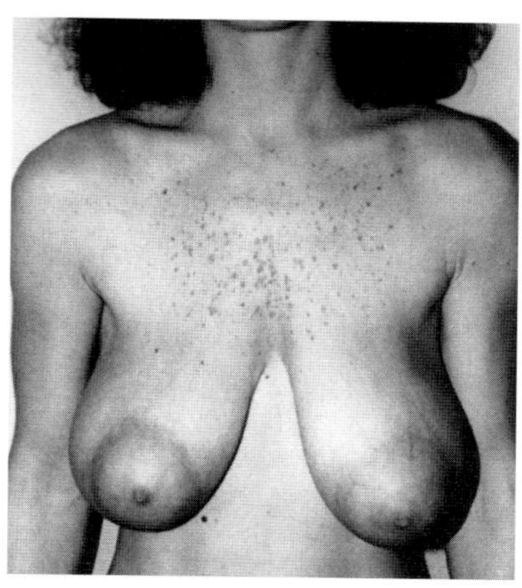
18-year-old patient whose breasts are hyperplastic with striae and marked ptosis

Skin thickness, quality, elasticity, and the presence of striae are also noted as are support, tightness, and mobility. Striae indicate the dermis is torn and stretched and are associated with reduced skin thickness and elasticity and diminished skin vascularity. Recurrence of breast ptosis is predictable when aesthetic corrections depend on thinned, stretched skin for contour and support. Striae are tears within the skin. The patient should understand that they cannot be eliminated, are a potential cause and predictor of ptosis recurrence, and increase the likelihood that additional corrections will be required. ***When striae are present, plans should be made preoperatively for increasing the stability of the underlying breast mound.*** Large breast volume and excessively mobile parenchyma with thin, inelastic skin can result in early loss of shape and recurrent pendulousness in patients having reduction or mastopexy procedures. Furthermore, if the breast parenchyma is thin or if the skin is thin and tight over the breast, when a breast implant is placed, particularly in a submammary position, the patient has an increased probability of implant rippling, palpability, visible folds through the skin, or even implant extrusion with the development of spherical capsular contracture.

INFRAMAMMARY CREASE AND AXILLARY FOLD

The position and extent of the inframammary crease are observed closely as well as its definition and symmetry. ***The inframammary crease is an important aesthetic landmark for surgical planning and nipple site determination; it is also an indicator of developmental breast abnormalities, ptosis, and asymmetries.*** The inframammary creases should be symmetric and distinct on both sides and circumscribe an arc beginning near the midline and continuing laterally to the lateral aspect of the breast and its juncture with the lateral chest wall and flow into the lateral breast line.

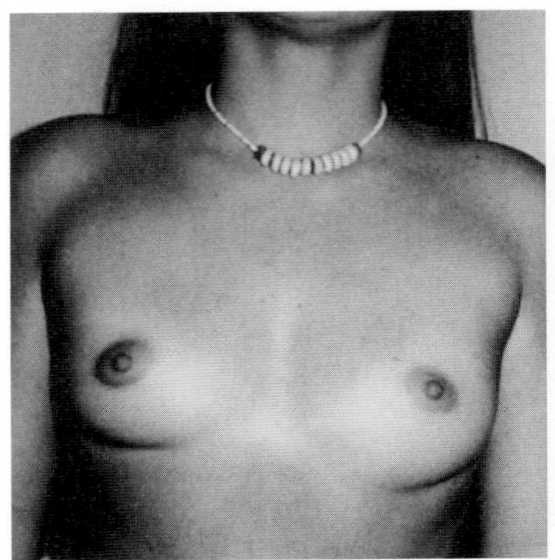

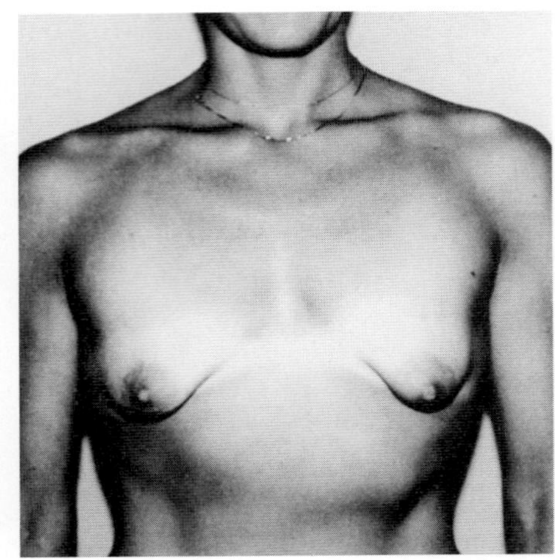

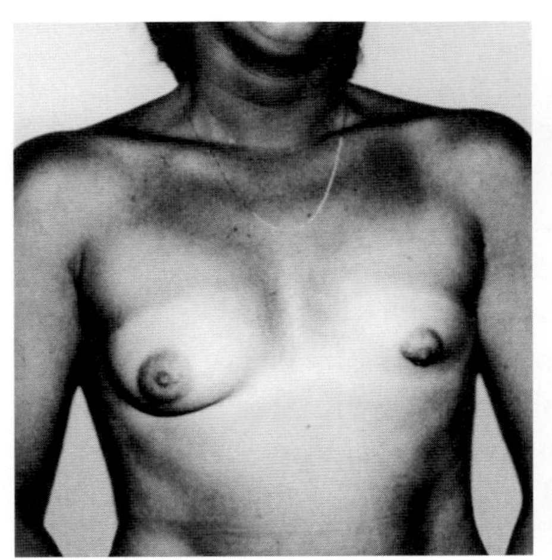

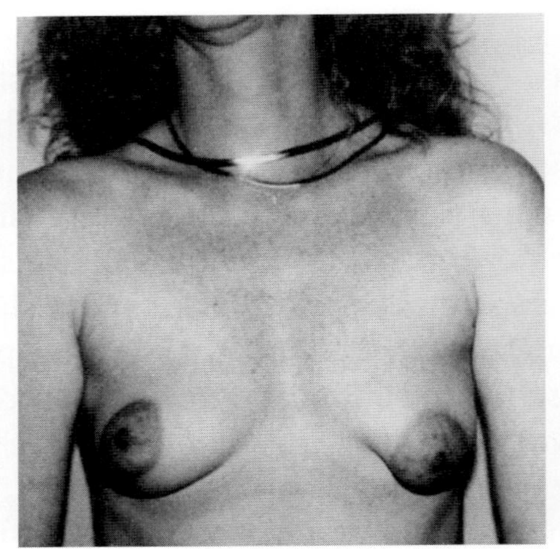

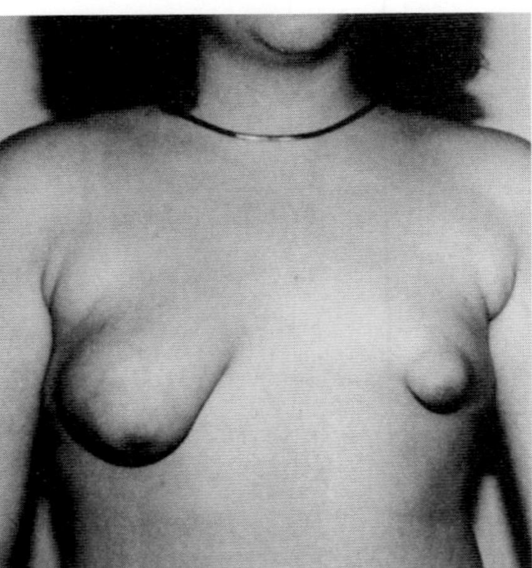

An inframammary crease that begins somewhat laterally indicates breast constriction that is often associated with tubular breast deformity as well as an upwardly displaced inframammary crease if the condition is marked. Women with this condition illustrate some of the possible deformities associated with the inframammary crease, including mild asymmetries of the crease, a constricted breast, and tubular breast deformity. These conditions often are associated with obvious breast asymmetries.

These conditions must be recognized and addressed when the surgical plan is developed. When there is a distinct inframammary crease located approximately 5 to 7 cm below the areola, placement of an incision here usually leaves an inconspicuous scar after aesthetic breast surgery. When there is no crease or it is constricted and high with a shortened areola-to-crease distance and the breast is hypoplastic, periareolar or axillary access is preferable for placement of a breast implant. In these situations the normal infra-areolar proportions and a more normal inframammary crease must be determined in the preoperative plan and a new, defined crease produced.

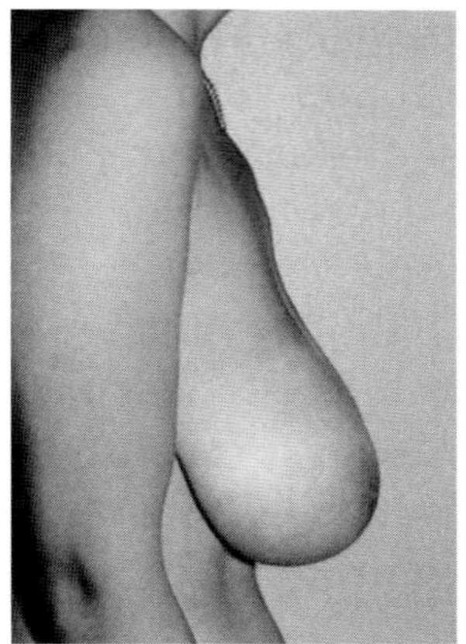
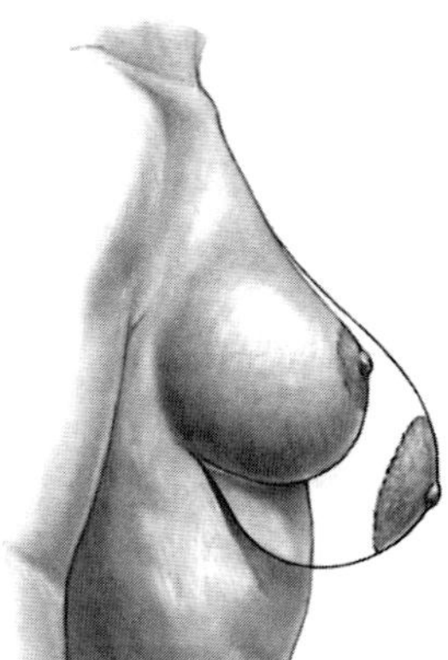

The lateral breast line is evaluated. Is it distinct or is it full? Does it end in the lateral chest and subaxillary region with fullness flowing onto the back? Loss of this fold is most often seen in women who request breast reduction. This area usually must be addressed by removing the lateral fullness and redefining the fold. The medial breast definition, often called breast cleavage, is evaluated. As the breasts get larger they usually extend laterally and inferiorly rather than medially. Cleavage is often accentuated by bringing the breasts together with a bra. Attempts to create cleavage by placing the implants close together can be very disappointing; if symmastia develops, cleavage may be lost altogether.

The fullness and extent of the axillary fold are also observed. Anterior axillary fullness and breast tissue can appear larger when reduction mammaplasty of the lower breast area is performed. Since these folds contain breast parenchyma, they should be included in the oncologic evaluation. Upper breast fullness is also noted. This area, frequently full in younger women, may be lost with aging and development of breast ptosis. ***Flatness in the upper breast should be addressed in the preoperative plan and can be improved by shifting breast parenchyma superiorly, transferring autologous tissue, or inserting a breast implant.***

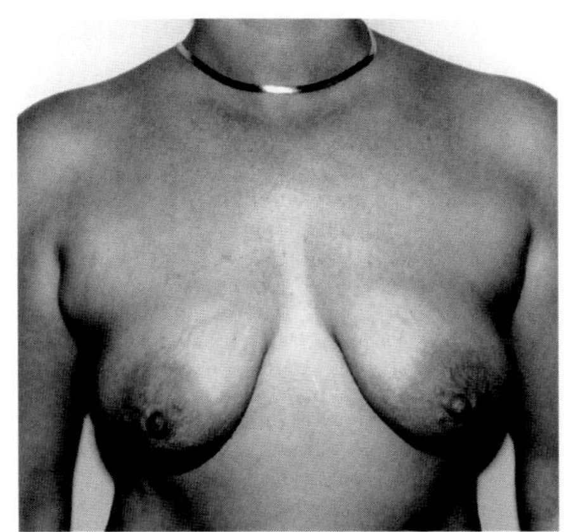

AREAS FOR FLAPS

To treat complications of aesthetic surgery or to supply additional tissue during breast reconstruction, the surgeon may at times need to use flaps of autologous tissue from local, regional, or distant sources. Primary areas for obtaining donor tissue include the back (latissimus dorsi musculocutaneous flap), upper and lower abdomen (transverse rectus abdominis musculocutaneous [TRAM] flap), occasionally the buttocks (inferior gluteus maximus musculocutaneous flap), and rarely the hips (Rubens flap). When one of these areas is being considered for autologous tissue, it must be checked for tissue availability and volume, scars, and suitability as a donor site. (Specific guidelines for evaluating the back, abdomen, and buttocks are detailed in Chapters 14 to 16.)

When discussing the options for breast reconstruction with a patient, the possible donor sites for flap procedures and the donor scar and resultant donor deformity and functional impact are described. Most patients have strong feelings about which areas they do not want violated and which donor sites they prefer to be used. Many prefer the added benefits conferred by a TRAM flap to achieve an abdominoplasty-like improvement of the abdominal wall. These preferences for choice of a donor site should be identified and incorporated into the surgical plan.

Oncologic Evaluation

While the surgeon evaluates breast aesthetics, he must also consider the breast as the source of distinct benign and malignant conditions that must be evaluated and diagnosed prior to a decision for aesthetic or reconstructive breast correction. The surgeon should be alert to the patient's age and risk status and current and past history of benign and malignant conditions. All further evaluation and planning should take the patient's oncologic status into consideration. The supraclavicular and regional axillary nodes are palpated, and a complete visual and physical examination of the breast is performed with the patient in sitting and recumbent positions and with her arms up and also leaning forward. ***The patient needs to be checked for all of the primary and secondary signs of breast cancer*** (see Chapter 10); this is the usual practice for all of my patients. Evidence of breast lumps or discrete or unexplained thickenings is recorded and investigated. The quality and condition of the breast and areola skin are evaluated as is the appearance of the nipple-areola. I check for inverted nipples as well as signs of breast or nipple-areola retraction. The patient is asked if she has noted any recent change or breast mass and, if so, to point it out. If the patient is 30 years of age or older and a breast operation is planned, a baseline mammogram is taken and assessed to screen for preexisting disease or breast irregularities prior to scheduling aesthetic breast surgery. If she has a family history of or is at high risk for breast cancer, a preoperative mammogram should be obtained even in women in their twenties. It is essential for the breast surgeon to develop a close working relationship with members of the breast management team, particularly the oncologic breast surgeon, who understands the complexities and significance of aesthetic and reconstructive breast surgery and can complement the skills of the breast surgeon. Fine-needle aspiration, stereotactic localization, ultrasound-guided biopsy, or open biopsy may be necessary to explain a suspicious lesion prior to an aesthetic procedure. The presence of fibrocystic change, mastitis, or cysts is not a contraindication to aesthetic breast surgery, although the surgeon must thoroughly investigate these conditions to check for possible malignancy. It is also important that the radiologist feel comfortable and be experienced in evaluating breasts after aesthetic and reconstructive breast surgery. For example, the breast imager should know that two additional displacement views will be needed to adequately view the breast tissue in augmentation patients who have breast implants. Certain internal scarring and tissue derangement are also to be expected after reduction mammaplasty.

HEALING AND SCAR EVALUATION

The type of healing exhibited by other incisions is checked, particularly for signs of hypertrophic scarring or widening of incisions. Breast biopsy scars and their location should be identified and detailed on the patient record; they can affect the vascularity of flaps and breast parenchyma and will influence the surgical plan, especially future incisions. At times these incisions can be used for approaches to the breast for implant placement, reduction, breast mass excision, or even mastectomy. The mastectomy scars in heavy cigarette smokers can exhibit characteristic changes; they appear widened and thin with evidence of delayed secondary healing. When such scars are observed, the breast surgeon should be alert to other potential healing difficulties if the patient is still engaging in the same level of cigarette smoke inhalation at the time of surgery. Scars at potential flap donor sites are also evaluated to determine if they will affect the design or safety of the proposed operation.

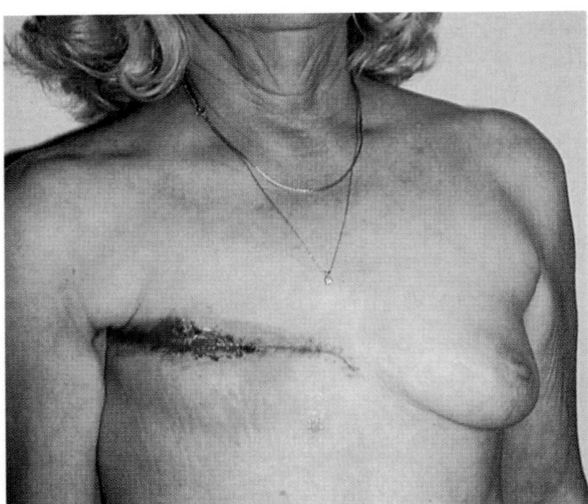

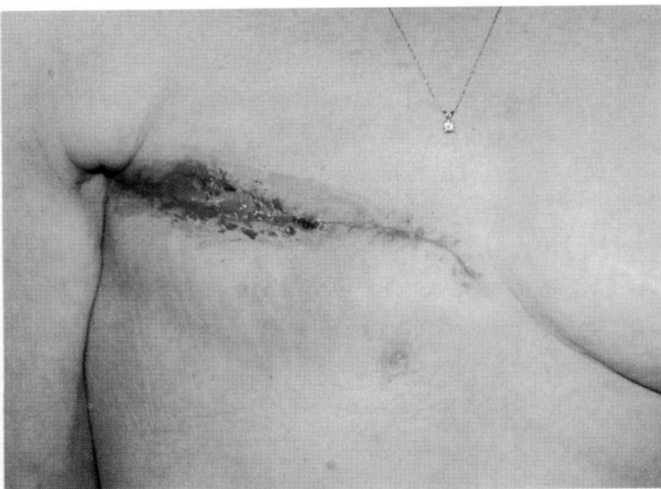

This 48-year-old woman exemplifies the wound-healing problems sometimes encountered in the heavy smoker. She had a 90 pack-year cigarette history and smoked three packs of cigarettes a day. (She had been smoking at this rate since age 18.) She presented 7 weeks after mastectomy for breast reconstruction. At that time her mastectomy scar had not healed, demonstrating the prolonged healing with associated wide scars that are characteristic of heavy smokers and indicating the poor healing potential for any breast reconstructive procedure, especially a TRAM flap, particularly if she continued smoking cigarettes.

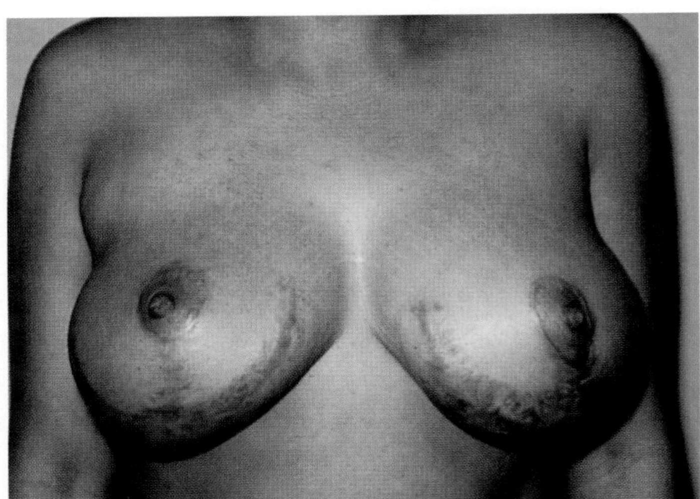

When there is evidence of hypertrophic scarring from previous operations, this healing problem is also considered. This 24-year-old patient was seen for secondary reduction mammaplasty complaining of hypertrophic and unaesthetically positioned scars. Management of her healing problem was a major consideration in planning the secondary procedure.

If possible, incision sites should be selected to minimize this problem, to hide or shorten the scars, or to place the scars at a distance from skin that is at risk for visible scarring. Endoscopic or video-assisted plastic surgery is helpful in reducing breast scar length. Healing of previous incisions will also influence the length and position of any new incisions and will help predict final scar appearance. Perhaps an old scar can be used for the procedure, and careful closure, postoperative pressure, tapes, and even intralesional steroids and postoperative silicone sheeting may help improve its appearance. When a breast implant is being used, it can sometimes be placed through the scars from previous biopsies or incisions to obviate the need for new scars in patients with wound-healing problems. Previous scars can even be used for a mastectomy to reduce scarring and optimize vascularity to the skin flaps.

Documentation

Photographic documentation is an important aspect of planning, recording, and evaluating aesthetic and reconstructive breast surgery patients. ***I use preoperative photographs during my initial consultations, during planning, and for reference during postoperative sessions with patients.*** Once the surgery has been completed, the patient can easily forget what she looked like before. These photographs remind the patient of the actual preoperative condition and appearance of her breasts and clearly demonstrate the extent of her former problem. They also provide me with an important source of information for critiquing my technique and results.

The patient's breast appearance can be recorded using Polaroid prints, 35 mm slides, or digital photography. Polaroid photographs provide immediate prints to show the patient during the initial consultation and for inclusion in the permanent record for review and discussion during postoperative visits. Digital photographs also provide immediate feedback and can be stored for ready review with the patient. It is also possible to manipulate or morph these digital images to provide a preview of possible breast changes. I continue to take 35 mm slides for top-quality case documentation. They are easily stored, can be magnified and projected at teaching conferences, can be digitized for high-quality images, and can be reproduced as high-quality prints.

To ensure an accurate and fair evaluation of surgical results, preoperative and postoperative views must be comparably positioned and exposed. The preoperative photographs taken today must parallel the postoperative photographs 10 years later. This means that the photographic recording system should be consistent and reproducible. Because I work in a number of examining rooms and several hospitals, I use a simple, transportable system that can be adapted to all of these settings. In my primary examining rooms I have a permanent lighting setup, which adds to the reproducibility of the photographs. Whatever system is chosen should permit the same preoperative and postoperative photographs without variations of camera, lens, film, positions, camera-subject distance, background, and exposure. Ideally, a single imaging site with modern computer digital imaging equipment will enhance documentation and archiving of results.

I use a 35 mm camera with a 105 mm macro lens and 100 ASA film for photographs of the patient's breasts and torso. (My personal choice has been Nikon equipment, although many other major suppliers also provide suitable high-quality equipment.)

An automated flash provides accurate exposure and sufficient light output for the lens to be a minimum of F-8 depth of field or smaller. This ensures an acceptable depth of field. The background should be smooth, consistent, and uncluttered and provide some contrast with the patient's skin. Doors, windows, diplomas, trophies, photographs, bookshelves, medical equipment, and mirrors in the background are distracting. To achieve this consistent background for patient photographs, one wall in each of our examining rooms is painted a standard light blue and is reserved for this purpose. To minimize shadows the patient stands about 2 feet in front of the wall. Photographic lights are also installed in these examination rooms. Professionally designed lighting with multiple flashes with diffusers is ideal; however, consistency of exposure, distance, and lighting is even more important.

STANDARD VIEWS

Standard preoperative views include one anteroposterior, two oblique, and two lateral positions. They are all taken with the lens set at a standard distance, and I move the camera in and out to get a properly focused subject at the standard distance. The 5-foot distance with the 105 mm lens includes the entire chest area for most patients. If the subject is unusually large, the photographs are taken at 6 feet. With the flash mounted on top of the camera, a horizontal format gives good breast definition and minimal shadows for the frontal view. The patient is asked to slip her clothing down below the umbilicus since the frame includes the chin and umbilicus.

Lateral and oblique views are taken in a vertical format with the flash positioned in front of the patient, thereby casting a shadow behind the subject rather than in front. Oblique views should show the closest breast on frontal view and the distant breast on profile.

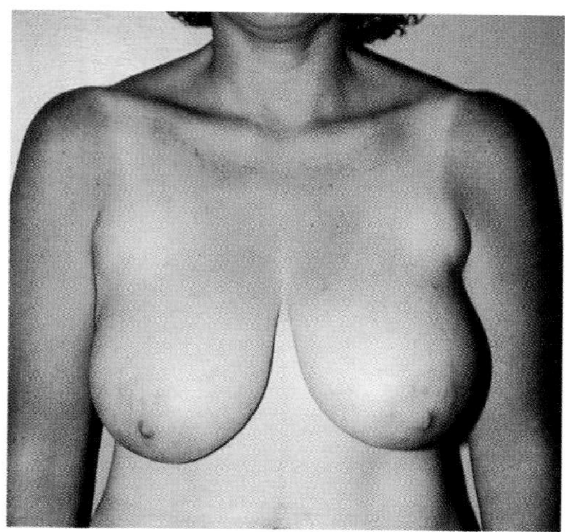

Frontal view

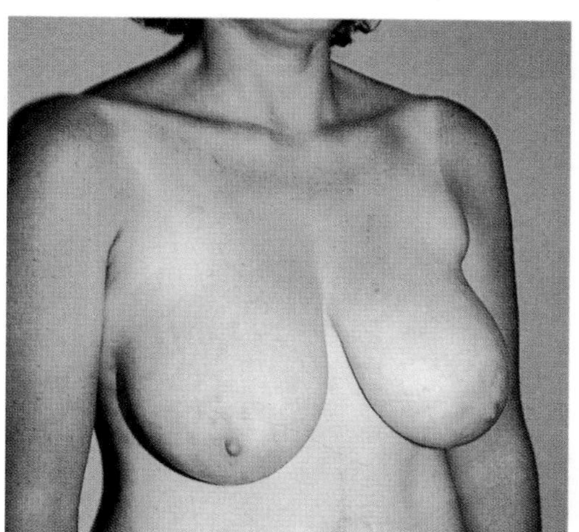

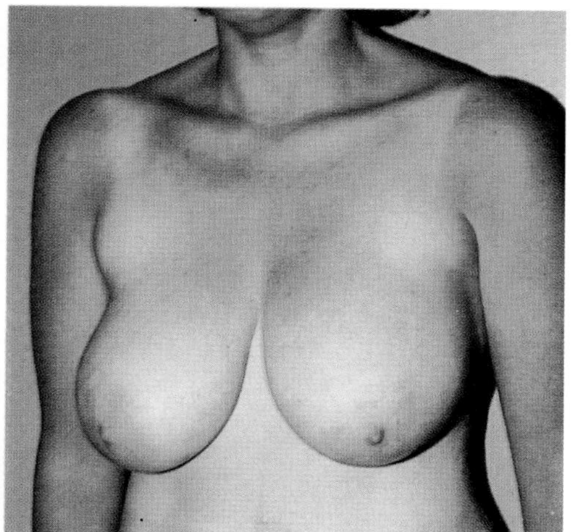

Oblique views

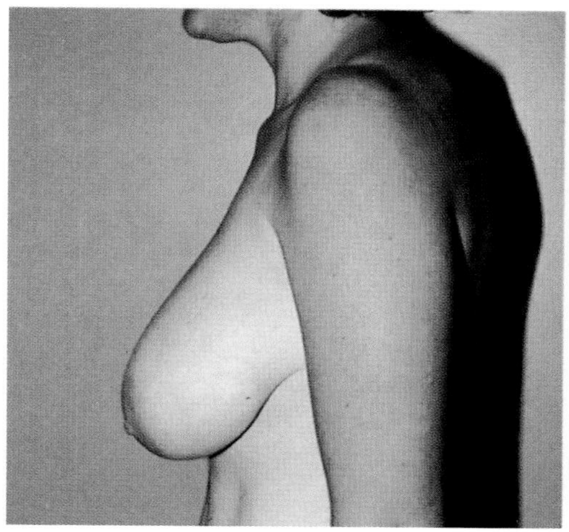

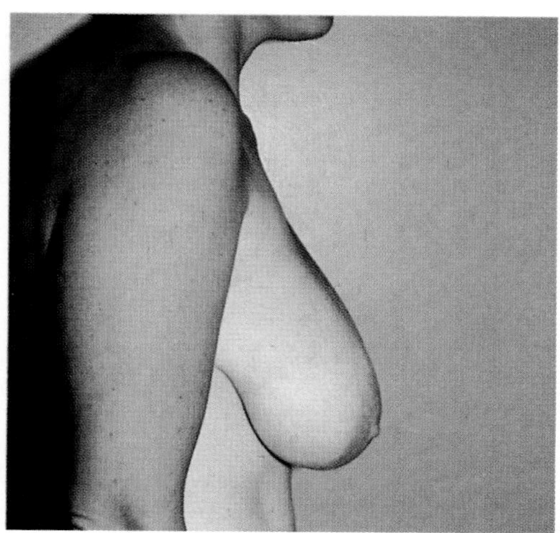

Lateral views

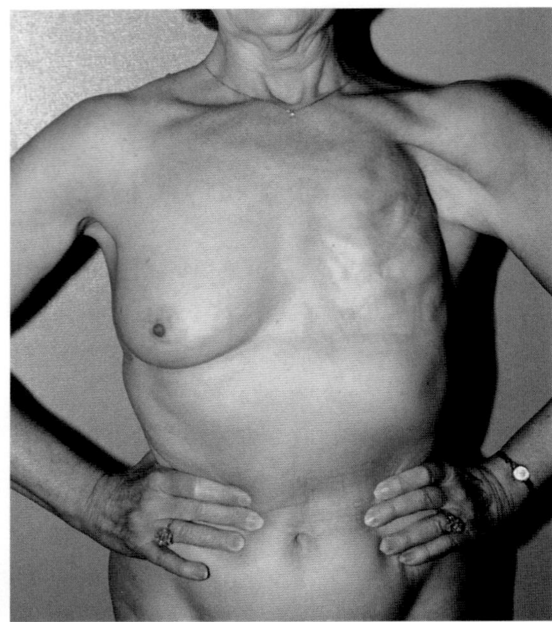

To accentuate pectoral muscle contractions and their effects the patient is asked to place her hands on her hips and push in. Another view of pectoral contractions is obtained by having the patient place her palms together below the waist and push in.

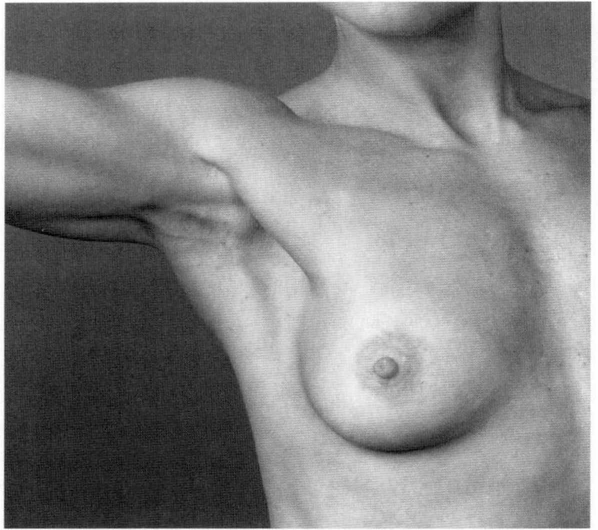

Axillary views picture the shoulder abducted 90 degrees, elbow flexed 90 degrees, and hand pointed upward in an oblique position.

DONOR SITE PHOTOGRAPHS

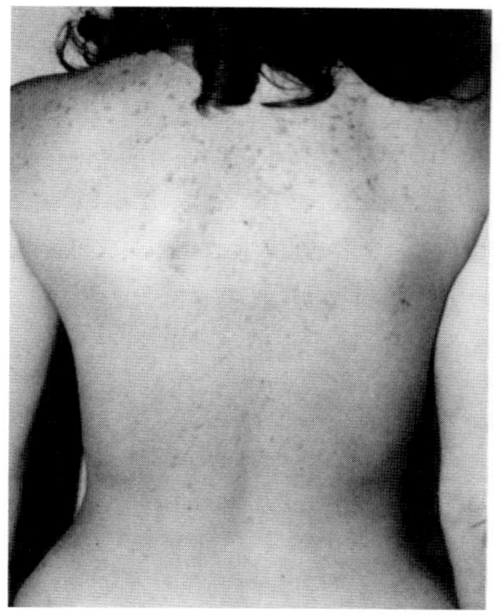

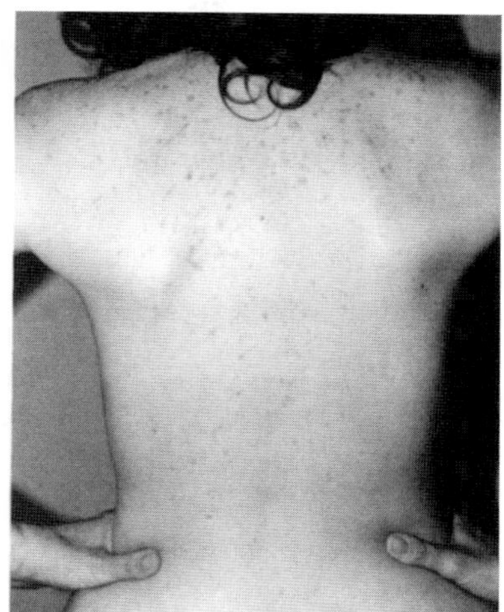

Patient positioning and camera-subject distances for photographing the latissimus dorsi donor site on the back are similar to those used for photographing the anterior chest wall down to below the posterior iliac spine. A view with the patient's hands on her hips, pushing in, can demonstrate muscle contractions and function, that is, the intact thoracodorsal nerve of the latissimus dorsi muscle. A lateral view with the hands elevated can document the lateral positions of the breast and latissimus donor site.

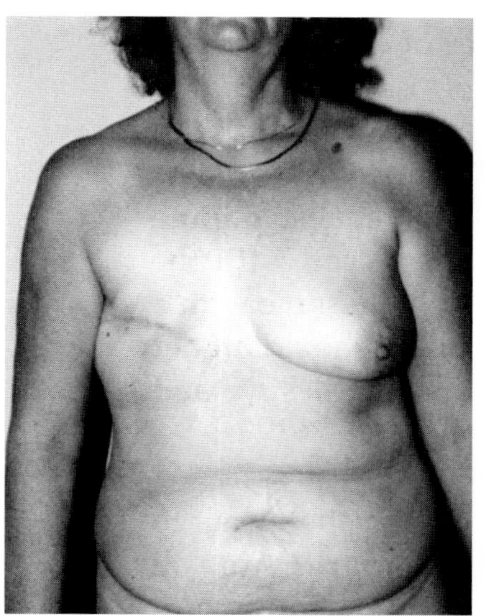

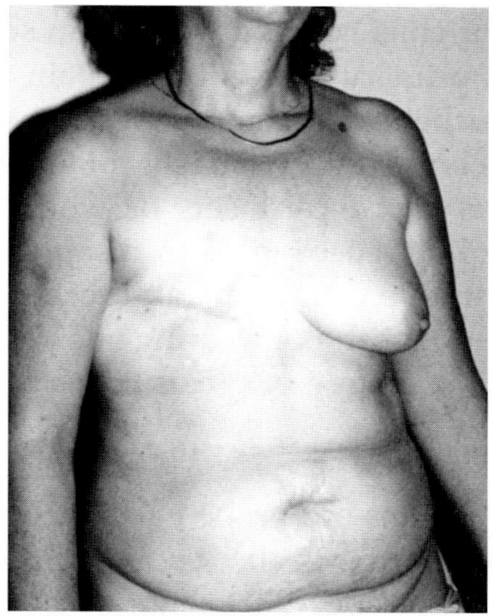

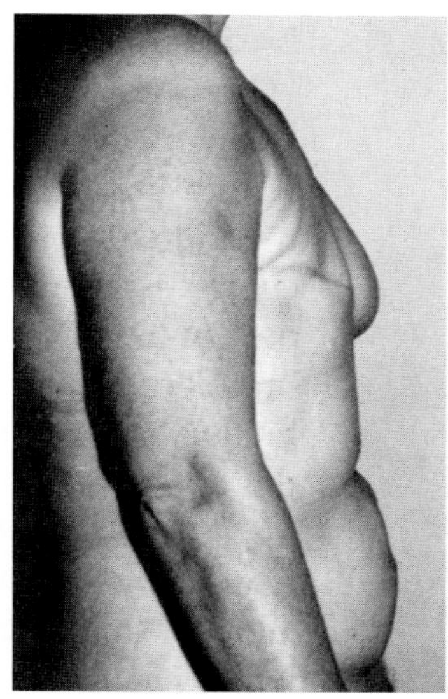

When photographing the abdominal wall donor site, I first obtain the standard breast views and then views of the abdomen and breast at a 6-foot camera-subject distance with the camera held vertically. The vertical frontal view is taken with the flash on the side of the deformity or, in cases of bilateral deformities, to the left of the deformity. In oblique views the flash is again directed to minimize shadows. These views always include both the breast and abdominal donor site area; a TRAM flap breast reconstruction cannot be effectively evaluated in preoperative and postoperative views without views of the entire torso area.

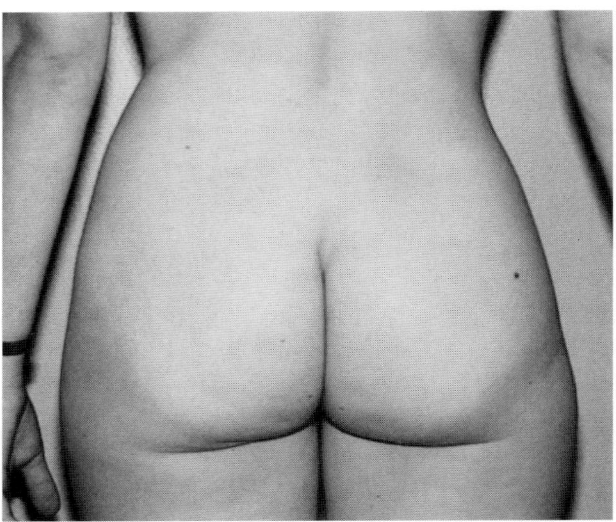

Donor site photographs for the gluteus free flap donor site should include the lower lumbar region as well as the upper thigh region. Oblique views are also helpful to demonstrate the length of the incision.

A full range of comparable-quality photographs provides a valuable record of preoperative and postoperative appearance. These photographs assist me in assessing the patient's deformity, discussing operative plans, documenting treatment, and evaluating results. They also lend credibility during consultations with patients and presentations to colleagues.

Clarifying Patient Expectations

Understanding patient expectations is the key to producing a surgical result that satisfies the patient. My approach to the patient places the responsibility on her to define her goals. At first she works through this without my input; afterward I guide her by direct questioning to better define her desires. In essence, I say, "You know your expectations better than anyone else. You will have to live with these changes so it is important that you give me a clear picture of what you want me to do. Now, tell me how you want your breasts to look and what you think I should do to alter them."

The patient is asked to actually point to her breasts and demonstrate exactly what she wants to change. Do you want them to be larger, fuller, smaller, flatter, less pointed, more uplifted? Do you want your breasts to look the same with a brassiere on as they do when not wearing one? When you look at your breasts, what is your chief concern, your main source of dissatisfaction? The mastopexy patient should lift her breasts to indicate the degree of ptosis correction that she desires and the appearance she wants. ***When the patient's primary goal is breast pain relief, I am particularly wary of advising aesthetic or reconstructive breast surgery, except in the case of breast reduction, where symptoms of back pain, shoulder grooving, and breast rashes can often be alleviated by reducing the weight of the breasts.*** Patients with an inordinate focus and a high level of concern over a relatively minor or practically unnoticeable deformity, patients who mention deformities that I cannot see, or women who request minute changes or revision surgery especially soon after an operation for minor asymmetries are particularly susceptible to disappointment, even with the best of improvements. ***Patients who express excessive disappointment over a relatively good result achieved by another surgeon may be impossible to satisfy and any additional surgery may further increase their stress.***

Any particular operative "no-no's" or restrictions such as scars and donor sites are probed and defined as are changes that she wants to avoid. What are her concerns about scar position and length? Is she willing to accept breast scars? What about a scar placed in the inframammary crease, the lower areola, or the axillary area? If the axilla frequently is exposed while playing tennis or sunbathing, a scar beneath the breast in the fold covered by a brassiere is perhaps the best solution. Does she object to having a breast implant inserted behind her breast? This is a particularly important question for the augmentation, ptosis, and breast reconstruction patient. The patient considering implant surgery is automatically supplied with a manual providing comprehensive information on these devices.*

It is helpful to get some idea of what the patient thinks about her current breast size; the size of her brassiere and the amount of padding it contains should be checked. ***I point out to the patient that brassiere sizes are not standardized and can vary with each manufacturer.*** Brassieres are shaped to fit natural breasts and may not fit an operated breast properly. The patient is also encouraged to bring in a brassiere of her desired size and any pictures or drawings that depict the basic form or look that she is requesting. These are

*Berger K, Bostwick J III. What Women Want To Know About Breast Implants. Reprinted from Berger K, Bostwick J III. A Woman's Decision: Breast Care, Treatment, and Reconstruction, 3rd ed. St. Louis: Quality Medical Publishing, 1998.

good indicators of the patient's desires and of the relative realistic nature of her expectations. I know that I have a problem when a patient's brassiere size is 40DD and she tells me that she wants to be a "34." In such cases it is in order to explain the lack of standardization of bra sizing and the relationship of cup size to chest diameter. The cup volume is larger when the chest diameter increases. A 40-inch chest diameter before a reduction will be 40 inches after the operation. Thus a change in breast size will not alter the diameter of the chest wall.

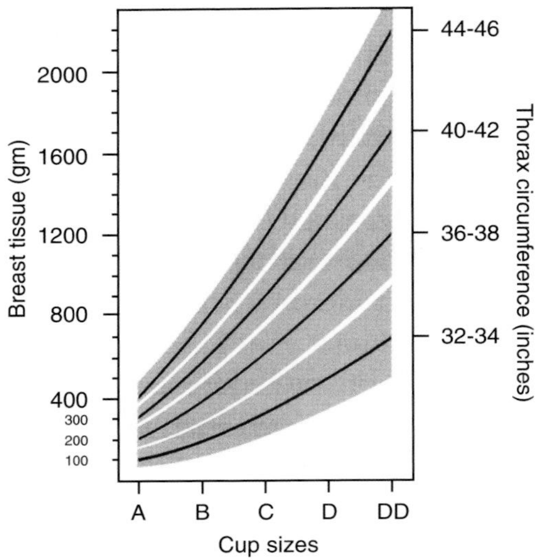

Relationship of breast volume, brassiere cup size, and chest circumference

No promises or guarantees of future breast size, especially brassiere size, are given; too much variation exists in sizes among manufacturers, and I do not offer such a guarantee. However, brassiere size can be of general help in conceptualizing breast volume changes and in understanding patient expectations.

Many patients, particularly breast reconstruction candidates, have a definite opinion about the timing of reconstruction and the particular surgical technique that they would like to have. The media has made the public aware of what can be accomplished with plastic surgery and the different breast surgery procedures. Additionally, support groups and other professional organizations inform the breast cancer patient of her options and possibilities for rehabilitation. We are dealing with a better educated and more assertive patient population that often has preconceived ideas about what plastic surgery can achieve. Many women consult with me because they want a specific procedure performed or technique used. If my judgment, experience, and training make me unwilling to do so (and sometimes that is the wisest decision on my part), they will go elsewhere until they find someone who will perform the operation that they have requested. Others come seeking secondary or reoperative surgery. I often suggest that they go back to the original surgeon who knows more of the specifics of the operation he performed. Nothing is wrong with these patient preferences, but they must be explored with the patient to determine the feasibility of the requested procedure for her particular physical problem. Sometimes her body type is inappropriate for the approach that she requests. Most patients do not have extensive knowledge that would enable them to judge what can realistically be achieved with breast surgery. Often it is possible to meet the patient's expectations with a less complex procedure than the one requested; she should always be informed of this simpler option. Patient expectations and requests sometimes appear bizarre or extreme because of information received from friends or the media. For instance, one patient came to see me with a photograph depicting the type of result she desired. The picture she gave me was of a thin woman with 100 cc breasts. Unfortunately, the woman I was examining weighed 180 pounds and had 42DD breasts and an ample protuberant abdomen; this was a truly impossible request.

Additional questions must be directed to the reconstructive breast surgery patient. Do you want to match an opposite breast? Are you willing to accept surgical alteration of your remaining breast if it will help obtain breast symmetry with the reconstructed breast? Are you willing to have breast implants? Most patients have heard about implants and have definite ideas about them. (Some feel strongly that they do not want these devices used because they do not want to add implant anxiety to breast cancer anxiety.) Do you object to a back scar, side scar, abdominal scar, or additional breast scar to improve the breast reconstruction? Some flaps require muscle transposition, and the functional implications of this transfer must be discussed. Are you willing to have a flap reconstruction if it will provide the optimal shape and breast fullness that you have requested? Alternatively, a woman may not want the additional scars associated with autologous tissue breast reconstruction. To help women understand the range of options available to them, I give my breast reconstruction patients written material to read and share with their families to help them make treatment decisions.* It provides details of operations, interviews with patients, and information on breast cancer and breast reconstruction.

*Berger K, Bostwick J III. A Woman's Decision: Breast Care, Treatment, and Reconstruction, 3rd ed. St. Louis: Quality Medical Publishing, 1998.

With cancer patients the breast surgeon needs to be aware of recommendations from referring physicians. The surgeon may have expressed a preference for a type of breast reconstruction for the mastectomy side and also may have given advice concerning the management of the opposite breast. These recommendations should be investigated with the patient and her other physicians. The age of the patient and her health and prognosis can also influence the choice of technique.

DIGITAL IMAGING

Digital imaging can be used to illustrate the results that can be achieved by surgical correction in addition to providing a system for archiving patient images. This technology, which can alter the preoperative image, is a relatively recent addition to our patient evaluation process. Although it is a useful tool to help the patient visualize potential changes, it also carries some hidden risks if it is not used cautiously and the patient forewarned that this is not an exact depiction or guarantee of a result. It is only being used to help the patient in her decision-making process.

Surgery with real tissues and real incisions can never be fully compared to computer-generated graphics. However, this digital imaging system can help the patient determine what areas need correction, what size and shape she would prefer, where the scars are to be placed and approximately what they will look like, and what techniques seem to meet her expectations for correction. Care should be taken to demonstrate average or even less than average results on the digital image so that the patient's expectations are realistic.

Not everyone will want to invest in a digital imaging system. Although this can be a helpful adjunct to patient consultation, similar results can be demonstrated by depicting the proposed changes on tracing paper placed over Polaroid preoperative views or by drawing a sketch of the proposed change to indicate (with the patient's input) the desired or expected breast appearance.

SURGICAL NOTES

As the patient explains her expectations, I take notes about each request and particular concerns that are identified. Any pictures or sketches that she brings as well as my sketches of what she desires are included in the record with my notes for later referral and further documentation.

Communicating

The entire sequence of patient consultation, evaluation, selection, and treatment is an extended dialogue. In the initial interview much of the information flows one way, from patient to doctor. By the time a decision has been made to recommend an operation for this patient, the balance begins to change; the surgeon becomes the source of information, advice, realistic expectations, and comfort. Now, specific information needs to be conveyed to the patient to address fears, answer her questions, develop a rational plan, and provide continuity of care with her other physicians.

THE DIPLOMATIC "NO"

Not every individual who comes for a consultation should be scheduled for an operation. Women seeking to mend an ailing relationship, succeed in a career, or bolster a sagging ego are poor candidates as are women who are psychologically troubled, have exaggerated, unrealistic expectations, or are obese, dangerously thin, or seriously or systemically ill. Sometimes the woman must be told "no." Before this decision is rendered, however, it is important to allow the patient to fully air her concerns and expectations and to thoroughly evaluate her situation. I try to deliver this negative decision without offending her but rather point out to her why I feel that an operation is not in her best interest. The skill lies in making her content with your decision.

I approach this problem by explaining to the patient that my primary duty to her as a physician is to advise and guide her in choosing the best course of action. If my evaluation indicates the advisability of a surgical procedure and if she feels comfortable with my decision and with me as her surgeon, then I might be able to proceed. Sometimes, however, I do not feel that an operation is in her best interest, that the risk is too great, that I have the particular skills to treat her problem, or that the timing is right for an operation (as in the case of the obese patient who needs to lose weight or the breast cancer patient who requires adjunctive therapy or more time to heal). In that case my only recourse is to either recommend that she not have an operation or that she see another doctor, better qualified and experienced, who can better meet her needs.

Not every patient and surgeon are a perfect match. ***Over the years I have come to trust my instincts and intuition to help me decide who is an appropriate candidate for surgery.*** If it just doesn't feel right, I say "no." This policy serves me well. ***The bottom line is that surgeons should like their patients, feel comfortable with them and their expectations, and feel confident that***

they could work with them if a complication develops. If the patient seems aggressive, questions every suggestion, denigrates previous surgeons, or blames others for her condition, I probably will be unable to help her.

DISCUSSING THE OPTIONS AND DEVELOPING A TREATMENT PLAN

For the woman who is a good candidate for an operation, the process continues. After assessing her specific breast deformity, I review her expectations with her in light of current, practical surgical options and what I feel is possible and appropriate in her particular situation. This is a challenge. To be effective this discussion should:

1. Achieve a balance between the patient's aesthetic appearance, psychological expectations, and oncologic considerations
2. Reconcile the patient's expectations with her age, body type, and physical condition
3. Address the patient's fear of and potential for developing breast cancer
4. Address the patient's concerns or questions about breast implants
5. Respond to the patient's questions about the different operative options
6. Emphasize the importance of individualizing her care

Now is the time for examining the options and deciding which operation is appropriate for the patient. I have found the best way to develop a plan is to attempt to define her expectations, visualize her ideal result, and then plan in reverse to determine the ideal operation to achieve this result. Digital imaging can be a useful adjunct for this planning process. First, we discuss the options for anesthesia. I explain to the patient that I ordinarily prefer to use general anesthesia to ensure that she is completely relaxed and carefully monitored by an anesthesiologist and to permit me to focus on the surgery without distraction. It is important to reassure the patient, address her concerns about general anesthesia, and explain the advances in outpatient anesthesia today that permit administration of short-acting agents as well as the use of drugs that minimize side effects such as dizziness, hangover, nausea, and vomiting. Furthermore, modern techniques for monitoring of Po_2, CO_2, blood pressure, temperature, and electrocardiographic changes make anesthesia much safer. She should be told that she will be able to talk to the anesthesiologist before her operation and to review her past experiences with anesthetic agents to ensure that the safest anesthesia will be used with minimal postoperative morbidity such as nausea and sedation.

For some primary aesthetic procedures such as breast augmentation, mastopexy, and small reductions, a local anesthetic supplemented by a continuously monitored sedative is appropriate. Local anesthesia is more difficult in secondary operations because of scarring around nerves that retards the uptake of the anesthetic agent. Generally, however, I feel that I achieve the best results with the patient under general anesthesia. I do perform some secondary reconstructive procedures using local anesthesia, especially for a hypesthetic breast that occurs frequently after a mastectomy. ***The prerequisite for any procedure using local anesthesia is effective communication and a patient committed to this experience.*** Ideally, the patient should be calm and not unduly anxious or frightened at the prospect of surgery. Nervous patients can become excited and hyperreactive, making a local procedure with the usual sedative agents uncomfortable and difficult.

Once the specifics of anesthesia have been discussed, I carefully review the preoperative images, pointing out any conditions such as breast asymmetries or hypertrophic scars. Since the patient often has not viewed herself in this manner, she gains a better understanding of the proposed surgical plan by assessing these pictures with my help. It is important that the patient and I agree on what we see. I also explain any contraindications to particular changes that she would like made, pointing out why her expected result cannot be achieved with her particular anatomic configuration. Sometimes I show the patient examples of possible complications if I am concerned that she does not grasp the seriousness of what she is contemplating and the potential problems associated with aesthetic and reconstructive breast surgery.

The rationale and realistic possibilities of each of the surgical procedures are explained and discussed. Along with the other choices, I always discuss the option of doing nothing. I explain that although in my judgment a particular procedure or approach will be best for the patient, my opinion may differ from what she expects or desires. The patient may say, “Do I have to have this operation?” I respond, “You don’t have to have any operation, but I feel this is the best for you if you choose to proceed.”

Most of the dissatisfied patients I have seen complain about poor communication with their doctors and results that deviate from their preoperative expectations. Many of these dissatisfied litigious patients say they wish that they had not had the operation in the first place. By carefully defining patient expectations and then discussing how and if they can be met, I allow the patient to participate in developing a treatment plan that combines what she wants with what is surgically feasible for her particular breast problem.

For example, the breast reconstruction patient should know from the beginning if a procedure on the opposite breast will be necessary or can be expected to achieve symmetry.

Photographs of other patients who have had breast surgery for similar problems are useful in exploring the various surgical options available to that patient. Selection of these examples is critical to avoid misleading the patient by showing her patients with unusually good results or idealized images. The patient should understand that these photographs or digital images do not guarantee that she will have the same quality of surgical correction. These patient photographs should be used for comparison, pointing out areas of similarity between their problems and her problem and explaining differences and potential difficulties. The images should show average or slightly less than average results that can be expected in her personal situation. Sometimes a potential patient is astonished by the scars associated with a good result. It is best to know this preoperatively so she can understand the sequelae, confront her misgivings, and make a truly informed decision as to whether to proceed.

Talking to other patients who have experienced similar deformities and who have had breast reconstruction or aesthetic breast surgery provides another positive source of information and support for the patient. My office staff keeps a list of women who have had a variety of procedures (especially breast reconstruction) and who are willing to speak with other women contemplating this operation. These women can help remind the patient that she is not alone or unique in her deformity or in her desire for correction. Women who have had similar operations can candidly discuss the advantages and disadvantages of the operation from an informed point of view, providing additional insights about pain, recovery, and expected breast appearance. By talking to another patient, the woman will understand that plastic surgery is not a magical panacea that offers immediate perfect results with no scarring. She can ask questions of another woman who has had this operation and actually see the scars resulting from the procedure. Selection of these postoperative patients is important; they should demonstrate "average" results, and the surgeon should explain that these results provide no guarantee that the patient will have the same level of satisfaction.

Timing

The appropriate timing of the operation and the number of procedures needed is another component of this doctor-patient dialogue. To avoid disappointment postoperatively, patients, particularly breast reconstruction patients, should be prepared for the possibility of at least two procedures to complete the reconstruction and to ensure proper breast shape and symmetry. Techniques that require more than two stages are often unacceptable to many patients. When the patient expects a two-stage procedure, she is more accepting of any shortcomings after the first stage, knowing that this is not a mark of failure but part of the plan. It is essential to remind the patient that she will have to live with her decision and her operation for the rest of her life; so it is important to take the necessary time now to ensure an optimal result. Timing of breast reconstruction is increasingly being coordinated with the breast management team because immediate breast reconstruction with autologous tissue is being performed more frequently by the oncologic surgeon and plastic surgeon.

Decisions for scheduling the operation must be individualized. The patient's psychological concerns, her age and maturity, her readiness to face surgery, the stress and emotional climate surrounding her deformity, and the quality of result that can be anticipated influence and determine the timing of surgery. The patient's social circumstances and lifestyle must also be factored in. She needs to know the specifics of the recovery process and how long she will be incapacitated. For most aesthetic breast operations, pain medications will be needed for 2 to 4 days; driving and normal activities will be curtailed and upper extremity exercise prohibited for a few weeks.

YOUNG PATIENTS

Younger patients are often distressed about variations in their breast size and shape. Normal breast development is essential to the healthy psychological growth of teenagers. Breast abnormalities in these patients can be corrected, but only if the patients are motivated and emotionally mature enough to undergo an operation. In my experience, breast reduction and correction of asymmetry and congenital absence of the pectoralis major muscle have been beneficial operations, even to patients in their early teens. One of my most appreciative patients was a 9-year-old girl with huge breasts who had a reduction mammaplasty. (See Chapters 7 and 9 for more detailed information on timing decisions.) Increasingly I am seeing younger patients who have experienced early puberty and are seeking reduction and correction of asymmetry. Many of my young breast reduction patients are 15 to 20 years old.

A good time to reconstruct the chest wall defect in a patient with Poland's syndrome is when anxiety about the deformity prompts the patient to request an operation. Patient cooperation is imperative. Many of the patients I have treated for this problem have ranged from 12 to 14 years of age. For males with Poland's syndrome who have an intact, functioning latissimus dorsi muscle, reconstruction at age 12 or 13 has been satisfactory. Females with Poland's syndrome who have an intact latissimus dorsi require individualized treatment. If possible, I prefer to wait until the breasts have fully developed so the reconstructed side will match a developed opposite breast and thorax. This is not always possible; sometimes the patient's psychological distress dictates earlier intervention.

I prefer delaying augmentation mammaplasty until the patient is at least 18 years old when breast growth is complete and she can make a more mature decision as to whether to undertake this operation with its long-term implications.

OLDER PATIENTS

I set no particular age restrictions for older patients as long as they are in good health and properly motivated to have an operation. Age alone is not a factor in deciding to operate on a patient who requests improvement in breast form. Some of my most satisfied patients who have had both aesthetic and reconstructive breast operations have been in their sixties and seventies. People are living longer and healthier today and often desire elective surgery to help them maintain their quality of life. However, our breast management team has observed that breast reconstruction can be a bit more difficult, complication rates higher, and postoperative pain greater for women over 65 years old.

BREAST RECONSTRUCTION PATIENTS

Timing decisions for breast reconstruction must accommodate adjunctive therapy for systemic breast disease, cancer phobia, and quality of life considerations. Although the trend today is toward immediate breast reconstruction, the choice between immediate and delayed reconstruction after mastectomy needs to be discussed. (See Chapters 11 and 17 for more detailed information on this topic.) Decisions about timing should be delayed until pathologic evaluation and staging of the patient's disease are completed. At that time the doctor and patient can weigh the different operative approaches and decide on the appropriate option. The patient's wishes, the stage of disease, and the timing of adjunctive therapy influence the timing of surgery. Today many women with larger or more advanced stages of breast cancer are getting premastectomy chemotherapy to shrink their tumors and possibly reduce local recurrences and permit less extensive surgery. Also more women are getting postoperative radiation, which may affect decisions regarding reconstructive surgery. These decisions must always be individualized. Some patients with advanced disease and a poor prognosis still request immediate reconstruction hoping to enhance their lives during the time they have remaining. Dilemmas about timing must be resolved by the patient, surgeon, and breast management team after assessing the alternatives.

Patient Education

A necessary component of communicating with the patient is providing information and access to community resources and educational materials that will help her understand her problem. Appropriate pamphlets, books, and articles related to the patient's problem should be available in the waiting room or library or the surgeon should be able to recommend a bibliography of suggested readings that she might want to pursue. The American Society of Plastic and Reconstructive Surgeons, Inc., has informative procedure-specific pamphlets available. Some surgeons use videocassettes. Although these can be helpful for some individuals, I have found that most patients would rather hear this information from their physician and members of the breast management team and then reinforce what they learn by reading about it in the privacy of their homes.

Information should also be provided about the various support groups that can assist the patient. Organizations such as the American Cancer Society, Reach to Recovery, and local support groups for women who have had mastectomies can be enormously helpful as can patient education materials.

Furthermore, the patient needs to understand that the plastic surgeon does not work in isolation but within the structure of the breast management team, a group of specialists who cooperate in providing her with the best care possible. The surgeon works closely with each of the members of the team in evaluating the patient and considering the most effective treatment. Despite the individual skills of the surgeon, this team backup is essential even for aesthetic breast surgery.

Postoperative Recovery

The necessity for good communication continues into the postoperative period. It is normal after surgery for the patient's breasts to be bruised, swollen, discolored, and painful. Anesthesia and pain-relieving drugs and sedatives can often make the woman feel depressed. She often will look at herself and think, "Why did I do this?" Postoperative depression and inappropriate concern that her breast appearance is permanent may upset the patient and cause her to request an immediate reoperation in the postoperative period. It is difficult at this point for the patient to see beyond the postoperative period to the final result. It is important to talk to the patient about these feelings and to anticipate them in advance. At this stage the patient needs to be reminded that her early postoperative appearance is normal and should not be a source of concern. The final psychological and aesthetic results of the operation will not become manifest immediately. It will take time; bruising will usually resolve in 2 to 3 weeks and swelling in 2 to 3 months. Complete healing may take 1 year and maximal sensory return possibly several years. In other words, it may take months until she feels normal and her final breast result becomes evident. Immediate reoperation is usually not wise except to correct obvious complications such as hematoma or to repair a defect associated with tissue necrosis. Ordinarily it is better to provide emotional support and advise her that any minor problem can be more accurately corrected later.

If there are any obvious shortcomings or unexpected results after surgery, the surgeon should acknowledge and point out these problems, if possible, before the patient mentions them. Or, if the patient does point out an asymmetry or other imperfection, the surgeon should not minimize the problem or her concern but address the problem and propose solutions. "Yes, there is an asymmetry, but this should improve with time. Give it a year to heal and then let's reexamine the situation. I assure you that if it still does not look right, then I will make the appropriate adjustments at that time to improve your appearance. Now, however, your tissues need adequate time to heal."

Medical-Legal Considerations

Most of the medicolegal problems I have witnessed stem from some missing link or breakdown in communication between the surgeon and the patient. That is why it is so important to devote time to establishing a close and meaningful relationship with the patient. In my experience, the most extreme cases of patient dissatisfaction involve:

1. Lack of or poor communication
2. A major disparity between the patient's expectations and the surgeon's expectations
3. Patient perception that the surgeon was uncaring or too busy to be bothered
4. Surgeon embarking on a complex or new procedure without sufficient training and experience
5. Patient perception that the surgeon or his office staff was unavailable or did not have enough time to spend with her
6. Surgeon who was unwilling to admit complications existed and address them openly and appropriately
7. Surgeon who reoperated frequently, inappropriately, and too soon after a complication
8. Surgeon who had not kept up with appropriate current techniques for this type of surgery and overlooked aesthetic or oncologic aspects
9. Poor patient selection
10. Patient who feels that the surgeon has abandoned her

Doctor-patient communication becomes even more important when a problem develops. In these situations the surgeon must double and redouble his time with the patient to let her understand his concern, willingness, and commitment to help her get through this situation and to achieve a result that meets her expectations. Early consultation in these situations can provide additional input as well as solace for the patient and her family.

INFORMED CONSENT*

Not until the latter half of this century did the courts and legislature add to the physician's duty of obtaining consent a new obligation of disclosure of information ("informed" consent). Physicians are now required to provide information in addition to obtaining consent because of the physician's fiduciary relationship with his patient—in other words, because the patient places confidence and trust in and relies on the judgment and advice of the surgeon.

*Modified from Sprung CL. Informed consent and the critically ill. Perspect Crit Care 1(1):61-72, 1988.

CONSENT TO OPERATION OR OTHER PROCEDURE

Date: ____________________ Time: __________ Patient: ________________________________

Diagnosis: ____

Procedure: ____

In conjunction with the procedure identified above, I understand the following:

Nature and purpose of procedure *(describe in laymen's terms):* ____________________________________

____

____

Material risks of procedure: Hematoma, infection, severe loss of blood, disfiguring scar, tissue loss, allergic reaction, cardiac arrest, and death. Other risks of procedure are: ______________________________

____

Likelihood of success: ☐ Good ☐ Fair ☐ Poor

☐ Unknown because: ____

Practical alternatives to procedure: ☐ None ☐ Other ______________________

____

Prognosis if procedure is rejected: ☐ Good ☐ Fair ☐ Poor

☐ Unknown because: ____

CONSENT: The procedure identified above has been explained to me, the material risks have been described, and all of my questions have been answered. I acknowedge that no guarantees have been made concerning the outcome of the procedure. I hereby consent to the performance of this procedure by Dr. __________ ____________________ and/or any assistants selected by this physician/surgeon. I also consent to the administration of anesthesia by a physician, anesthesiologist, and/or any assistants selected by, and acting under the direction and supervision of, this physician.

I realize that during the procedure the physician/surgeon may become aware of conditions which were not apparent before the start of the procedure. I therefore consent to any additional or different operations or procedures the physician/surgeon considers necessary or appropriate to treat, cure, or diagnose such conditions.

____________________ Witness	____________________ Patient Signature
____________________ Signature of Physician/Surgeon	____________________ Signature of Person Authorized to Consent for Patient* Relationship to Patient: ☐ Parent ☐ Guardian ☐ Spouse

*When the patient is a minor (under 18 years of age), the signature of a person authorized to consent for the patient is required. A parent or guardian may consent for a minor.

Most states require that patients be told the diagnosis, the nature of the proposed procedure, the risks and benefits of the procedure, and the consequences of not having the procedure. A surgeon may not be required to disclose risks that the average patient is likely to know. Several standards have been used by courts to evaluate a physician's duty to disclose information and each state has specific informed consent statutes. The professional standard of care is based on the custom of surgeons practicing in the community, and more than ever this is now based on a national standard of care provided by a properly trained physician. A second standard, that of material risk, requires a surgeon to disclose information that a reasonable person in the patient's position would consider material to a decision. Whether a risk is material is determined by its frequency and severity and may be defined by the state statute. If the risks are minor, the surgeon should inform the patient of common risks. If a serious injury could occur, however, the patient should be informed of all but extremely remote risks.

The elements of informed consent include disclosure of new information, competency, understanding, voluntariness, and decision making. Ideally, there should be mutual participation by the patient and doctor. The surgeon provides information to a competent patient who understands the information and who after being fully informed weighs the benefits of the proposed procedure against the risks; compares them to the benefits and risks of alternative procedures or treatments, including not having the procedure; and then agrees or refuses to have the procedure or treatment. Informed consent for procedures involving alloplastic implants, especially breast implants, must include information supplied by the manufacturer as well as that mandated by the United States Food and Drug Administration.

Informed consent forms are used to document that informed consent has occurred. Although a signed form provides evidence that some consent was obtained, it does not necessarily substantiate that the consent was informed. That is why a verbal explanation is crucial to the informed consent process.

Surgeons have become increasingly concerned about legal liability. In recent years there has also been growing emphasis on the rights of patients to direct the course of their lives. Physicians should recognize the right of patients to influence their care. ***To avoid legal difficulties, informed consent must be viewed as a means to foster trust rather than a way to avoid liability.*** As surgeons, we need to be aware of the elements of informed consent and the legal requirements.

Preoperative Instructions for Breast Surgery

ARRIVAL
Make plans to arrive 60 minutes prior to scheduled time of your procedure unless otherwise instructed.

POSTOPERATIVE MANAGEMENT AND TRANSPORTATION
If you are staying in a hotel nearby or going home, plan to have someone stay with you for the first postoperative night. Your *postoperative transportation must be prearranged.* It is best for the person responsible for your transportation to stay during the procedure. If this is not possible, the person responsible for driving you home must arrive in the department 1½ hours after the scheduled time of your operation.

MEDICATIONS
Do not take aspirin, aspirin products, or vitamin E for 4 weeks prior to surgery as these may promote bleeding. Also, medications containing ibuprofen may have effects similar to aspirin if taken on a regular basis just prior to your surgery. *See accompanying list.*

If you are taking such medications or any other medication for pain or arthritis or anticoagulants, please notify your surgeon. You may take Tylenol or products containing acetaminophen. *All drug allergies must be noted prior to surgery.*

ANESTHESIA
If you will be receiving general anesthesia, IV regional block, or monitored anesthesia, you *must* observe the following instructions:

Night Before Surgery
- Eat a light supper the night before surgery.
- *Do not eat or drink anything after midnight, not even water!*
- Do not take any drugs (medicine or alcohol) except those prescribed by your physician.
- Bathing either the night before or the morning of surgery is permitted.
- Notify your physician the day before your scheduled surgery if there is any change in your physical condition (i.e., temperature, nausea, vomiting, diarrhea, or extreme pain).

The Morning of Surgery
- *Do not eat or drink anything!*
- Brush your teeth but do not swallow any water.
- You may apply light facial makeup if you wish, but *no* mascara, eye shadow, eyeliner, or false eyelashes.
- Do not wear your contact lenses.

ATTIRE

- Wear casual clothing such as a jogging suit or loose-fitting clothing that buttons in front. *Do not* wear panty hose, high heels, or many layers of clothing.
- Do not worry about bringing a bra. We will supply one for you.
- Leave all jewelry and valuables at home.

HOME CARE AFTER SURGERY

- Before leaving you will receive verbal and written instructions for your postoperative care. Included in this information will be general instructions regarding diet, medication, bathing, and activity restrictions in addition to those specific to your procedure.
- After your surgery, have on hand easily digested foods such as ginger ale, crackers, Jell-O, and canned soups.

RECUPERATION

Plan to be off work _____ to _____ days after surgery, especially if your work consists of heavy lifting or vigorous activity.

Postoperative Instructions for Breast Surgery

PAIN AND MEDICATIONS

A. Your greatest discomfort will be within the first 24 to 48 hours after your operation. During this time, take your prescribed pain medication according to the instructions on the bottle. It is helpful to take the pain medication with crackers or toast to avoid nausea; it is not advisable to take medication on an empty stomach. After the first 24 to 48 hours your discomfort should decrease and the pain medication should be taken less frequently and then only as needed.

B. If you are given any additional prescriptions by your surgeons, take the medication as instructed on the bottle.

C. Remember to avoid aspirin and ibuprofen for 2 weeks after your operation. Tylenol is permitted.

DIET

Easily digested foods such as ginger ale, Jell-O, and canned soups are usually tolerated well during the first 24 hours after surgery. If you have no nausea, you may resume your usual diet.

WHAT TO EXPECT AFTER SURGERY

A. After surgery you can expect some breast soreness, swelling, and bruising.

B. You may also notice drainage on your dressings for a few days.

C. Rarely are there major complications following breast surgery, but you should contact your physician if you have:
   - Severe pain that does not respond to the prescribed pain medication taken as directed
   - Excessive pain or swelling in one or both breasts (Report this especially if there is accompanying redness, warmth, or hardness.)
   - Thick, odorous drainage or bleeding that does not subside

DRESSINGS

A. Dressings consist of Steri-Strips (small tapes directly over the incision), a strip of yellow gauze, and a white gauze pad. The outer white gauze pad and the yellow gauze may be removed 48 hours after your operation, but the Steri-Strips should be left in place. It may be necessary to keep a gauze pad inside your bra for a few days since some drainage will occur.

B. Over the gauze you will wear a bra or tube top. Depending on your operation and your surgeon's preference, you may also be wrapped in an Ace bandage. You may remove the Ace bandage the following day. Unless otherwise instructed, you should wear the bra or tube top for 2 weeks, day and night. (You may bathe without the bra.)

C. You will see stitches under the Steri-Strips. Depending on your surgeon's preference, these will be removed 1 to 2 weeks after surgery. You will be given an appointment date and time or a number to call and make an appointment.
D. Special instructions will be given to you by your doctor if you have any kind of dressing or drainage apparatus other than those mentioned above.
E. After nipple reconstruction, dressings consist of medicated yellow gauze held in place with Steri-Strips and gauze dressing. If soiled, the outer white gauze pad may be removed the day after surgery; the stint stays on until your next appointment. It may be necessary to keep the gauze pad on inside your bra or tube top since drainage is expected. The gauze will also serve as protection over the stint.
F. Keeping the incision covered with a gauze pad under your undergarments is usually more comfortable. After the expected drainage diminishes, some patients feel more comfortable wearing no undergarments around the household.

ACTIVITY

A. Have someone help you with showers, baths, etc. when you are taking the pain medication.
B. You may need to stay off work for 2 to 3 days after your operation until some of the soreness has subsided.
C. Limit arm use to routine daily activities such as brushing your teeth, eating, and combing or shampooing your hair. Avoid vigorous arm motion that requires pushing, pulling, and lifting heavy objects.
D. Once you heal and the soreness subsides, let pain be the deciding factor. If it hurts, don't do it!
E. Check with your surgeon before you resume jogging, aerobics, or any vigorous exercise program. Usually physical activities may be resumed 3 weeks postoperatively and sports activities in 4 to 8 weeks.
F. If you are not taking pain medication, you may drive a car 4 to 5 days postoperatively. If it hurts, however, don't drive. Please exercise caution and good judgment in this matter.

You may shower or bathe the next day after surgery, but do not soak your breasts in water and leave the nipple area dry until your next appointment. Remove outer gauze dressings as described above. Do not remove the Steri-Strips over the stitches. The Steri-Strips are water resistant and usually stay in place without difficulty until the first postoperative visit. If Steri-Strips happen to unpeel on their own, don't worry; replace them or simply protect the area with a piece of gauze.

Patient Evaluation and Treatment: Case Examples

PATIENT WITH BREAST HYPOPLASIA

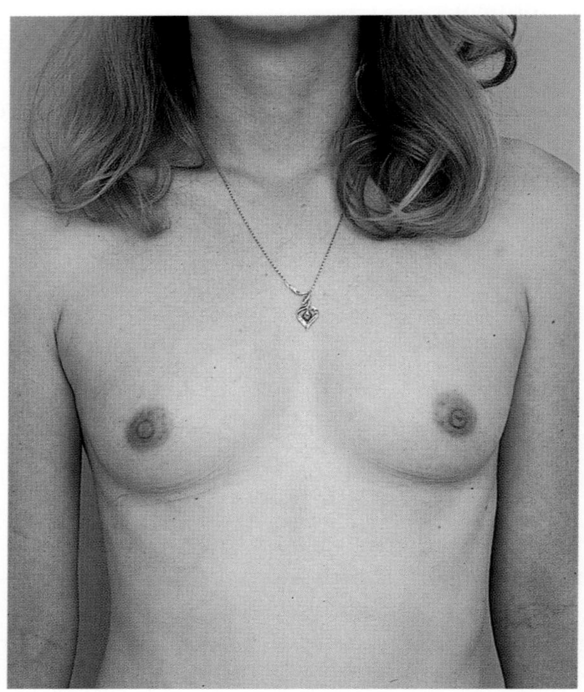

Her concern that her breasts were disproportionately small prompted this 24-year-old woman to request breast augmentation. She was very sensitive about her appearance, was particularly embarrassed when wearing sportswear and swimwear, and felt uncomfortable wearing a padded brassiere. She was athletic and highly weight conscious. When she lost weight, as she was prone to do, her breasts became even smaller and felt more nodular.

Motivations

Her emotional and psychological distress motivated her to seek corrective surgery. She desired breasts that were of normal size and in proportion to her body habitus. Several of her friends who had breast augmentation suggested that she consider this option. She was highly motivated to have breast augmentation to enlarge her breast size, improve her feelings about her appearance, and give her more self-assurance.

Medical History

This patient's general health status is excellent. A tonsillectomy was the only operation she had undergone. She has no systemic diseases or allergies and no family history of breast cancer. Breast development began at 12 years of age and she describes it as minimal with no additional breast enlargement since the age of 15 years. She barely fills a size 34A bra. Her mother is 50 years old and her father 52; they are both in good health, even though the father has previously had a coronary angioplasty.

Physical Examination

The physical examination confirms her good health. Breast examination reveals small symmetric breasts with an estimated weight of 100 gm. Although asymmetry is minimal, the left breast is approximately 20 gm larger than the right. Skin quality is good and without striae. She has no breast tenderness; however, the breasts are mildly nodular. She has a poorly developed inframammary fold and the areolar diameter measures 38 mm.

Discussion of Options

General

1. Do nothing. This approach is unacceptable to the patient since she desires larger breasts.
2. Gain weight. The patient is very active physically and wants to maintain her current state of health and level of nutrition. She does not want to gain weight and is convinced that it would have little effect on her breast size.

Surgical Choices

The patient desires a breast augmentation that does not produce visible scarring, maintains breast sensation and function, and minimizes the potential for capsular contracture. Choices include axillary, inframammary, or periareolar incisions, subglandular or subpectoral implant placement, standard open vs. endoscopic technique, and round or anatomic-shaped textured- or smooth-surface implants. The inframammary approach is ruled out because of the patient's poorly defined inframammary fold.

Treatment of Choice

Endoscopically assisted axillary subpectoral breast augmentation with a smooth-surface implant is recommended because it offers the best likelihood of a satisfactory result with a minimal scar. The axillary approach eliminates a visible breast scar, whereas the subpectoral placement minimizes potential problems with palpability and capsular contracture. The smooth-surface implant is chosen over the textured-surface implant because the patient is thin and has little subcutaneous tissue to cushion and mask possible ripples or texturing that may be evident with a textured-surface device.

Treatment Plan

1. Make 2.5 cm transverse incisions in the midportion of the axillary hair in a high axillary crease.
2. Develop subpectoral pockets with endoscopically assisted division of the medial and lower pectoralis major fibers to create satisfactorily positioned pockets for breast implants.
3. Insert 275 cc smooth-surface implants and inflate with normal saline solution to 300 cc; make further adjustments to provide the best symmetry.

AUGMENTATION MAMMAPLASTY WORKSHEET

PATIENT DATA

Name: Barbara Paddington
Age: 24 Height: 5'4" Weight: 120
Married: ____ Single: X
Nulliparous: X Pregnancies: 0
Children: ____ Nursing: ____

ONCOLOGIC INFORMATION

Family history of breast CA: 0
Prev. breast cancer: 0
Prev. breast surg.: 0
Mastodynia: 0
Fibrocystic chg.: 0
Breast disease: 0
Mammogram: NA
Masses: R 0 L 0
Biopsies: R 0 L 0

MEDICAL INFORMATION

Systemic disease: 0
Diabetes: 0
Bleeding problems: 0
Allergies: Pollen
Medications: Birth control pills
Smoking (pk-yr): 0
Alcohol/wk: Three drinks/wk.
Other: ____

PHYSICAL EXAMINATION

Chest wall:
Pectus defor.: 0 Scoliosis: 0
Asymmetries: R ____ L >20 gm
Constriction: R ____ L ____
Tubular: R ____ L ____
Striae: R ____ L ____
Breast scars: 0
Neurologic exam:
Normal: X Problem: ____

INFORMED CONSENT

Verbal explan.: X Signed form: X
Bleed sheet: X Preop. mamm.: No
FDA info.: X Mfg. info.: X

EXPECTATIONS Larger, fuller breasts to size 34B+ or -C

SPECIFIC DESIRES

To achieve: Fuller, more rounded breasts with more upper fullness
To avoid: Visible scars, capsular contracture

SYMPTOMS Embarrassed by small breast size

MEASUREMENTS AND PLAN

Chest circum.: 34"
Bra size: 34A
Breast width:
R 12 cm L 12 cm
N → infr. cr.:
R 4 cm L 4 cm
SN → N:
R 18 cm L 18 cm
Vol.: R 150 gm
L 150 gm

Other: ____

PLANNED AUGMENTATION

R 275 cc L 275 cc
Type of implant: Smooth X Textured ____

TECHNIQUE

Endoscopic: X
Subpectoral:
Incision: Inframam. ____ Periareol. ____ Axillary X
Subglandular:
Incision: Inframam. ____ Periareol. ____
Mastopexy: R ____ L ____

IMPRESSIONS AND NOTES Well informed; good candidate

PLAN Endoscopic axillary subpectoral breast augmentation with 275 cc round smooth-surface saline implants with anterior fill valve

Postoperative Result

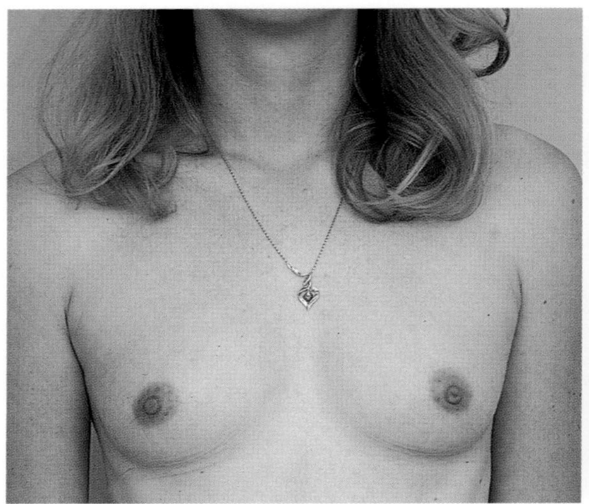

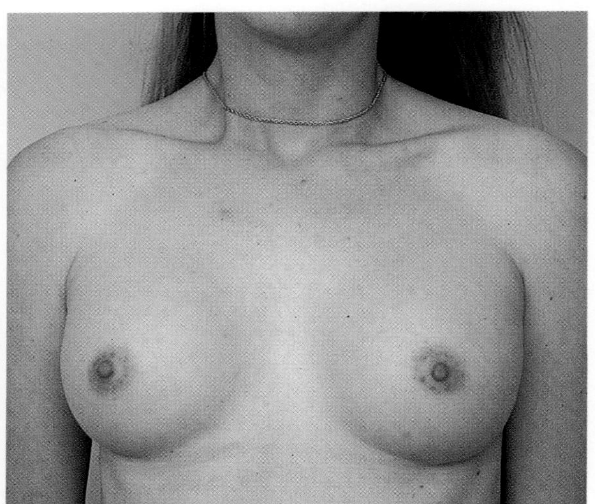

The patient was delighted with her new breast appearance. The procedure was performed on an outpatient basis, and when she returned at 1 week, primary healing without complications was noted. She began lower extremity exercises and fast walking at 1 week but waited 6 weeks to resume upper extremity exercises. She was comfortable with the improvement in her body image and her overall appearance. She now wears a size 34C brassiere. The axillary scars were somewhat erythematous for about 8 months and then faded until they were barely visible. Sensation below the areola was decreased for about 3 to 4 months but has returned to normal. After 3 months she resumed all preoperative activities. She reports that she feels much better about her appearance and that she no longer feels self-conscious in her clothing.

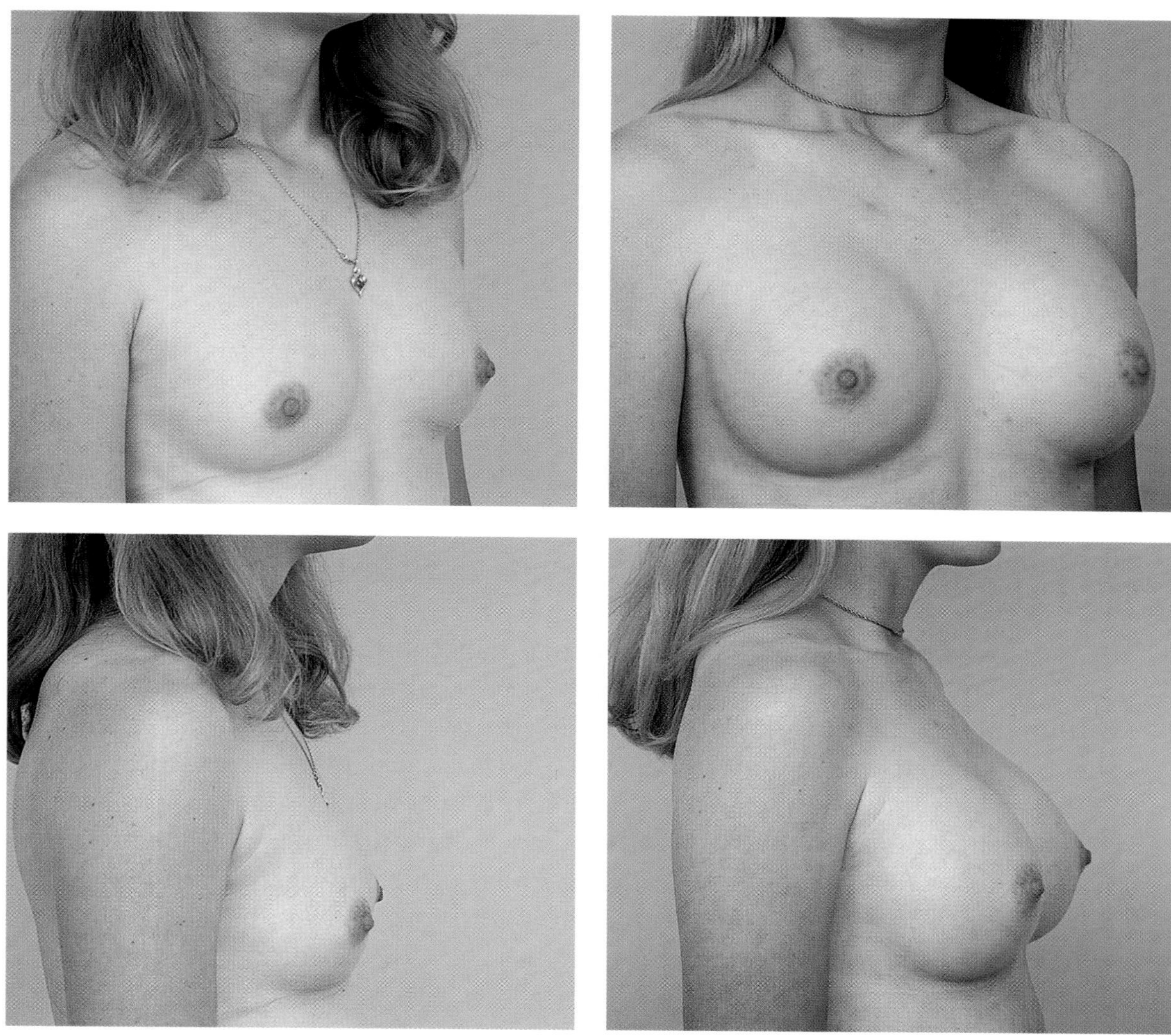

PATIENT WITH BREAST HYPERPLASIA

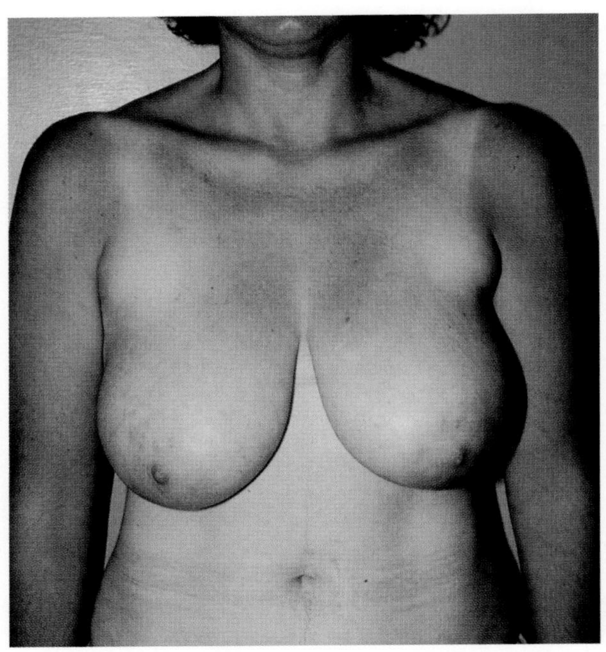

This young woman requested breast reduction as a solution for problems associated with her heavy breasts. She was a senior in college, a physical education major, and a sports enthusiast. Her breasts were uncomfortable, and she complained of the emotional and psychological problems associated with her large breasts. She was embarrassed by people who focused on her breasts when they spoke to her rather than looking into her eyes. She was self-conscious and had difficulty finding sports attire for jogging and swimming. As a runner who had competed in marathons, she felt that her breast size impeded her progress in sports activities.

Physical symptoms included pain in her shoulders and arms. She had difficulty in finding clothing to fit. Usually she had to purchase two different sizes of outfits, one large size for jackets and blouses and a smaller one for skirts and slacks. She also experienced some irritation under her breasts and pain caused by the necessarily tight support from the underwire brassieres she required. Her breasts were also painful during menstruation. Weight loss had not been a feasible solution because she said her breasts only looked larger as the rest of her body became slimmer. She was reluctant to diet because she feared that her already disproportionate figure would become even more so if she lost weight.

Motivations

She was motivated to have breast reduction to relieve the weight and discomfort of her breasts, to look thinner and more attractive, to facilitate her participation in sports activities, and to enable her to fit comfortably and appropriately in sports attire appropriate for those activities.

Medical History

This patient is 22 years old and has a history of good health. She has had no previous operations, no systemic diseases, no allergies, and no history of breast cancer in her family. Breast development began at 11 years and was completed at 15 years. She now wears a 36DD brassiere. Her mother is 48 years old and healthy and her father is 52 years old and in good health.

Physical Examination

Physical examination reconfirms the impression of general good health gathered from the medical history. Examination of the patient's breasts reveals full breasts estimated at 1000 gm weight with mild asymmetry; her right breast is slightly more ptotic and is 50 gm larger than the left breast. Her skin is of good quality with minimal striae. Her breasts are tender on palpation, and although dense, they reveal no prominent masses. The undersides of her breasts are moist and covered with a mild rash, but no infection is found. Her areolae are distended; their diameter is 6.5 cm. The results of a neurologic examination are normal. Examination of her shoulders demonstrates grooving from her brassiere.

Discussion of Options

General

1. Do nothing. This option is unacceptable to the patient because her large breasts represent a serious problem to her.
2. Lose weight. The patient has tried this alternative, but it was difficult for her because of the limits her large breasts posed on physical activity and because her breasts did not diminish proportionately with her body weight.

Surgical Choices

The patient desires a significant reduction but wishes to maintain lactation function and sensation potential. The choices include the vertical mammaplasty techniques, the superior pedicle techniques, and the inferior pedicle techniques. A free nipple graft is ruled out because of the patient's desire to breast-feed when she has children.

Treatment of Choice

The superior pedicle technique is chosen for this patient because of its potential for a larger reduction, thereby creating a smaller breast through removal of lower ptotic breast tissue with more likelihood of a permanent result with less recurrent ptosis.

Treatment Plan

1. Right breast: Estimated volume of 1050 gm. Left breast: Estimated volume of 1000 gm. Reduce breasts to 400 gm; remove 650 gm from right breast and 600 gm from left breast.
2. Position nipple-areola upward just above the inframammary crease and decrease areolar diameter from 6.5 to 4.0 cm.
3. Elevate nipple-areola on a superior parenchymal pedicle.
4. Remove hypertrophic breast tissue inferiorly and laterally to effectively eliminate ptosis and to narrow breast base with inverted T incisions.
5. Remove tissue from depths of breast to reduce breast projection.

REDUCTION MAMMAPLASTY WORKSHEET

PATIENT DATA
Name: Joan Decker
Age: 22 Height: 5'5" Weight: 130
Married: ____ Single: X
Nulliparous: X Pregnancies: ____
Children: ____ Nursing: ____

ONCOLOGIC INFORMATION
Family history of breast CA: 0
Prev. breast cancer: 0
Prev. breast surg.: 0
Mastodynia: 0
Fibrocystic chg.: 0
Breast disease: 0
Mammogram: 0
Masses: R 0 L 0
Biopsies: R 0 L 0

MEDICAL INFORMATION
Systemic disease: 0
Diabetes: 0
Bleeding problems: 0
Allergies: 0
Medications: 0
Smoking (pk-yr): 0
Alcohol/wk: Occasional beer
Other: —

PHYSICAL EXAMINATION
Chest wall:
Pectus defor.: 0 Scoliosis: 0
Asymmetries: R +50 gm L ____
Constriction: R 0 L 0
Tubular: R 0 L 0
Striae: R Minimal L Minimal
Breast scars: ____
Neurologic exam:
Normal: OK Problem: ____

INFORMED CONSENT
Verbal explan.: X Signed form: X
Bleed sheet: X Preop. mamm.: 0
FDA info.: ____ Mfg. info.: ____

EXPECTATIONS
Reduction to size B bra

SPECIFIC DESIRES
To achieve: Small, symmetric breasts, good support
To avoid: Long, thick scars

SYMPTOMS
Heaviness, back/shoulder pain, moisture under breasts

MEASUREMENTS AND PLAN
Chest circum.: 36"
Bra size: DD
Breast width:
R 22 cm L 22 cm
N → infr. cr.:
R 12 cm L 12 cm
SN → N:
R 26 cm L 26 cm
Vol.: R 1050 gm
L 1000 gm

PLANNED REDUCTION
Resection: R 650 gm L 600 gm
Areolar diameter: R 6 cm L 6 cm
Lateral folds: 0
Abdominal excess: 0

TECHNIQUE
Vertical pedicle: ____
Superior pedicle: X
Inferior pedicle: ____
Free nipple graft: ____

Liposuction: SAL: ____ UAL: ____

IMPRESSIONS AND NOTES
Good candidate, athlete

PLAN
Superior pedicle technique

Postoperative Result

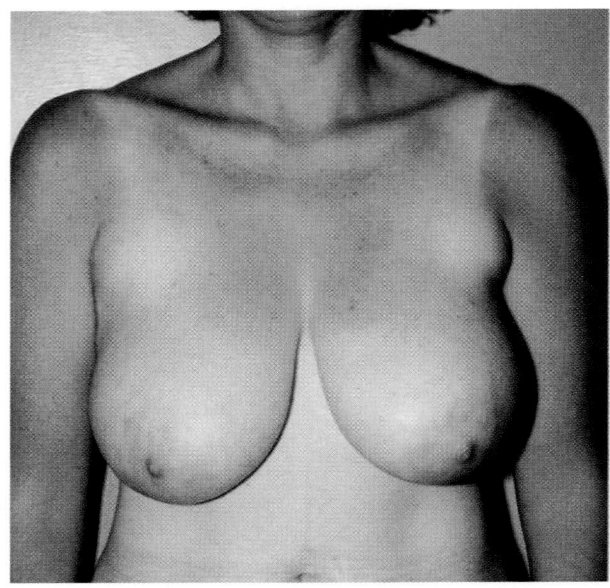

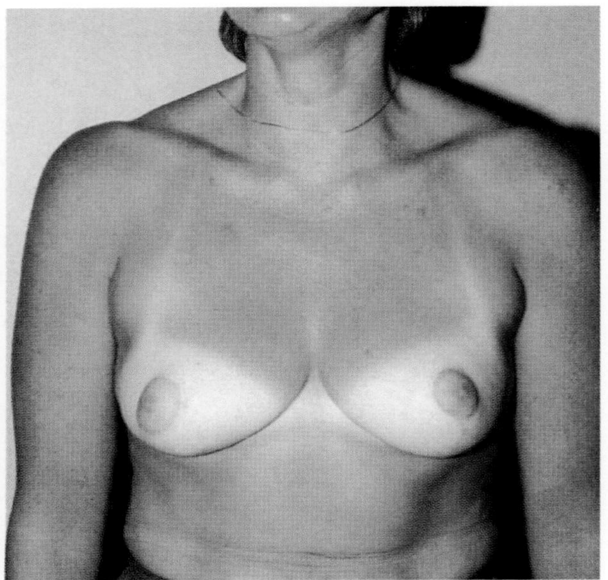

The patient was pleased with her new breast proportions. She returned to lower extremity exercises and fast walking in 1 week and waited 6 weeks to resume overhead arm activity. She found the positive effects on her body image led to increasing physical activity to the point of training for another marathon, and as she enthusiastically reported, 1 year following her reduction and especially with increased training she was able to clock a 30-minute improvement in her marathon time.

Her scars were erythematous for the first year, but they gradually faded during the second year. Nipple sensation was somewhat diminished for the first month after surgery. After a period of paresthesia, nipple-areola sensation returned.

She is presently employed as a high school science teacher and coach and is participating actively in sports and is even competing in triathlons. She has subsequently lost 10 pounds in addition to the 2+-pound breast reduction. Her weight loss has had little noticeable effect on her surgically reduced breasts; even though they did get somewhat smaller, they were still in proportion to her general body weight.

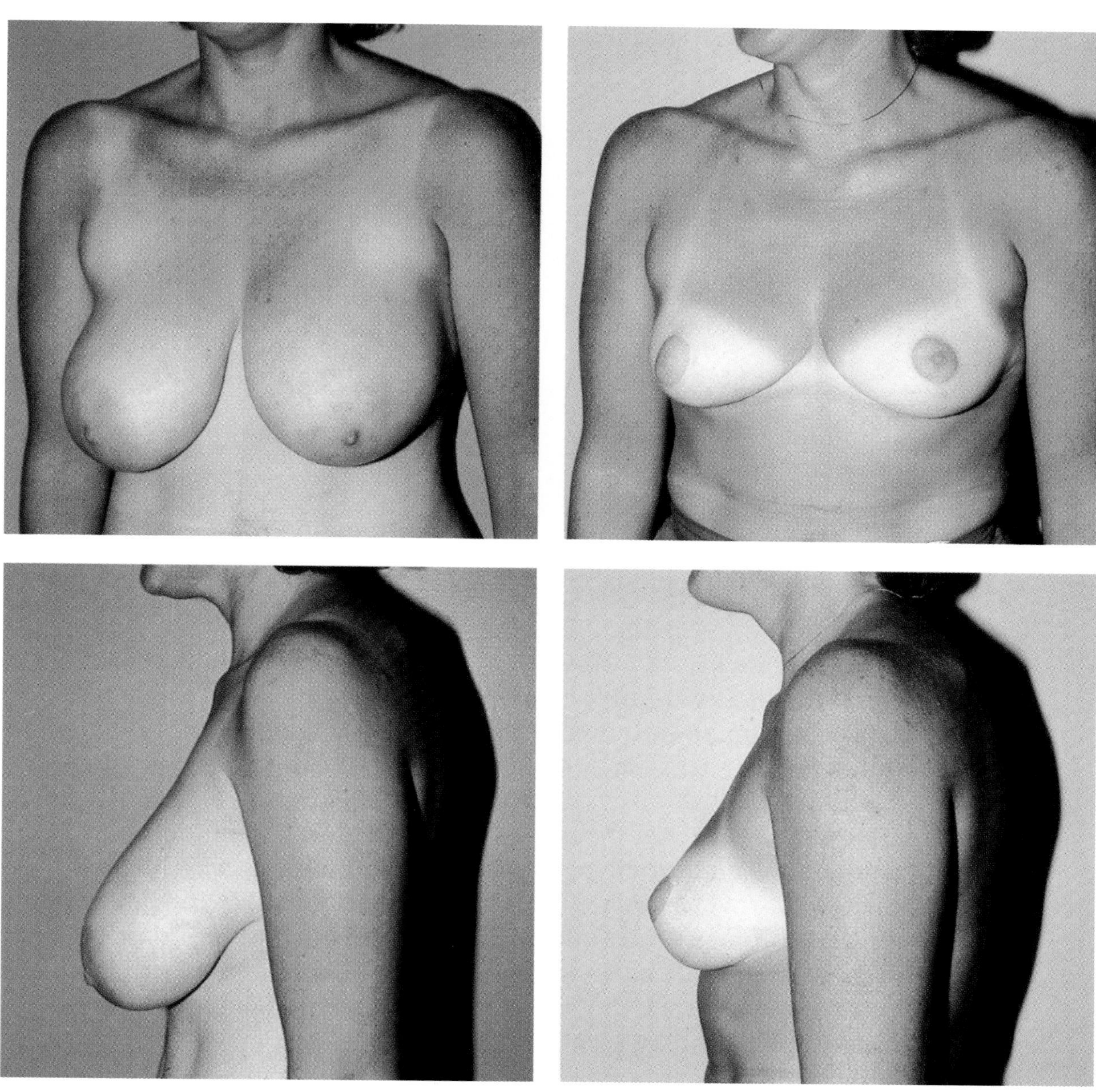

PATIENT WITH CARCINOMA OF THE RIGHT BREAST

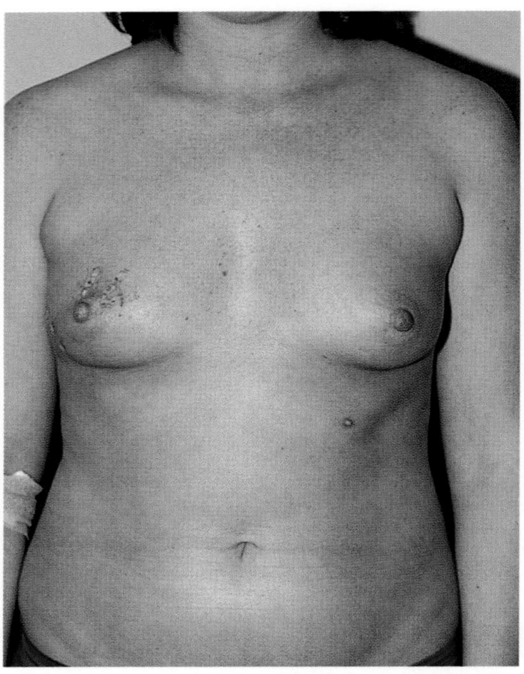

This young woman discovered a small mass in the central lateral portion of her right breast during her monthly breast self-examination. Mammography revealed a suspicious mass and multiple areas of calcification in her breast. A biopsy identified a 1 cm diameter infiltrating ductal carcinoma of the breast and multiple areas of ductal carcinoma in situ extending to the margin of the resection. Because of the extensive calcifications and ductal carcinoma in situ, a total mastectomy with skin-sparing incisions was advised and immediate breast reconstruction was suggested. The patient concurred with her surgical oncologist's recommendation for the skin-sparing mastectomy and was relieved that the option of immediate breast reconstruction was also available because she did not want to experience breast loss. She wanted to have minimal breast scars and to avoid a mastectomy deformity. She had concerns about breast implants and did not want them used for her reconstruction.

Medical History

This 34-year-old woman has enjoyed good health. She does not smoke cigarettes and avoids alcohol consumption. She has had no previous operations, no history of systemic disease, no allergies, and no family history of breast cancer. Breast development began when she was 9 years old and was completed by age 15. She wears a size 36B brassiere. Her mother is 58 years old and her father is 62 years old; they are both in good health.

Physical Examination

Physical examination confirms that she is a healthy young woman with cancer confined to her right breast region. There is a well-healed biopsy scar in the lateral aspect of her right breast but no axillary adenopathy and no additional positive findings on breast examination. The mild fullness in the lower abdomen will provide sufficient tissue for a breast reconstruction with autologous tissue. Her skin is of good quality and there is no breast tenderness and no striae. Her areola is 4 cm in diameter and she has a well-defined inframammary fold. Results of a neurologic examination are normal.

Discussion of Options

General

1. Lumpectomy vs. mastectomy
2. Skin-sparing mastectomy vs. traditional transverse extended incision
3. Sentinel node vs. axillary lymph node dissection
4. Immediate vs. delayed reconstruction
5. Autologous vs. implant reconstruction

Reconstructive Choices

The patient desires an aesthetic, natural breast restoration with minimal breast scars and good axillary contour. She does not want a breast implant and would like her abdomen reduced with the TRAM flap procedure. She also wants nipple-areola reconstruction but not at the expense of additional scars. She requests that her opposite breast not be modified, but be used as the model for the reconstructed breast. Although the patient has indicated a preference for the TRAM flap, the other reconstructive approaches are reviewed, including a latissimus dorsi flap with tissue expansion, microsurgical transfer from the abdomen, buttocks, or thigh, and a unipedicle TRAM flap. A latissimus dorsi flap with tissue expansion would produce the symmetry desired, but the patient does not want a back scar and desires abdominal contouring. Microsurgical tissue transfer of the thigh or buttock tissue is ruled out because the patient objects to these donor sites and associated scars. An abdominal tissue free flap would also be an acceptable alternative; however, the patient would still need extensive abdominal dissection for the abdominoplasty she requested.

Treatment of Choice

A right contralateral pedicled TRAM flap immediate breast reconstruction was done after a total skin-sparing mastectomy and sentinel node biopsy. The areola site was replaced with TRAM flap skin. The TRAM flap met the patient's criteria for an autologous tissue reconstruction that would produce a warm, natural-feeling breast symmetric with her opposite breast without modifying it. It also provided the abdominoplasty that she wanted. The nipple was reconstructed with a C-V flap to avoid additional breast scars and produce the moderate-sized nipple required for symmetry. The areola was tattooed 2 months after nipple restoration.

Treatment Plan

1. Periareolar and lateral incision for right total skin-sparing mastectomy
2. Axillary incision for sentinel node biopsy
3. Immediate reconstruction with contralateral unipedicle TRAM flap
   a. Define model for breast reconstruction by determining opposite breast size and dimensions and dimensions and size of mastectomy specimen.
   b. Confirm intraoperatively vascularity of superior epigastric pedicle with Doppler probe.
   c. Define and preserve inframammary fold and lateral and medial breast margins.
   d. Create upper abdominal tunnel and transfer flap to breast.
   e. Position flap at 90 degrees.
   f. Deepithelialize flap after positioning and trimming to provide optimal symmetry.
   g. Close areolar circle with purse-string suture.

BREAST RECONSTRUCTION WORKSHEET

PATIENT DATA

Name: Carol Fulton

Age: 34 Height: 5'5" Weight: 130

Married: X Single: ______

Nulliparous: ______ Pregnancies: 0

Children: ______ Nursing: ______

ONCOLOGIC INFORMATION

Family history of breast CA: 0

Prev. breast cancer: 0

Prev. breast surg.: Recent lateral biopsy

Gen. surgeon: Melanie Jones

Oncologist: Catherine Sears

Gen. surgeon's recom.: Skin-sparing mast. and immed. reconstr.

Breast Cancer:

R: X L: ______ Bilateral: ______

Type cancer: R IDC L ______

Positive nodes: R ? L ______

Therapy:

Rad. mast.: ______ Mod. rad.: ______

Skin-sparing mast.: X

Lump/radiat.: ______ Chemo.: 0

Hormonal: 0 Radiat.: 0

Opposite Breast: R ______ L 0

Mastodynia: 0 Fibrocystic chg.: 0

Mammogram: Recent

Masses: R 0 L 0

Biopsies: R 0 L 0

MEDICAL INFORMATION

Systemic disease: 0

Diabetes: 0

Bleeding problems: 0

Allergies: 0

Medications: 0

Smoking (pk-yr): 0

Alcohol/wk: 0

Other: —

PHYSICAL EXAMINATION

Breast Exam:

Scars: R 2 cm lat. L 0

Scars: Back 0 Abdomen 0

Chest Wall:

Pectus defor.: 0 Scoliosis: 0

Muscle Function:

Lat. dorsi: OK Other: Abd. wall OK

Neurologic Exam: Normal

INFORMED CONSENT

Verbal explan.: X Signed form: X

Bleed sheet: X Preop. mamm.: X

FDA info.: X Mfg. info.: X

EXPECTATIONS Skin-sparing mast., immed. breast reconstr., abdominoplasty

SPECIFIC DESIRES

To achieve: Treatment of breast cancer and immed. reconstr.

To avoid: Breast implants

Timing of Procedure: Immed.: X Delay: ______

MEASUREMENTS AND PLAN

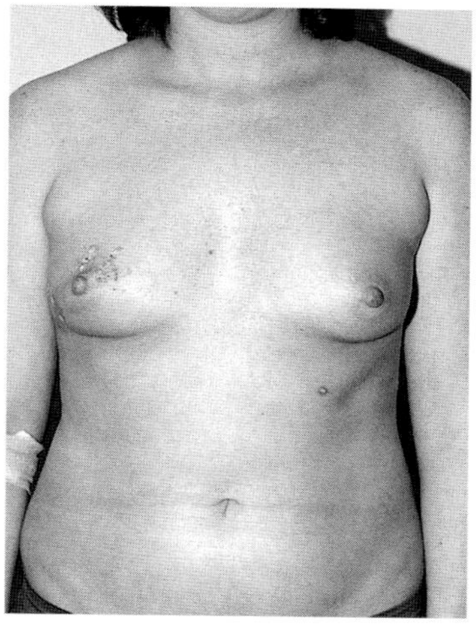

Chest circum.: 36"

Bra size: C

Breast width:

R 22 cm L 22 cm

Clav. → N-A: 22 cm

N-A → infr. cr.: 30 cm

Opposite Breast:

Estimated preop. vol.: 600 gm

Ptosis: Pseudo: 0 Mild: 0 Mod.: 0 Major: 0

Striae: R 0 L 0

Planned Change: Nothing: ______

Reduction: ______ Augmentation: ______

Mastopexy: ______ Prophylactic mastectomy: ______

Reconstructive Breast:

Clavicle to infr. cr.: 22 cm

N-A: 0

Skin quality: OK Rad. injury: 0

TECHNIQUE

Avail. tiss.: ______

Tiss. expan.: ______

Latiss. dorsi: ______

TRAM: Unipedicle lower

Microsurgery: ______

Lateral tissue to remove: ______

Tissue deficiency: ______

Abdominal excess: ______

IMPRESSIONS AND NOTES Motivated, candidate for immed. TRAM

PLAN Unipedicle right TRAM after skin-sparing mast.

Postoperative Result

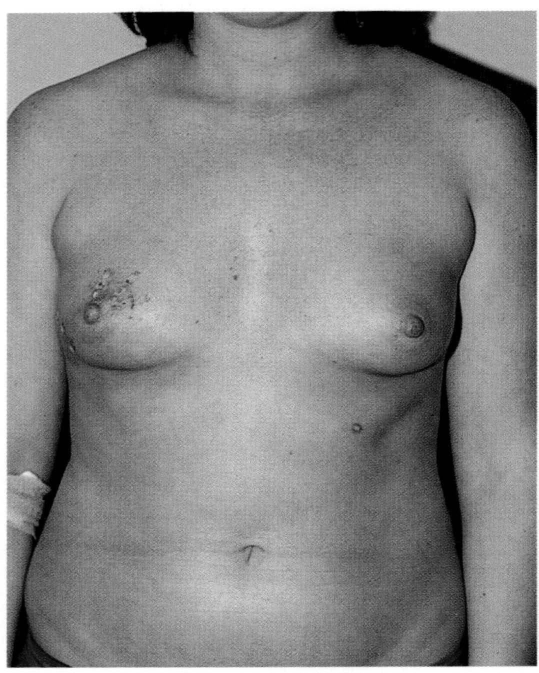

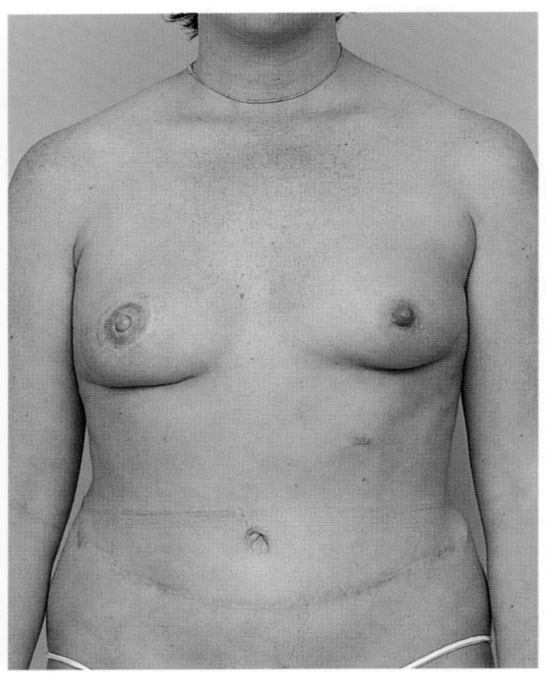

The patient had immediate reconstruction with a unipedicle TRAM flap after skin-sparing mastectomy. She had one positive node and required a right axillary node dissection in addition to the skin-sparing mastectomy. She was hospitalized for 4 days following the procedure. After recovering at home for 6 weeks, she returned to work with restrictions on activity level. She began chemotherapy 1 month following the operation, and her nipple was reconstructed 6 months following the completion of chemotherapy and 8 months following the mastectomy. When her nipple was reconstructed, liposuction of the upper and lateral abdominal areas and the mons pubis region was performed. The areola was tattooed 2 months after nipple reconstruction. At 3 years she had no evidence of recurrence and was delighted with the results of her breast reconstruction and her slimmer abdominal contour. Her breasts are symmetric and warm and sensation is beginning to return. She has resumed full physical activity and has experienced no restrictions or abdominal wall weakness when she swims, jogs, rides her bicycle, and works out at her health center.

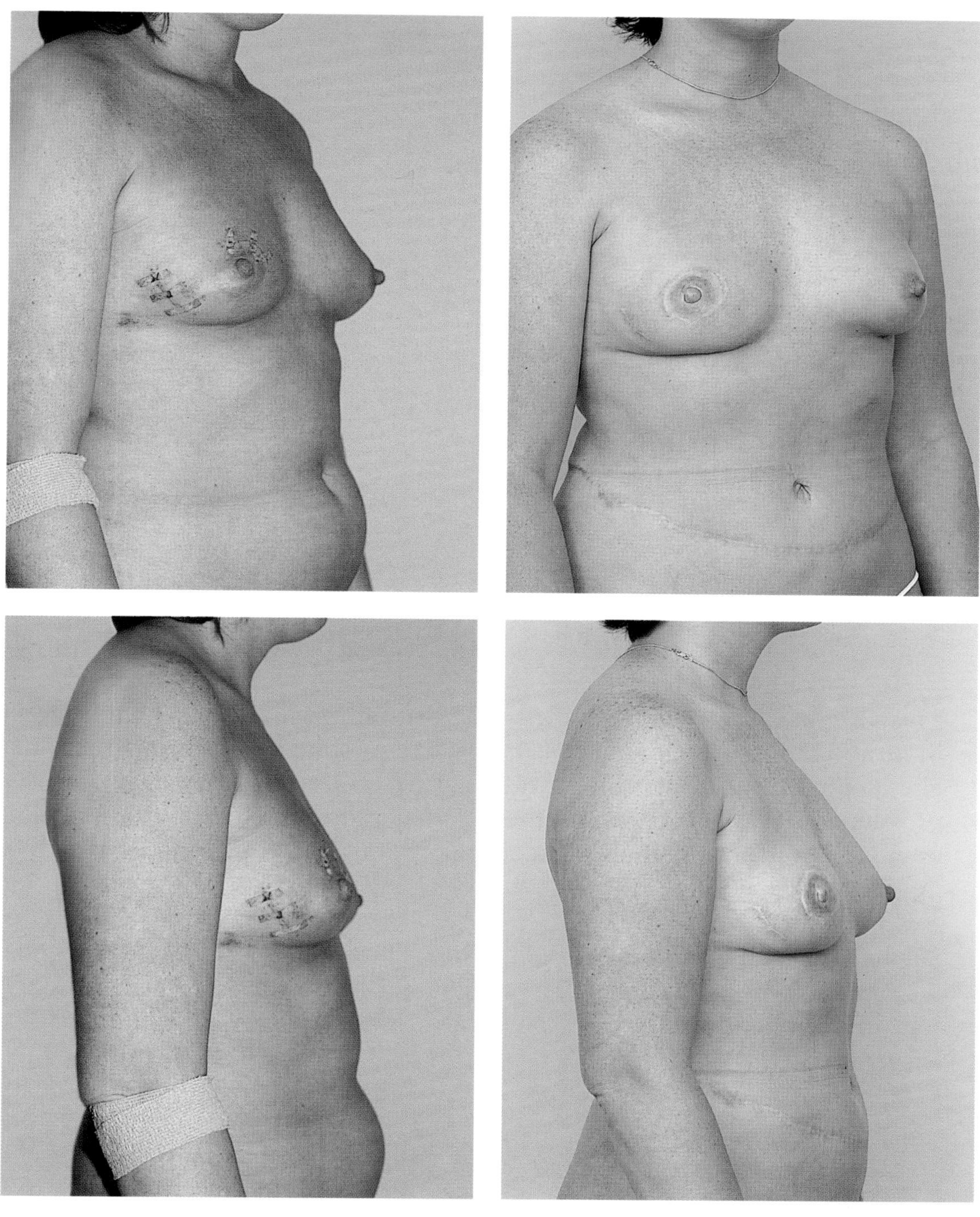

PATIENT WITH MODIFIED RADICAL MASTECTOMY DEFORMITY

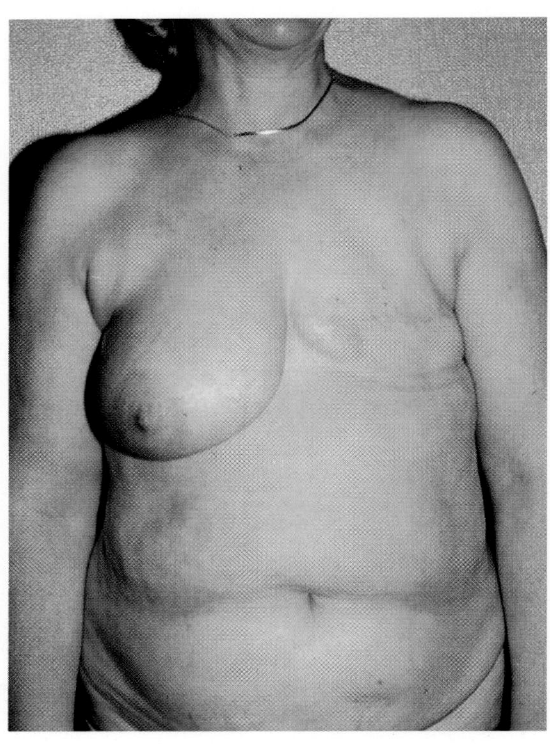

This 48-year-old woman had a left modified radical mastectomy for stage I infiltrating breast carcinoma 1 year before requesting breast reconstruction. She had a large, full opposite breast that necessitated a large, heavy breast prosthesis for balance. Despite the external prosthesis, there was marked asymmetry. The woman also had a large abdomen and desired an abdominoplasty.

She had physical symptoms of pain in her right shoulder and heaviness and discomfort in her right breast. The weight and size of the external prosthesis was irritating, uncomfortable, physically tiring, and severely limited her leisure activities.

Motivations

She is motivated to have breast reconstruction and specifically requests a TRAM flap technique to avoid breast implants and to contour her abdomen. She also desires a small reduction of her opposite breast.

Medical History

The patient is 48 years old and has enjoyed good health prior to the diagnosis of breast cancer. She has no family history of breast cancer and does not want a prophylactic mastectomy. A mammogram of her right breast reveals no calcifications or suspicious masses. She wears a 40DD brassiere. Her mother is 72 years old and well; her father died of heart disease at 69 years of age. She has borne three children and has no abdominal scars from previous operations. She had never smoked cigarettes and had no indications of arthritis, collagen or vascular diseases, or any systemic illness.

Physical Examination

Physical examination reveals a generally healthy but overweight woman who has recently had a left modified radical mastectomy; her right hypertrophic breast has an estimated volume of 1200 gm. Her abdomen is protuberant and has a generous panniculus. There are no abdominal scars. Her skin is of good quality but has some striae. Examination of her right breast reveals no dominant masses. A mild rash is evident beneath the right breast, but it is not associated with infection. Her right areola is 7 cm in diameter and shows no evidence of rash.

Discussion of Options

General

1. Do nothing. This is not acceptable to the patient because of her mastectomy deformity, heavy opposite breast, and excess abdominal tissue.
2. Lose weight. The patient has unsuccessfully tried losing weight but was limited in her physical activity because of her deformity and the imbalance it produced.

Reconstructive Choices

The patient desires breast restoration and an abdominoplasty. Because her opposite breast is large and ptotic, she also requests some breast reduction and elevation. Although the patient has requested a specific technique, we reviewed all possible options to make sure that her request was realistic. Possible choices include tissue expansion, a latissimus dorsi flap with tissue expansion, microsurgical tissue transfer from the abdomen or buttocks, and a bipedicle TRAM flap. A reduction of the opposite breast is planned to accompany the technique chosen. Tissue expansion is ruled out because it would be difficult to achieve the required volume needed for a large breast reconstruction to match her somewhat reduced, ptotic breast. The patient also desires an abdominoplasty. The patient would have a better chance for a symmetric reconstruction with a latissimus dorsi flap combined with tissue expansion. However, the patient prefers an autologous tissue reconstruction, does not want a back scar, and requests an abdominoplasty. Microsurgical tissue transfer from the abdomen or buttocks would provide tissue similar to that of the pedicle TRAM flap; however, a suitable abdominoplasty would require just as extensive a dissection as a TRAM flap. A bipedicle TRAM flap would permit an autologous well-vascularized breast reconstruction for symmetry with a reduced opposite breast, and the donor site could be managed as the abdominoplasty that this patient desires.

Treatment of Choice

A left bipedicle TRAM flap technique is chosen for this patient because it is a less extensive procedure than a free flap and is a reliable and safe operative option that can meet this patient's expectations, providing a symmetric autologous tissue breast reconstruction and the abdominoplasty that she desires.

Treatment Plan

1. Define model for breast reconstruction by determining final desired volume and contour for right breast.
2. Plan lower TRAM flap with sufficient skin and fat to provide symmetry with opposite breast.
3. Confirm superior epigastric pedicle intramuscular position with a Doppler scan and elevate bipedicle TRAM flap.
4. Reduce right breast from 600 to 800 gm with a superior parenchymal technique.
5. Excise mastectomy scar and elevate mastectomy flaps.
6. Create a medial subcutaneous tunnel from chest to abdomen.
7. Position bipedicle TRAM flap obliquely.
8. Deepithelialize a portion of TRAM flap to provide subcutaneous fill.
9. Trim deep surface of flap to contour it to match reduced opposite breast.

BREAST RECONSTRUCTION WORKSHEET

PATIENT DATA

Name: Georgia Brown

Age: 48 Height: 5'5" Weight: 160

Married: X Single: ____

Nulliparous: ____ Pregnancies: 3

Children: 3 Nursing: X

ONCOLOGIC INFORMATION

Family history of breast CA: 0

Prev. breast cancer: L (5/82)

Prev. breast surg.: MRM (5/82)

Gen. surgeon: Richard Jones

Oncologist: Robert Sears

Gen. surgeon's recom.: No prophylactic mastectomy needed

Breast Cancer:

R: ____ L: X Bilateral: ____

Type cancer: R ____ L IDC

Positive nodes: R ____ L 0

Therapy:

Rad. mast.: ____ Mod. rad.: X

Skin-sparing mast.: ____

Lump/radiat.: ____ Chemo.: 0

Hormonal: 0 Radiat.: 0

Opposite Breast: R X L ____

Mastodynia: 0 Fibrocystic chg.: 0

Mammogram: Needs

Masses: R 0 L ____

Biopsies: R 0 L ____

MEDICAL INFORMATION

Systemic disease: 0

Diabetes: 0

Bleeding problems: 0

Allergies: 0

Medications: Tylenol

Smoking (pk-yr): 0

Alcohol/wk: 3 drinks/wk

Other: —

PHYSICAL EXAMINATION

Breast Exam:

Scars: R 0 L TVS

Scars: Back 0 Abdomen 0

Chest Wall:

Pectus defor.: 0 Scoliosis: 0

Muscle Function:

Lat. dorsi: OK Other: Abd. wall OK

Neurologic Exam: Normal

INFORMED CONSENT

Verbal explan.: X Signed form: X

Bleed sheet: X Preop. mamm.: X

FDA info.: ____ Mfg. info.: ____

EXPECTATIONS Balance, smaller right breast, abdominoplasty

SPECIFIC DESIRES

To achieve: Smaller, symmetric breasts

To avoid: —

Timing of Procedure: Immed.: ____ Delay: X

MEASUREMENTS AND PLAN

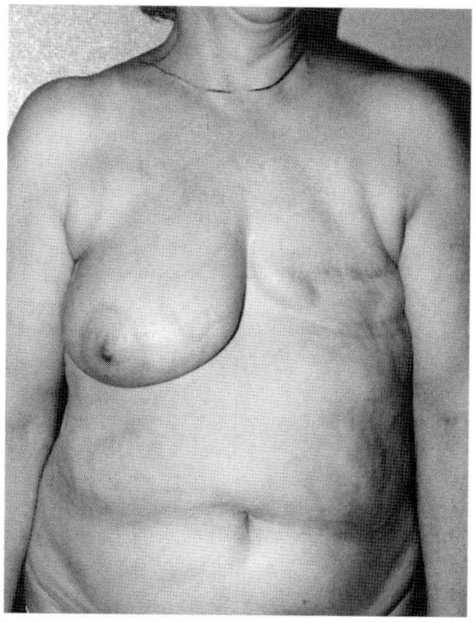

Chest circum.: 40"

Bra size: DD

Breast width:

R 24 cm L 16 cm

Clav. → N-A: 28 cm

N-A → infr. cr.: 14 cm

Opposite Breast:

Estimated preop. vol.: 1200 gm

Ptosis: Pseudo: ____ Mild: ____ Mod.: X Major: ____

Striae: R Mild L ____

Planned Change: Nothing: ____

Reduction: X Augmentation: ____

Mastopexy: ____ Prophylactic mastectomy: ____

Reconstructive Breast:

Clavicle to infr. cr.: 22 cm

N-A: 0

Skin quality: OK Rad. injury: 0

TECHNIQUE

Avail. tiss.: ____

Tiss. expan.: ____

Latiss. dorsi: ____

TRAM: Bipedicle lower

Microsurgery: ____

Lateral tissue to remove: ____

Tissue deficiency: ____

Abdominal excess: ____

IMPRESSIONS AND NOTES Motivated, good candidate for TRAM

PLAN Bipedicle left lower TRAM, right superior pedicle reduction

Postoperative Result

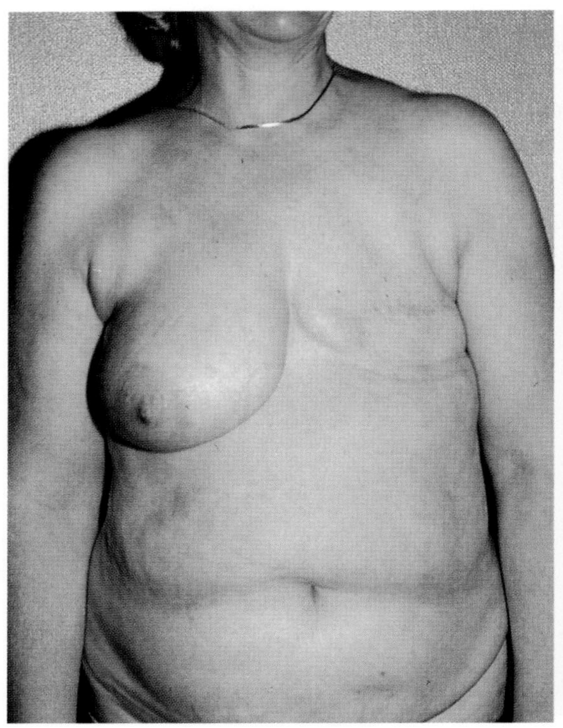

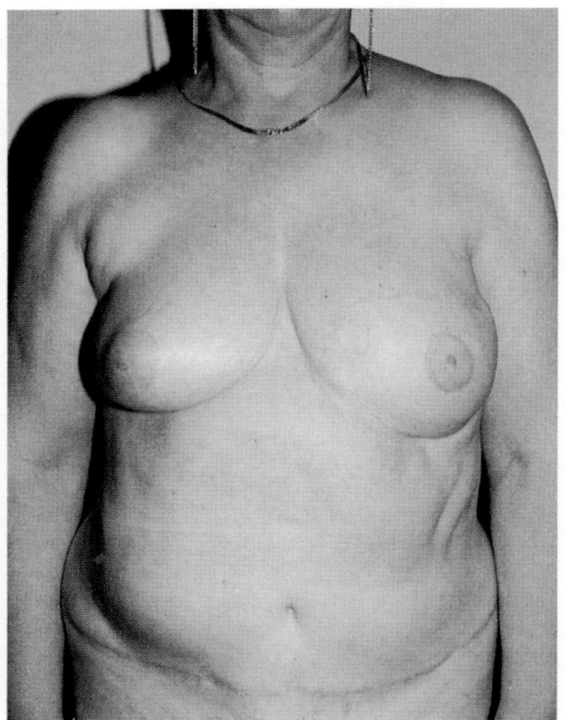

The patient focused as much on her slimmer abdomen as on her new breast. She was out of bed the day after her operation and the drains were removed 3 days later. She was discharged 6 days after the operation. The TRAM flap healed primarily without evidence of fat necrosis or skin loss. The abdomen remained flat. The nipple-areola was reconstructed with nonspecialized tissue 3 months later, and the nipple-areola was tattooed 2 months after this procedure. Four years have elapsed since her breast reconstruction. Her scars have matured and faded, and there is no evidence of recurrence. The patient is delighted with her choice of reconstruction method and the reduction of her opposite breast.

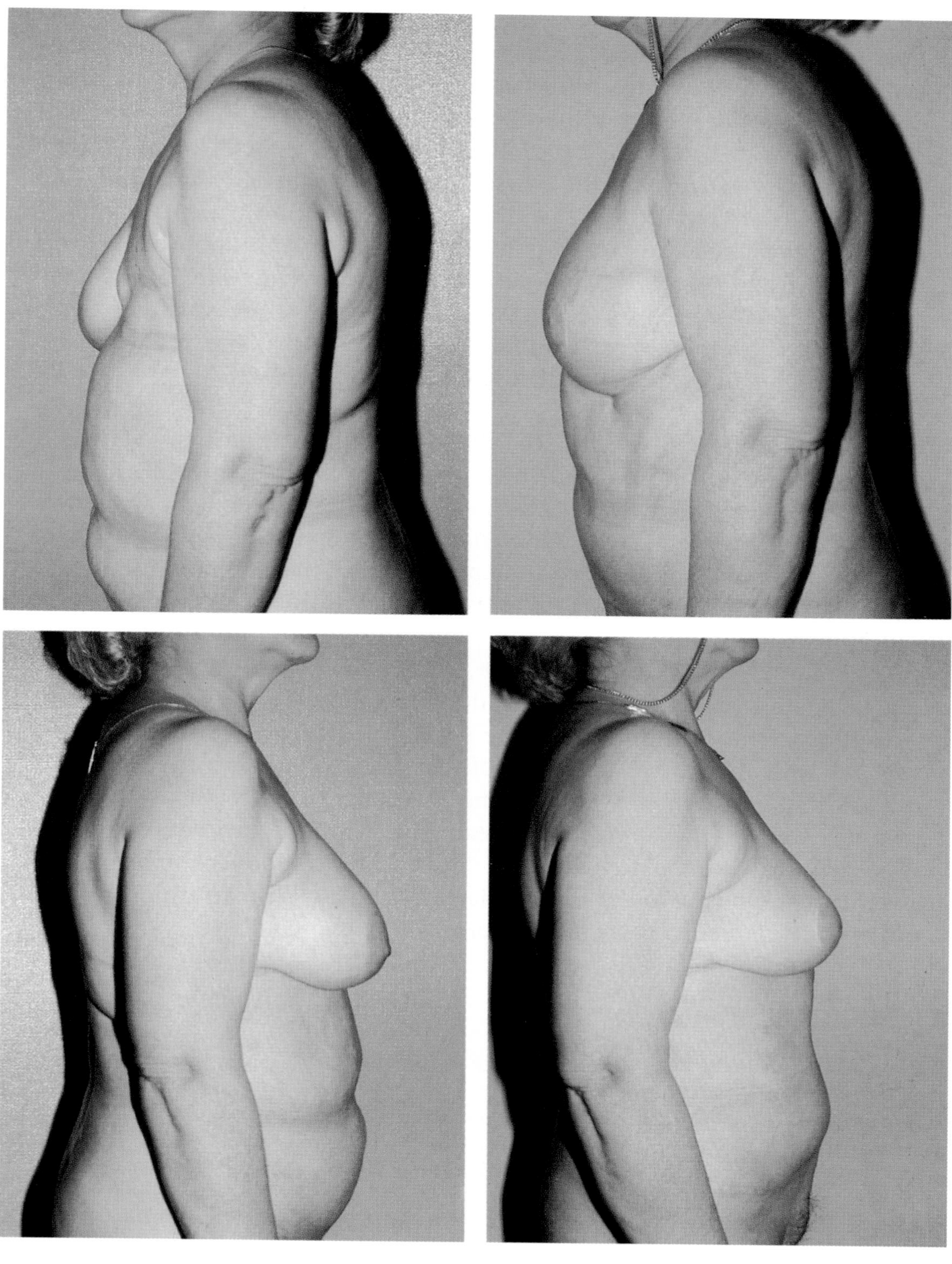

Closing Thoughts

Women have a deep psychological attachment to their breasts. Oncologic concerns compound the other emotionally charged issues. The breast surgeon who operates on a woman's breasts must have the necessary experience and knowledge to recommend and perform the proper procedure at the proper time to achieve the best results and to manage potential complications that could have profound effects. The aesthetic breast surgeon must fully understand that the patient seeking a cosmetic breast procedure today may later come to him as a breast reconstruction patient. The incidence of breast cancer is increasing among women, and knowledge of reconstructive and aesthetic techniques must be integrated. Many of the same techniques can be used for aesthetic or reconstructive breast surgery. Frequently these techniques are combined with a reconstructive procedure on one breast and an aesthetic procedure on the other breast.

Good communication cements the doctor-patient relationship. We would be doing ourselves and our patients a disservice if we attempted to short-circuit this dialogue. As caregivers, we can better understand the psychological overtones by listening to our patients and responding with sensitivity and empathy. We cannot rely on the patient's intuitive ability to know that we are concerned about her well-being. This confidence can only be established through ongoing discourse.

The ultimate goal of this communication, of course, is to create the optimal patient experience and to achieve the results the patient can most comfortably live with. This is the very basis of what we do. Through effective communication, we are able to understand the patient's expectations and motivations so that the appropriate treatment plan and procedures can be selected to produce the desired result. This goal cannot be accomplished unless we are responsive to the patient's feelings and establish an atmosphere in which she feels free to voice her concerns.

REFERENCES

Beale S, Lisper HO, Palm B. A psychological study of patients seeking augmentation mammoplasty. Br J Psychiatry 136:133, 1980.

Bennett AE, ed. Communication Between Doctors and Patients. London: Oxford University Press, 1976.

Bennett G. Patients and Their Doctors: The Journey Through Medical Care. London: Baillière Tindall, 1979.

Berger K, Bostwick J III. A Woman's Decision: Breast Care, Treatment, and Reconstruction, 3rd ed. St. Louis: Quality Medical Publishing, 1998.

Bird B. Talking With Patients, 2nd ed. Philadelphia: JB Lippincott, 1973.

Bostwick J III, Eaves FF III, Nahai F. Endoscopic Plastic Surgery. St. Louis: Quality Medical Publishing, 1995.

Carlson G, Bostwick J III. Aesthetic surgery for benign disorders of the breast. World J Surg 13:761, 1989.

Carlson GW, Bostwick J III, Styblo TM, Moore B, Bried JT, Murray DR, Wood WC. Skin-sparing mastectomy: Oncologic and reconstructive considerations. Ann Surg 255:570, 1997.

Cole NM. Informed consent: Considerations in aesthetic and reconstructive surgery of the breast. Clin Plast Surg 15:541, 1988.

Gifford S. Emotional attitudes toward cosmetic breast surgery: Loss and restitution of the "ideal self." In Goldwyn RM, ed. Plastic and Reconstructive Surgery of the Breast. Boston: Little, Brown, 1976.

Goin JM, Goin MK. Changing the Body: Psychological Effects of Plastic Surgery. Baltimore: Williams & Wilkins, 1981.

Goin MK, Goin JM, Gianini MH. The psychic consequences of a reduction mammaplasty. Plast Reconstr Surg 59:530, 1977.

Goldwyn RM. The dissatisfied patient. In Goldwyn RM, ed. The Unfavorable Result in Plastic Surgery: Avoidance and Treatment, 2nd ed. Boston: Little, Brown, 1984, pp 11-17.

Goldwyn RM. The Patient and the Plastic Surgeon. Boston: Little, Brown, 1981.

Goldwyn RM. Patient selection: The importance of being cautious. In Courtiss EH, ed. Aesthetic Surgery: Trouble—How To Avoid It and How To Treat It. St. Louis: CV Mosby, 1978, pp 14-16.

Goldwyn RM. The woman and esthetic surgery. In Norman MT, Nadelson CC, eds. The Woman Patient. Medical and Psychological Interfaces, vol 1. Sexual and Reproductive Aspects of Women's Health Care. New York: Plenum, 1978, pp 271-280.

Goldwyn RM. High hopes and malpractice. Arch Surg 111:1042, 1976.

Goldwyn RM. Ingredients for failure. In Goldwyn RM, ed. The Unfavorable Result in Plastic Surgery: Avoidance and Treatment. Boston: Little, Brown, 1972, pp 2-4.

Goldwyn RM. The consultant and the unfavorable result. In Goldwyn RM, ed. The Unfavorable Result in Plastic Surgery: Avoidance and Treatment. Boston: Little, Brown, 1972, pp 5-7.

Hart D. The psychological outcome of breast reconstruction. Plast Surg Nurs 16:167, 1996.

Klassen A, Jenkinson C, Fitzpatrick R, Goodacre T. Patients' health-related quality of life before and after aesthetic surgery. Br J Plast Surg 49:433, 1996.

Lasser T, Clarke WK. Reach to Recovery. New York: Simon & Schuster, 1972.

Lejour M. Vertical Mammaplasty and Liposuction. St. Louis: Quality Medical Publishing, 1994.

Millard DR Jr. Principalization of Plastic Surgery. Boston: Little, Brown, 1986.

Morello DC, Converse JM, Allen D. Making uniform photographic records in plastic surgery. Plast Reconstr Surg 59:366, 1977.

Nelson GD, Krause JL, eds. Clinical Photography in Plastic Surgery. Boston: Little, Brown, 1988.

Regnault P, Daniel RK, eds. Aesthetic Plastic Surgery: Principles and Techniques. Boston: Little, Brown, 1984.

Rohrich RJ, Beran SJ, Kenkel JM. Ultrasound-Assisted Liposuction. St. Louis: Quality Medical Publishing, 1998.

Sarwer DB, Bartlett SP, Bucky LP, LaRossa D, Low DW, Pertschuk MJ, Wadden TA, Whitaker LA. Bigger is not always better: Body image dissatisfaction in breast reduction and breast augmentation patients. Plast Reconstr Surg 101:1956, 1998.

Schlebusch L. Negative bodily experience and prevalence of depression in patients who request augmentation mammaplasty. S Afr Med J 75:323, 1989.

Sheen JH, Sheen AP. Photography. In Aesthetic Rhinoplasty, 2nd ed. St. Louis: Quality Medical Publishing, 1987, pp 147-163.

Shipley RH, O'Donnell JM, Bader KE. Personality characteristics of women seeking breast augmentation. Plast Reconstr Surg 61:369, 1977.

Strombeck JO, Rosato FE, eds. Surgery of the Breast: Diagnosis and Treatment of Breast Diseases. Stuttgart: Georg Thieme, 1986.

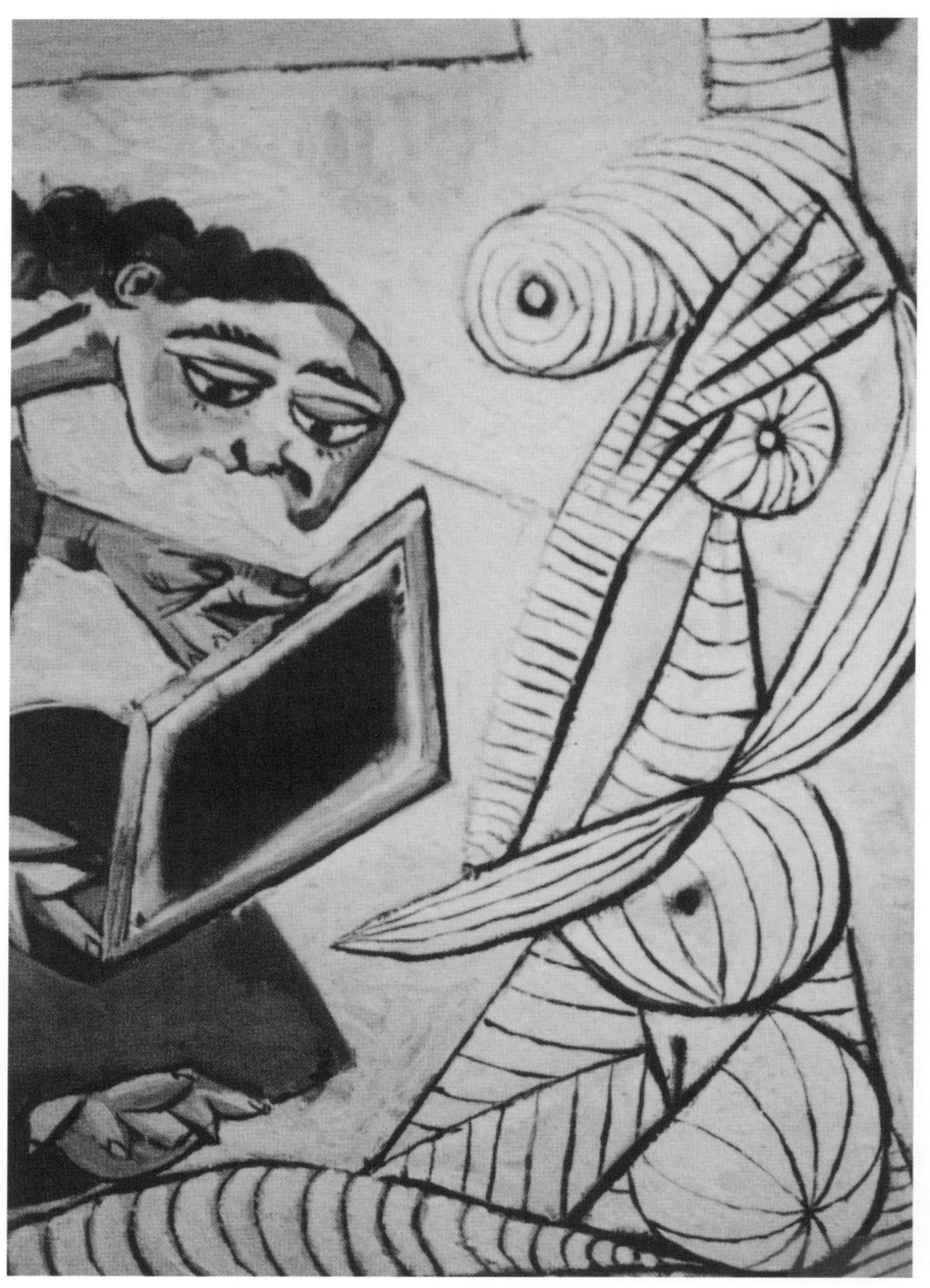

2 Anatomy and Physiology

Key Topics

Embryology

Skin

Breast Composition and Function

Parenchyma

Fascia

Cooper's Ligaments

Musculature

Blood Supply

Venous Drainage

Nerve Supply

Lymphatics

Nipple-Areola

Observations

Most breast surgeons readily acknowledge that a thorough grounding in anatomy and physiology is prerequisite to performing surgery. Most would also admit, however, that they prefer to focus on the surgical maneuvers that they perceive to be more exciting. Today's complex breast surgery procedures, however, do not afford that luxury. They stress form and function and frequently incorporate muscle and musculofascial flaps—some with microvascular transfer. New techniques of minimally invasive surgery require an even more detailed knowledge of anatomy. Any deficits in anatomic and physiologic knowledge will soon become apparent to the surgeon and his patient. There are no shortcuts. When augmentation mammaplasties were subglandular and reduction mammaplasties were planned as a pattern on a single dermal pedicle, this knowledge, while important, was not as crucial as it is with today's more sophisticated procedures. They often involve deeper anatomic structures and tissue planes, are more dependent on the underlying blood and nerve supply and various parenchymal segments, and utilize muscles and submusculofascial flaps and planes. Knowledge of anatomy is essential for safety and also to satisfy the patient's expectations for preservation of function and sensation. More patients are requesting secondary procedures; these women's scarred breasts present an anatomic conundrum. The anatomic and vascular changes subsequent to previous operations must be carefully considered in any surgical plan. Breast irradiation increases the challenge since tissues are affected at a molecular level. Respect for the anatomic roadmap is essential to avoid potential complications inherent in reoperative breast surgery. Without this direction the surgeon can fail to recognize potential problems until too late. The surgeon must know the basic anatomy and be able to visualize in his mind's eye the underlying structures and their inherent relationships.

Three-dimensional visualization of the breast and chest wall based on anatomic and physiologic constructs is mandatory to successfully perform present-day procedures and to meet the exacting demands of the future.

Embryology

Breast growth begins with differentiation of the cutaneous epithelium of the pectoral region during the eighth to tenth week of embryonic development. By the sixth week of intrauterine life a milk ridge can be identified extending from the axilla to the groin. The human breast develops in the anterolateral pectoral region, primarily at the level of the fourth intercostal space. Supernumerary breasts can persist anywhere along this milk line from the axilla to the groin; most often they occur just below the inframammary crease on the lower left chest wall.

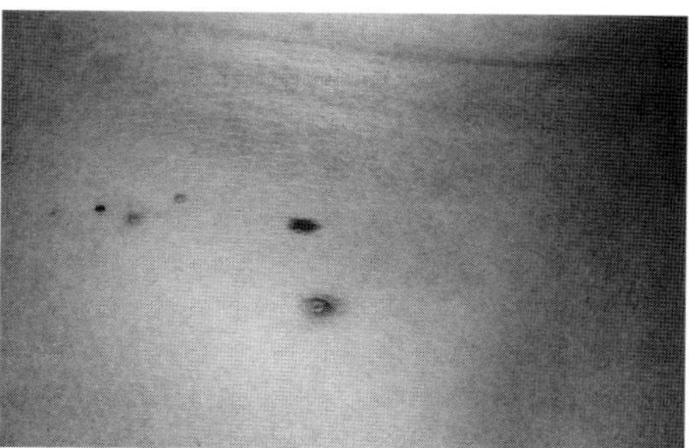

A supernumerary nipple is common in the inframammary area and is often confused with a nevus. It can function during pregnancy and lactation and can be the site of breast carcinoma.

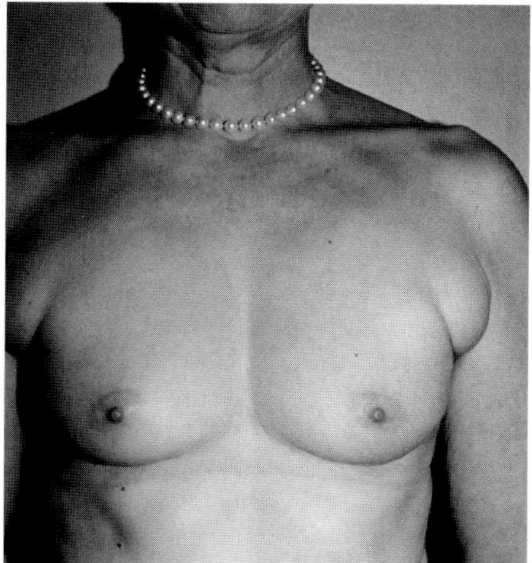

An axillary breast can present as axillary fullness. It, too, can be the site of breast cancer. These axillary breasts are unsightly and distressing to the patient; supernumerary nipples may also occur in this location.

Immediately after birth an infant's breasts exhibit some activity and can even secrete milk because of the high levels of hormones circulating in the mother. After the newborn period, however, breast activity subsides until puberty. Today, puberty is occurring sooner in many young women, sometimes as early as 7 to 9 years of age. This early onset can speed the development of breast problems in girls who are emotionally and psychologically unprepared to handle them or cope with the necessary treatment. These young women and their parents should be advised to wait as long as possible, ideally until growth ceases, before surgical intervention so they will be better psychologically prepared and to avoid additional operations.

Before the onset of puberty the nipple is located at the fourth intercostal space in the male and female. When a breast bud first appears, it is palpable just under the nipple-areola as a localized small, firm breast disk. Breast buds can be tender and sensitive, but this is a normal condition and should not be a source of concern. I have seen a number of partial breast deformities and even complete absence of a breast as a result of biopsy or excision of a normal breast bud because the parents and physicians feared that this was a tumor.

The female breasts begin to develop between the ages of 9 and 14 years. At this time the breast bud develops into a conical structure with some projection. Although both breasts usually grow simultaneously at puberty, one can develop a few months before the other. Temporary developmental differences or permanent asymmetries may occur, and these are first noticeable shortly after breast development begins. If the breast buds have been incised such as during a thoracotomy, girls can develop significant deformities during puberty. When one breast begins developing weeks to months before the other, patience is advised until the other breast starts to grow. Adolescents are most concerned and sensitive psychologically about their breast development. Although some mild breast asymmetries are normal and should be expected, when they are marked and the patient and parents become concerned, surgical correction may be requested. ***Generally it is best to delay correction of a breast asymmetry until development is complete, usually when the girl is 14 to 16 years old, when full vertical height has been attained, and when progressively larger brassiere sizes are no longer needed.*** When asymmetric breasts are treated at this early age, the patient and parents must be informed that various factors such as weight loss or gain, pregnancy/lactation, endogenous or exogenous hormones, and aging may produce additional breast asymmetry over time and that will require further operations.

Certain types of asymmetry will not improve with time. In cases of unilateral hypoplasia or aplasia and Poland's syndrome, the asymmetry can actually increase with time, often developing early and requiring operative correction. When the patient has a constricted breast with an inframammary fold that originates more laterally and higher on the chest wall or a tubular protrusion of the central breast and nipple-areola, these are permanent conditions and will not be remedied by time.

Breast hypertrophy can also develop just after the onset of puberty. Basically, two manifestations of hypertrophy concern the teenager and her parents: giant virginal hypertrophy and, more frequently, teenage breast hypertrophy. In my experience, extensive endocrine workups do not reveal abnormalities in these young patients with breast hypertrophy. Hormonal therapy has not proved helpful, and surgical reduction of their large breasts is the only realistic option for these patients.

Skin

As a skin appendage, the breast is closely related to the skin, and its quality, thickness, and elasticity affect breast appearance. The skin enveloping the breast is subject to hormonal, expansible, weight, gravitational, and aging influences, and after breast development it can become stretched, especially in the lower breast area and the areas of relative breast fullness, with thinning skin and loss of elasticity. Striae, actual tears and separations of the thinned dermis with thinning of the epidermis, are often noted in the supra-areolar and periareolar regions in skin that is inherently thin and has stretched rapidly or extensively or after weight loss or postpartum involution. The thickness and elasticity of the breast skin are important in obtaining immediate and lasting surgical results. When the skin is thin and inelastic with striae, it will not provide optimal support for the weight of the breast or the addition of an implant over the long term. In these situations it is likely that normal postoperative stretching after a mastopexy will precipitate the recurrence of ptosis earlier than is usually expected. In such a case some other method for supporting the breast is needed combined with resection of breast parenchyma in the lower pole to minimize the pull of gravity. The nipple-areolar skin has a thinner dermis than the remainder of the breast skin. Central breast skin thinness and absence of elastic containment for the breast parenchyma are associated with a constricted breast and can lead to the development of a central breast protrusion, the tubular and tuberous breast.

BLOOD SUPPLY

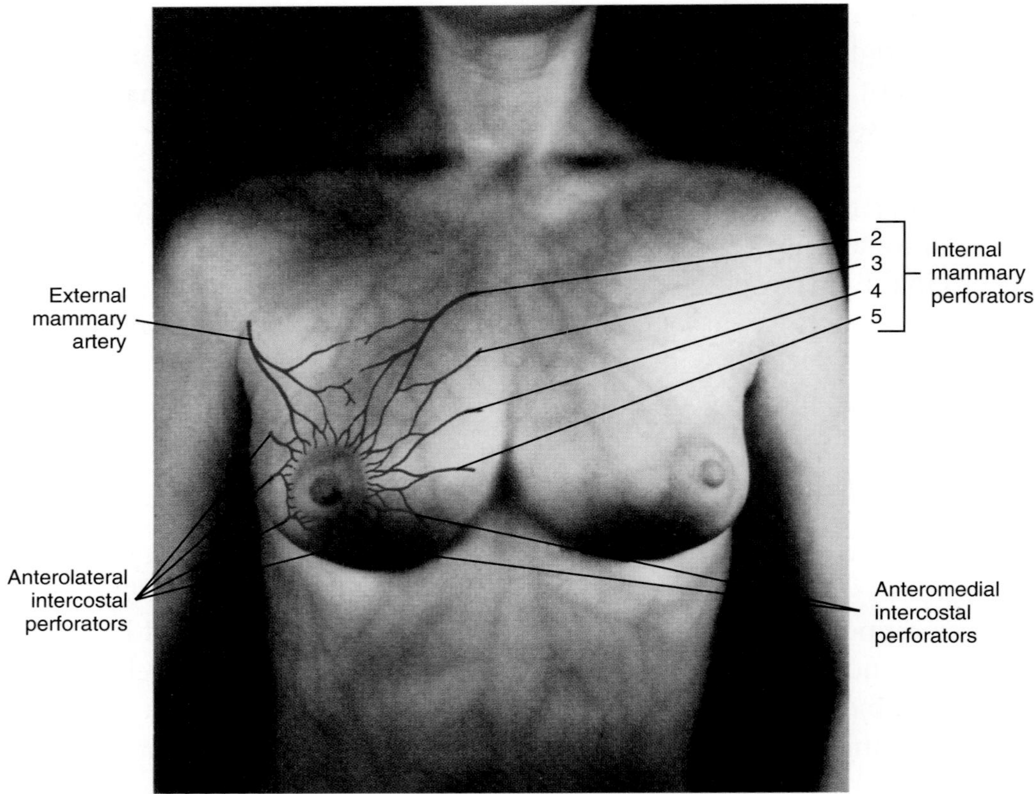

The blood supply to the breast skin originates primarily from the subdermal plexus with communications to the underlying anteromedial intercostal and chest wall breast parenchymal perforators and the subjacent breast parenchyma. When flaps of breast skin are required for an operation, the viability of these flaps is determined by their length, the quality and presence of the subdermal plexus, the quality of the microcirculation, and the presence of specific inflow vessels such as the medial breast perforators. Skin incisions can interrupt the subdermal blood supply and diminish or interrupt blood flow, leading to flap necrosis. The blood supply to the skin of the central breast area focuses on the nipple-areola, and the blood supply from the subdermal plexus around the nipple-areola is enhanced in this region.

NERVE SUPPLY

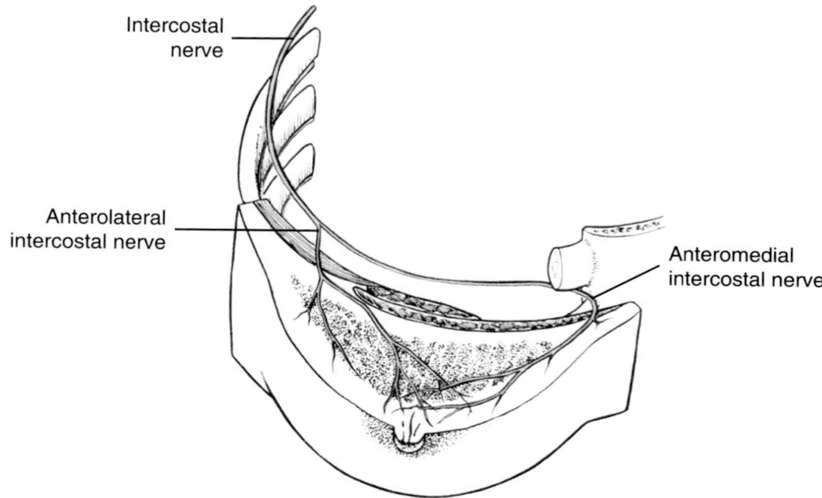

The sensation of the skin of the breast is segmental and derives from the dermatomes of breast development. ***The innervation of the central breast and the nipple-areola is primarily from the T3-T5 branches of the anterolateral and anteromedial intercostal nerves.*** Any breast reduction technique selected should preserve at least one of these branches to ensure that breast sensation is maintained. The lower fibers of the cervical plexus also contribute to the innervation of the important upper breast area. Skin-sparing mastectomy and free nipple-graft reduction techniques generally preserve more sensation. Skin incisions interrupt sensory nerves and thus decrease sensation. ***Nipple-areola sensation should be documented before any operation that could potentially diminish it is undertaken.***

Injury to the segmental nerves in the anteromedial and anterolateral regions during breast procedures can result in areas of hypesthesia or actual anesthesia. When there is partial injury to the nerves, the reinnervation is accompanied by paresthesias, dysesthesias, and increased sensitivity of the involved areas. I have found that this hypersensitivity is diminished when the patient uses sensory reeducation with frequent massage of the affected areas.

Breast Composition and Function

Originating from the ectoderm, the breast is basically a specialized skin gland with breast parenchyma extending up to the subdermal level. Breast parenchyma in the adult covers a large area of the anterior chest wall, extending upward to just below the clavicle and downward to below the usually well-defined inframammary crease. Medially some breast tissue (the cleavage) reaches to the midline and even over the sternum, and laterally it extends lateral to the lateral breast fold and to or beyond the edge of the latissimus dorsi muscle. Breast parenchyma also reaches into the axilla; the axillary tail of the breast actually penetrates through axillary pectoral fascial foramina, and breast parenchyma is present in the axillary fat pad.

Studies have demonstrated the limitations of surgical procedures designed to completely remove all breast parenchyma. Despite the thoroughness of surgical ablation, some breast tissue is left behind and can be detected microscopically, even after a radical mastectomy. Residual breast parenchyma is left after both therapeutic and prophylactic mastectomies; therefore some risk of neoplasia remains.

Breast shape and contour are influenced by the volume of breast parenchyma, the amount and location of the subcutaneous fat and intraparenchymal fat, the bony contour of the chest wall, its muscular covering and thickness, and the tightness and elastic quality of the skin. The fascial attachments of the breast to the underlying chest wall also influence breast appearance.

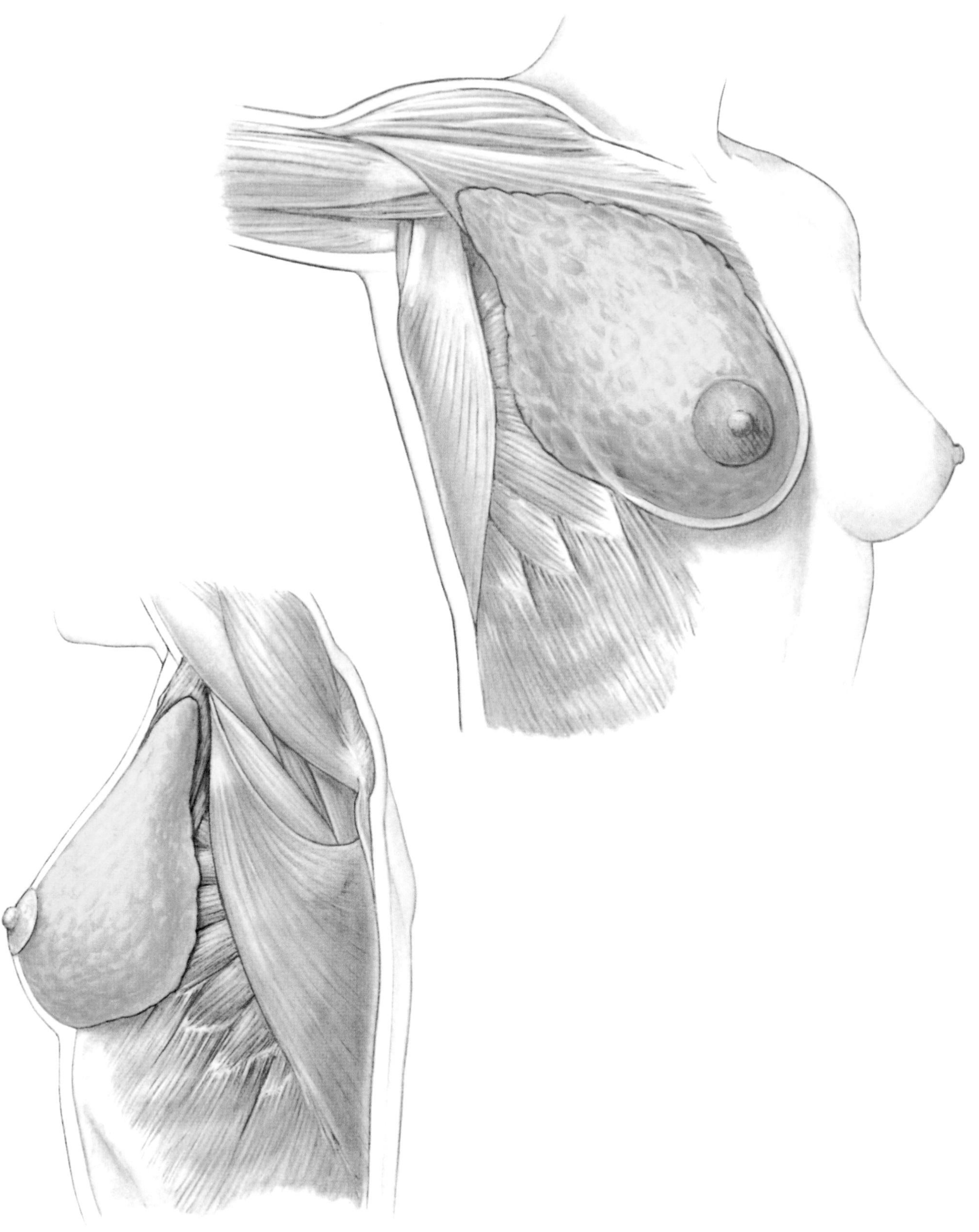

Parenchyma

The actual glandular, secretory, milk-producing component of the breast is situated within a connective and fatty tissue stroma. These glandular and stromal tissues respond to systemic hormonal and genetic influences. About 20 main lactiferous ducts connect and drain the individual breast lobules to the nipple. The breast lobules are distributed radially about the breast; each of these breast lobules is composed of hundreds of potentially secretory acini and each has a separate interlobular duct connecting to the lactiferous ducts.

The nipple is a focused part of the parenchyma from a functional and sensory perspective. Contained within the nipple are special lactiferous ducts that act as conduits for glandular secretions.

The breast, lactiferous ducts, and breast lobules normally contain bacteria because the ducts provide a conduit for bacteria to enter the breast through the nipple. Bacteria can usually be cultured from the breast tissue, most commonly *Staphylococcus epidermidis.* The presence of bacteria helps to explain the incidence of infection after mastectomy and the presence of *Staphylococcus epidermidis* in cultures of most breast capsules surrounding breast implants. Most findings concerning the etiology of capsular contracture around breast implants implicate infection as a probable causative factor. For this reason I recommend systemic antibacterial therapy when breast implants are used or the breast parenchyma is divided. Subpectoral implant positioning probably disturbs fewer ducts than subglandular implant placement because it does not separate the parenchyma from the pectoralis major fascia.

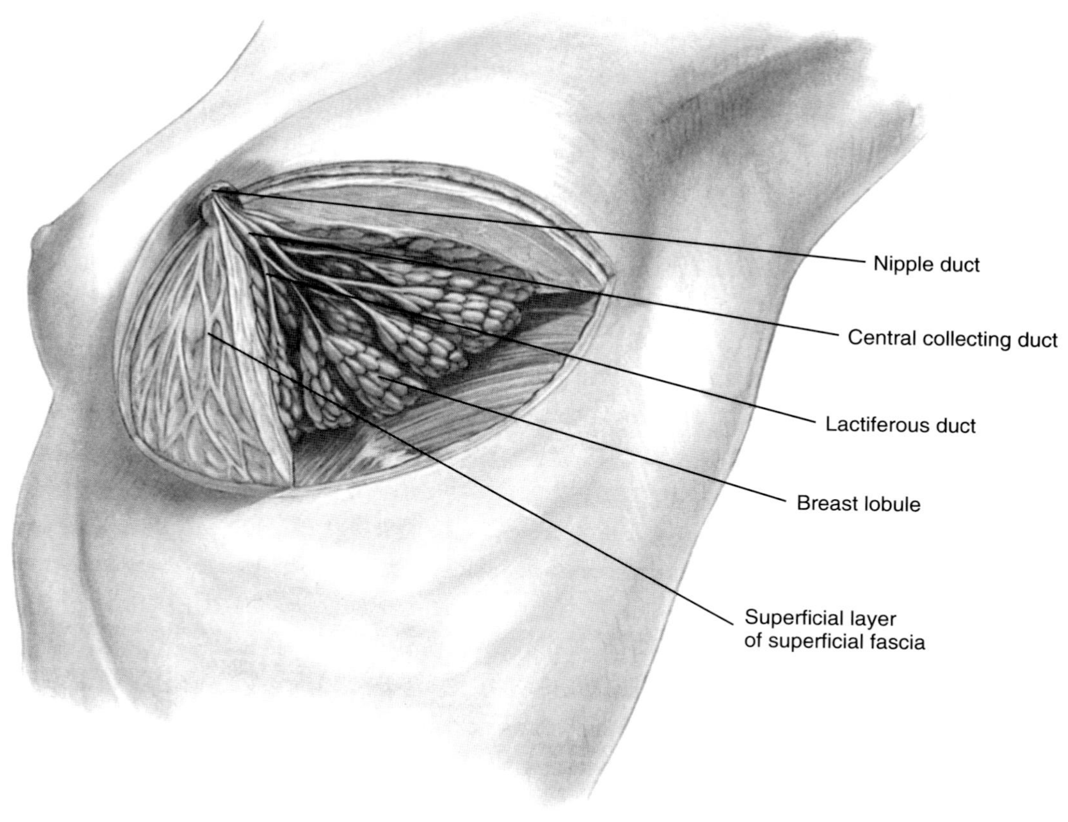
Nipple duct
Central collecting duct
Lactiferous duct
Breast lobule
Superficial layer
of superficial fascia

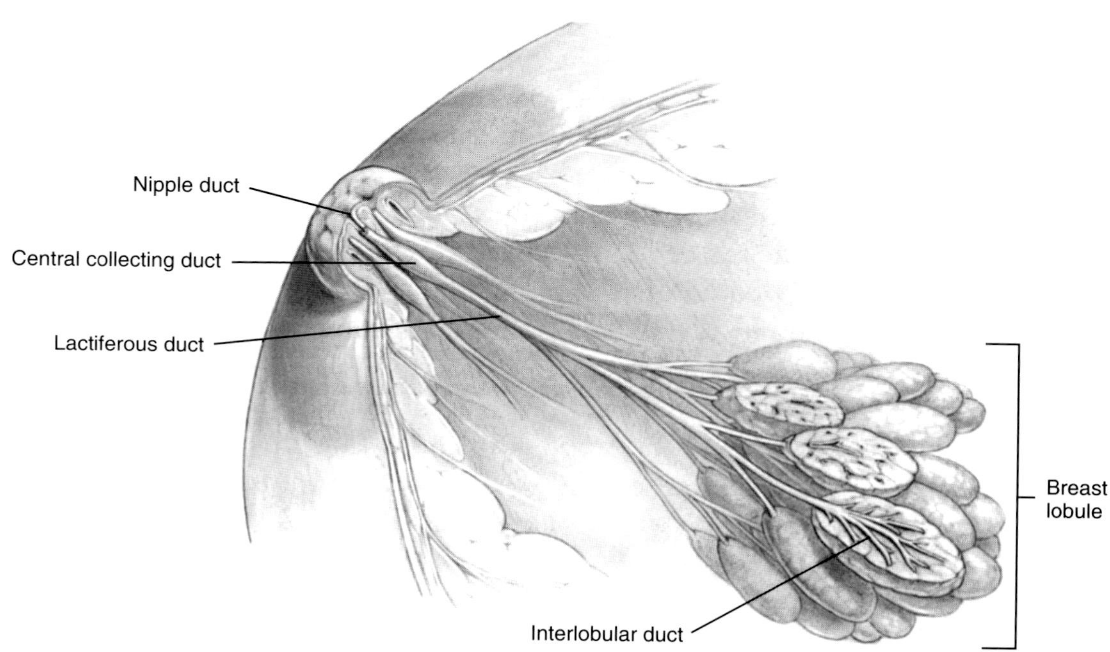
Nipple duct
Central collecting duct
Lactiferous duct
Breast
lobule
Interlobular duct

FAT CONTENT

The amount of fat within the breast varies; this fat is responsible for most of the bulk, contour, softness, consistency, and shape of the breast. It is selectively deposited within the breast and is influenced by genetic and hormonal factors. The percentage of body fat also influences the amount of breast fat, although some women seem to selectively deposit more fat within their breasts. The breast with considerable fat content feels soft, whereas the breast with a predominance of stromal and glandular components is often firm, irregular, and nodular. Patients who undergo a significant weight loss often notice a change in the consistency of their breasts as they begin to feel the nodularity of the normal breast tissue that previously was undetectable or not palpable within the fatty tissue. Women who experience cyclic fibrocystic changes notice that this condition diminishes with the onset of menopause, and their breasts often are less lumpy. When estrogens are administered after menopause, the breast parenchyma can proliferate and nodularity can persist. The breast fat component increases as the glandular components subside after lactation or atrophy after menopause. Breasts of postmenopausal women have more fat and are easier to evaluate on mammography. Liposuction of the breasts in these women lowers the fat content and their breasts appear more dense on mammography. Before 40 years of age women's breasts are more glandular and dense and contain less fat. It is generally harder to detect the early signs of breast cancer in these women. Breast liposuction can reduce the fat content of the parenchyma. It is difficult to predict the amount of fat that can be removed preoperatively.

BLOOD SUPPLY

The blood flow and supply of the breast parenchyma are affected by an individual's age, health status, microcirculation, and endocrine activity. ***Blood flow to the breast parenchyma decreases after menopause and with the aging process, at which time the breast becomes primarily fatty tissue with only atrophied strands of glandular tissue present.*** Many women maintain hormonal levels with supplemental exogenous estrogens. Operated breasts that would heal primarily with excellent blood supply in a healthy premenopausal woman may show evidence of decreased blood supply, potential fat necrosis, and loss of breast and nipple-areola flaps in the postmenopausal woman with increased fat and poorly vascularized breasts. Conditions that further compromise the microcirculation, such as diabetes mellitus, generalized atherosclerosis, advanced age, collagen vascular diseases, radiation therapy, and cigarette smoking, also contribute to a decreased blood supply.

Fascia

The breast develops and is contained within supporting layers of superficial fascia. Specifically, the superficial layer of this superficial fascia is located near the dermis and is not always distinct from it. The superficial layer of the superficial fascia is the outer layer covering the breast parenchyma and is most clearly defined in thin patients whose skin is mobile over a more fibrous parenchyma. A variable amount of subcutaneous fat is present between the dermis and the actual breast parenchyma. In some thin individuals the breast parenchyma is not separated from the subdermis by a fat layer, whereas in others the subcutaneous layer is well established. Some identifiable breast tissue is located in the subcutaneous tissue and can be identified microscopically after a mastectomy even with thin skin flaps remaining. Therefore, at this level, sharp dissection is necessary during mastectomy.

Because the breast is an ectodermal derivative attached to the skin by these fascial layers, it does not have a distinct superficial plane, making it difficult to completely separate the breast from the skin. The subdermal plexus of blood vessels that supplies the breast skin is situated on the deep surface of the dermis in close approximation to the subcutaneous fat and the outer layer of the superficial fascia. ***This layer of subdermal blood vessels must be left intact to maintain breast flap viability.*** Incisions into the dermis undersurface can devascularize the breast flaps. ***This is even more important with the skin-sparing mastectomy technique, which requires longer flaps and has an increased incidence of skin flap necrosis.*** When striae are present, the dermis is thinned and the subdermal plexus lies under the thinned dermis and the epidermis. These layers and anatomic components of the superficial breast area have distinct implications for breast flap survival, the completeness of mastectomies, and the techniques used for breast reconstruction, especially for immediate breast implant coverage.

More distinct is the superficial fascia's deep layer on the deep posterior surface of the breast; it is identifiable on the deep surface of the breast when the breast is elevated during a submammary augmentation mammaplasty. A loose areolar area is interposed between the deep layer of the superficial fascia and the deep fascial layer that covers the pectoralis major, the adjacent rectus abdominis, the serratus anterior, and the external oblique muscles.

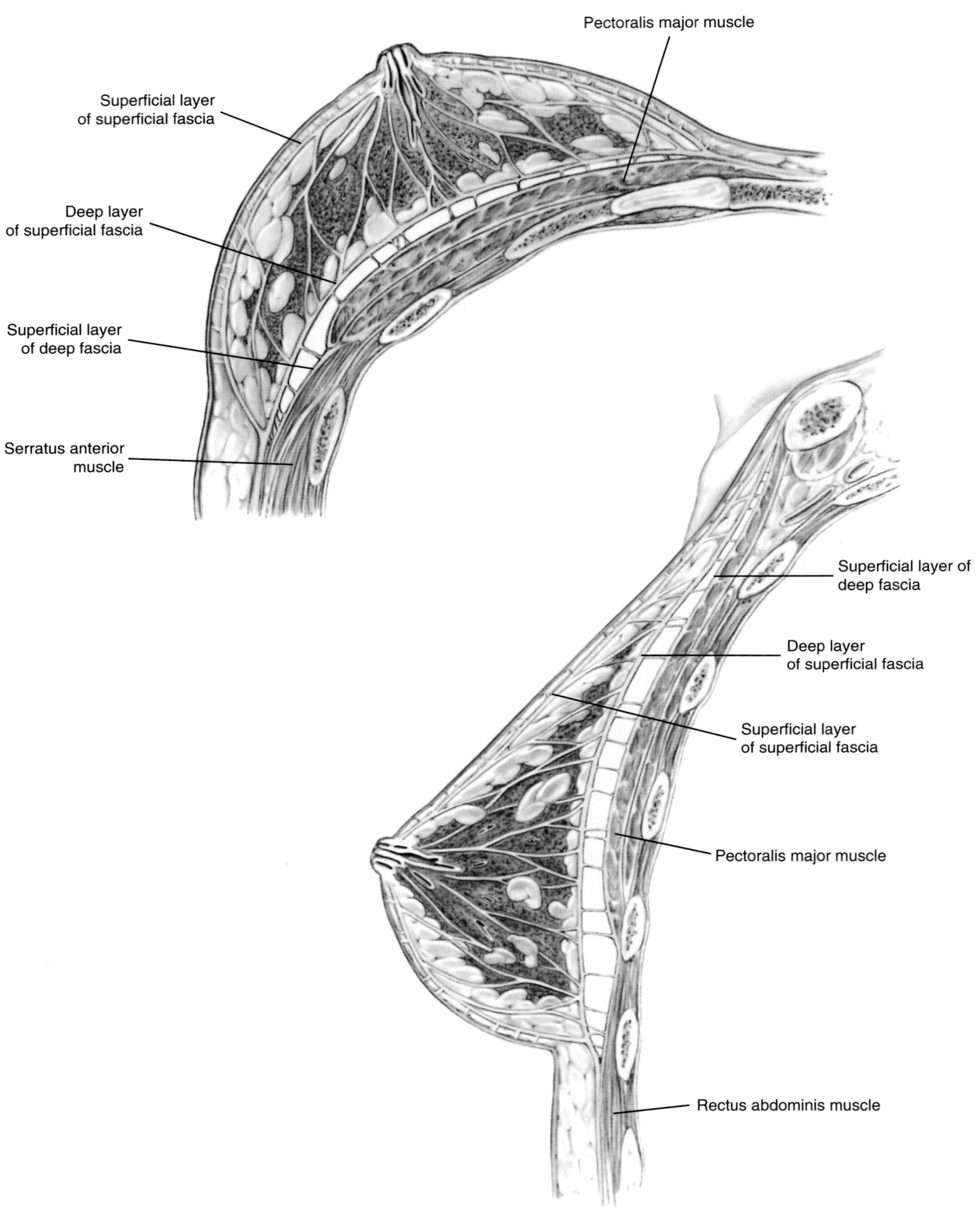
Pectoralis major muscle
Superficial layer
of superficial fascia
Deep layer
of superficial fascia
Superficial layer
of deep fascia
Serratus anterior
muscle
Superficial layer of
deep fascia
Deep layer
of superficial fascia
Superficial layer
of superficial fascia
Pectoralis major muscle
Rectus abdominis muscle

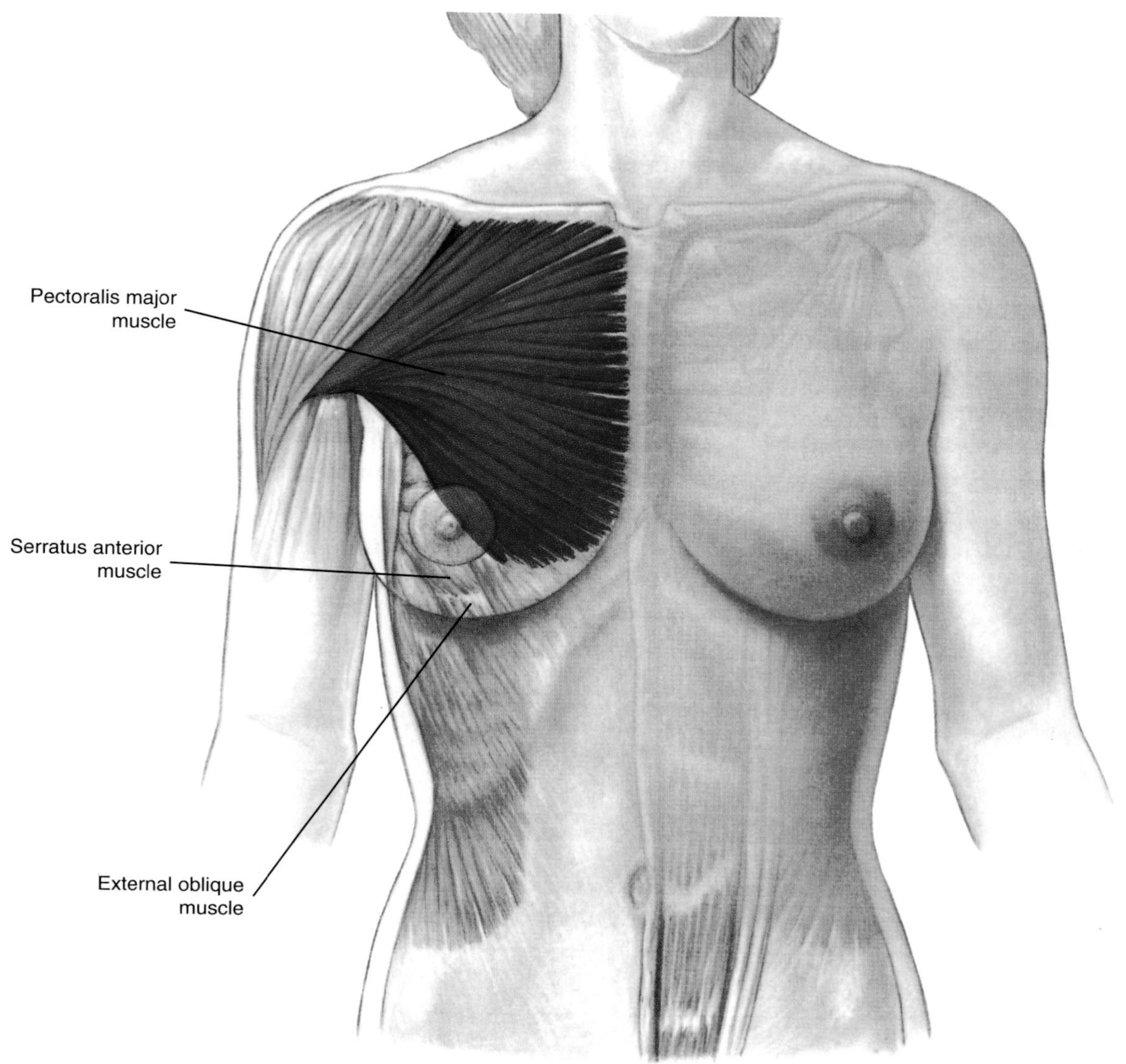

The superficial layer of the deep muscle fascia covers the outer layer of musculature of the chest wall and overlays the outer surface of the pectoralis major, the medial serratus anterior, the upper portions of the rectus abdominis, and the external oblique muscle in the lower central breast. This fascia is better defined, more substantial, firmer, and less elastic over the lower breast area than in the upper breast area over the pectoralis major muscle. It is thinner over the muscular portions of the pectoralis major and serratus anterior. ***The lower fascia is inelastic; if not released properly during submusculofascial dissections for submuscular implants, it can constrict an underlying implant or resist expansion and descent of an implant, contributing to an unacceptable result.***

The posterior surface of the breast parenchyma is covered by the deep layer of the superficial fascia. This layer is separate and distinct from the superficial layer of the deep fascia that covers the pectoralis major muscle and the serratus anterior muscle. This deep layer of the superficial fascia is penetrated by fibrous attachments and support (Cooper's ligaments) as well as vessels, nerves, and lymphatics extending from the deeper structures to the breast parenchyma. Some microscopic portions of breast parenchyma, including microscopic breast ducts, can also be identified extending through the outer layer of the deep fascia and within the subjacent muscles. The deep layer of the superficial fascia is better defined when the breast parenchyma is mobile over the superficial layer of the deep fascia. This is most often seen in the ptotic or hypertrophic breast. When the breast is excessively mobile, the connecting fascial attachments between these two layers become attenuated and appear as areolar tissue. It is this plane that is separated and the breast parenchyma elevated for subglandular breast augmentation. When there is loss of support and elasticity of the breast attachments to the deep fascia, methods used to increase support and maintain a corrected ptotic breast by suturing the breast parenchyma to the fascia at a higher level have not been documented to be successful over time. When there is poor skin elasticity, poor deep support, and breast ptosis, one strategy to improve this condition is to transfer the glandular tissue by rotating the lower breast parenchyma to the upper breast region and suturing it to minimize the upper breast flatness.

Suspensory Ligaments of Cooper

Connective tissue (Cooper's ligaments) extends from the deep fascia to the dermis and runs throughout the breast parenchyma, attaching to the dermis of the overlying skin. These suspensory ligaments also reach to the posterior layer of the superficial fascia and connect onto the deep muscle fascia. Because these deep attachments are not taut, they allow greater breast mobility on the deep fascia during motion and activity. These suspensory ligaments can be stretched and elongated by pregnancy, by aging, or by weight fluctuation. Loss of elasticity in these connective tissues contributes to breast ptosis and excess breast mobility.

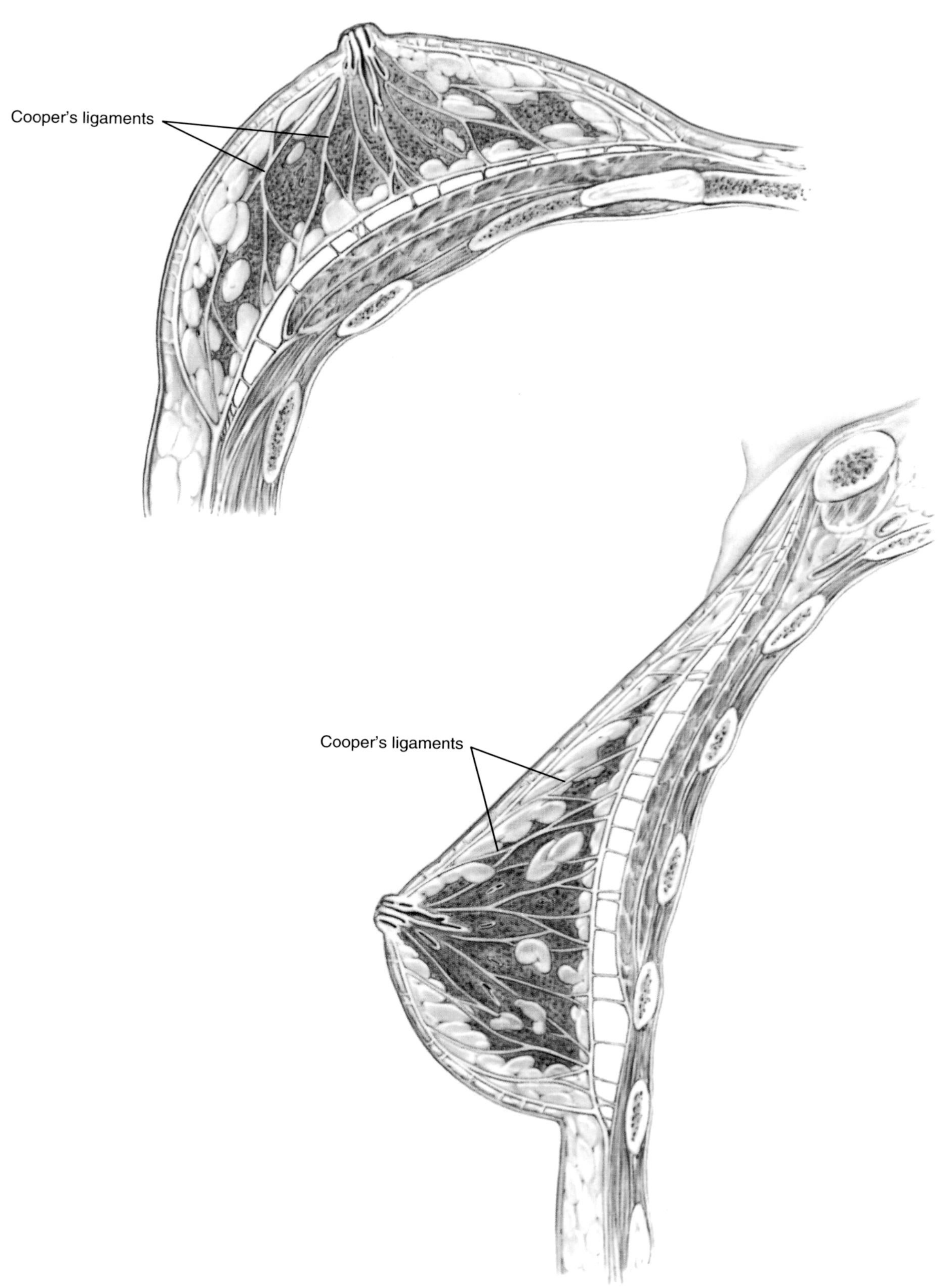
Cooper's ligaments
Cooper's ligaments

Musculature

The breast is situated over the deep fascia and underlying musculature of the anterolateral chest wall. ***The central upper and medial portions of the breast lie over the pectoralis major muscle. The lower portion of the breast covers the anterolateral serratus anterior muscle digitations laterally, the upper external oblique muscle origins and its fascia, and the fascia over the upper origins of the rectus abdominis muscle inferomedially.*** The breast parenchyma extends laterally to the lateral margin of the latissimus dorsi muscle, and the upper lateral breast parenchyma extends into the axilla. Upper breast parenchyma approximates the clavicle, and the cleavage at the lateral sternum defines the extent of the breasts medially.

A substantial portion of the breast's blood supply, innervation, and lymphatic drainage passes up through these underlying muscles. An intact musculofascial layer ensures maximal blood supply to the breast and can act as a biologic barrier between the breast parenchyma and a breast implant after aesthetic and reconstructive breast surgery. The blood vessels from the muscle into the breast are analogous to musculocutaneous perforators in other parts of the body since the breast is derived from specialized skin components. Many of the current techniques in aesthetic and reconstructive breast surgery rely on an accurate knowledge of the musculature deep to the breast and its blood supply from the internal mammary and intercostal system perforators.

PECTORALIS MAJOR AND MINOR MUSCLES

The *pectoralis major* muscle is a primary muscle of the upper chest and extends from broad origins over the anteromedial chest to insert onto the upper portion of the humerus. It is located just beneath the upper medial breast area and provides the primary fill for the infraclavicular area. In women who work out to build up their breasts the upper pectoralis major muscle becomes enlarged, resulting in upper breast fullness, not lower breast fullness. A variable thickness of subcutaneous tissue and some breast parenchyma also contribute to the infraclavicular contour. When overdeveloped, as often seen in weight lifters, this muscle can project as a prominence in the upper chest. This muscle forms the anterior wall of the axilla and is the major component of the anterior axillary fold. The deep fascia of the pectoralis major muscle becomes the axillary fascia and then continues across the axilla to become the investing fascia for the latissimus dorsi muscle. This deep layer of pectoralis major fascia is attached to the axillary fascia over the deep axillary sheath; these attachments contain and support the axillary contents and preserve the characteristic axillary concavity between the anterior and posterior axillary folds.

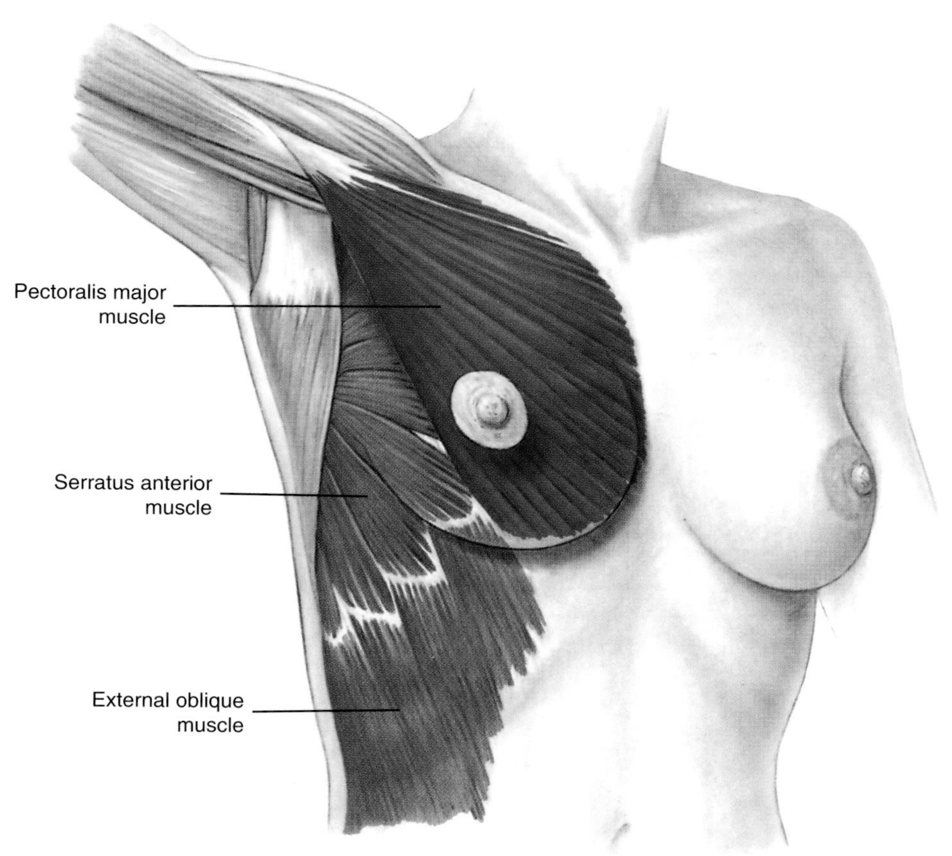
Pectoralis major muscle
Serratus anterior muscle
External oblique muscle

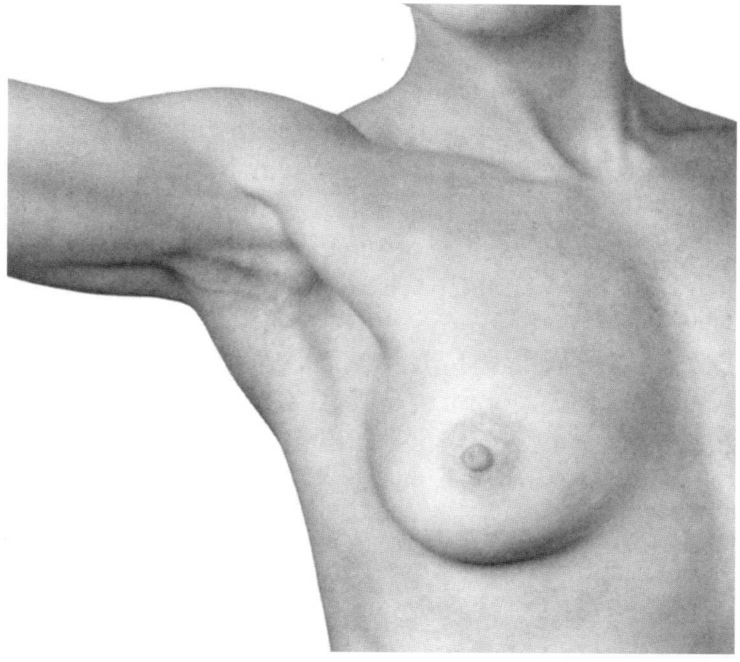

The pectoralis major muscle originates from the medial sternal half of the clavicle and from the lateral aspect of the sternum and costochondral region, from the sternal notch down to the sixth or seventh costal cartilages. It also originates from the medial cartilages of the second through the sixth or seventh ribs and below from the external oblique and rectus abdominis fascia. The sternal and clavicular portions of the pectoralis major are usually distinct embryologically and morphologically and are separated by a fascial interval. In patients with Poland's syndrome the lower portion may be missing. The superficial layer of the deep fascia also extends from the external surface of the pectoralis major muscle across the sternum and joins the fascia above the opposite muscle.

The pectoralis major muscle fibers converge spirally toward the axillary region and form a broad origin for a double-laminated 5 cm tendon of insertion that attaches to the lateral lip of the intertubercular sulcus of the upper humerus about 10 cm distal to the head of the humerus. The insertion of the pectoralis major is anterior to the coracobrachialis muscle and is covered by the anterior portion of the deltoid muscle. Fascial laminae also attach to the tendon and the axillary fascia. The axillary vessels lie below the coracobrachialis muscle, which serves as a landmark when reattaching or reconstructing the anterior axillary fold and the insertion of the pectoralis major muscle.

The pectoralis major muscles function primarily to assist in arm adduction and medial rotation. The functional deficit caused by removal of the pectoralis major muscle or denervation is not, however, significant. ***Many women experienced minimal or no functional impairment following a radical mastectomy when the pectoralis major and minor muscles were excised and the latissimus dorsi muscle was denervated.*** Patients' cosmetic rather than functional concerns prompted surgeons to develop the "modified" radical mastectomy to preserve the pectoralis major muscle. When a breast implant is placed beneath the pectoralis major muscle, contractions of the muscle can be noticeable in some individuals, which is aesthetically displeasing. To minimize this contraction and resulting deformity the lower and inferomedial pectoralis major muscle origins can be detached. The lateral portion of the pectoralis major muscle can be selectively denervated to further reduce muscle hyperactivity and thin the muscle. A high release of pectoralis major muscles can enhance cleavage but may allow breast implants to show through the divided muscle. When there is excess medial dissection, breast implants can touch, resulting in symmastia, a major aesthetic concern and difficult to correct. During medial dissection care must be taken to avoid or specifically control both ends of divided major internal mammary artery perforators. Releasing the lower pectoralis major muscle fibers allows more aesthetic breast implant positioning because the pectoralis major muscle does not restrict the level at which the implant can be placed. During video-assisted breast surgery the pectoralis major muscle is approached from its deep surface, and its fascial connections to the pectoralis minor are separated. It is selectively divided about 1 cm from its origins, usually from the level of the nipple to its most lateral lower extent.

The *pectoralis minor* muscle is located just beneath the lateral upper portion of the pectoralis major muscle. It originates from the anterolateral surfaces of the third to sixth ribs and inserts into the coracoid process of the scapula. This muscle is not a major muscle for breast reconstruction; however, it is strategically located in relation to important structures and can help provide lateral muscular cover for a breast implant. The pectoralis minor covers the second portion of the axilla and is an important landmark for the axilla and its lymph nodes during axillary lymph node dissection. Its lateral margin separates the superficial from the deep axillary nodes. The pectoral nerves to the pectoralis major muscle are closely related to the pectoralis minor muscle. Some course through it, whereas others course lateral and medial to the pectoralis minor muscle.

Nerve Supply

The medial and lateral pectoral nerves innervate the pectoralis major muscle. The clavicular portion of the muscle fibers is supplied by C5-C6 and the sternal muscle fibers by C7-C8. The names of these nerves are derived from their respective cords of origin from the brachial plexus rather than from their position in relation to supply of the pectoralis major muscle. Two to five or more filaments of these pectoral nerves lead into the pectoralis major muscle. Some of these motor nerve filaments to the pectoralis major muscle course through the pectoralis minor muscle and are excised or can be ignored if this muscle is resected during an axillary dissection or radical mastectomy. Pectoralis major muscle denervation at the time of axillary lymph node dissection causes atrophy of the muscle and infraclavicular flattening.

The medial pectoral nerve fibers provide motor innervation to the lateral and lower portion of the pectoralis major muscle. Selective interruption of these nerve fibers can reduce the activity of the pectoralis major muscle, bothersome contractions, and a pulling sensation over the upper portion of a subpectoral breast implant without significantly compromising function or producing a noticeable atrophy in the upper breast area.

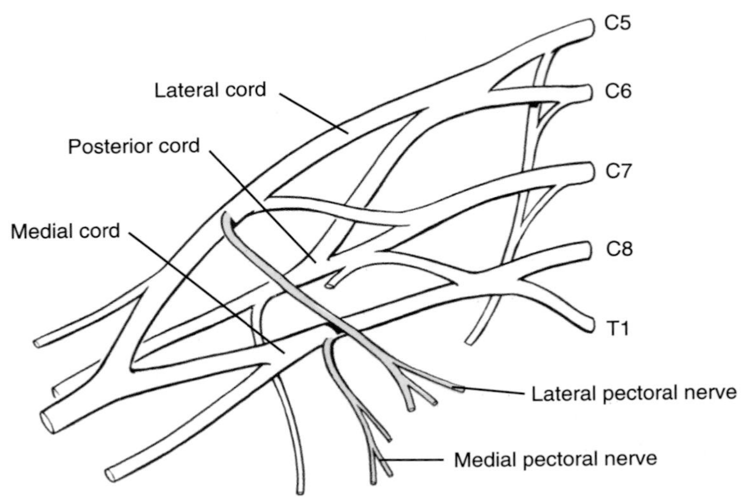

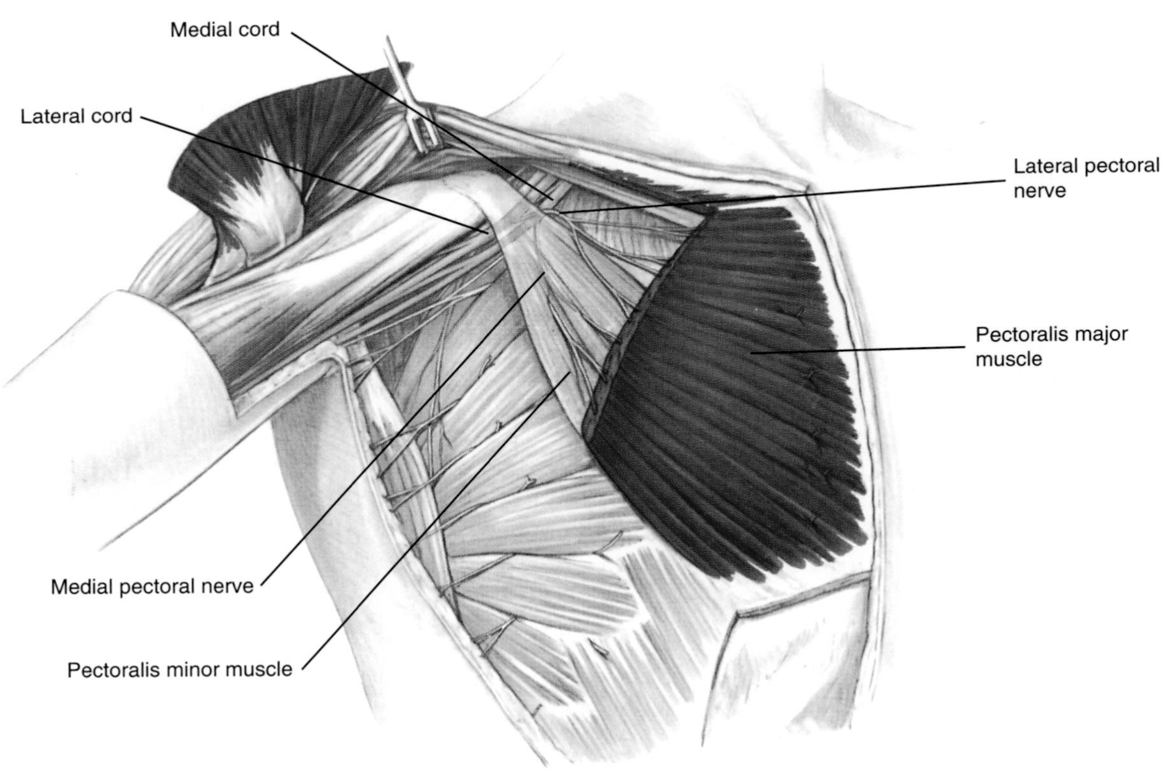

A standard radical mastectomy divides the pectoral nerves and excises the pectoralis major and minor muscles. Excision of these muscles causes an infraclavicular hollowness and loss of the anterior axillary fold. The ribs show through the thin skin that outlines the underlying skeletal structures, and the heart can be seen beating through the intercostal muscles when the radical mastectomy is on the left side. A split-skin graft was commonly used in the past for closure of the radical mastectomy. The resulting infraclavicular hollowness was often as distressing to the patient as her missing breast.

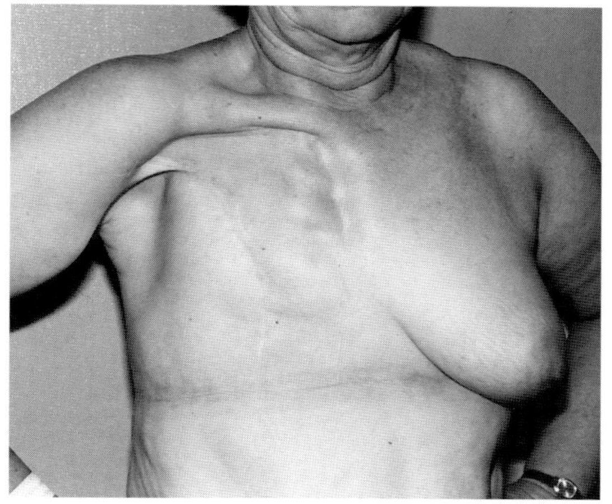

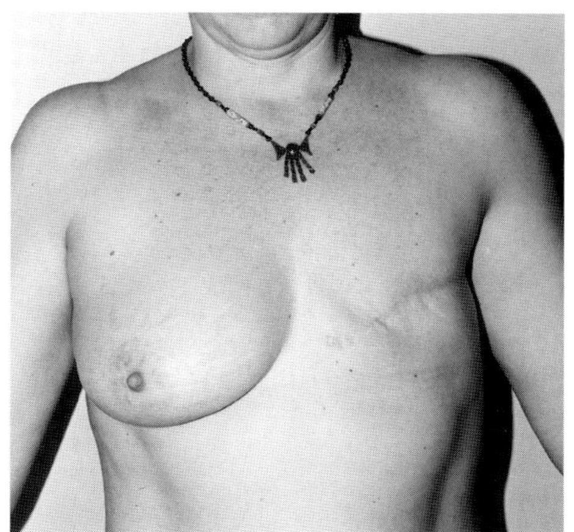

A modified radical mastectomy excises the pectoralis minor muscle and can remove these motor nerves to the pectoralis major muscle. During an axillary dissection these nerves and the pectoralis minor muscle must be preserved to maintain pectoralis major function and bulk. It is difficult, however, to remove the lymph nodes at the apex of the axilla without sacrificing the pectoral nerves. Most oncologic surgeons believe that a representative sampling of the axillary lymph nodes can be obtained without taking the pectoralis minor muscle and the pectoral nerves. Sentinel node biopsy, in which the sentinel node or nodes are sampled and a full axillary dissection performed only if these nodes are found to contain metastatic breast cancer, offers further promise for limiting dissection in this area and preserving innervation (see p. 119).

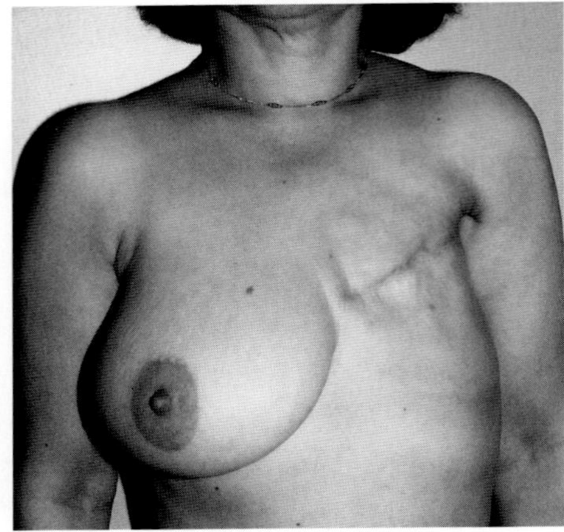

Division of the pectoral nerves during a modified radical mastectomy results in muscle atrophy and decreased pectoralis major muscle thickness. At least 70% of the muscle bulk is generally lost 4 to 6 months following motor nerve division. This loss of bulk can simulate the appearance of a radical mastectomy in the infraclavicular area. This is especially noticeable if a significant thickness of the subcutaneous tissue is removed from the infraclavicular region. During immediate breast reconstruction the reconstructive surgeon must take note of this upper breast region and plan a strategy to fill and restore it to its natural contour. This upper area is usually easier to correct with autologous tissue rather than with a breast implant. The anterior axillary fold is preserved even when the muscle is atrophic and deficient. These areas of pectoralis major muscle atrophy and infraclavicular hollowness must be addressed if breast reconstruction is to be satisfactory.

Patients with Poland's syndrome have a congenital absence of the pectoralis major muscle, usually the sternal component, as well as breast and areolar hypoplasia. This condition can also be associated with absence of the latissimus dorsi and serratus anterior muscles, hand syndactylies, and other extremity deformities.

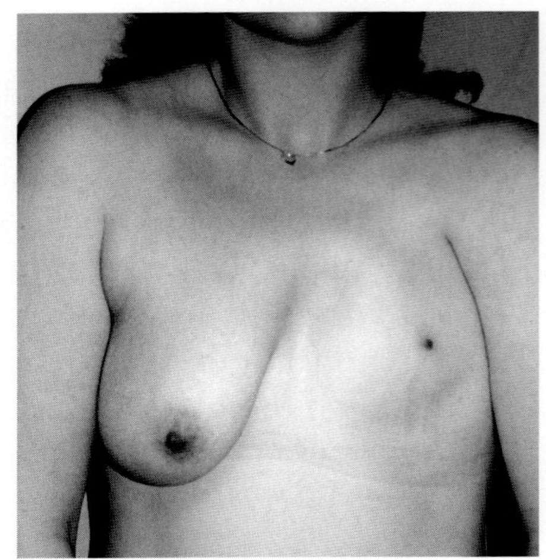

Blood Supply

The blood supply of the pectoralis major muscle is derived from numerous sources and nourishes the muscle as well as the overlying breast parenchyma and breast skin. The arteries coursing into the pectoralis major muscle contribute the dominant blood supply. Significant communication and collateralization of these vessels also exist within the muscle. If one or more of these vessels is excised or occluded, the flow from the others fills from the collaterals and can supply its secondary areas. Medial internal mammary artery perforators provide significant flow to the pectoralis major muscle. Internal mammary arterial flow usually comes from above but can change with upper occlusion. ***The second intercostal internal mammary perforator is usually the largest vessel entering the pectoralis major muscle and overlying breast parenchyma.*** With the superior medial pedicle breast reduction technique, excellent blood flow comes from these large perforators.

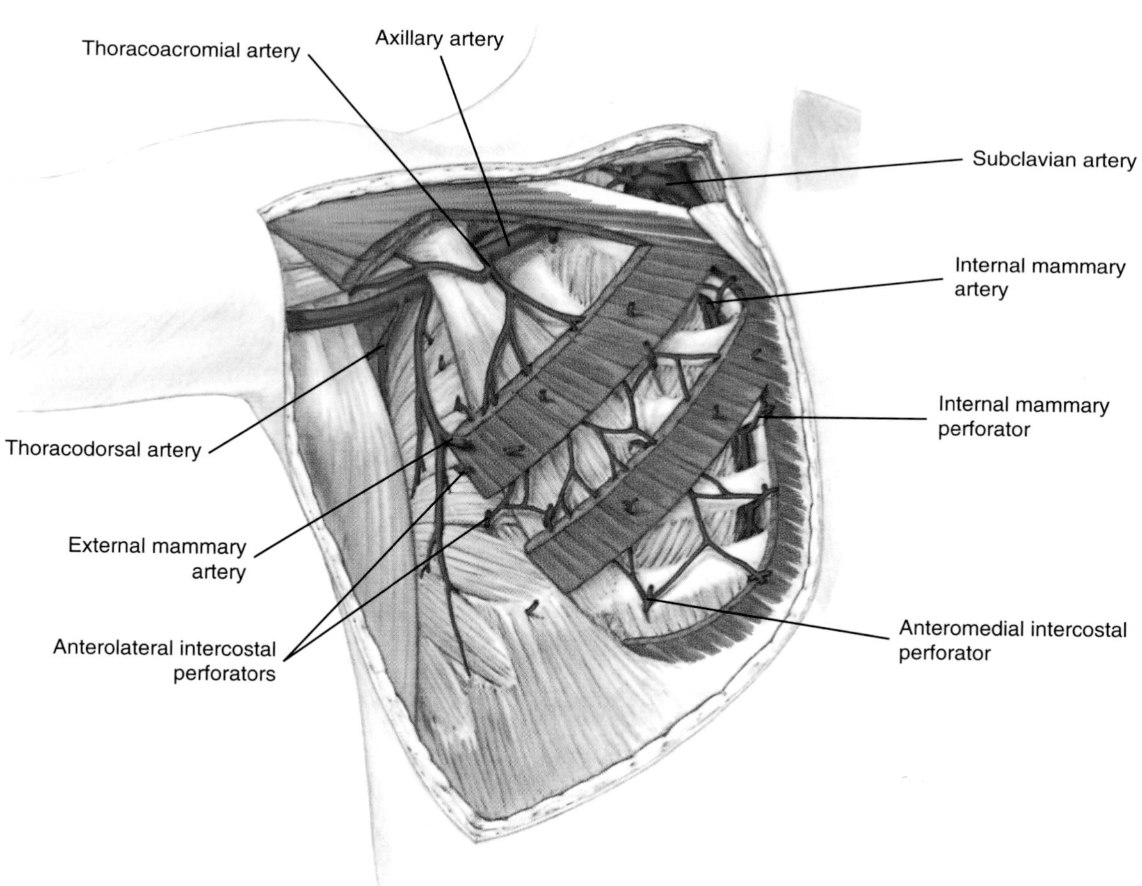

The thoracoacromial artery, a major branch of the axillary artery, enters the deep surface of the pectoralis major muscle near its upper lateral portion and sends branches and flow throughout the muscle. Perforating vessels from the thoracoacromial artery enter the deep surface of the breast. It is a substantial vessel, 2 to 3 mm in diameter, and can nourish the entire pectoralis major muscle along with the overlying skin and breast. It is also the primary pedicle for the pectoralis major musculocutaneous flap that is used for reconstruction of the head and neck area.

Another major group of vessels, branches of the internal mammary artery, enters the pectoralis major muscle from the intercostal spaces medially. Large direct perforators from the internal mammary artery continue through the muscle and its fascia to enter the overlying medial breast. The entire pectoralis major muscle, skin, and breast can also be nourished by these internal mammary vessels from the internal mammary artery.

The second intercostal arterial perforator is the largest of these perforators. It is located high and medial and is preserved during breast augmentations and reductions, thus maintaining a major component of blood flow to the breast from its medial aspect. This arterial supply provides the most direct flow to the upper inner quadrant and central parenchyma of the breast. Because of the major collateralization within the breast, it can supply the entire breast parenchyma when there is normal microcirculation. The other three major perforators of the internal mammary artery, the third, fourth, and fifth, are also major sources of inflow into the breast and should be preserved during aesthetic breast surgery. When the pectoralis major muscle is released, both ends should be adequately controlled to prevent postoperative hematoma.

Another group of vessels, the anteromedial intercostal perforators, enters through the costal origins of the pectoralis major muscle through the fourth, fifth, and sixth intercostal spaces. These vessels supply the lower portions of the pectoralis major muscle and then course superficially to supply the breast and overlying skin.

The anterolateral intercostal perforators course anteriorly and enter at the junction of the lateral pectoralis major muscle through the intercostal spaces at the medial aspect of the serratus anterior muscle. Branches of these arteries supply the pectoralis major muscle, and their primary flow enters the deep surface of the breast along with the accompanying veins and nerves. These intercostal perforators are segmental vessels that communicate with the aorta posteriorly and the internal mammary artery anteriorly. ***These perforating vessels can supply most if not all of the breast and are a primary source of blood supply for inferior and central pedicle breast reduction.*** For this reason the inferior pedicle breast reduction techniques should preserve the parenchyma's attachment to the underlying musculofascial layer.

SERRATUS ANTERIOR MUSCLE

The serratus anterior muscle is a broad flat muscle of the posterolateral and anterolateral chest. It originates from extensive costal attachments of the anterolateral aspects of the first through the eighth or tenth ribs. A thick layer of deep fascia covers these segmental muscular digitations that are densely and broadly attached to the chest wall. The muscle passes backward posteriorly deep to the latissimus dorsi muscle to insert onto the deep medial surface of the scapula.

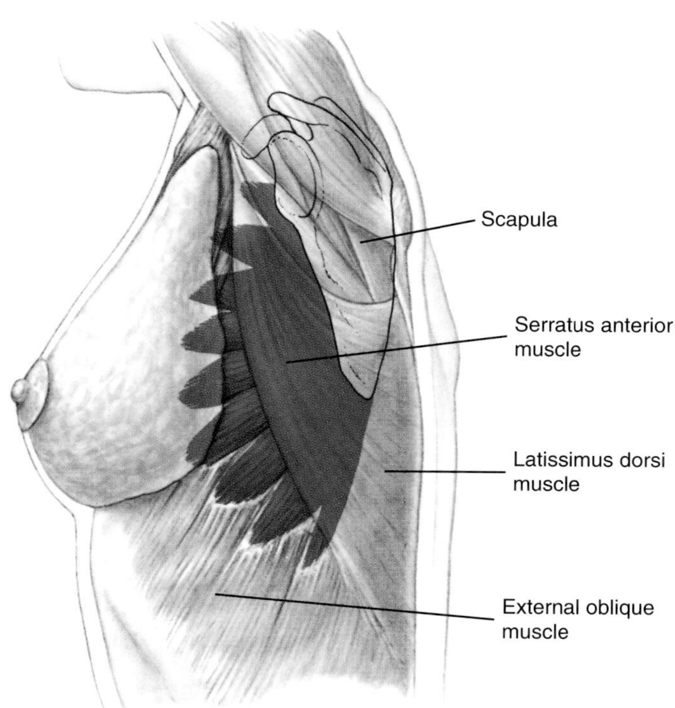

The serratus anterior muscle holds and stabilizes the scapula to the chest wall, assists in rotating the scapula laterally, and draws the scapula forward around the chest. It is important for reaching and pushing movements of the arm. It also assists in respiration. The muscle and its fascia are beneath the lateral and inferior portions of the breast. The fascia of the serratus anterior is rather dense and substantial in its lower portions and is continuous with the pectoralis major fascia. Above, toward the axilla, the serratus anterior fascia becomes thinned and is associated with the pectoralis minor muscle. When a musculofascial dissection proceeds bluntly from the pectoralis major laterally beneath the lower breast area, it goes below the lower serratus anterior fascia and elevates some of the serratus anterior muscle. Sharp dissection is necessary to elevate the full thickness of the serratus anterior off its numerous adherent costal origins beneath the lateral breast. Blunt dissection laterally from the pectoralis major in the upper breast often pushes out through the thin fascia over the pectoralis minor muscle and upper serratus anterior muscle, and the dissecting finger or instrument will go on top of this fascia to the subglandular position of the upper outer breast. ***Developing subpectoral pockets for breast augmentation with blunt dissection usually elevates minimal or little serratus anterior muscle with some of its fascia.*** Although the serratus anterior forms a distinct layer for musculofascial coverage, it is not as thick and substantial as that provided by the pectoralis major muscle and fascia. The serratus anterior goes deep to the latissimus dorsi and the outer fascia is under the latissimus dorsi. Because of the movement of the scapula, this fascial interval has loose areolar tissue and is an excellent plane for separating these structures during elevation of a latissimus dorsi flap.

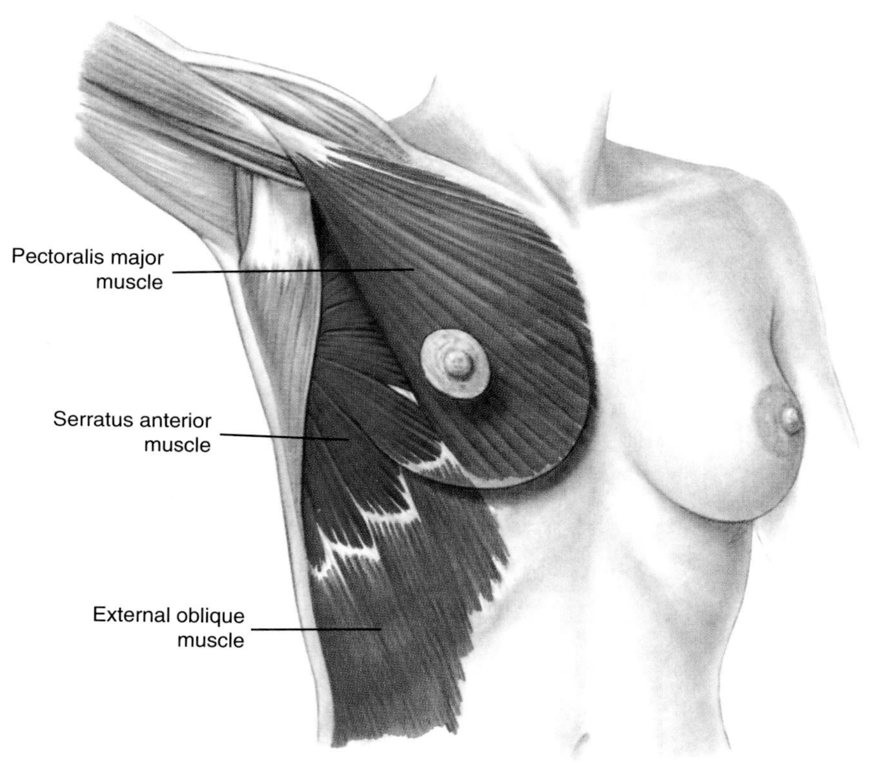
Pectoralis major muscle
Serratus anterior muscle
External oblique muscle

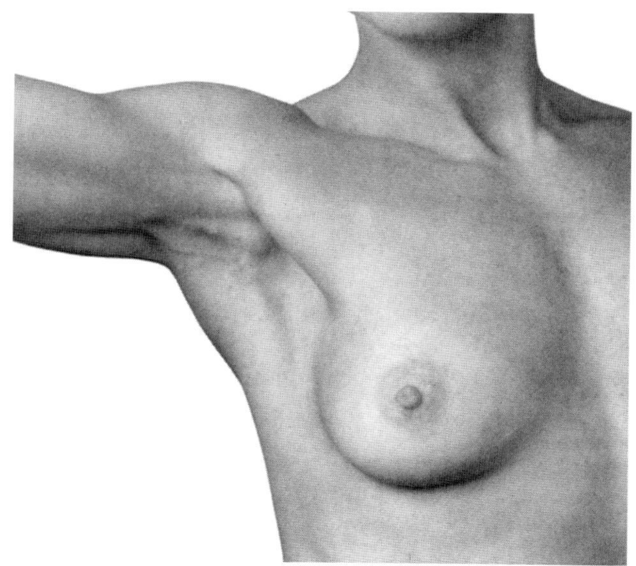

Nerve Supply

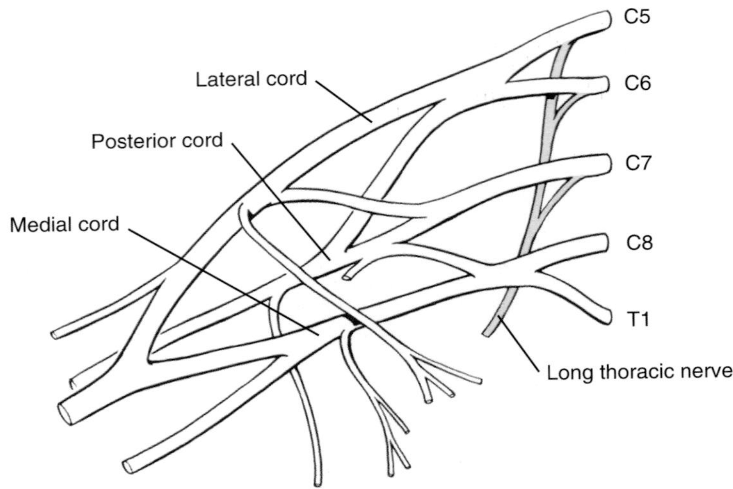

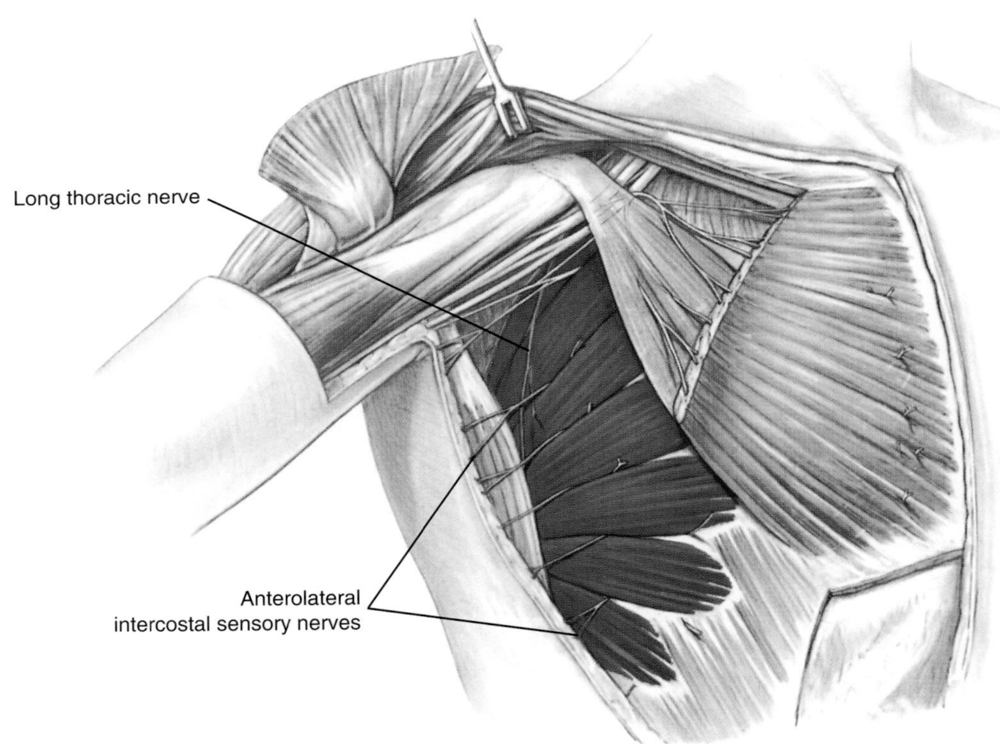

The long thoracic nerve from the posterior roots of C5-C7 supplies most of the innervation to the serratus anterior muscle. This nerve is situated laterally and is covered by the external serratus fascia, but it is superficial to the external surface of the serratus anterior muscle in the midaxillary line.

The long thoracic nerve is preserved during a mastectomy and axillary dissection. Its location is carefully observed so that it is left intact during elevation of the serratus anterior muscle and fascia for breast implant coverage and latissimus dorsi flap elevation. Injury to this nerve weakens or paralyzes the serratus anterior muscle, releasing the scapula and allowing it to move upward and outward to assume a "winged" appearance because the serratus anterior muscle can no longer hold the scapula firmly to the chest wall posterolaterally.

Blood Supply

Segmental intercostal arteriovenous perforators penetrate the anterolateral and lateral serratus anterior muscle digitations at each intercostal space laterally. A few branches of these lateral intercostal perforating arteries join on the outer surface of the serratus anterior muscle and merge into one or more superficial serratus branches; others branch upward to the lateral margin of the latissimus dorsi muscle; still others enter the lateral breast and subcutaneous tissues of the lateral chest wall. ***These external serratus vessels form a collateral branch that connects to the thoracodorsal vessels, which joins a continuation of the thoracodorsal artery near its entrance into the latissimus dorsi muscle about 10 cm below the axillary artery.*** When the thoracodorsal artery is divided or occluded, the flow in these vessels on the outer surface of the serratus anterior muscle provides a significant portion of the blood supply to the latissimus dorsi muscle. More detailed information on the serratus anterior branch and its surgical implications is presented in Chapter 14.

Segmental anterolateral intercostal vessels and nerves penetrate the serratus anterior muscle near the lateral edge of the pectoralis major muscle supplying the breast parenchyma and its overlying skin. The fourth and fifth anterolateral intercostal nerves initially course deep a few centimeters above the pectoralis fascia; then they continue anteriorly upward through the breast parenchyma. These nerves contribute to the innervation of the nipple-areola, as do the third and fifth anterolateral intercostal nerves and the third through the fifth anteromedial intercostal nerve branches. Anterolateral intercostal nerves, three through six, also innervate the skin of the breast. Anteromedial sensory nerves accompany the internal mammary perforators to provide sensation for the medial aspect of the breast and presternal region. There is considerable overlap of these nerve territories. Other primary breast skin innervation is provided by upper clavicular fibers from the cervical plexus.

RECTUS ABDOMINIS MUSCLE

The rectus abdominis muscle is a long strap muscle that extends the entire length of the anterior abdomen from chest to pelvis. Arising from the pubic line, it has three slips of insertion into the fifth, sixth, and seventh costal cartilages.

The rectus abdominis insertions can reach up to the third or fourth costal cartilages and share close attachments with the lower medial pectoralis major muscle origins. The upper rectus abdominis areas of insertion are covered by the lower inner aspect of the breast and the well-defined strong rectus fascia. ***This fascial covering of the upper medial rectus abdominis is the most dense fascia found deep to the breast. It is inelastic and therefore expands poorly.*** Before an implant can be placed beneath this fascia, it must first be released and mobilized sufficiently so that it will not restrict the breast implant positioning or impede tissue expansion. The rectus abdominis muscle is covered by the anterior rectus sheath in the chest area and is enclosed by the rectus sheath below the costal margin in the abdominal area.

Segmental motor nerves from the lower six or seven thoracic intercostal nerves supply the rectus abdominis muscle. Its blood supply comes primarily from the superior and inferior deep epigastric vessels and secondarily from an upper costal marginal branch and segmental intercostal perforators. The upper blood supply is from the lower internal mammary arterial perforators. There is collateral flow between the internal mammary arteries deep to the sternum. (See Chapter 15 for more information on rectus abdominis muscle anatomy.)

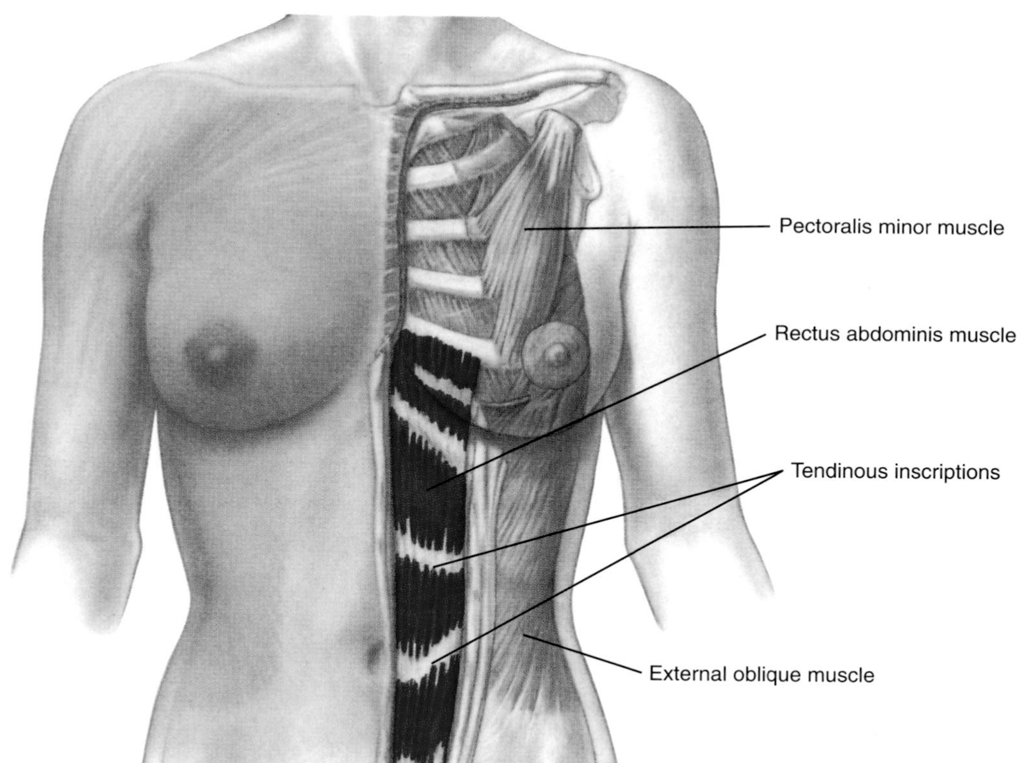
Pectoralis minor muscle
Rectus abdominis muscle
Tendinous inscriptions
External oblique muscle

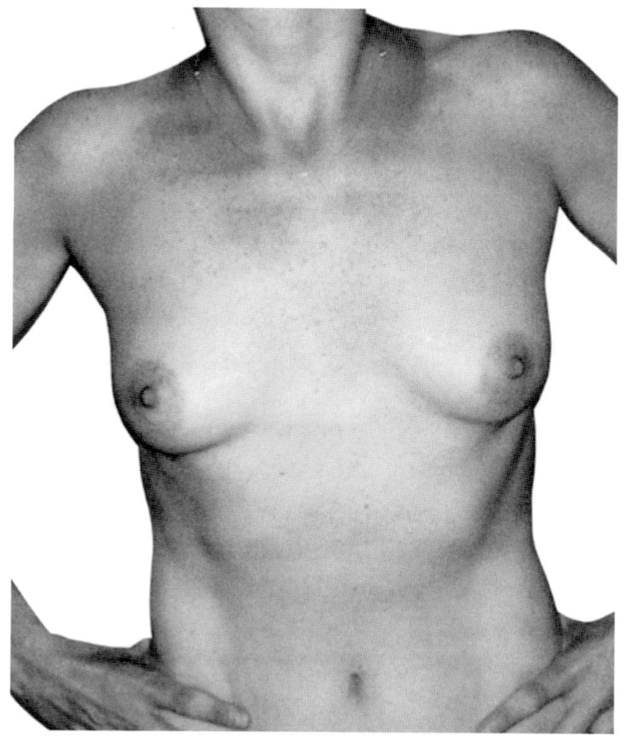

EXTERNAL OBLIQUE MUSCLE

The external oblique muscle contributes to anterior abdominal wall strength and support and is important for abdominal wall support after a TRAM flap procedure (see Chapter 15). It arises from the outer surfaces of the lower anterior and lateral ribs and curves around the lateral and anterior parts of the lower thorax and abdomen. These segmental slips of origin are closely related to the serratus anterior origins in the lower breast area and the origins of the lateral latissimus dorsi muscle further down on the chest.

The external oblique muscle fibers and outer fascial layer insert on the iliac crest and into the medial abdominal fascial aponeurosis, contributing a major portion of the anterior rectus sheath. Segmental motor nerves from the lower six thoracic spinal nerves innervate the external oblique muscle; its blood supply is primarily segmental from the corresponding intercostal arteries, which interconnect with deep collaterals to the central deep epigastric system and superficially into the complex vascular supply to the skin of the abdominal wall.

The portion of the external oblique muscle underneath the lower breast is of interest in aesthetic breast surgery and breast reconstruction primarily for its contribution to the musculofascial cover for a breast implant. The upper abdominal external oblique muscle can also be elevated to give additional coverage and support for breast implant cover in the lower breast region. The external oblique fascia is relatively unyielding. An implant placed behind the unreleased external oblique muscle and its fascia will generally not expand or stretch this fascia and may fail to "settle" down postoperatively, causing the implant to rest too high. Any mobile or ptotic breast parenchyma can slide over it to a lower position. If the breast implant is trapped by the lower musculofascial layer, the breast will have a "double-bubble" contour. Since release of the lower fascia beneath the breast can minimize this unflattering definition of the inframammary fold by a breast implant, I have found that it is sometimes best to place the lower portion of the breast implant in the subglandular or subcutaneous position.

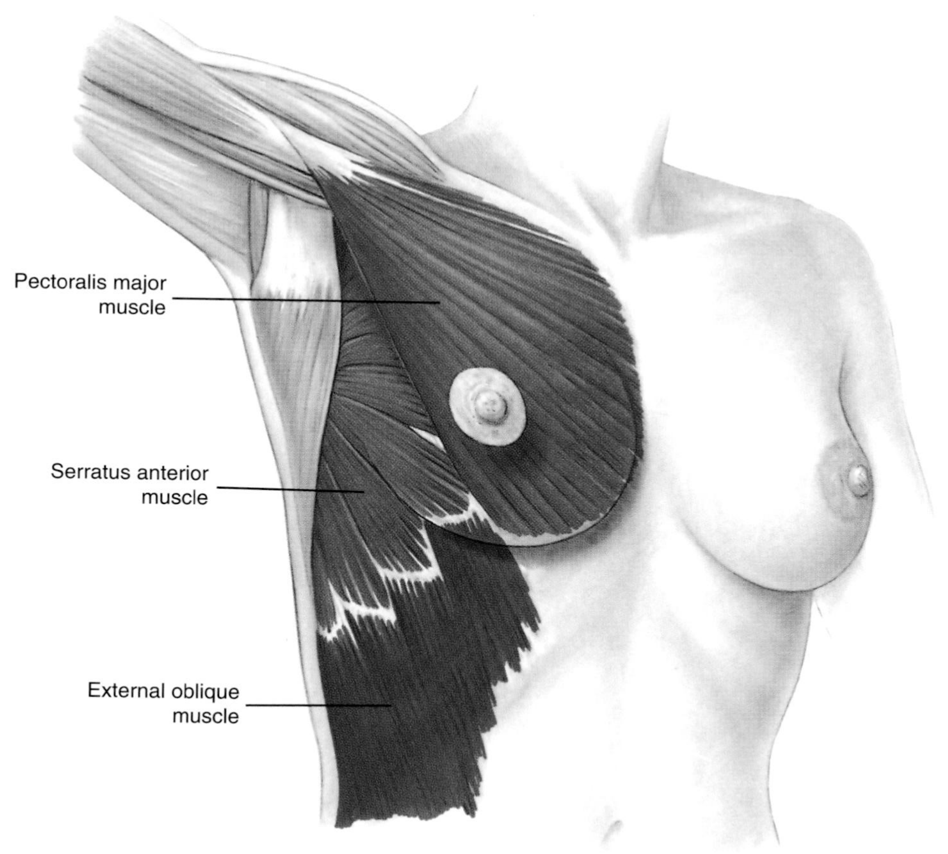
Pectoralis major muscle
Serratus anterior muscle
External oblique muscle

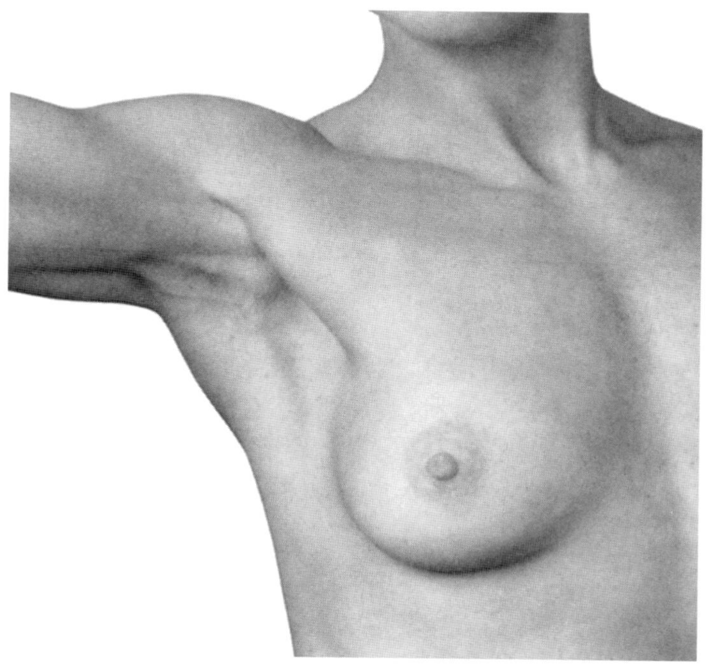

Blood Supply to the Breast

The blood supply of the breast parenchyma is closely related to the blood supply of the underlying muscles; knowledge of both is crucial when planning aesthetic and reconstructive breast operations. The blood supply to the breast is also primarily responsible for the blood supply to the overlying skin via perforators and the subdermal plexus. The principles applicable to muscle and musculocutaneous flaps also contribute to an understanding of the blood supply to the breast because the breast is essentially a skin derivative and its blood supply is analogous to musculocutaneous flaps (see Chapter 14).

The blood supply to the breast comes from numerous arterial sources. ***A substantial collateralization of arterial flow is present within the breast, making it possible for the entire normal breast to survive on a fraction of its usual total arterial input, provided that the breast parenchyma incisions do not transect a major portion of the blood supply to a particular segment.*** However, if all the arterial flow to a segment of the breast is divided, necrosis of portions of the breast, and especially the fat, will result.

The external mammary artery is a major artery entering the upper lateral portion of the breast. It originates from the axillary artery and enters the breast in the lower axillary region. ***This vessel is large, about 2 to 3 mm in diameter, and can nourish the entire breast under normal circumstances.*** During a total mastectomy, when the remainder of the breast is elevated and the other arterial supply is divided, an intact external mammary artery can provide good flow to vascularize the breast parenchyma.

The pectoralis major musculocutaneous flap, elevated on its thoracoacromial pedicle, will nourish the pectoralis major muscle and the overlying breast. Significant perforating arteries from the pectoralis major muscle enter the upper, central, and lower breast tissue. These vessels are preserved during submusculofascial augmentation mammaplasty, but many are divided during subglandular dissection and breast parenchyma elevation. Because the subglandular dissection may create a layer of poorly vascularized fascia, there is speculation that this approach is more prone to low-grade infection from *Staphylococcus epidermidis* and therefore to capsular contracture.

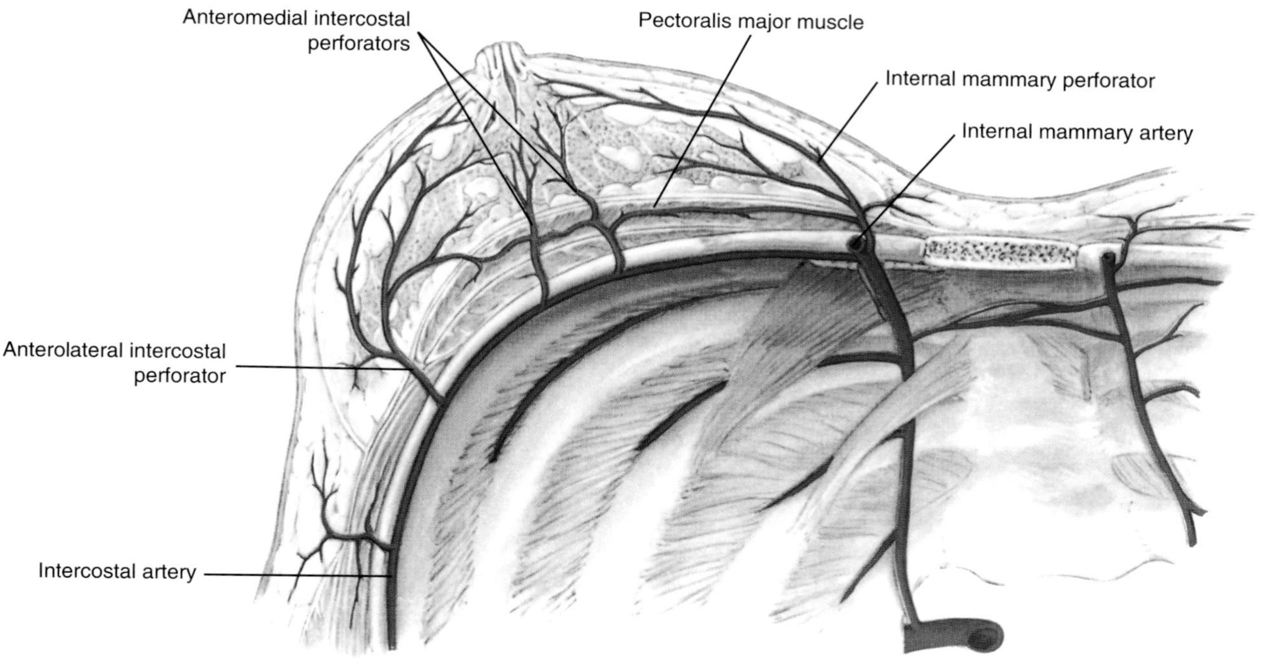

Anteromedial intercostal perforators
Pectoralis major muscle
Internal mammary perforator
Internal mammary artery
Anterolateral intercostal perforator
Intercostal artery

Second internal mammary perforator
External mammary artery
Internal mammary perforator
Anterolateral intercostal perforator
Anteromedial intercostal perforator

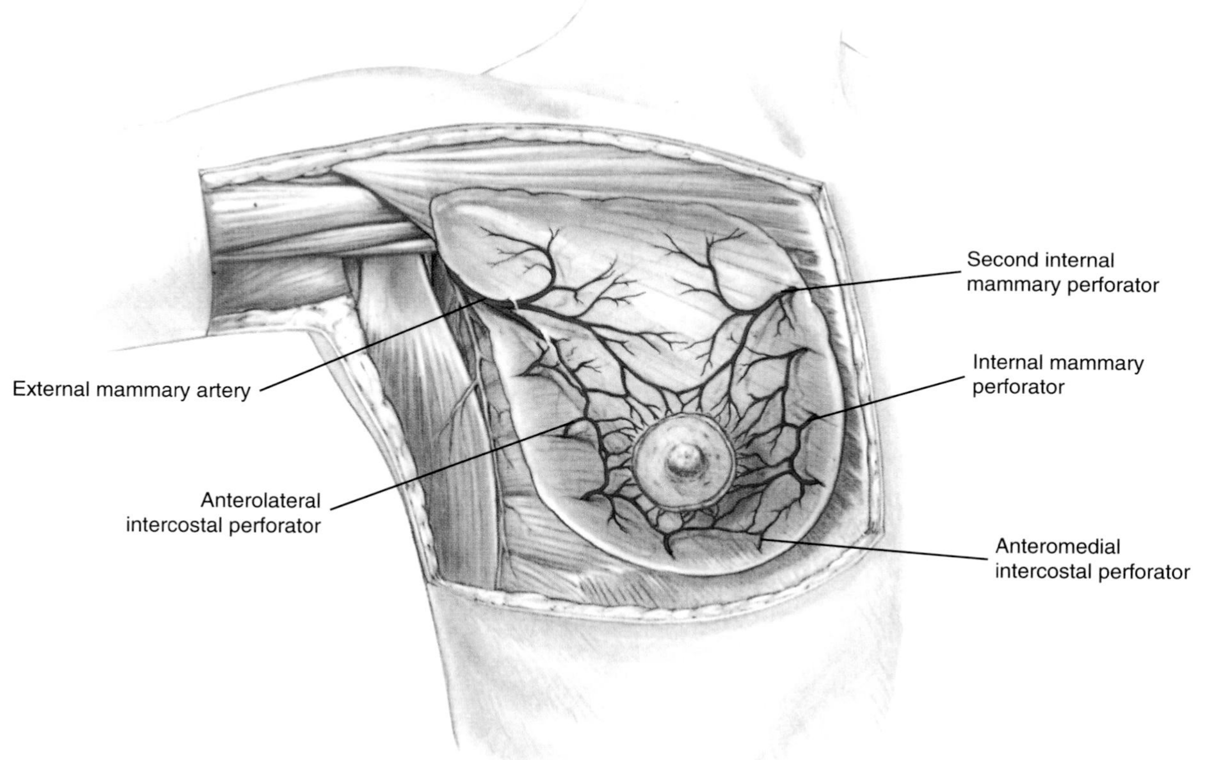

The internal mammary segmental perforating vessels of the internal mammary artery provide another primary source of arterial inflow. These vessels penetrate the breast via perforators through the medial intercostal spaces through the intercostal muscles and through the pectoralis major muscle origins between the second and sixth intercostal spaces. The internal mammary perforators go to the pectoralis major muscle, the breast, and the overlying skin. Preservation of these perforating vessels to the breast skin during a total mastectomy helps ensure adequate blood supply to the skin. The second and third internal mammary perforators are also the largest, providing the primary blood flow into the upper medial breast area. Although the size of the internal mammary artery and the internal mammary perforators vary in each individual, the upper perforators are usually dominant. These upper vessels are usually not divided during a submusculofascial blunt dissection. I try to preserve them by avoiding detachment of the pectoralis major at the second and third intercostal space when doing a submusculofascial augmentation mammaplasty. ***During superomedial pedicle breast reduction the upper medial and central breast parenchyma is preserved to ensure continued inflow from these important sources and to preserve a natural fullness and a satisfactory cleavage in the upper medial breast.***

The intercostal perforators also provide a major source of blood flow to the breast. These large arterial perforators are accompanied by sensory nerves and veins perforating through the intercostal spaces at the lateral margin of the pectoralis major muscle through serratus anterior muscle digitations. They primarily supply the lateral breast segmentally from the third through the sixth intercostal spaces. Additional lateral intercostal perforators enter the lateral breast parenchyma at the lateral margin of the latissimus dorsi muscle. They send branches to the latissimus dorsi muscle as well as to the lateral breast and the lateral breast subcutaneous tissue and skin.

Blood flow to the central and lower breast is also supplied by another group of intercostal perforators that enters the lower medial and central aspect of the breast parenchyma from the nipple level (fourth interspace) downward. These perforators, often 1 to 2 mm in diameter, are a primary source of blood supply to the central breast in inferior central pedicle reduction mammaplasty. Some of these intercostal perforators branch upward through the lower fibers of origin of the pectoralis major muscle. These anteromedial and anterolateral arteries have branches that course upward through the breast tissue to the nipple-areola. Others enter centrally through digitations of the external oblique muscle origins. These lower intercostal pectoralis major perforators communicate within the muscles with the other major vessels in the intramuscular network. They then enter the breast and develop further communications with vessels from the internal mammary artery, external mammary artery, and pectoralis major perforations from the thoracic aorta.

The nipple-areola receives substantial blood flow from its underlying breast parenchyma. In addition to the deep blood supply, it is nourished by a periareolar plexus of arteries and veins, a special arrangement of the subdermal plexus; this rich nourishing blood supply allows the nipple-areola to be based on the underlying breast parenchyma or on a dermal flap.

Venous Drainage of the Breast

A superficial subdermal venous plexus just superior to the superficial fascia and a deeper venous system closely related to the deeper parenchymal and muscular arteries provide the venous drainage of the breast. Superficial veins originate and form around a periareolar vascular venous plexus; these veins interconnect across the midline, draining superiorly and medially. This superficial venous system connects with the deeper veins of the breast through the breast parenchyma. Their subcutaneous pattern is effectively visualized with infrared photography. Recent studies of the venous drainage of the breast demonstrate the presence of valves that direct the blood flow from the superficial to the deep system.

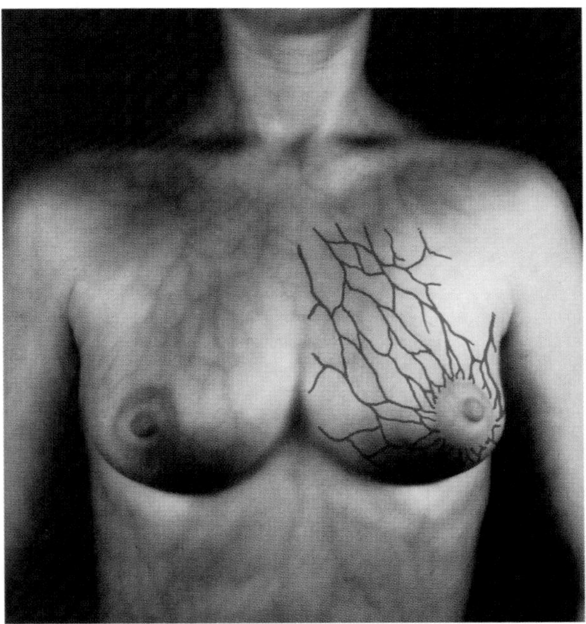

The deep venous drainage of the breast generally parallels the arterial supply. Internal mammary perforators drain to the innominate vein through the internal mammary veins. Deeper vessels drain into the pectoralis major muscle and also into the external mammary vein and from there toward the axilla and the axillary vein. Veins also accompany the intercostal arteries to the azygos and vertebral veins and on into the superior vena cava.

Venous drainage of the nipple-areola has both superficial and deep components. I prefer to keep both of these intact by preserving a deepithelialized portion of dermis about the periphery of the nipple-areola and also by preserving the nipple-areola on the breast parenchyma.

Nerve Supply to the Breast

Perception of breast sensation has two aspects: the general sensitivity to touch with two-point discrimination of pressure, vibration, heat, and cold similar to that of the rest of the body and the unique special sensual responsivity characteristic of central breast and especially nipple-areolar stimulation. Skin sensation to touch, temperature, and pressure can be preserved even if the specific sensation to the nipple-areola is diminished or absent. The abundant sensory innervation of the skin of the breast has considerable overlap and comes from the intercostal segmental nerves entering from medial, midlateral, and lateral directions.

Supraclavicular filaments from the cervical plexus extend downward beneath the platysma muscle to innervate the upper portions of the breast skin collateralization. They enter the subcutaneous tissue and supplement innervation of the upper breast, perhaps below to the nipple-areolar region. The extent of this innervation is best determined by the area of sensation of the upper flap after an extensive mastectomy removes the medial and lateral nerves. More sensation is retained in skin-sparing mastectomy, possibly because no medial incision divides these nerves. This upper cervical plexus innervation should be considered when planning a local block of the breast.

The lateral intercostal nerves along the lateral edge of the latissimus dorsi provide sensory innervation for the lateral portions of the breast. Significant overlap exists among these nerves, the anterolateral and anteromedial nerves, and the clavicular nerves coming down from the cervical plexus.

Primary sensory nerves of the breast skin also enter from the third to the sixth anterolateral intercostal nerves. These nerves pass through the interdigitations of the serratus anterior muscle at the lateral margin of the pectoralis major muscle. They course superficially from the intercostal nerves beneath the lower portion of the ribs.

The second anterolateral intercostal nerve, known as the intercostobrachial nerve, courses across the axilla and through its contents to supply the upper medial arm. It is often divided during axillary dissection, resulting in anesthesia and paresthesia of the upper medial arm. Surgeons try to spare this nerve during axillary dissection. It can also be damaged during endoscopic axillary augmentation mammaplasty if the dissection goes deeper in the axilla rather than superficially to the lateral margin of the pectoralis major muscle. Painful neuromas often develop after the anterolateral cutaneous nerves are divided over the serratus anterior muscle, especially after mastectomy but also after breast augmentation or reduction. These nerves and neuromas can be caught up in the scar of the mastectomy or in an implant capsule. Resection of these neuromas and coverage with an implant or interposition of a flap will occasionally but not predictably alleviate these symptoms.

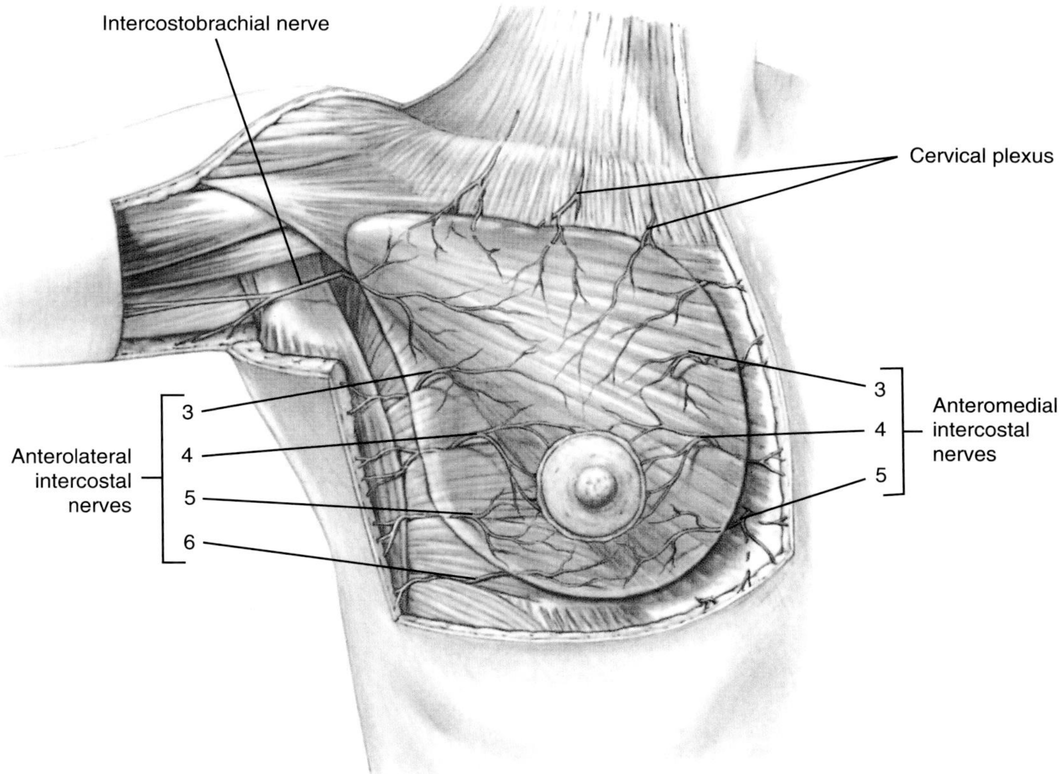

The second to sixth anterior medial intercostal segmental nerves supply the medial breast and presternal area and enter the breast parenchyma with the internal mammary perforators. The medial branches are the sensory nerves of the presternal region. They also extend to the central breast, and their third, fourth, and fifth segmental nerves contribute to nipple-areola sensation along with those from corresponding anterolateral branches.

Lymphatics of the Breast

Lymphatics of the breast extend throughout the parenchyma, facilitating both deep and superficial lymph drainage. ***Individual lymphatics drain each of the lobules and the lactiferous ducts.*** Central lymphatic collaterals comprise the periareolar lymphatic plexus and accompany the venous plexus in this area. Deep direct lymphatic connections penetrate through the deep fascia into the underlying muscles, especially the pectoral major muscle. Primary lymph efferents pass from the breast's upper outer quadrant, around the pectoralis major muscle, and to the deep pectoral nodes. Some also communicate directly with the subscapular nodes. The lymph then drains to the central axillary group of lymph nodes and from there to the apical nodes of the axilla and on to the supraclavicular nodes. The internal mammary perforators are accompanied by medial lymph channels that drain to the parasternal nodes. The total gland supplies lymph to these medial nodes.

The lymphatics can be conduits for the local spread of breast cancer to the regional nodes. Since lymphatics drain each lobule and duct, when breast cancer cells penetrate the basement membrane, they spread as the tumor extends into the lymphatics and vessels. Removal of the axillary lymph nodes at the time of mastectomy removes gross and microscopic breast cancer contained within these lymph nodes, provides staging information, and is an excellent prognostic indicator of the likelihood of both local recurrence and systemic spread. However, removal of the lymphatics of the axilla can also predispose the patient to lymphedema of the upper extremity because the lymphatics draining the arm also course through the axillary lymphatic conduits. Lymphedema can occur immediately following mastectomy or months to years later. It can be aggravated by infection, especially streptococcal infection. Long-term antibiotic coverage specific for *Streptococcus* is indicated for these women. Radiation therapy in the area of axillary lymph node removal also strongly predisposes the patient to lymphedema of the upper extremity.

The option of sentinel node biopsy holds promise for women in whom a node dissection is required. ***It has been shown that axillary spread of a breast cancer is initially to the "sentinel" lymph node or nodes. Identification of this node or nodes and a histologic evaluation for metastatic breast cancer cells can help determine if the remainder of the axillary lymph nodes should be removed.*** With sentinel node identification and biopsy the number of axillary lymph node dissections can be limited to those with breast cancer metastasis.

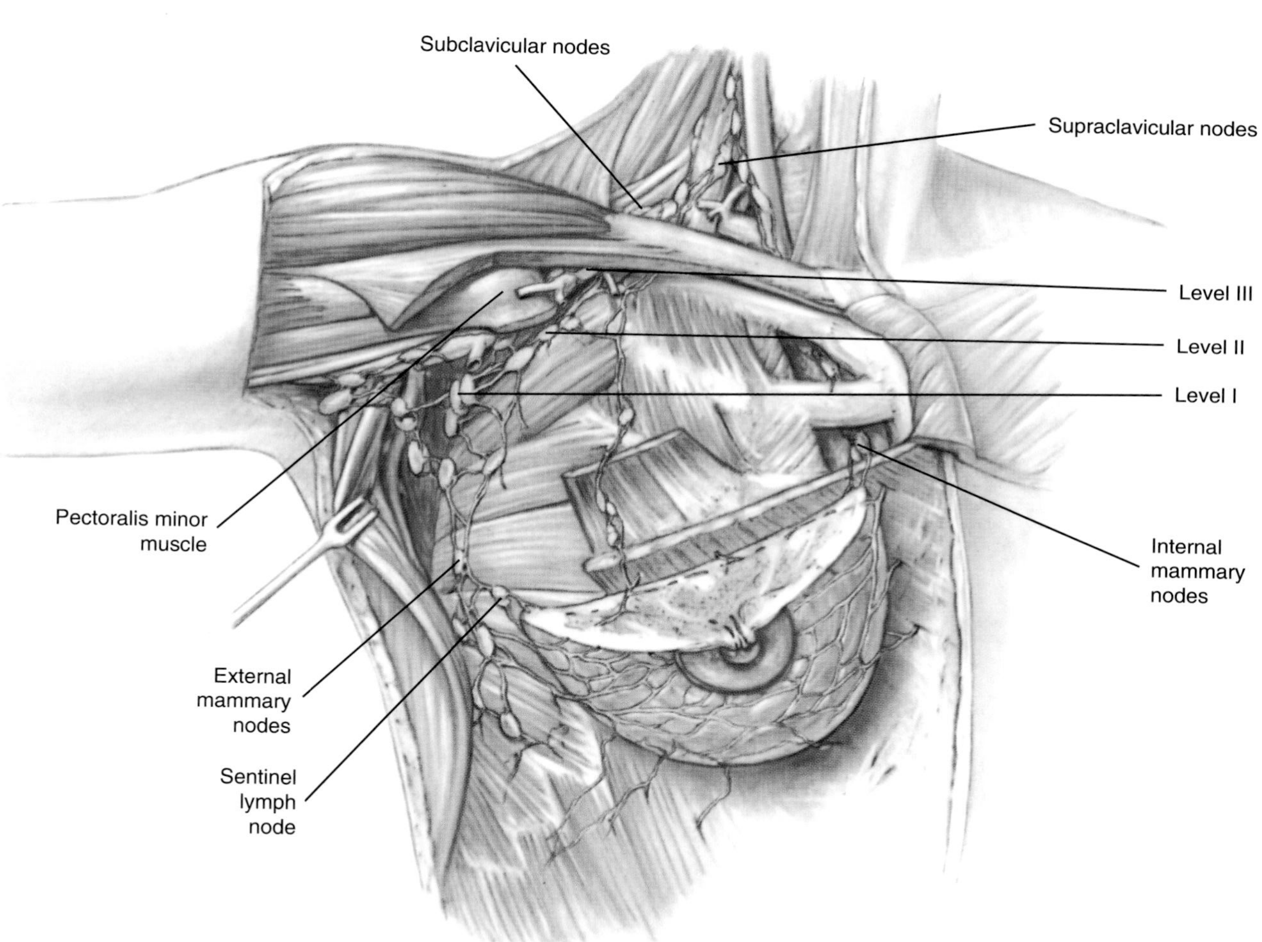

Nipple-Areola

The nipple-areola is the aesthetic, functional, and sensory focus of the breast. Its enhanced blood supply and collateral vascular and neurologic network contribute to an anatomic structure that is resilient after reduction and augmentation procedures. Its limits, however, have to be understood and respected to ensure predictable results without compromising nipple vascularity, sensation, and function.

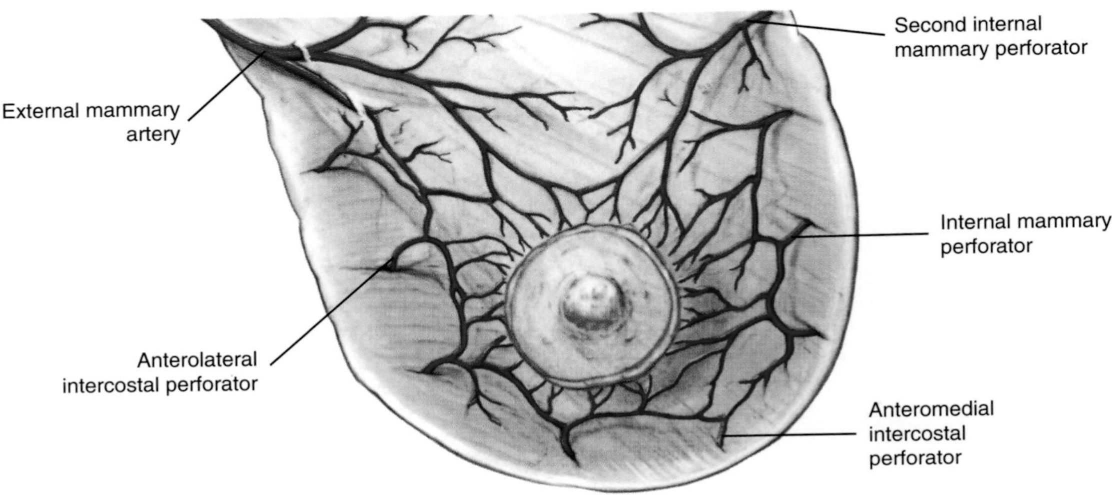

Breast reduction procedures that leave the nipple-areola attached to a well-vascularized underlying breast parenchyma ensure nipple-areolar survival because the blood supply is both parenchymal and subdermal. This parenchymal blood supply contributes additional flow to the nipple-areola while maintaining central breast tissue and underlying lactiferous ducts and nerves—thus preserving sensation and future lactation potential. In superior and inferior central pedicle techniques for reduction mammaplasty, the nipple-areola remains attached to the underlying breast parenchyma as well as to the nipple ducts. These techniques provide a reliable source of blood flow to the nipple-areola. A dermal and subdermal blood supply can also support the nipple-areola.

The blood supply to the nipple-areola is related to the blood flow in the breast parenchyma beneath the nipple-areola as well as a normal functioning superficial periareolar vascular plexus. When intact, well-vascularized breast parenchyma is preserved, good blood flow is maintained to the nipple-areola. A rich subdermal plexus surrounds the nipple-areola and contributes the necessary blood supply to support the viability of the nipple-areola after reduction mammaplasty or subcutaneous mastectomy.

Contained within the nipple are specialized lactiferous ducts and accompanying muscles that assist with lactation and breast-feeding. The areola also contains muscles that cause erection of the nipple-areola and assist in lactation. Present within the mature areola are Montgomery's glands that appear as small bumps on the areolar surface and lubricate the areola, particularly during lactation. These glands can enlarge, usually in younger women taking supplementary hormones or in association with pregnancy or lactation. Some patients need to be assured that these lumps of Montgomery's glands are normal; they should not be removed or biopsied. A nipple-areolar rash, however, is a concern and can represent Paget's disease, an indicator of underlying breast cancer. The nipple does not normally produce a spontaneous discharge, although most women can express some material from it. ***If the nipple bleeds spontaneously, it is usually located in and exudes from a specific lactiferous duct that should be localized and treated.*** Radiographic localization of the specific duct is important for a definitive diagnosis. The problem is often traceable to an intraductal papilloma, which should then be removed; however, the bleeding source can be breast cancer. (See Chapter 10 for more information on breast disease.) A chronic infection can develop in the lactiferous ducts and the collection system beneath the nipple-areola. Excision of the central breast ductal area is usually curative. This condition should be treated and controlled before aesthetic breast surgery is attempted, especially augmentation mammaplasty, to decrease the risk of postoperative infection, implant extrusion, or capsular contracture.

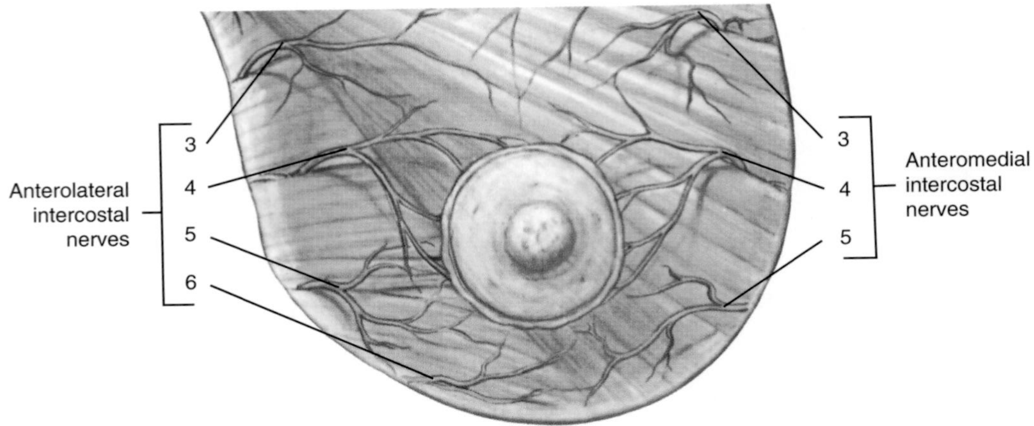

The nerve supply of the nipple-areola is derived primarily from the fourth anterolateral and anteromedial intercostal nerve, although the adjacent third and fifth intercostal nerves contribute to its sensation as well as the supraclavicular nerves. The loss of one of these nerves usually will not render the nipple-areola anesthetic. The fourth anterolateral intercostal nerve enters laterally through the fourth interspace and runs medially under the deep fascia for a few centimeters. It then courses upward through the breast parenchyma to supply the nipple-areola and the adjacent area. The third and fifth anterolateral nerves as well as the third through the fifth anterior medial intercostal nerves contribute to nipple-areola sensation. The fact that nipple-areola sensation involves a number of nerves with overlapping sensory zones helps explain how nipple-areola sensation is preserved in a high percentage of women after reduction mammaplasties despite the use of different techniques. Techniques that preserve underlying breast parenchyma of the nipple-areola and the deep attachments to the chest wall (central and inferior pedicle) as well as medial attachments (superior central pedicle or superior medial pedicle) of the upper breast usually preserve nipple sensation. Nipple-areola sensation should always be mentioned to the patient and assessed before aesthetic breast surgery. Patients differ widely in their subjective feelings about sensation in this area. Some women say that they have no sensation of the nipple-areola preoperatively, whereas others relate that their nipples are exquisitely sensitive and place a high priority on sensation preservation.

REFERENCES

Arey LB. Developmental Anatomy, 7th ed. Philadelphia: WB Saunders, 1965.

Baruchin AM, Rosenberg L. Axillary breast tissue: Clinical presentation and surgical treatment. Ann Plast Surg 36:661, 1996.

Carramenha e Costa MA, Carriquiry C, Vasconez LO, Grotting JC, Herrera RH, Windle BH. An anatomic study of the venous drainage of the transverse rectus abdominis musculocutaneous flap. Plast Reconstr Surg 79:208, 1987.

Clemente CD, ed. Gray's Anatomy of the Human Body, 30th ed. Philadelphia: Lea & Febiger, 1985.

Cooper AP. On the Anatomy of the Breast. London: Longmans, 1840.

Courtiss EH, Goldwyn RM. Breast sensation before and after plastic surgery. Plast Reconstr Surg 58:1, 1976.

De Cholnoky T. Accessory breast tissue in the axilla. NY State J Med 51:245, 1951.

Goldman LD, Goldwyn RM. Some anatomical considerations of subcutaneous mastectomy. Plast Reconstr Surg 51:501, 1973.

Guiliano AE, Guenther JM, Kirgafi DM, Morton DL. Lymphatic mapping and sentinel lymphadenectomy for breast cancer. Ann Surg 220:391, 1994.

Hoffman GW, Elliott LF. The anatomy of the pectoral nerves and its significance to the general and plastic surgeon. Ann Surg 205:504, 1987.

Hoffman S. Reduction mammaplasty: A medicolegal hazard? Aesthetic Plast Surg 11:113, 1987.

Hollingshead H. Textbook of Anatomy, 3rd ed. New York: Harper & Row, 1974, pp 77-178.

Kaye BL. Axillary breasts: An aesthetic deformity of the trunk. Clin Plast Surg 2:397, 1973.

Letterman G, Schurter M. Suggested nomenclature for aesthetic and reconstructive surgery of the breast. Part I: Breast reduction. Aesthetic Plast Surg 7:187, 1983.

Letterman G, Schurter M. Suggested nomenclature for aesthetic and reconstructive surgery of the breast. Part II: Augmentation mammaplasty and mastopexy. Aesthetic Plast Surg 9:293, 1985.

Letterman G, Schurter M. Suggested nomenclature for aesthetic and reconstructive surgery of the breast. Part III: Gynecomastia. Aesthetic Plast Surg 10:55, 1986.

Letterman G, Schurter M. Suggested nomenclature for aesthetic and reconstructive surgery of the breast. Part IV: Congenital anomalies of the breast. Aesthetic Plast Surg 13:59, 1989.

Mathes SJ, Nahai F. Reconstructive Surgery: Principles, Anatomy, and Technique. St. Louis: Quality Medical Publishing, 1997.

Miller LB, Bostwick J, Hartrampf CR, Hester TR, Nahai F. The superiorly based rectus abdominis flap: Predicting and enhancing its blood supply based on an anatomic and clinical study. Plast Reconstr Surg 81:713, 1988.

Newman M. Supernumerary nipples. Am Fam Physician 38:183, 1988.

Pearl RM, Johnson D. The vascular supply to the skin: An anatomical and physiological reappraisal—Part II. Ann Plast Surg 11:196, 1983.

Rouviere H. Anatomy of the Human Lymphatic System. Ann Arbor: Edwards, 1938, pp 10-16.

Wood WC, Scandalakis JE. Anatomic Basis of Tumor Surgery. St. Louis: Quality Medical Publishing, 1999.

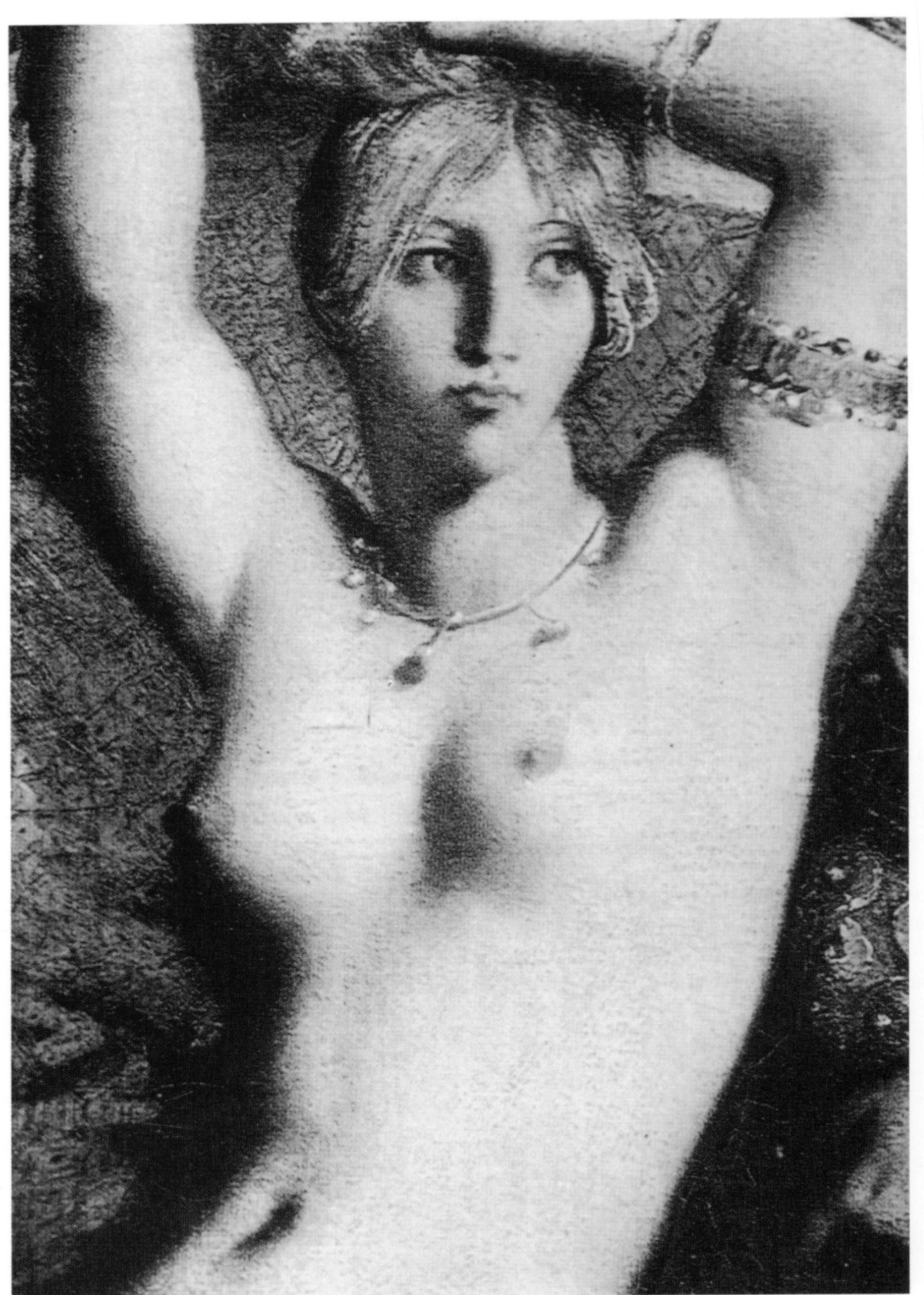

3 *Applied Aesthetics*

Key Topics

Aesthetic Concepts

Breast Shape

Nipple-Areolar Position and Appearance

Breast Flow

Breast Cleavage

Symmetry

Breast Ptosis

Applying Breast Aesthetics to Surgery

Adjustments for Different Body Types

Aesthetic Placement of Incisions

Assessing the Result

Observations

Breast surgery is an artistic endeavor, an exercise in right-brain creativity. Clarification of patient expectations and knowledge of individual anatomic characteristics are critical to the surgical plan, but ultimately it is an internalized vision of what is normal and aesthetically pleasing that guides the scalpel. I visualize the most attractive breasts for the patient and then work backward in planning the actual breast surgery, selecting reliable techniques that will help attain a result that will meet her expectations and mine. I know of no shortcuts to teach this aesthetic judgment. It exists in different degrees in each of us and is manifest in the creativity, skill, and artistry of the surgical results we produce. Techniques and technologic innovations are not the answers but rather the tools to be guided by personal artistic vision and careful preoperative assessment.

Breast Aesthetics

Aesthetics in breast surgery is a desirable but elusive goal. Although standards of beauty exist and define the ideal breast, these standards cannot always be approximated through surgery. The sculptor may reshape his clay with abandon until he achieves the desired effect; the surgical artist, however, is limited in his search for the perfect, the normal, the well-formed breast by the nature, limitations, and viability of the materials he molds. ***To be successful the surgeon's plan must anticipate the expected alterations in breast appearance, form, and shape that invariably result from wound healing, maturation, and settling of the tissues after the operation.*** He must also accommodate changes associated with placement of foreign bodies or movement of autologous tissues. His tools are tissue, muscle, and skin, and every incision or transfer of tissue results in scars and changes that cannot be erased. Furthermore, each patient heals in a unique manner. The surgeon must understand how each procedure affects healing and the result as it "ages." After breast implant surgery the tissue ages differently than after breast reduction operations, which in turn mature differently than after autologous flap procedures. Unilateral procedures, particularly with implants, also produce longitudinal aging disparities. The surgeon's primary goal is to understand the patient's aesthetic ideal and to plan a procedure that will meet patient expectations as closely as possible; her psychological well-being is closely tied to the success of the operation and the excellence of the result. To create breasts that approximate this aesthetic norm while satisfying the patient's aesthetic expectations, the surgeon must develop a concept of the normal, attractive breast with knowledge of the anatomic landmarks and proportions that contribute to it. Only then can a surgical approach be planned for the individual patient with an idealized goal in mind.

Breast aesthetics are based on two senses: the visual and the tactile. A woman's breasts must not only look good, but they must be sensitive and feel normal. Softness, warmth, smoothness, mobility on the chest wall, and sensitivity to touch, particularly in the central breast and nipple-areolar region, are all important aspects of the normal breast. Observable visual aesthetic characteristics of symmetry, flow, contour, and proportion combine with the sensual to produce attractive breasts.

BREAST SHAPE

STAGES IN BREAST DEVELOPMENT

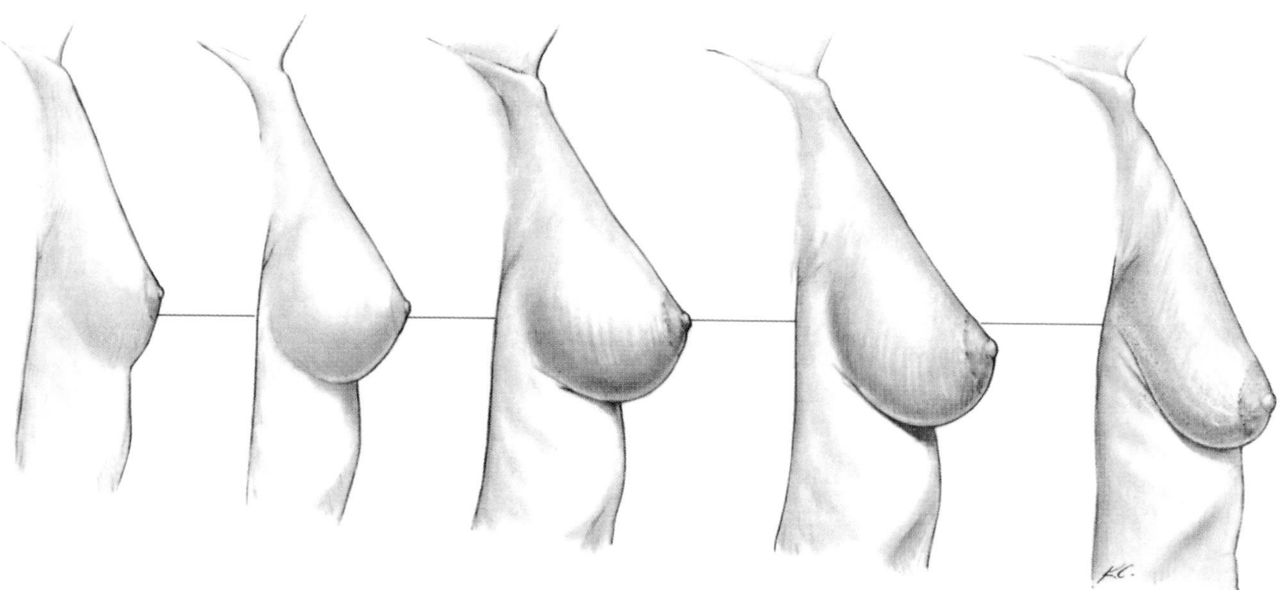

Breast development is usually complete when the young woman attains her final height, somewhere between the ages of 13 and 16 years. Normal aesthetic development leads to fully rounded, hemispherical, symmetric pubertal breasts. At that time, reflecting the influences of individual genetic, hormonal, gravitational, and postural changes, the upper portion of the breast usually becomes less convex, appearing flattened as the breast parenchyma settles, and the lower portion of the breast becomes fuller. The breasts gradually assume a more mature look by settling downward and laterally with relatively more tissue retained in the lower outer quadrant of the mature breast. This general direction of change in form continues with the aging process as the breasts develop additional glandular ptosis that is reflected in a general settling of the breast and an upper pole breast flattening with stretching and descent of the gland and nipple-areola.

After the breasts have fully developed, their shape is influenced by the quality and elasticity of breast skin, the volume and position of breast parenchyma, the changes associated with aging, and the quality of musculofascial support. A number of life factors contribute to variations in what we consider "normal" breast shape. For example, women with thin, inelastic skin or women who have lost breast parenchyma volume are prone to striae and may lose breast skin support, thereby developing early ptosis, especially if the musculofascial attachments (Cooper's ligaments) also become attenuated and inelastic.

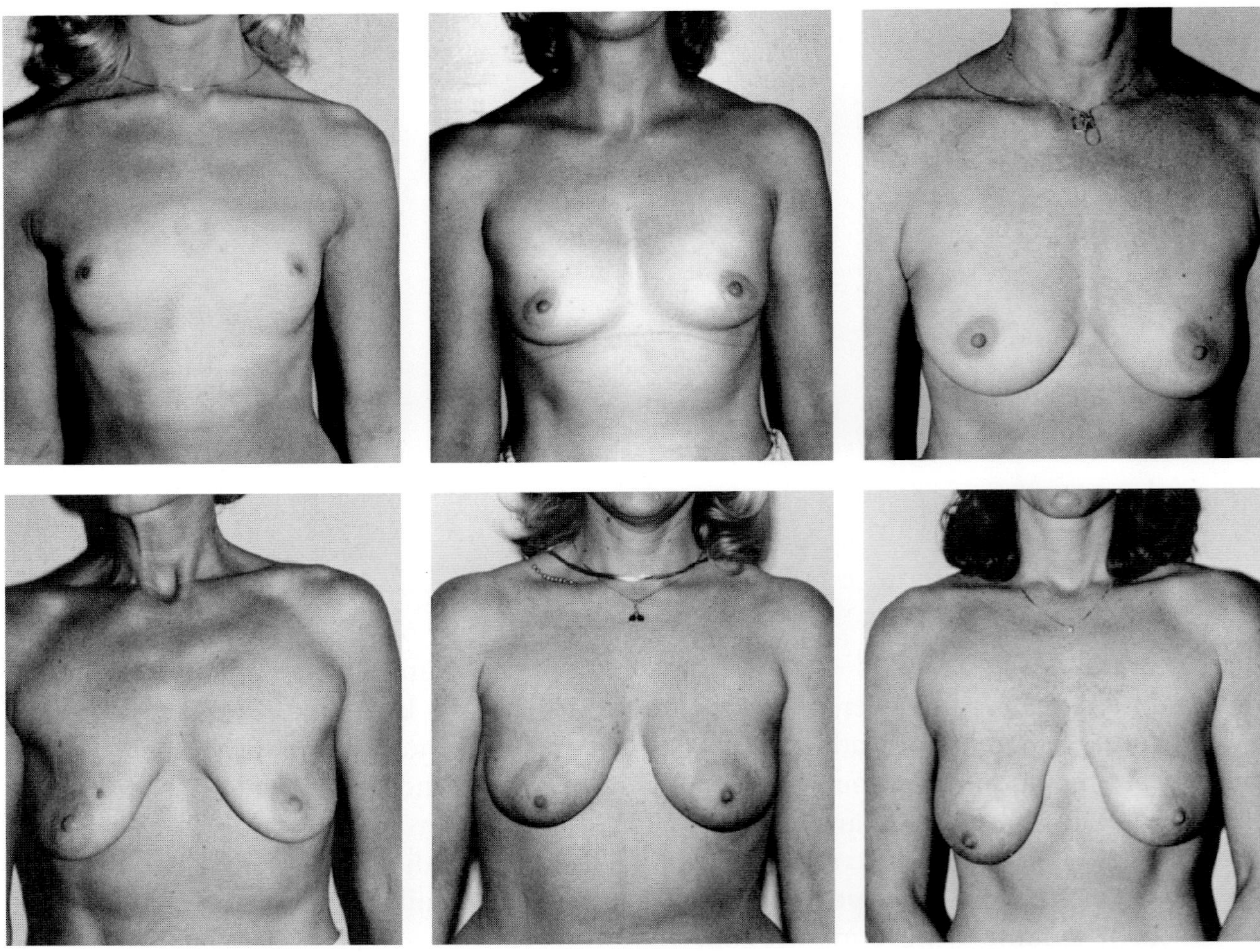

Cyclic breast volume changes may produce stretching, which can lead to a premature aged appearance. Pregnancy and lactation expand both the parenchyma and the overlying breast skin and stress the musculofascial ligaments. The skin's expandability, resiliency, and elasticity may also be affected by varying degrees of tightening when these cycles are completed and by the effect of high hormonal levels that weaken the fascial support and allow it to stretch. Fluctuations in weight (affecting body and breast parenchyma fat content) also change breast volume as well as the ratio of volume to skin and deeper fascial support and can therefore lead to changes in the normal "ideal" breast shape. ***As breast size increases, the nipple-areolar position progressively moves inferiorly and laterally.***

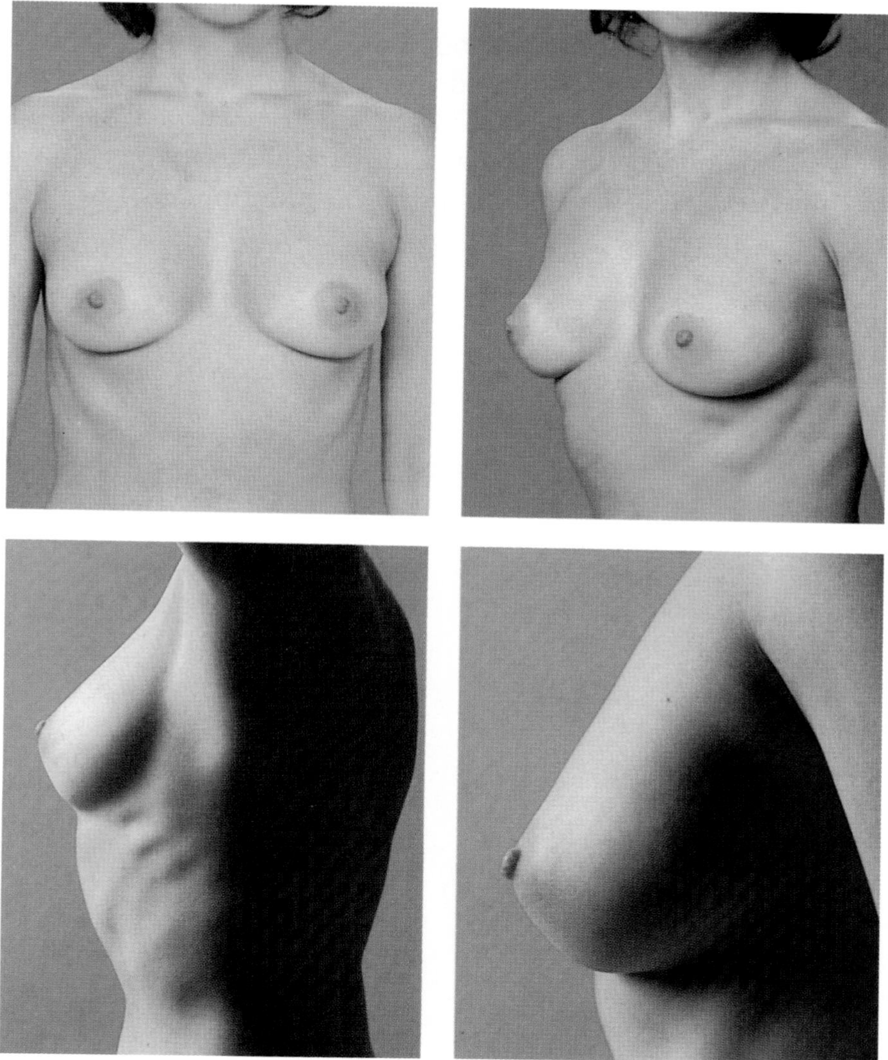

The breast surgeon needs to have an ideal model to work from in analyzing each patient, fully recognizing normal breast variations. This ideal breast shape exhibits elastic skin cover and support, strong, deep fascial attachments, and a breast volume in the range of normal, generally between 300 and 500 gm. An understanding of breast proportions is essential. On frontal view the breast is less full above the areola in the upper pole and fuller below, especially lateral to the areola in the lower pole. The breast is located over the anterior lateral chest with a lateral inclination of 45 degrees. Breast volume and contour are in harmony with the proportions of the chest, torso, and buttocks. Laterally, ideal breast appearance would again reflect good cutaneous and fascial support with the breast parenchyma positioned above the inframammary crease, a subtle fullness above the areola, and a roundness and convexity below.

NIPPLE-AREOLAR POSITION AND APPEARANCE

Lines of contour all flow to the nipple-areola, the focal point of the breast. Nipple-areolar position, size, color, texture, inclination, and symmetry are related to and define breast form and function. Reference points for determining nipple-areolar location extend from the sternal notch and midline to the umbilicus, the midclavicular point and the midbreast line, and from the midbreast line to the midclavicular point to the anterior superior iliac spine.

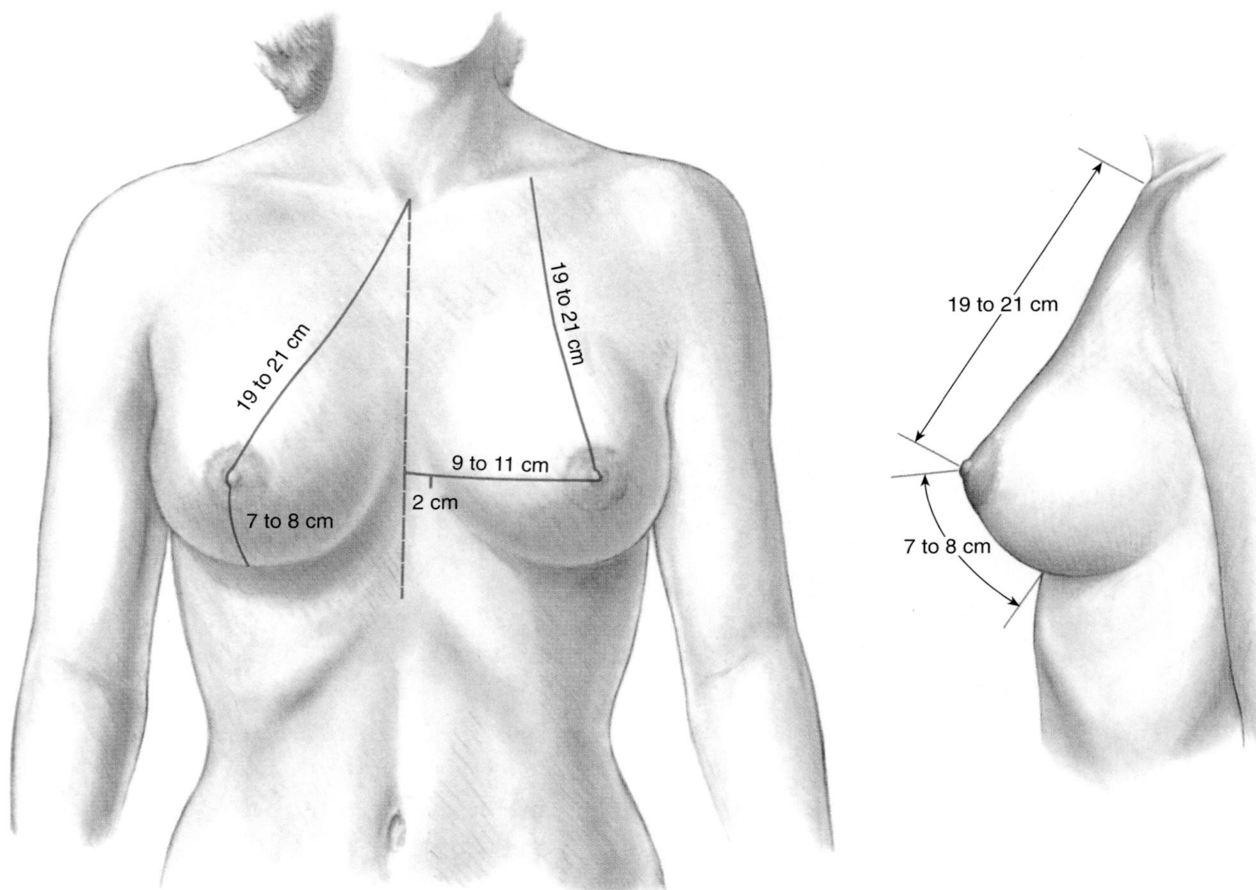

The nipple is situated on the midbreast line approximately 19 to 21 cm from the midpoint of the clavicle. This breast line begins at the midclavicular point and continues through the nipple to the inframammary crease. A horizontal line at the level of the nipple further defines the upper and lower breast quadrants. When a person is upright, approximately two thirds of the breast volume is below this transverse line and one third above it.

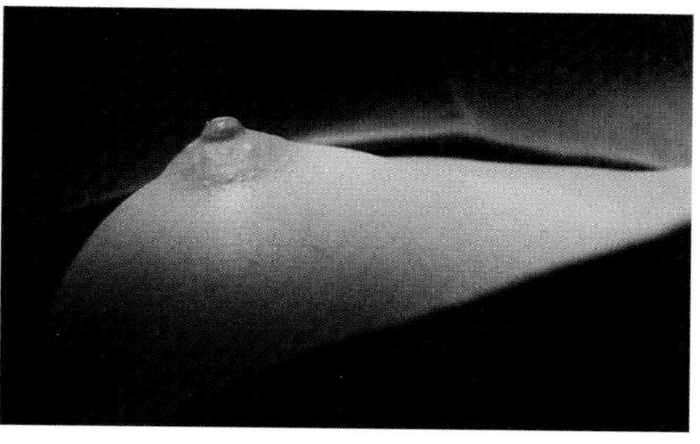

The nipple has a normal 10% to 15% medial and slight upward inclination, and it is usually situated 9 to 11 cm from the midsternal line and approximately 13 cm from the midaxillary line, usually the lateral extent of the breast. The distance from the nipple to the inframammary fold is 7 to 8 cm, depending on breast size, volume, maturation, and degree of ptosis. The vertical measurement over the breast from the clavicle to the inframammary crease is 26 to 29 cm; the lateral width is approximately 18 to 22 cm from midline to lateral breast line; and the breast base, providing coverage of the underlying musculofascial layer, is 11 to 14 cm. An areolar diameter of 35 to 45 mm is usually judged attractive, as is a nipple diameter of 5 to 8 mm and a nipple projection of approximately 4 to 6 mm.

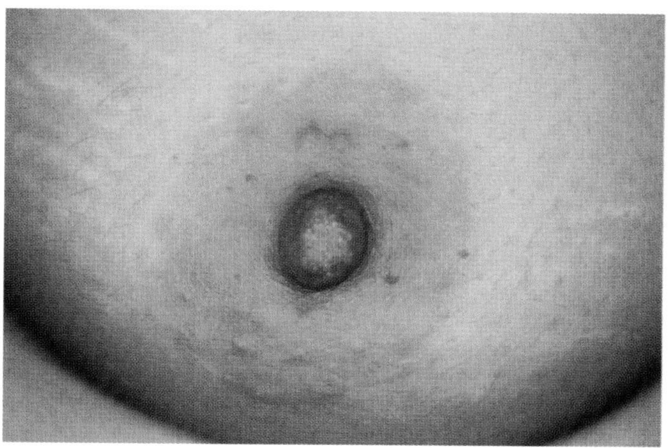

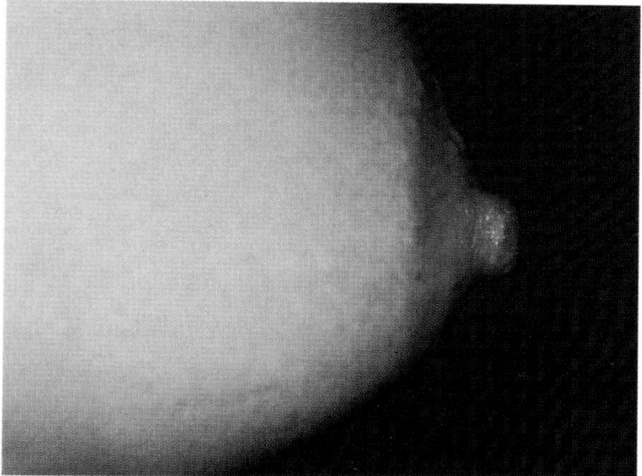

The areola projects from the breast mound. The areolar diameter in relation to the overall breast size varies; it can become stretched disproportionately from mammary hypertrophy. Areolar diameter is a consideration in planning a reduction mammaplasty; many patients have a preference for areolar diameter and this should be elicited during preoperative planning. With a tight skin envelope and a medially and laterally constricted breast, associated with less support centrally because of the thin dermis of the areola, central protrusion of breast parenchyma can produce a tubular breast deformity. The nipple protrudes centrally from the areola; its projection increases when it is erect. Large areolae containing a significant portion of breast parenchyma are commonly seen in patients with tubular breasts.

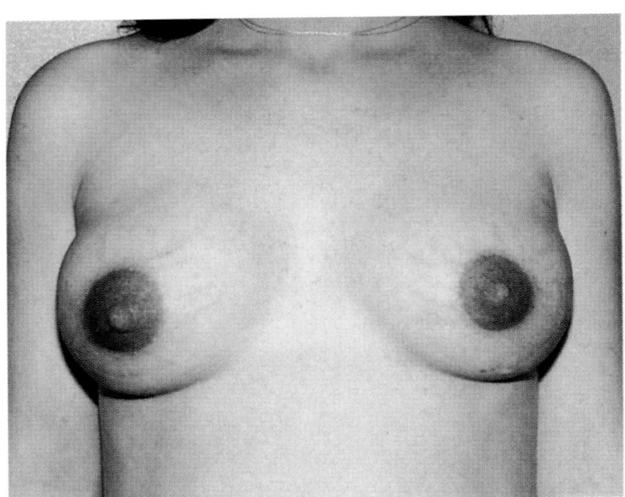

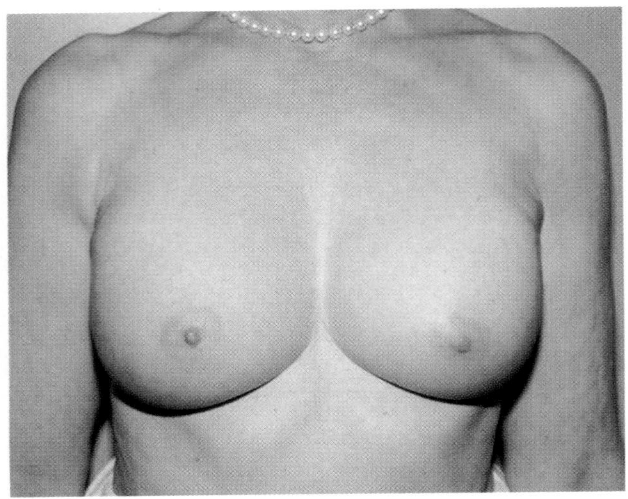

The areola has distinct coloration and skin textures that are subject to hormonal and genetic influences as well as the natural changes associated with aging. Characteristically the areolar pigmentation is darker than that of the surrounding skin. Nulliparous women have a light brown or even pinkish areola. The color usually darkens with hormonal and solar exposure as well as during pregnancy and after delivery and usually lightens several months after lactation but not to its original shade. It has a firm texture with a corrugated surface produced by the muscles and Montgomery's glands within. Areolar pigmentation often decreases after menopause and the natural withdrawal of estrogen and progesterone. The nipple is frequently more deeply pigmented than the areola.

BREAST FLOW

The breasts are an aesthetic mixture of soft curves and flowing lines. Situated on the chest wall in an anterolateral position, the breasts flow gently from the clavicles onto the chest wall, over the upper abdomen, and from the axilla—key anatomic juncture points. From above, the breasts flow from the clavicle and contribute fullness along with that supplied by the axillary fold, which consists of the pectoralis major muscle and tendon, axillary breast tissue, and subcutaneous tissue. Flow continues from the clavicle downward to the breasts and projects forward to the nipple-areolae, which are inclined slightly upward and outward. As breast size increases, this nipple-areolar position progressively moves inferiorly and laterally.

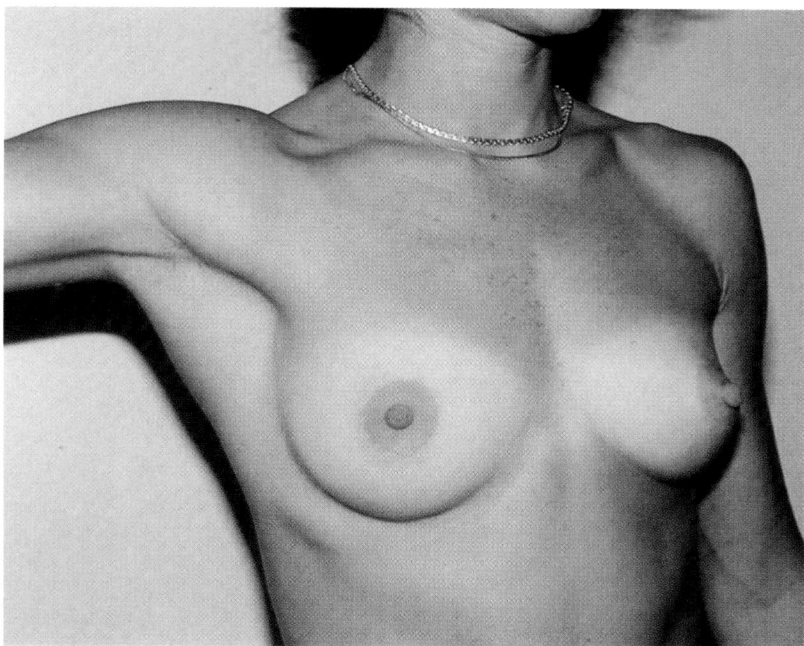

Below the areola, breast fullness and convexity increase, and then the breast curves downward to a slightly concave inframammary juncture with the upper abdomen at the inframammary line or fold. This breast-abdomen juncture, the inframammary crease, begins medially near the sternal midline and curves gently downward to the midbreast line; it then curves upward slightly and diffuses near the anterior axillary line at the lateral breast border and the lateral chest and may be continuous with the lateral breast line. ***A more lateral takeoff of the inframammary crease is a forme fruste of constricted breasts.*** The ideal breast profile has a smooth breast projection in balance with posterior buttock projection. The breast profile from the clavicle to the second and third ribs is practically vertical with a subtle suggestion of fullness. In thinner women there is a distinct lateral breast crease near the anterior axillary line, which is lost when increased body fat fills this area and creates lateral chest fullness.

Breast projection begins at the level of the second and third ribs, flowing downward and outward to the nipple located at the level of the fourth and fifth rib interspaces. The areola projects slightly from the surrounding breast tissue, and the nipple projects centrally and more prominently. The nipple is above the level of the inframammary crease, which is usually located at the sixth and seventh rib interspace; breast flow downward to this crease is slightly convex. Age, gravity, breast volume, and decreased elasticity contribute to a gradual lowering of the breast landmarks relative to the underlying musculoskeletal system over time as a woman gets older and experiences normal physiologic changes. The extent of this descent depends primarily on the volume of the breast and the elasticity of the tissues.

BREAST CLEAVAGE

As the breasts enlarge, fullness usually develops inferiorly and laterally. With increased volume, the influence of gravity, and the development of ptosis, the breasts appear to diverge and fall away from the midline laterally and inferiorly. Additionally, when a woman is supine, the breasts flow laterally, sometimes even beyond the actual chest wall.

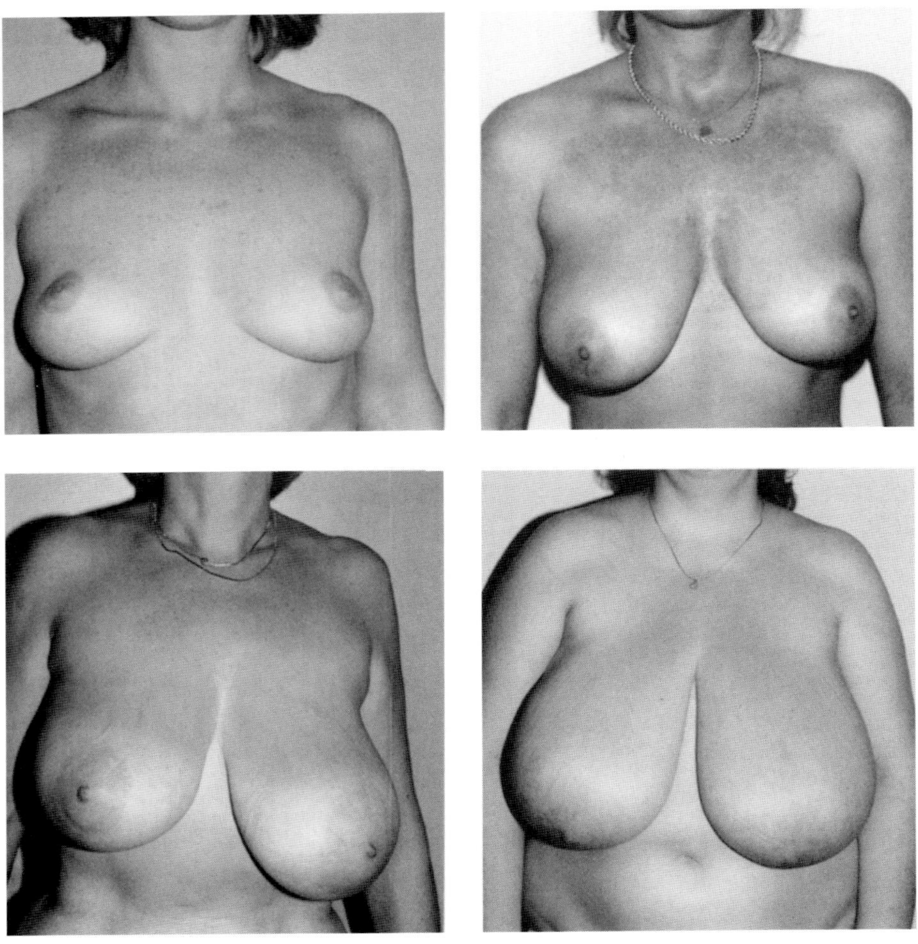

Cleavage is an aesthetic goal for many women seeking breast surgery; they desire the appearance of a full cleavage that will be evident in low-cut clothing or bathing suits. Many women do not understand that this type of cleavage does not usually exist naturally unaided by artificial devices such as underwire, push-up, or "Wonder" bras. This is even true for women naturally endowed with an abundance of upper breast tissue. Most photographs of women with full cleavage are taken while their breasts are artificially pushed upward and medially with brassieres or other supports. Women who desire a full cleavage without these supports are often disappointed with aesthetic and reconstructive breast operations unless it is pointed out that this cleavage is the product of substantial support combined with medial breast flow. Breast implants may be used to provide upper breast fullness; however, these are not always a natural-appearing solution, particularly in cases where the normal breasts flow over these devices.

SYMMETRY

Symmetry is key to aesthetic breast appearance. Ideally, breasts should be comparable in size, shape, and degree of ptosis. Most individuals feel that their bodies are not "right" unless they are balanced and symmetric.

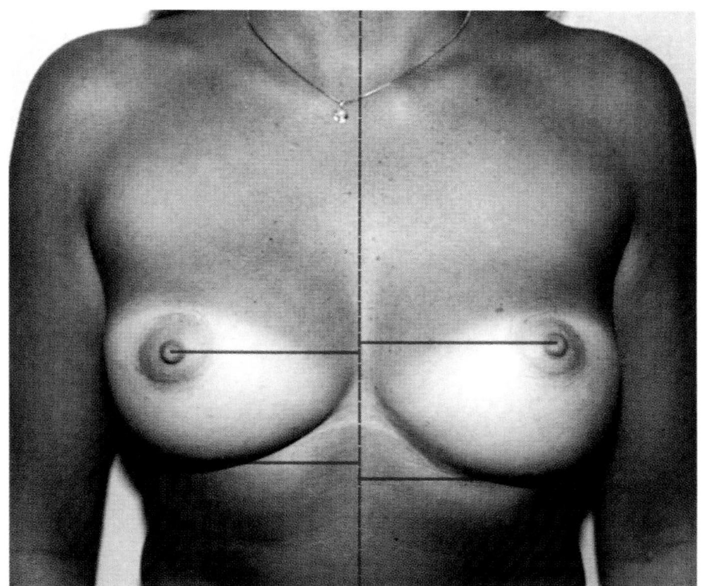

Perfect symmetry, however, rarely if ever exists in nature and is even more of a rarity after breast surgery. It is normal for some asymmetry to be evident in paired body structures, and the breasts are most likely to be naturally asymmetric. In fact, it is the unusual woman who does not demonstrate some breast, nipple-areolar, or chest wall asymmetry. For example, one side of the trunk is usually larger than the other. Additional disparities may be seen in muscle development or in the underlying skeleton in the costal region, particularly when there is scoliosis or other curvature of the spine. These natural asymmetries should be pointed out to the patient, discussed, documented during the preoperative evaluation, and included in the development of the treatment plan. Even when a woman's breasts appear symmetric at some point in time, longitudinal healing and aging will accentuate any minor asymmetries that are present.

BREAST PTOSIS

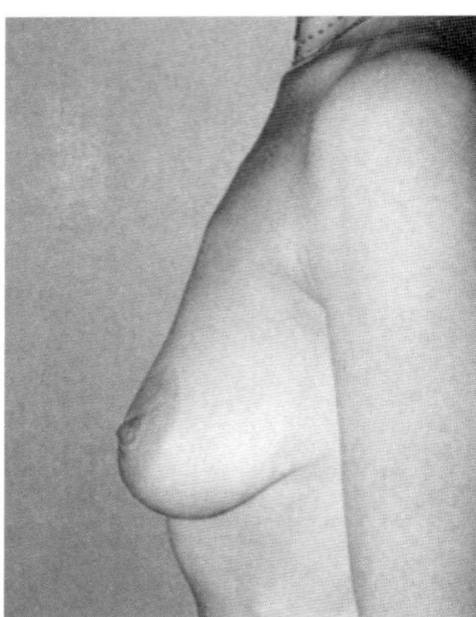
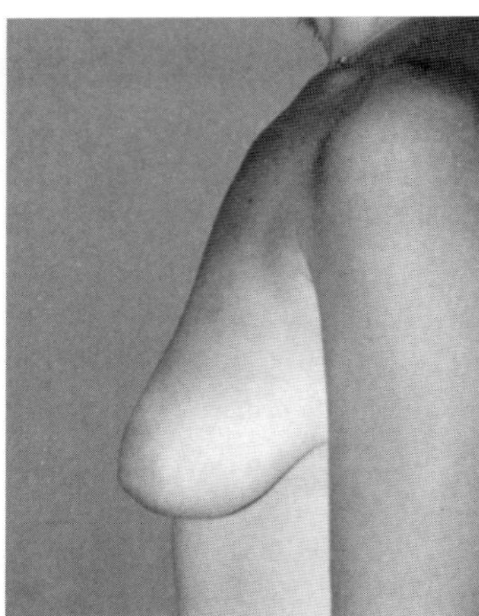

Some breast ptosis is a normal, desirable component of the mature breast since it contributes to natural contour, mobility, and definition. The nipple position relative to the breast parenchyma also affects the aesthetics of breast ptosis. Ptosis becomes undesirable when the nipple points downward and the breast parenchyma predominates below the areola and droops on lateral view considerably beneath the inframammary crease. This degree of ptosis gives the breasts an aged appearance. Most women accept the increased lower breast fullness but object to the upper breast flatness and desire a visible nipple position. Providing additional upper fill with breast implants or with a pedicle flap of lower breast parenchyma is a consideration for these patients.

Applying Breast Aesthetics to Surgery

Surgical modifications and postoperative breast appearance are evaluated based on the surgeon's and patient's aesthetic standards. Are the breasts symmetric? Are the size and proportions correct? Are the breasts softly contoured with appropriate flow and definition? Are the incisions and scars hidden? Is breast appearance natural? Is the patient satisfied? Are her expectations met? There is nothing more frustrating than a result hailed by the surgeon as an aesthetic triumph that the patient views as a failure. That is why it is so important for the surgeon to understand patient expectations and to attempt to incorporate them as much as possible into the operative plan.

What happens when the general body proportions are not ideal, when the surgeon is faced with a patient who is shorter, heavier, or thinner than the mean? How do you modify your approach, adapt aesthetic standards to individual patients, and produce attractive, symmetric breasts proportionate to the patient's body type and compatible with her aesthetic ideals?

ADJUSTMENTS FOR DIFFERENT BODY TYPES

Breast shape and size should be proportional to individual body type. Body proportions and body fat content will vary, however, and those variations require alterations in the surgical planning process. To explore the possibilities for surgical modification, let us consider five different body types.

SLENDER, ANGULAR BODIES

Tall, thin women with a low percentage of body fat present a surgical challenge. Frequently any asymmetries are accentuated by smaller breasts that lack the layer of subcutaneous fat necessary to "soften" underlying irregularities. Usually structures of the breast and adjacent areas are more sharply defined in these slender patients, and even the slightest breast irregularity or change in symmetry or appearance is more noticeable. The thin skin is often elastic and not attenuated by underlying volumetric expansion. Such skin tends to retract when incised, is expanded with difficulty, and may heal with widened scars, with the younger, thicker dermis stimulating wound healing and scar proliferation and hypertrophy. Accordingly, procedures using hidden or minimal scars are preferred. These patients often lack lower breast overhang at the inframammary crease and have minimal breast projection; therefore there is little potential for hiding scars either in the periareolar region or in the inframammary region. The axilla is often an acceptable area for placing incisions in these women. ***The axillary skin usually heals better than other areas and with less hypertrophy.***

Aesthetic Procedures

A slender, angular body contour is most often seen in young nulliparous patients. In breast augmentation for women with this body type who are 5 feet to 5 feet 8 inches in height and weigh 100 to 120 pounds and who have a chest circumference of 32 to 35 inches, I usually find that implants ranging in size from 200 to 300 cc with a diameter of 11 to 13 cm provide attractive breasts in proportion to their bodies. Because their breast parenchyma and subcutaneous tissue are so thin, any capsular contracture or implant irregularity is visible and palpable in the upper and lower poles of the breast. Therefore I prefer to place the breast implants beneath the pectoralis major muscle to minimize the chance of seeing or feeling the implant, which may produce a rippled appearance. I also prefer the axillary incision because it often heals better without leaving conspicuous breast scars, which pose possible problems such as scar hypertrophy. Since these women may be athletic and have strong pectoralis major muscles, additional softening and expansion are obtained by releasing the lower and medial pectoral muscle origins and by dividing the medial pectoral nerve fibers to provide selective lateral pectoral muscle denervation, thereby reducing lateral tightness and muscle contractions over the breast implant.

Patients with this body configuration must have realistic expectations as to what breast surgery can achieve. Their narrow chests and thin bodies limit the diameter and therefore the size of the breast implants that can be placed during breast augmentation. Breast implants are selected according to the base dimensions of the breast as well as chest wall circumference. Relatively large implants will extend the breasts too far laterally beneath the arms and create an unnatural upper fullness. When the implants remain soft, they can create the appearance of glandular ptosis.

When these women have breast reductions, which is unusual, their narrow chests and full breasts are prone to scars that can extend beyond the newly shaped and reduced breasts. The newer, short scar reduction techniques are particularly useful in these patients.

Augmentation: Case Example

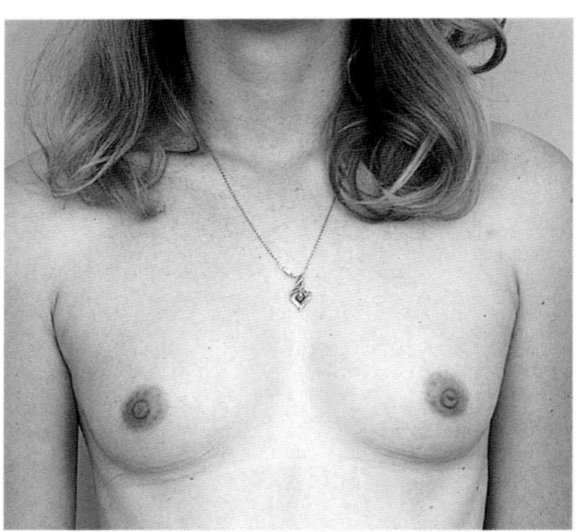

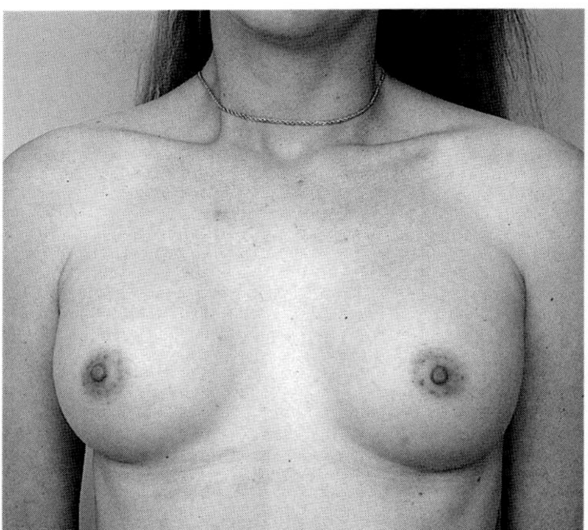

This 5-foot 5-inch athletic, weight-conscious patient weighs 110 pounds. She has a relatively narrow chest circumference of 34 inches. She was dissatisfied with her breast size and desired a breast augmentation without visible breast scars. Her chest width and proportions limited the size of breast implant that could be used to 275 cc. She had an endoscopically assisted subpectoral axillary breast augmentation with 275 cc smooth-surface saline implants that were inflated to 300 cc. She is shown 1 year postoperatively. Her augmented breasts exhibit a general fullness compared to their preoperative appearance, but they also look too firm and exhibit no ptosis. This type of result is frequently seen in patients of this body type who have limited, rather tight skin.

Reconstructive Procedures

Unilateral reconstructive implants are often not satisfactory for individuals with a slender, angular body type because they frequently have opposite breasts that are small, flattened, and difficult to match. In these cases it is often useful to place bilateral implants to give better and more lasting upper breast symmetry.

Following mastectomy, these women often have tight skin and little tissue to recruit laterally or from the thin upper abdomen. They are, however, excellent candidates for tissue expansion. If autologous tissue is needed for these thin patients, the gluteus maximus musculocutaneous flap is often the best donor source because these individuals tend to have minimal excess tissue available in the lower abdomen. Rarely is the latissimus dorsi flap or the TRAM flap useful for these women because the donor tissue volume is limited and the scars are not easily hidden.

Modified Tissue Expansion: Case Example

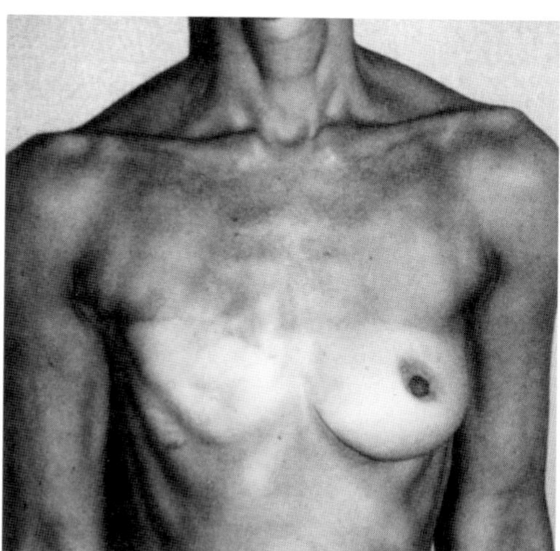

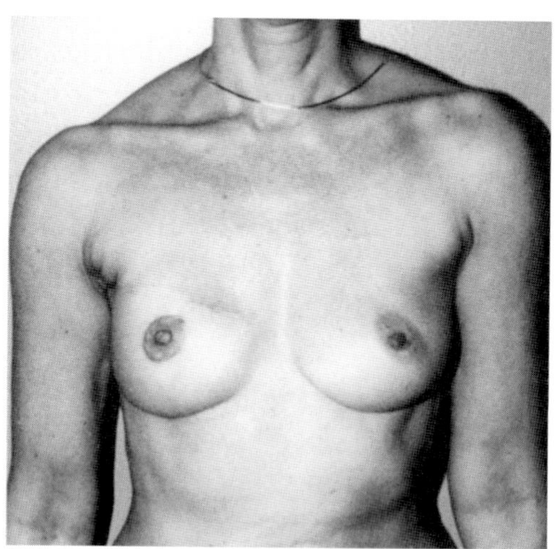

This 48-year-old woman is 5 feet 6 inches tall and weighs 120 pounds. Her left breast was atrophic and she had recently undergone a modified radical mastectomy on the right side for stage I breast carcinoma. A satisfactory breast reconstruction was accomplished with a 190 cc implant after modified tissue expansion to match her opposite breast. The implant was placed through the previous incision to avoid additional scars.

SOLID, COMPACT BODIES

Some women have bodies that are fuller and more compact with greater amounts of body fat. Body lines are rounder, and if breasts are to be proportional, they must be rounder with a suggestion of fullness below. For women 5 feet to 5 feet 6 inches tall and weighing 110 to 150 pounds, a breast volume of 300 to 600 cc produces attractive, proportional breasts for their bodies.

Aesthetic Procedures

Aesthetic procedures for women with this configuration are somewhat more forgiving. Women with this body type frequently desire breast reduction. The scars can be better hidden by the inframammary fold and by their somewhat wider chest and fuller breasts. The additional tissue also provides more coverage for breast implants, thereby ensuring a softer result.

When planning breast augmentation, I always keep in mind the percentage of augmentation in addition to the amount of increased projection. Fuller breasts initially require larger, wider implants to produce the same relative improvement as that produced in a more slender, angular woman with smaller breasts. A 300 cc implant produces a remarkable change in a 100 cc breast, increasing its size by a factor of 3; however, it only doubles the size of a 300 cc breast. These women have better defined inframammary folds, and a scar in this position is better concealed. The more abundant subcutaneous tissue softens the appearance of underlying capsular contractures or implant texture, ripples, and irregularities. Such women have fuller abdomens and buttocks and frequently desire proportionately fuller breasts. They should be advised, however, that larger breasts will tend to make them look heavier and that large, wide implants may produce inappropriate fullness laterally. These patients occasionally request standard liposuction or ultrasound-assisted liposuction of their torso and thighs to improve their overall appearance and body contour.

Augmentation: Case Example

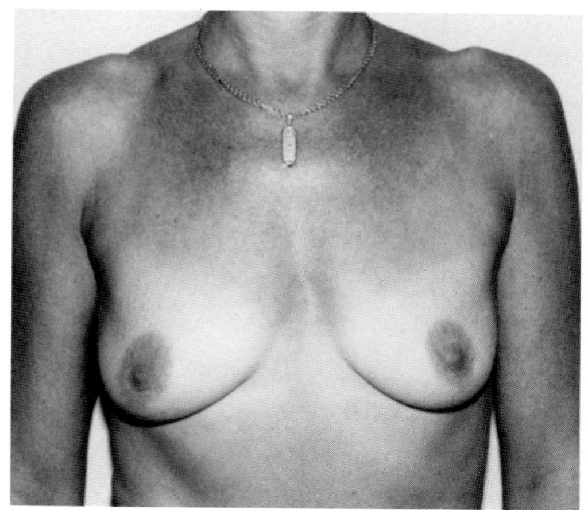

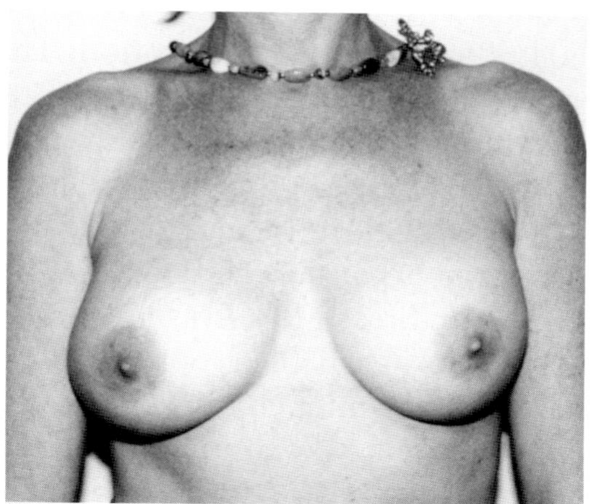

This 5-foot 4-inch patient who weighs 140 pounds requested larger breasts. Because of her thicker subcutaneous layer and more compact body, implants of 380 cc were placed using an inframammary approach. The inframammary scars are nicely hidden in the shadows beneath the patient's fuller breasts.

Reduction: Case Example

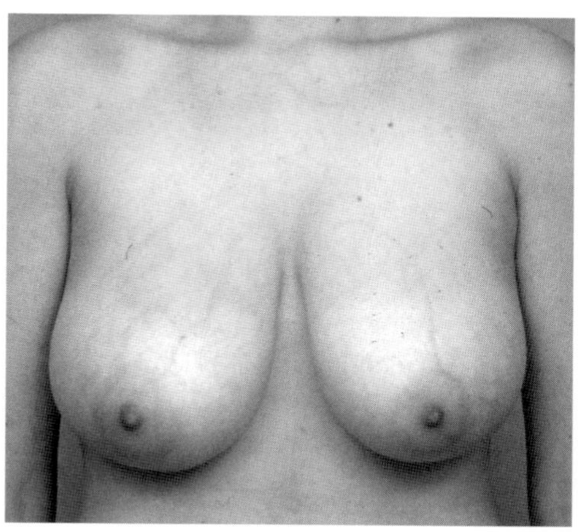

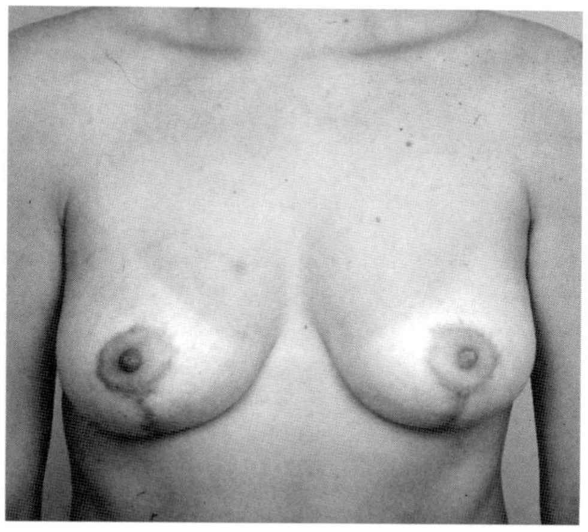

This young woman complained about her large breasts and the back and shoulder pain and breast irritation that they caused. She was only 5 feet 2 inches tall but weighed 140 pounds. She requested breast reduction to relieve these symptoms. A vertical approach was chosen after liposuction was done to reduce the breast centrally and laterally followed by resection in the central lower breast region. With this approach, her scars were limited to the periareolar area with a vertical extension that was less visible in the lower portion of her breast. She is shown before the operation and 1 year later.

Reconstructive Procedures

Women with solid, compact bodies are more frequently encountered as candidates for breast reconstruction. They tend to be older with more mature bodies that have accumulated additional body fat over time. Usually they have more lower abdominal tissue available, which makes them better candidates for a TRAM flap than their more slender counterparts. They also frequently have a larger, more ptotic opposite breast, decreasing the likelihood that tissue expansion and breast implants alone will be sufficient to create a symmetric breast. Realistically, these women will require more extensive interventions when their opposite breasts are full or ptotic. Augmentation, mastopexy-augmentation, or even reduction may be needed for the opposite breast, especially with implant breast reconstruction. Sometimes an upper abdominal flap or even a latissimus dorsi flap placed low on the reconstructed breast can be useful to gain increased ptosis and lower breast fullness. Additional donor scars on the lower abdomen or back and corrective scars on the reconstructed breast and the opposite breast accompany these procedures, but since there is often abundant tissue available for transfer, these donor sites are not as tight and are more easily concealed.

Tissue Expansion: Case Example

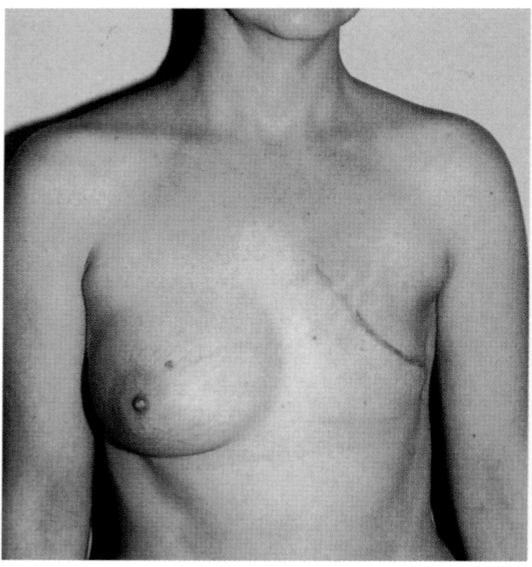

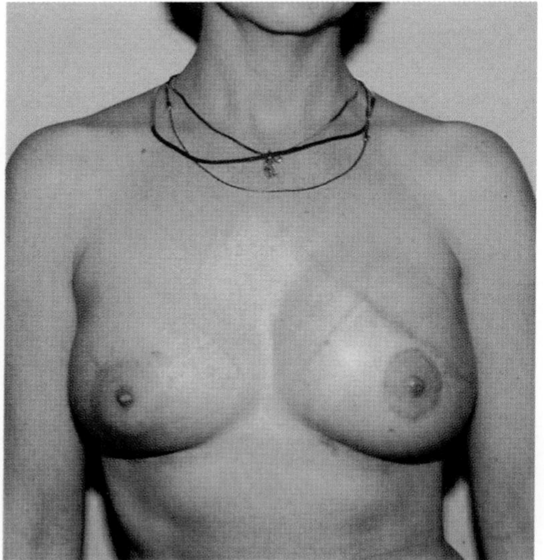

This patient is 5 feet 6 inches tall and weighs 148 pounds. She had a left modified radical mastectomy followed by adjunctive chemotherapy for 8 months prior to breast reconstruction. She desired a right breast augmentation. Her left breast was reconstructed with tissue expansion to match her augmented breast. The permanent tissue expander implant was positioned and inflated over a 2-month period. After overinflation it was deflated to approximate the size of her augmented right breast. At a second procedure the tissue expander was replaced with a permanent implant, and the nipple-areola was reconstructed. A nipple-areola tattoo was done 3 months after the second procedure. Breast augmentation permitted creation of a larger, fuller right breast that was more proportional to the patient's body type. It also made a symmetric breast reconstruction possible with tissue expansion, providing increased fullness in her upper breast region.

Immediate TRAM Flap After Skin-Sparing Mastectomy: Case Example

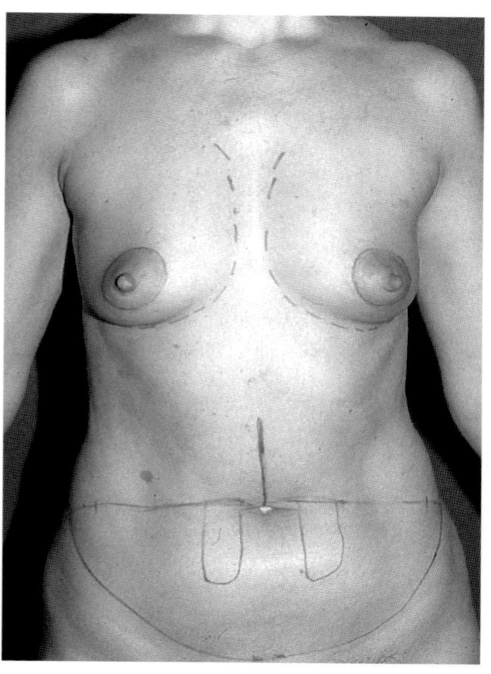

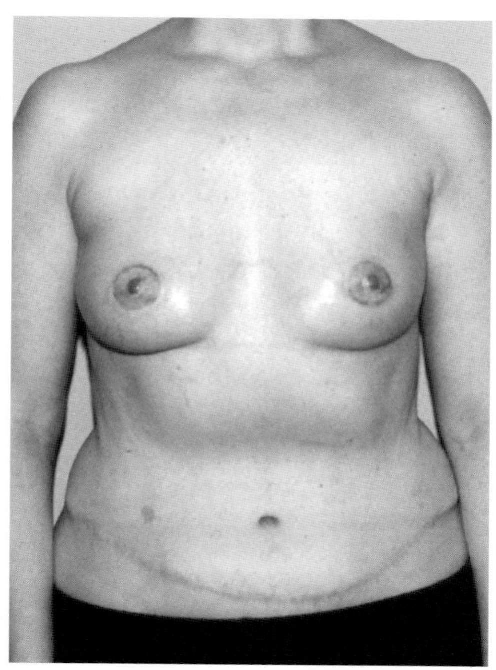

This 39-year-old woman had extensive bilateral ductal carcinoma in situ and was advised by her oncologist to have bilateral total mastectomy with skin-sparing incisions. She requested immediate breast reconstruction but did not want implants used, preferring an autologous tissue reconstruction with her lower abdominal tissue. Her areolae were large and the mastectomies and bilateral reconstructions were done through the areolar sites. The skin over the TRAM flap was used to replace the skin removed in the central breast region. The patient is shown 2 months following the nipple-areola reconstruction and areolar tattoo. The nipple reconstruction was done with local C-V flaps.

OVERWEIGHT, ROUNDED BODIES

In women who have a high percentage of body fat and pronounced body roundness accentuated by a full abdomen, wide chest, and excess weight, the breasts have less projection and require more tissue volume to exhibit an acceptable feminine shape. It is more difficult to attain significant aesthetic improvement in these patients because of their excess adipose tissue. To obtain an attractive breast contour with sufficient projection for patients desiring breast enlargement, greater breast volume with larger, wider implants is required. In heavier patients who are 4 feet 10 inches to 5 feet 8 inches tall and weigh 120 to 180 pounds, breast volume should be at least 300 to 600 cc and sometimes more to produce an attractive proportional appearance in which the breast base dimensions are in balance with the chest wall circumference.

Aesthetic Procedures

During augmentation mammaplasty, because of the relatively larger distance between the clavicles and abdomen, larger broad-based implants are often chosen to produce an acceptable increase in breast size in women with overweight, rounded bodies. These implants also tend to fill out the chest area, thereby accentuating the overall impression of being overweight.

Breast reductions in these individuals can effectively lift and remove breast tissue from a relatively protruding abdomen. The woman who has not considered the result of this reduction on her body proportions may believe that her abdomen has grown. The overall appearance of these women can be improved with abdominal contouring. Liposuction or abdominoplasty can provide the needed overall improvement in appearance and may be indicated when the newly reduced breasts no longer conceal the true abdominal appearance.

These patients also tend to have fullness laterally, making their breasts actually blend into the thicker tissues of the lateral chest wall. Lateral folds often extend to the back as well. For breast reduction, areas of lateral fullness should be addressed directly through a lateral extension of the lower inframammary fold incision or via a separate axillary approach. Other strategies for reducing the lateral upper chest are liposuction and direct open excision at the time of breast reduction. Liposuction of the lateral area is usually done to shorten the horizontal scar and to define the lateral breast crease. I tell the patient that she may eventually want to have her back suctioned for further contouring.

Frequently these patients also have excess tissue in the axillary breast area. These areas can be excised in combination with axillary augmentation. If not treated, these areas will appear proportionally larger after breast reduction. I generally use liposuction or ultrasound-assisted liposuction to reduce the volume in these areas.

Reduction: Case Example

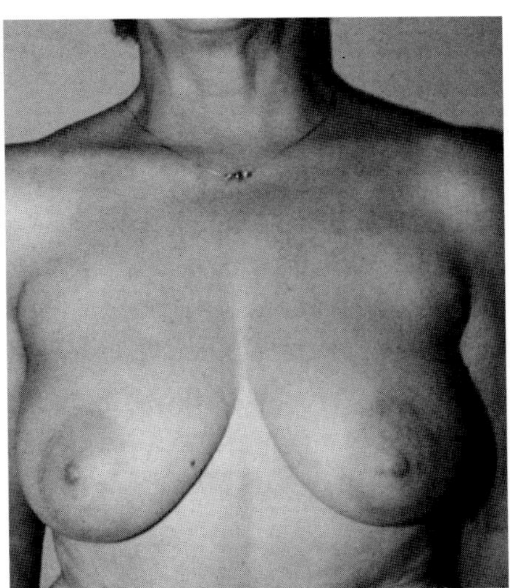

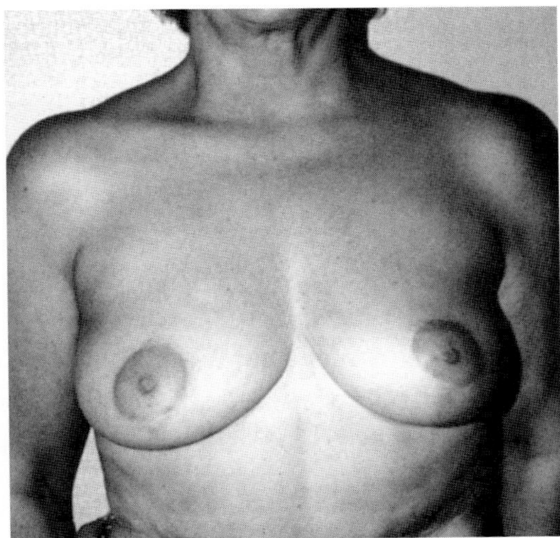

This 52-year-old woman's heavy breasts precipitated her request for breast reduction. She is 5 feet 6 inches tall and weighs 155 pounds. Her abdominal wall protruded following a weight gain after two pregnancies. A superior pedicle technique was selected to remove 400 gm from each side. She is shown 2 years following the breast reduction.

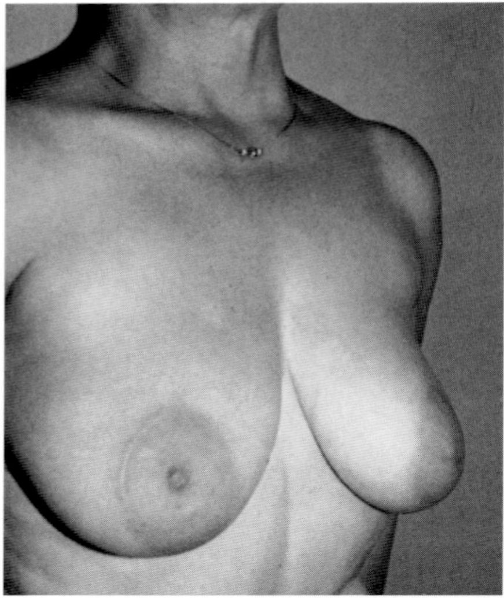 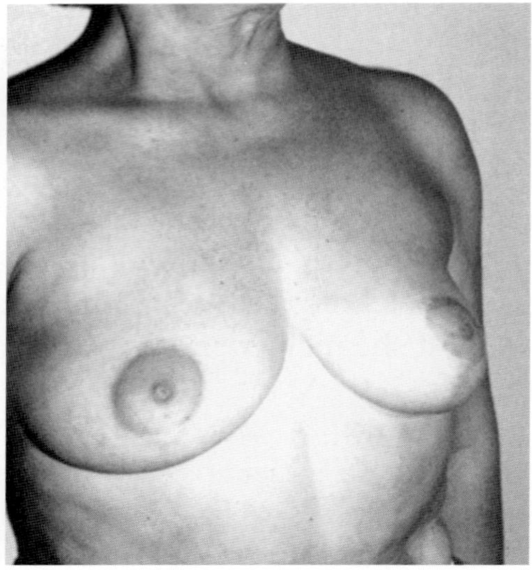

Note that her upper abdomen has become more prominent following surgery. This upper abdominal prominence could have been reduced with liposuction at the time of the initial reduction mammaplasty or even liposuction of the entire abdominal wall.

Reconstructive Procedures

Reconstructive procedures in patients with overweight, rounded bodies are often complex and challenging. Excess soft tissue deficits often require replacement with autologous tissue, usually a TRAM flap. Frequently a tissue deficit exists beneath the clavicle as a result of removing the fatty upper breast tissue during mastectomy. Often an implant alone or an implant subsequent to expansion does not fill this upper breast area. A latissimus dorsi muscle flap alone is only a temporizing method; it atrophies later. Adding a deepithelialized vascularized tissue flap with its overlying subcutaneous tissue from the back, abdomen, or buttocks is the best strategy for providing infraclavicular fill.

Women with this body configuration should have realistic expectations for reconstructive surgery. ***The amount of ptosis that implants and expanders can provide is limited.*** The TRAM flap is frequently used, but the abdominal wall donor site remaining after removal of the lower abdominal tissue is compacted and shortened. Thus a vertically shorter abdomen will result in increased girth. These subtle changes after the TRAM flap can accentuate the woman's overweight appearance.

TRAM Flap: Case Example

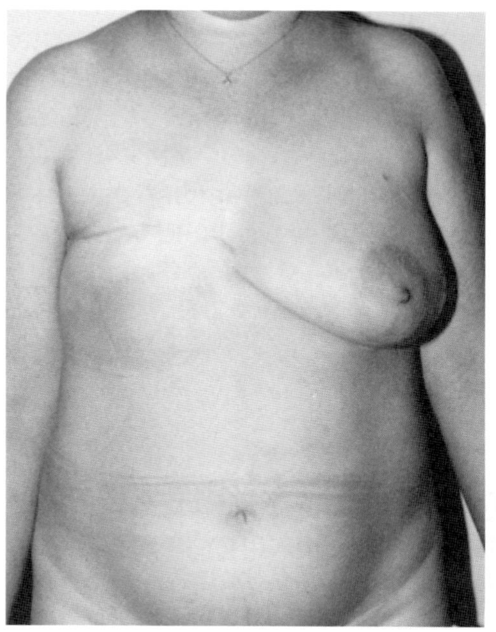

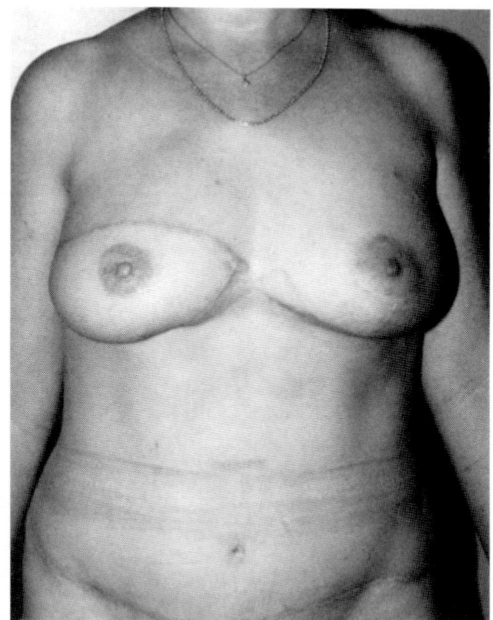

This 45-year-old woman is 5 feet 6 inches tall and weighs 152 pounds. She had a right modified radical mastectomy, a heavy, mildly ptotic left breast, and excess lower abdominal tissue. A satisfactory breast reconstruction was accomplished with a right bipedicle TRAM flap. Her nipple-areola was reconstructed 3 months following breast reconstruction and her lower lateral abdomen was contoured with liposuction. The autologous tissue breast reconstruction and abdominoplasty associated with the TRAM flap contribute to breast symmetry and an overall improved appearance.

ANOREXIC BODIES
Aesthetic Procedures

The ultra-thin, anorexic patient (body fat level often below 10%) is not a candidate for aesthetic surgery. Her mental condition and body image misperceptions should be managed and improved with psychiatric therapy rather than with breast implants, reduction, or mastopexy. There are some women, however, who resemble anorexics in their slenderness but are generally in good health and do not exhibit some of the deviant dietary behavior and psychological problems associated with this eating disorder. These patients aspire to a thin, aesthetic ideal, and because they are ardent exercisers and dieters, they have a gaunt appearance similar to that of the anorexic. These women have a low body fat content but may be well adjusted. Augmentation or mastopexy-augmentation is reasonable for these patients with the same precautions as those described for the slender patient discussed earlier.

Reconstructive Procedures

Anorexia is seen less frequently in patients seeking breast reconstruction, particularly if these women have had chemotherapy to treat their cancer. Most women who have chemotherapy gain 15 to 20 pounds and are trying to get their weight down to their preoperative norm.

Again, the ultra-thin patient is similar to the slender, angular patient described earlier, only to an extreme degree. Textured implants with surface ripples or irregularities are likely to be noticeable and palpable in this woman because of the deficiency of subcutaneous tissue necessary to soften any irregularities, asymmetry, or capsular contracture.

OBESE BODIES

The obese patient (40% or greater weight than normal) often is dissatisfied after aesthetic and reconstructive breast surgery. Any procedure performed on these patients is more extensive and associated with more complications. The potential for healing, circulatory, and scarring problems is significantly increased. Even the best result is usually not acceptable. Caution should be exercised in accepting these high-risk individuals for aesthetic surgery. They often have high levels of expectation with correspondingly low levels of satisfaction. Even if their breasts can be improved, the overall appearance may still be unattractive.

Aesthetic Procedures

Breast augmentation is rarely requested by the obese patient. Because of the thick subcutaneous tissue of the abdomen and chest, an implant's projection, even the largest available (600 to 1000 cc), can literally become "lost" in the excess tissue, making an attractive augmented contour impossible.

Breast reduction in the obese woman, while seemingly indicated because of weight and associated inframammary skin-to-skin contact, is in fact often not gratifying. The excess volume often extends laterally, even onto the back, and requires not only breast reduction but lateral and posterior liposuction or excision to improve the contour. ***A reduction sufficient to alleviate the symptoms of heaviness often leaves the patient with a disproportionately large abdomen, poorly fitting clothes, and an overall less "feminine" appearance.*** Abdominoplasty or liposuction should not even be considered until there has been significant weight loss. I prefer that she lose enough weight so that she is within 30 pounds of the ideal normal weight for someone of her size and frame. When weight loss occurs after a reduction has been performed on an obese patient, additional breast volume loss can occur, even to the point of causing breast atrophy, which then requires implants for correction.

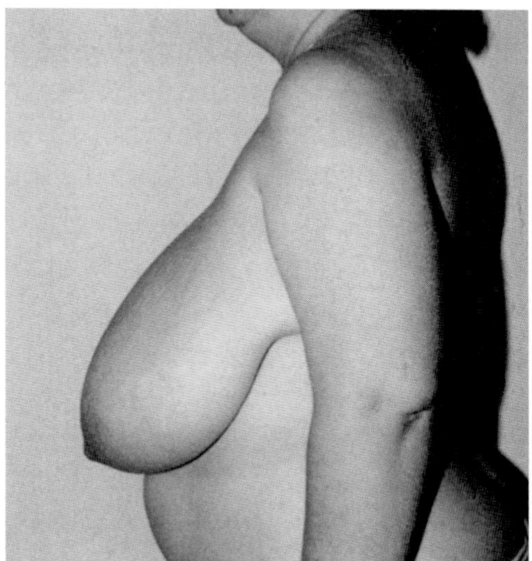
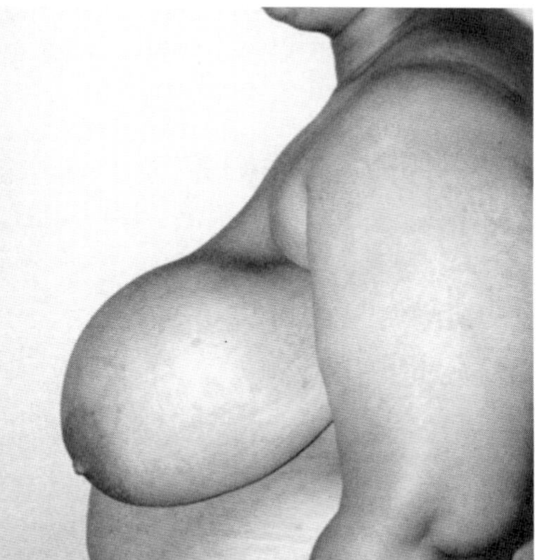

In my experience, it is generally a mistake to perform aesthetic breast surgery on the obese patient. Usually she has already tried many other strategies for losing weight and improving her appearance and is counting on aesthetic breast surgery to produce the magical transformation that dieting and willpower could not. This is simply not possible. Furthermore, operative risk is increased as is the possibility of systemic complications such as cardiac, pulmonary and deep vein thrombosis, and pulmonary embolus. If there is to be a chance of meeting patient expectations, obese patients should lose weight before having aesthetic breast surgery.

Reconstructive Procedures

Breast reconstruction in the obese woman is fraught with disappointments and complications. Breast implants and tissue expansion are often insufficient reconstructive tools because these women have extreme volume deficits with an associated loss of subcutaneous tissue. Flaps of autologous tissue from the abdomen are the most frequent source of tissue. ***TRAM flap reconstruction can be reliably performed in a premenopausal overweight nonsmoker if the tissue is taken just over the muscle in zone I and the flap is oriented to the midabdominal level.*** Tissue loss or fat necrosis is likely when the woman is a cigarette smoker or postmenopausal and obese. The presence of striae tends to increase the risk of TRAM flap vascular compromise.

Although I do not recommend aesthetic surgery for the obese patient, exceptions are sometimes made for the breast reconstruction patient. When an obese woman has a mastectomy, symmetry is lost and she feels unbalanced. Since obesity is also associated with breast cancer, these patients are at a high risk for developing breast cancer in the opposite breast. ***Implants are not good for breast reconstruction in the obese patient; autologous tissue is preferred.*** These patients usually have an abundance of lower abdominal tissue, and their overall appearance and torso proportions are improved by transferring the lower abdominal excess to the upper chest region. Since the TRAM flap can only be used one time, this is a factor when considering a prophylactic mastectomy with bilateral reconstruction.

TRAM Flap: Case Example

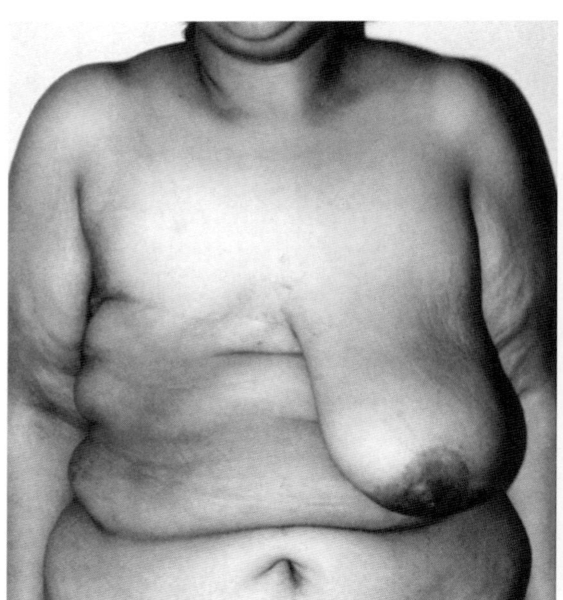

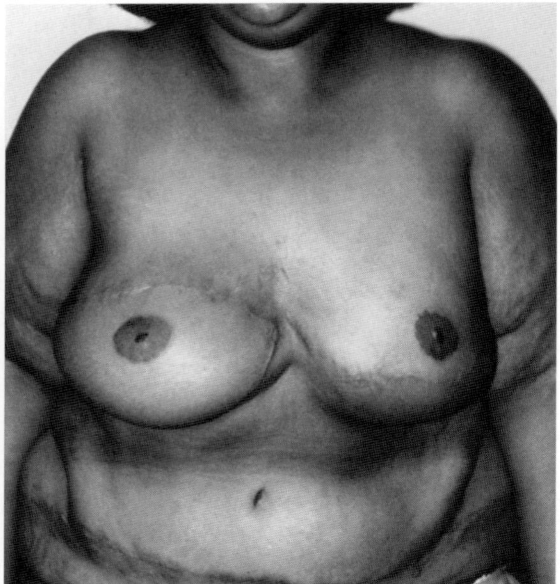

This 36-year-old woman is 5 feet 2 inches tall and weighs 220 pounds. She had a right modified radical mastectomy for stage I breast carcinoma with multicentric areas of intraductal carcinoma. She was in good general health. She requested a left total mastectomy and her general surgeon agreed with this choice. A bilateral lower TRAM flap reconstruction was successful in obtaining an adequate volume of tissue for breast reconstruction. However, she has not lost weight, and her body image and appearance show very limited improvement.

Aesthetic Placement of Incisions

Visible scars detract from the aesthetic appearance of the breast. If possible, incisions should not be placed in the upper hemisphere of the breast or the inner lower breast because these areas are not usually covered by clothing.

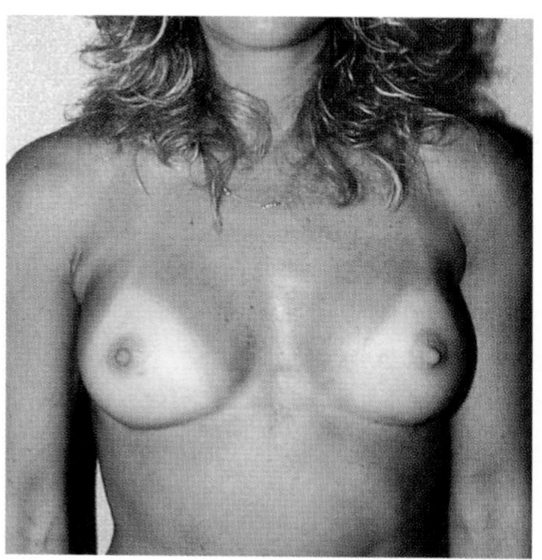

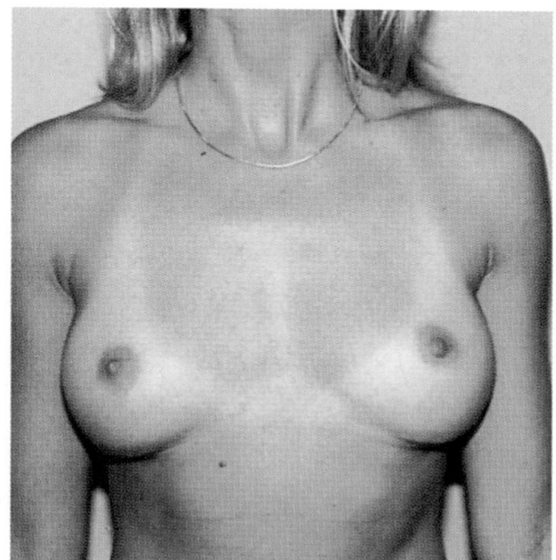

Rather, incisions should be planned out of the line of vision, camouflaged in the folds, shadows, or normal contour juncture lines, and if possible, covered by the patient's brassiere.

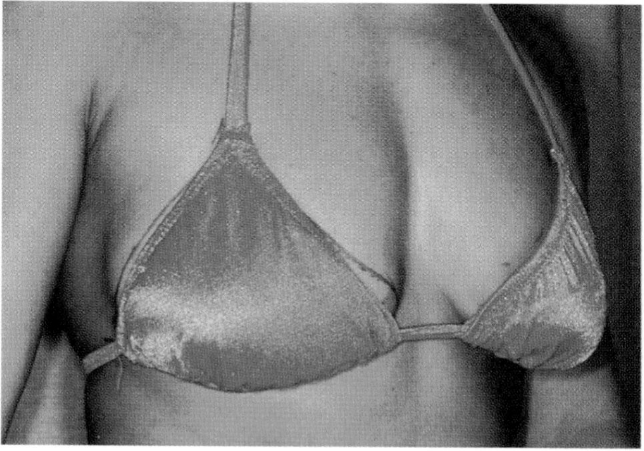

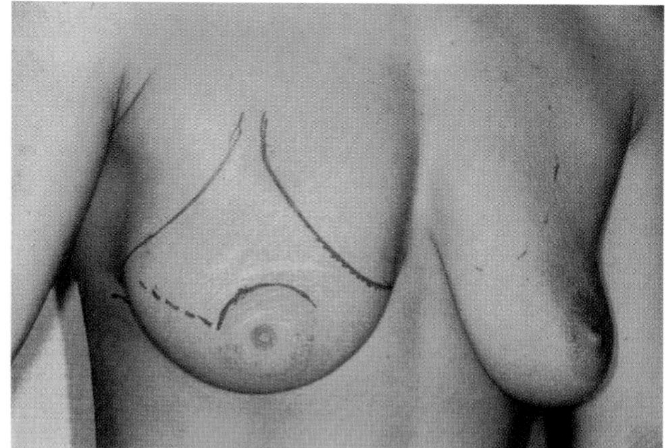

Patients usually accept biopsy and mastectomy scars that conform to these principles, as seen here when the total mastectomy incisions were planned within the confines of the patient's bikini.

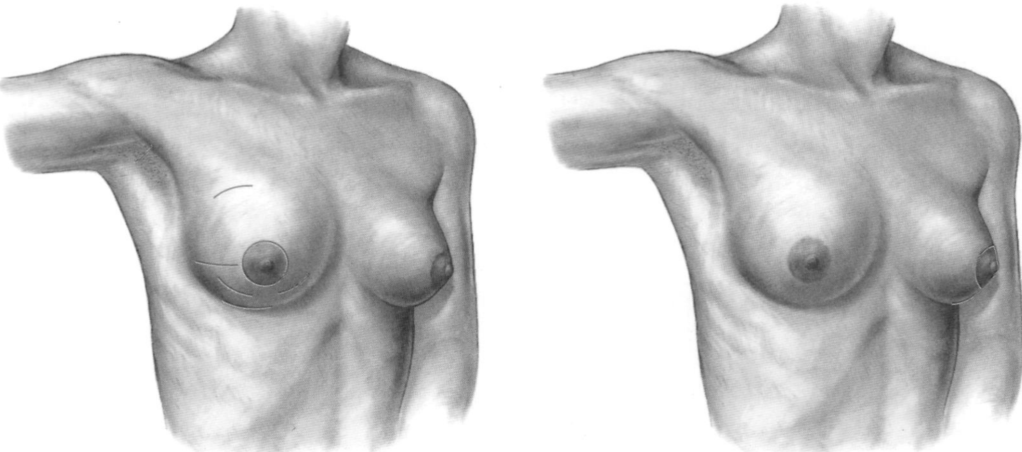

This goal can also be accomplished by positioning the mastectomy and biopsy incisions in an arc from the nipple-areola and extending them medially and laterally to the inframammary crease juncture. Incisions in this category include those around the areola at its juncture with the breast skin, radial incisions in this arc, inframammary incisions, and incisions in the lower arc parallel to the areola. The resulting scars usually heal well and are concealed in the breast shadows. These incisions should be as short as possible to avoid hypertrophy at the medial and lateral extremes of the inframammary crease. Incisions in the axilla, back, and lower abdomen provide adequate access to the breast and to tissue donor sites for breast reconstruction. A vertical incision from the areola to the inframammary fold heals predictably well and gives excellent access for mastopexy, reduction, and mastectomy.

The special characteristics and qualities of breast skin should be considered when planning breast surgery incisions. The skin, particularly in young individuals and often in those with heavier pigmentation, is subject to hypertrophic scarring. ***The risk of hypertrophic scarring increases as the midline is approached; the presternal area is particularly susceptible to this problem.***

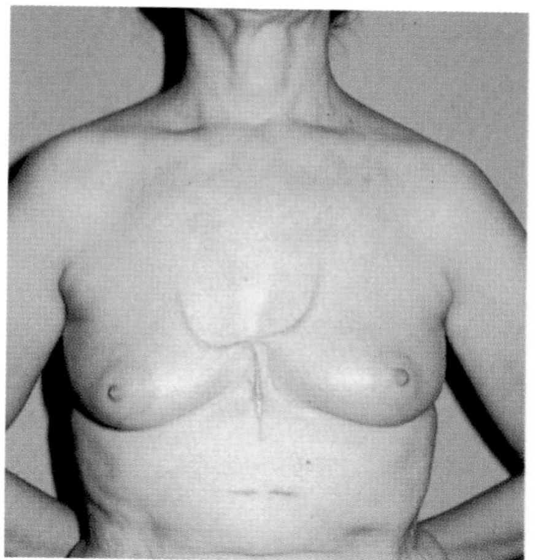

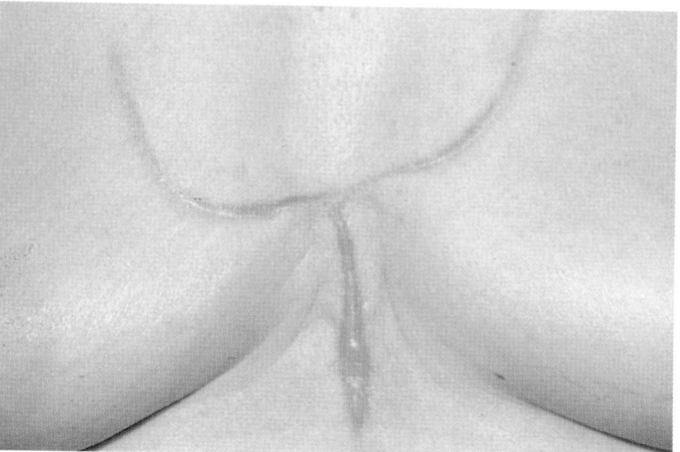

It is not advisable to extend a scar across the midline of the sternum during breast reduction unless there is no alternative for removing the extra breast skin. ***The "forbidden" triangle—the xiphoid through the nipples up to the acromion—heals unpredictably and often with scar hypertrophy.*** This area is also prone to keloid formation; in some individuals keloids may develop in this area spontaneously. The etiology of this special healing problem is unknown; it varies with each individual's pattern of healing and may be associated with tension produced from the gravitational pull of the breasts. Because of the possibility of keloids, scars and incisions should be avoided here.

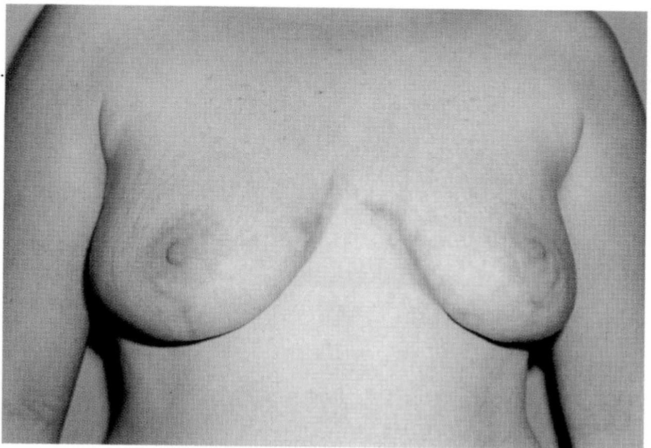

Horizontal incisions in the inframammary fold can also become hypertrophic, and the surgeon should try to avoid extending them medially to the presternal region. Vertical incisions from the inframammary fold up to the lower areola usually are not as susceptible to scar hypertrophy.

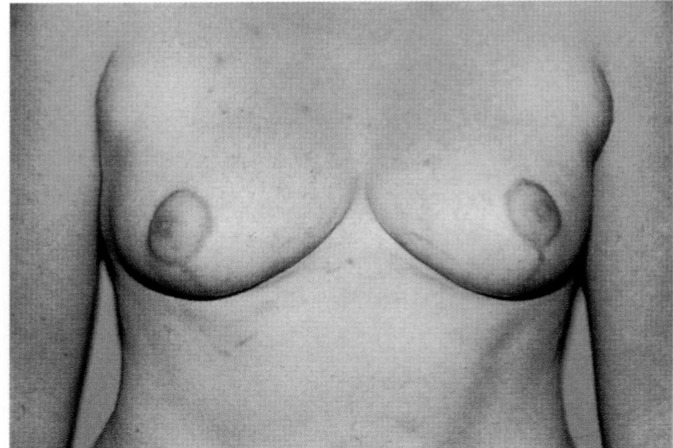

Less visible scars can be obtained by shortening them, avoiding tension, and avoiding the inframammary crease incision.

The areola usually heals without hypertrophic scarring; however, if the patient has a distinct tendency to hypertrophic scarring or keloid formation, the periareolar incision should not be the first choice for an augmentation mammaplasty incision. If a keloid develops, it is very noticeable.

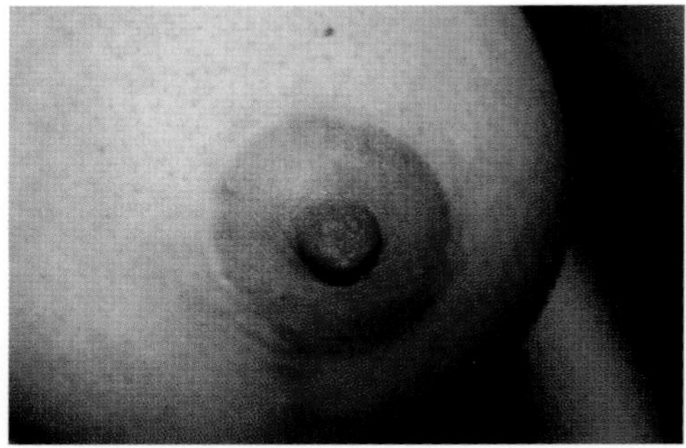

An intra-areola scar heals without pigment, but even if it has healed well, it can still appear as a noticeable white line when the adjacent areola is heavily pigmented.

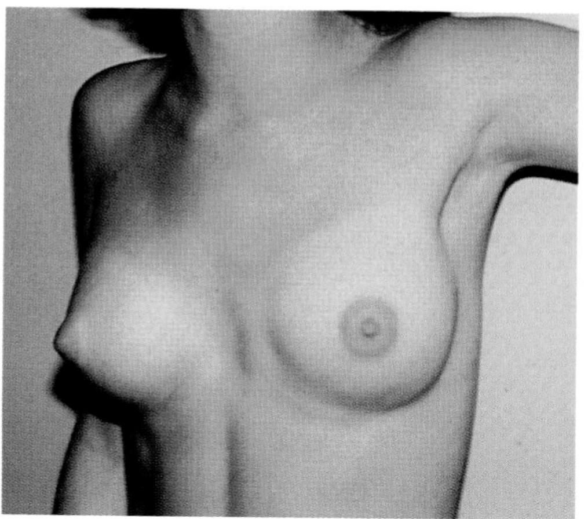

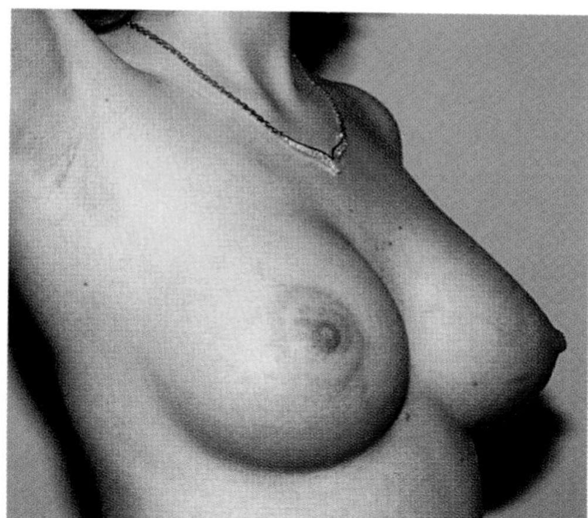

The axillary skin, particularly in the hair-bearing areas, is relatively exempt from hypertrophic scarring. An axillary incision should be considered for patients with a tendency to this healing problem because the short transverse axillary scar is usually not hypertrophic and breast scars are avoided. This is particularly useful for women requesting breast augmentation who have a tendency to hypertrophic scarring or do not have a specific inframammary fold.

The quality, visibility, and acceptance of scars are also affected by the technique of closure and method of postoperative support. Skin tension at the time of closure produces widened scars and contributes to scar hypertrophy. Breast shape should be controlled primarily by volume manipulation and contouring of underlying tissues rather than by tight skin closure. The skin's greatest strength is the dermis, and therefore it should be relied on for wound support of deep dermal structures. Ordinarily suturing of internal breast flaps is not advised. Wounds are generally closed in two layers: a deep dermal suture of 3-0 or 4-0 polyglycolic acid and a superficial closure with a fine absorbable polyglycolic acid or a pull-out polypropylene suture.

When areas of undue tension exist, I sometimes support the wound for the first 3 to 4 days with several skin staples. These do not leave marks if removed before 6 days. They reduce tension by pushing the edges of the wound together rather than pulling them together as do dermal sutures.

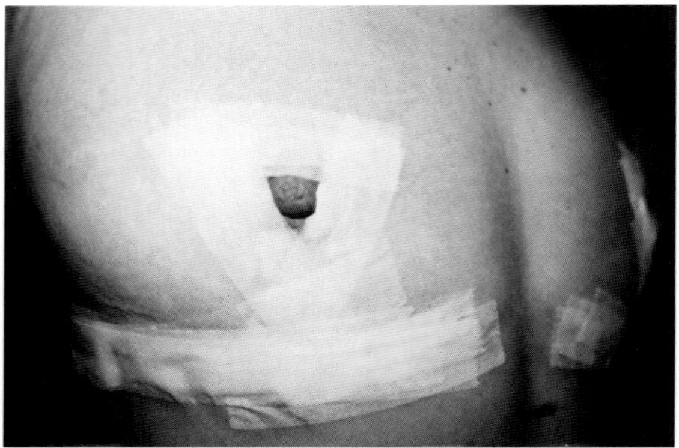

Postoperative support of incisions with surgical tape is important. For the first few days the tape seal provides a moist interface with the skin edges to promote epithelialization across the incision interface. I place the tapes longitudinally rather than across the incision. Tapes placed across the incision can cause blistering and shearing if there is postoperative swelling or edema. Later a single layer of surgical tapes supports the wound, minimizes spreading and widening of the incisions, and provides some pressure to resist scar elevation and hypertrophy. When concerned about scar hypertrophy or spreading, I recommend the application of Steri-Strips for several months or until the wound has matured, faded, and no longer has the propensity to thicken.

Assessing the Result

A good surgeon compares the physical reality of the breast he has formed to the internalized aesthetic ideals that directed the surgical plans. The final breast appearance represents the realization of the patient's expectations and the surgeon's artistry. The symmetric, softly contoured breasts should be proportionate to the woman's body to produce the optimal natural appearance. We are all too familiar with the "postsurgical look" characterized by undue breast projection, excessive supra-areolar fullness, extension of the breast beyond normal boundaries, or scars. Ideally, breast scars will not be visible, but if this is impossible, the residual should be inconspicuous, flat scars concealed within natural skin lines or breast shadows and creases.

Mathematical models and patterns meant to reduce operations to formulas are simply unsuccessful; they cannot possibly encompass the individual anatomic variations that we encounter daily in surgical practice. The surgeon must be able to conceptualize the ideal breast for a particular patient and work through the limitations and possibilities in view of the individual's anatomy to attain that ideal. The patient's desires must be incorporated throughout this planning process. The ultimate goal is breasts that are aesthetically pleasing to both patient and surgeon.

REFERENCES

Bostwick J III, Eaves FF III, Nahai F. Endoscopic Plastic Surgery. St. Louis: Quality Medical Publishing, 1995.

Bouman FG. Volumetric measurement of the human breast and breast tissue before and during mammoplasty. Br J Plast Surg 23:263, 1970.

Crosby JF Jr. Aesthetics: The ideas and ideals of beauty. In Masters FW, Lewis JR Jr, eds. Symposium on Aesthetic Surgery of the Nose, Ears, and Chin, vol 6. St. Louis: CV Mosby, 1973.

Cruz-Korchin NI. Effectiveness of silicone sheets in the prevention of hypertrophic breast scars. Ann Plast Surg 37:345, 1996.

Fredericks S. Skeletal and postural relations in augmentation mammaplasty. Ann Plast Surg 1:44, 1978.

Goldwyn RM, ed. Plastic and Reconstructive Surgery of the Breast. Boston: Little, Brown, 1976.

Grossman AJ, Roudner LA. A simple means for accurate breast volume determination. Plast Reconstr Surg 66:851, 1980.

Holman PD, Hetter GP, Peterson RA. Aesthetic concepts of augmentation mammaplasty: Breast dynamics in plastic surgery. In Owsley JW, Peterson RA, eds. Symposium on Aesthetic Surgery of the Breast. St. Louis: CV Mosby, 1978.

Kuzbari R, Deutinger M, Todoroff BP, Schneider B, Freilinger G. Surgical treatment of developmental asymmetry of the breast. Long-term results. Scand J Plast Reconstr Surg Hand Surg 27:203, 1993.

Letterman G, Schurter M. Suggested nomenclature for aesthetic and reconstructive surgery of the breast. Aesthetic Plast Surg 10:55, 1986.

Linn CF. The Golden Mean, Mathematics and the Fine Arts. New York: Doubleday, 1974.

Loughry CW, Sheffer DB, Price TE Jr, Bartfai RG, Morek WM, Lackney MJ, Bolyard BR. Right and left breast volume and volume distribution comparisons in normal and tumor-containing breasts. Cancer Detect Prev 10:215, 1987.

Penn J. Breast reduction. Br J Plast Surg 7:357, 1978.

Price CI, Eaves FF III, Nahai F, Jones G, Bostwick J III. Endoscopic transaxillary subpectoral breast augmentation. Plast Reconstr Surg 94:612, 1994.

Sarwer DB, Bartlett SP, Bucky LP, LaRossa D, Low DW, Pertschuk MJ, Wadden TA, Whitaker LA. Big is not always better: Body image dissatisfaction in breast reduction and breast augmentation patients. Plast Reconstr Surg 101:1956, 1998.

Sheffer DB, Price TE, Loughry CW, Bolyard BL, Moret WM, Varga RS. Validity and reliability of biostereometric measure of the human female breast. Ann Biomed Eng 14:1, 1986.

Wallace AF. The surgery of beauty. Trans Med Soc Lond 98:17, 1981-82.

Westreich M. Anthropomorphic breast measurement: Protocol and results in 50 women with aesthetically perfect breasts and clinical application. Plast Reconstr Surg 100:468, 1997.

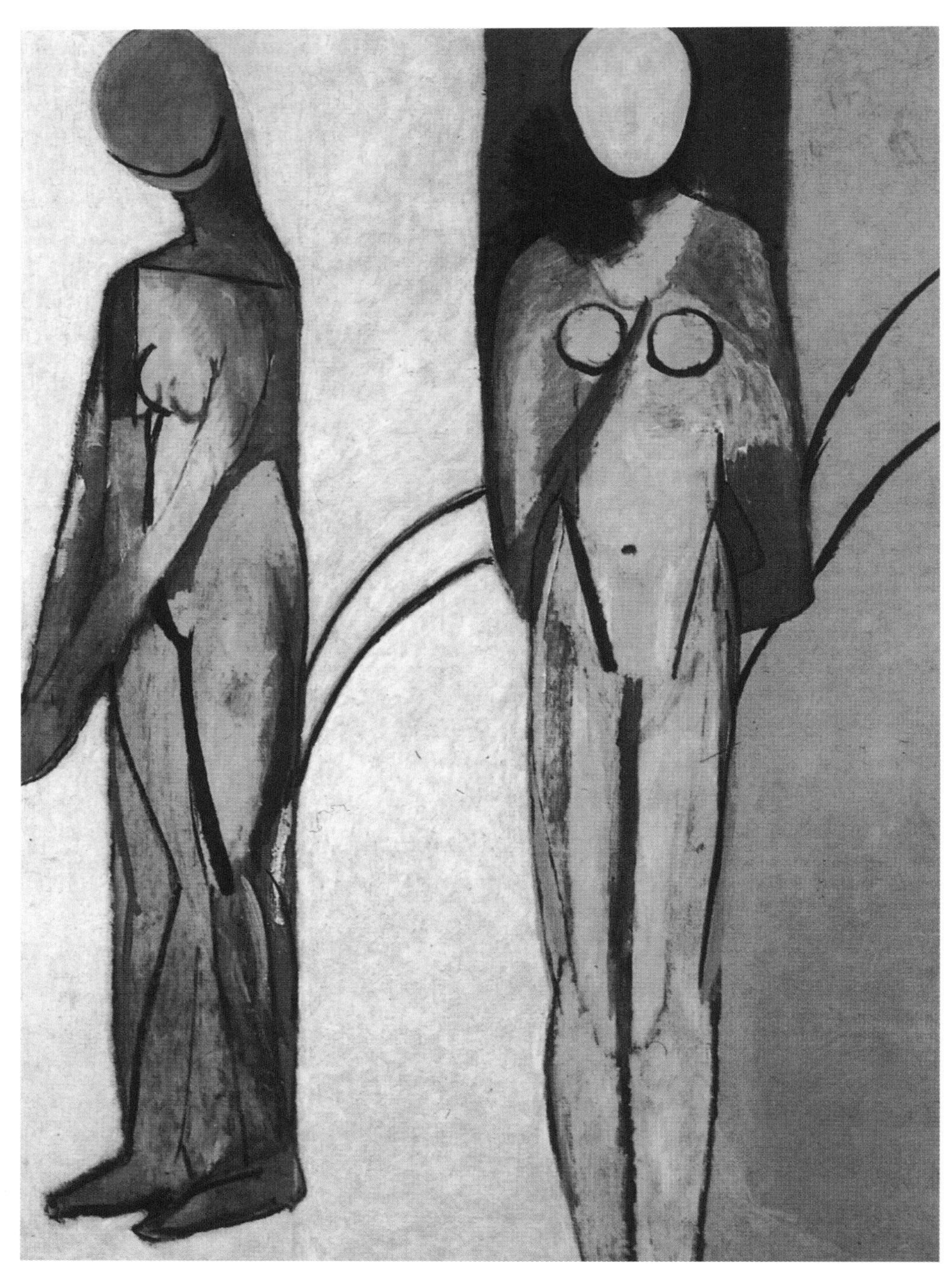

4 *Essentials of Endoscopic Breast Surgery*

Felmont F. Eaves III, M.D.
John Bostwick III, M.D.

Key Topics

Equipment Requirements

The Optical Cavity

Placement of Access Sites

Contour Constraints

Conversion to Open Dissection

Initial Dissection

Guidelines for Endoscopic Applications in Breast Surgery

Observations

Endoscopic techniques have greatly expanded the options we can now offer our patients and have infused a new high-tech dynamic into the practice of plastic surgery of the breast. Both aesthetic and reconstructive breast surgery procedures are amenable to an endoscopic approach, including augmentation mammaplasty and reconstruction with implants, expanders, and autologous tissue. Better visualization, improved control of dissection and hemostasis, shorter incisions, and reduced morbidity are all recognized benefits. Through small access incisions aesthetically positioned in the axilla, inframammary fold, areolar border, or existing scars, muscles can be manipulated, elevated, and divided and breast tissue can be inspected, biopsied, and excised. Minimally invasive approaches can also be used to facilitate mastectomy, particularly for gynecomastia, TRAM flap delay or revision, and implant and expander insertion and explantation. Additionally, endoscopic procedures may be used to complement other operations such as skin-sparing mastectomy. Tissue harvest remains one of the most promising applications. With the use of video-assisted surgery we can now harvest autologous tissue to reconstruct deformities after partial and total mastectomy or to provide a protective layer for breast implants and expanders. This new technology has enhanced our ability to provide creative solutions to ongoing aesthetic and reconstructive challenges.

Endoscopic breast surgery is equipment dependent, requiring a more complex operative setup and greater dependence on technology. Although the endoscope projects a brightly illuminated, enlarged image, this image must be visualized on a separate video monitor. The surgeon must operate with long instruments that do not provide the tactile reinforcement of standard open surgery and require excellent eye-hand coordination. ***Thus it is essential that the surgeon performing endoscopic procedures and his/her support staff have the necessary training as well as the equipment and skill to perform these procedures.*** Familiarity with methods for troubleshooting as well as a thorough understanding of safety measures is also necessary. This technologic dependence mandates a working knowledge of equipment and instrumentation. Understanding these basics will shorten the learning curve and establish a baseline for expanding the range of applications. As with any technology, system malfunction is always a possibility, and the more the surgeon understands about the system, the easier it is to prevent and correct problems.

This chapter provides a brief overview of pragmatic information that the surgeon needs to incorporate minimally invasive procedures into a breast surgery practice. It reviews equipment and instrument needs, preoperative system troubleshooting, optical cavity requirements, and access site placement and provides guidelines for the use of the endoscope in various breast surgery applications as well as practical suggestions to help the surgeon adopt these techniques safely and successfully. Specific endoscopic applications are described in detail in pertinent chapters throughout the book.

EQUIPMENT AND INSTRUMENT REQUIREMENTS

The equipment necessary for endoscopic breast surgery can be divided into general endoscopic equipment already available in most hospital or surgery center operating rooms and items specific to endoscopic breast surgery that may have to be purchased.

General equipment requirements for endoscopic surgery

- Endoscopic system/cart assembly
- Camera
- Light source
- Monitor
- Video recorder
- Still image system
- Fiberoptic light cables
- Electrocautery generator and cords
- Laparoscopic scissors (disposable or reusable)
- Endoscope warmers
- Defogging solution

The equipment listed above is generally widely available because it is used in laparoscopic, gynecologic, thoracoscopic, and other specialty endoscopic procedures. Existing video endoscopic systems are usually sufficient for plastic surgery procedures. ***At a minimum the video endoscopic system includes a video camera attached to the endoscope, a light source with associated cables, and a monitor on which to view the endoscopic image.*** Additional peripheral tools such as video recorders and image systems can be used for procedure review, teaching, and documentation. Endoscope warmers or defogging solutions are extremely helpful to minimize condensation on the objective lens of the endoscope.

Specific equipment requirements for endoscopic breast surgery

- Straight and curved endoscopic retractors with 10 mm cannulas
- Compatible 10 mm, 30- and 45-degree Hopkins rod endoscopes
- Curved suction-cautery instruments (2-3)

This equipment is generally specific to endoscopic plastic surgery and therefore may not be available in the operating room. For the majority of endoscopic breast procedures a standard straight-blade endoscopic retractor is satisfactory and is paired with a 30-degree downward-directed rigid endoscope. For endoscopic latissimus dorsi harvest a retractor with a longer, curved blade can be coupled with a 45-degree downward-viewing scope. This helps the surgeon negotiate the contour constraints posed by the chest wall.

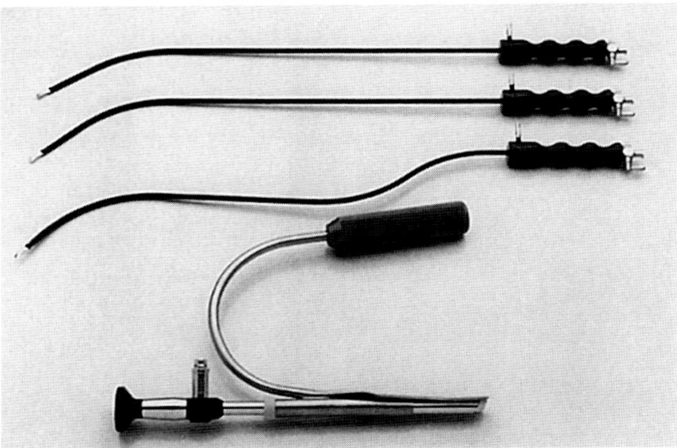

Suggestions for an instrument starter set for endoscopic breast surgery are pictured above.

Endoscope

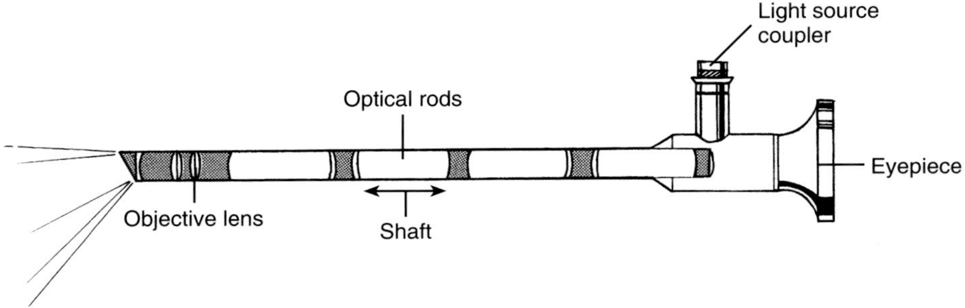

Hopkins rod design endoscopes are most suited to plastic surgery procedures. These endoscopes are rigid tubes with interspersed glass lenses and air pockets. It is a fixed-focus lens system designed for the simultaneous bidirectional transmission of light. The distal tip of the scope is composed of the objective lens that is bonded to the casing of the endoscope. Almost any objective angle between 0 and 120 degrees can be produced. Because of the upward tilt placed on the endoscopic retractor during breast surgery, a 30-degree downward-viewing angled endoscope usually produces an appropriately directed view. The shaft of the endoscope extends from the objective lens to the light source coupler and contains the glass lenses and fiberoptic bundles encased in a metal sleeve. Larger endoscopes have more fiberoptic bundles and therefore allow greater light transmission. ***Because the optical cavities encountered during breast surgery are relatively large and the tissues reflect relatively low levels of light, a larger endoscope (10 mm) that accommodates more fiberoptic bundles is generally necessary for adequate illumination.*** Flexible endoscopes are composed of flexible fiberoptic cables for both incoming and outwardly directed light. Because these instruments are more expensive and offer less clear visualization in larger optical cavities, they are not generally used for breast surgery.

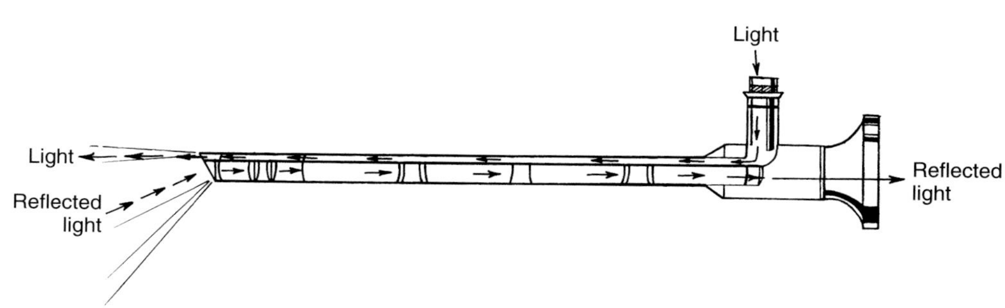

At the light source coupler the incoming light is directed distally down a dedicated fiberoptic pathway and out the objective lens. Reflected light is channeled proximally from the objective lens past the light source, through the neck of the endoscope, and then projected onto the eyepiece. The camera system couples to the eyepiece. Many newer systems dispense with the eyepiece per se, opting instead for a direct coupler system to connect the camera to the endoscope.

Light Sources

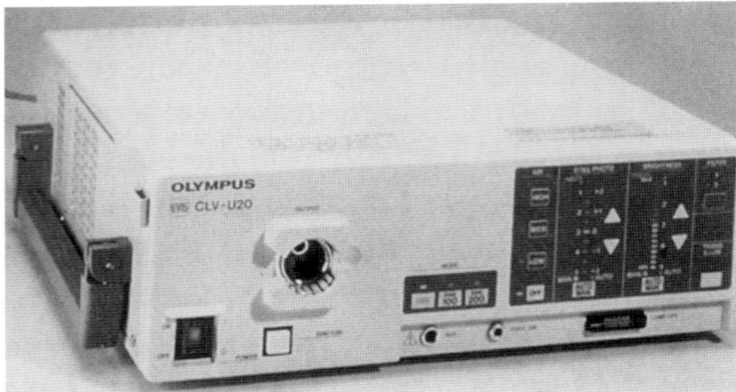

The light source (e.g., xenon bulb) is directed down the fiberoptic connecting cable to the endoscope. Light sources often have a standby mode that increases the life of the bulb. They also have controls to adjust the output source to obtain optimal surgical illumination.

Video Camera

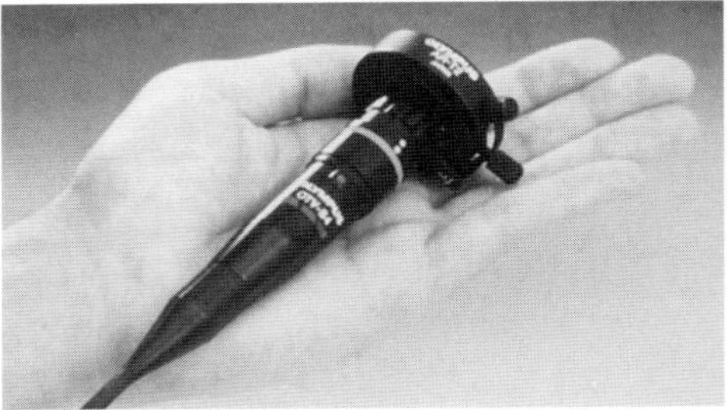

Placement of the video camera on the eyepiece of the endoscope has dramatically altered the operating room setup and influenced the positioning of the surgeon and assistants. A clear, brightly illuminated image on a large video screen allows the surgeon to choose the most comfortable and efficient position for operating while viewing a strategically located monitor.

The assistants view an identical image on the same monitor or on a secondary monitor that can be positioned anywhere in the operating room. The video image can be reproduced an infinite number of times and is easily recorded for procedural review or documentation.

Whether a standard eyepiece coupler or direct coupler system is used, the camera will have a head that attaches to the endoscope, a cord that connects to the camera chassis, and a focusing ring near the endoscope connection. Because the camera lenses have a wide angle and deep depth of field, once the focus ring is adjusted, it usually does not require attention during the remainder of the procedure.

Video Monitors

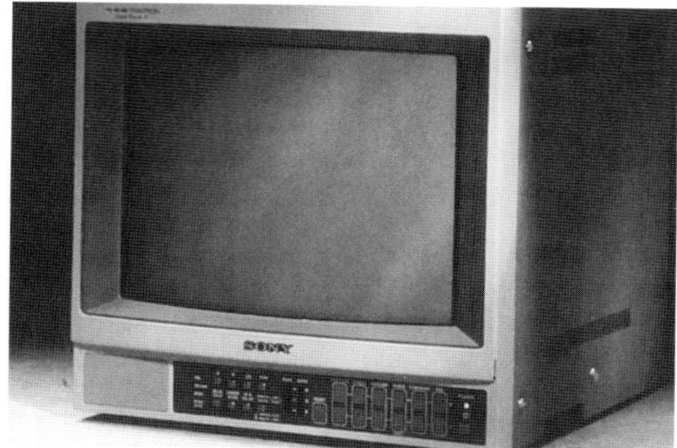

The video monitor is the final component of the video endoscopic system. In general high-resolution monitors are placed on endoscopic carts. Monitors are available in a range of sizes, but generally larger monitors are superior for operative visualization. The monitor is routinely located on the top of the endoscopic cart at the surgeon's eye level. Some operating rooms have monitors mounted on ceiling brackets. Secondary monitors are useful to allow surgical assistants, scrub personnel, and the anesthetist to follow the progress of the procedure. They also permit the surgeon to move to the opposite side of the operating table without having to relocate the equipment.

Electrocautery

The electrocautery source may be located either on the endoscopic cart or on a separate stand, depending on existing equipment and surgeon preference. The blended current is better for endoscopic dissection and coagulation in most instances. If a foot pedal is used, the pure cut current is often deactivated to prevent accidental activation, which could cause excessive bleeding. A bipolar cautery is now available for endoscopic delivery.

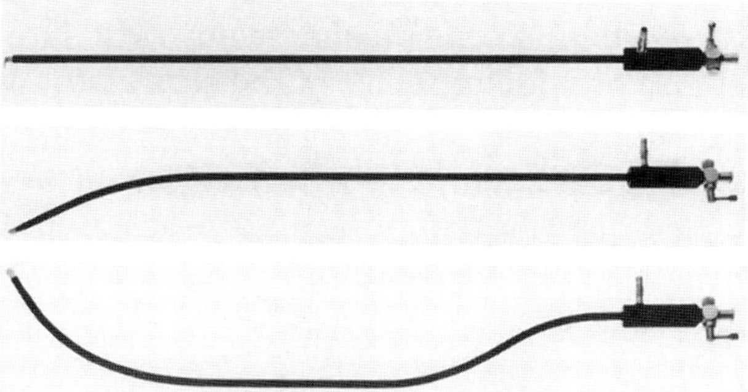

The shafts of reusable suction-cautery units may be configured in a variety of shapes during the manufacturing process to accommodate the various curves that must be negotiated during subcutaneous dissection. These instruments are not malleable because of the characteristics of the metal shaft.

Most endoscopic instruments with the appropriate conductive capability and external insulation can be used for electrocautery. Suction-cautery instruments consist of a hollow, electro-conductive tubular shaft, the lumen of which is open distally and in line with a connector proximally to which suction or irrigation tubing is secured. The shaft is insulated to allow the conduction of electrical current to the uninsulated tip. The suction-cautery instrument may have an integrated stopcock to allow intermittent or continuous suction. Alternate methods for endoscopic tissue dissection include laparoscopic ultrasonic instruments and laser systems.

Endoscopic Cart

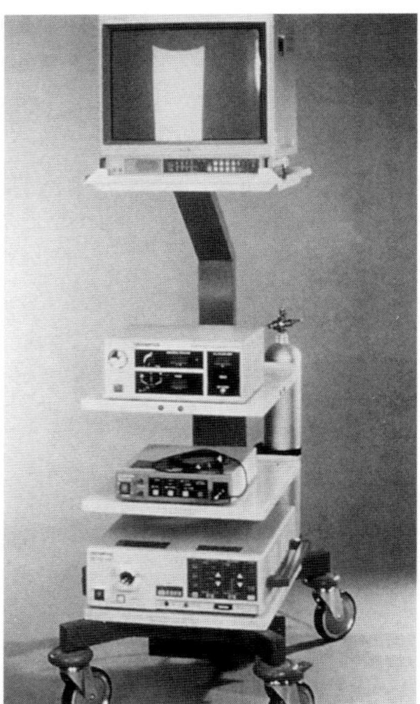

The camera box, light source, video monitor, video recorder, and insufflator are frequently assembled on a rollable endoscopic cart. This cart can reduce instrument clutter and provide mobility of the entire unit without requiring reassembly of the components. Some carts come with a lockable cabinet door for security. Others are equipped with fan systems to improve ventilation and expedite heat dispersal from the electronic equipment. Others may have a movable arm on which the monitor is located to aid in optimal monitor positioning.

The endoscopic cart is positioned to allow clear, unrestricted viewing of the video monitor by the surgeon and the operating team. The distance between the operating table and the cart is limited by the length of the light cord. If necessary for optimal viewing by either the surgeon or assistants, secondary monitors can be positioned as necessary. ***Prior to bringing the patient into the operating room, the electronic equipment is turned on to verify that all components are functioning in good order.*** The nurse should inspect the endoscope, fiberoptic light cord, electrocautery cords, and camera during this preoperative check. In addition, the insulated shaft of the suction-cautery units should be carefully inspected to detect any break in insulation that could cause unintended tissue coagulation.

Endoscope Warmers and Antifogging Solutions

A fogged image can be one of the most annoying problems associated with endoscopy. Fogging occurs secondary to condensation of humid air within the optical cavity onto a cool endoscope objective lens or less commonly between the eyepiece and the camera. Fogging of the distal objective lens occurs unless the scope is kept warm or antifogging solution is applied to the objective lens. Warming is accomplished by placing the distal end of the endoscope in a warm water lens warmer or water bath. Electric lens warmers are available as well. To be most effective the endoscope must be returned to the warmer whenever it has been removed from the body during the course of the procedure. If the camera head and endoscope are sterilized by a soaking method, removing the instruments from the bath several minutes before assembly allows adequate time for the lens surfaces to fully dry. This will prevent fogging at the endoscope-camera interface.

As an alternative or adjuvant to endoscopic warming, antifogging solutions are applied directly to the objective lens of the endoscope with a soft foam applier or gauze. Antifogging solutions also function as effective lens cleaners should body fluid obscure the lens. Besides the specifically marketed antifogging solutions, soapy surgical solutions such as a povidone-iodine surgical scrub can function as convenient and inexpensive antifogging solutions. Antifogging solution is reapplied as needed during the course of the procedure.

Preoperative System Checks

The entire system must be checked before the operation is begun. The free end of the light cord is passed out of the sterile field and plugged into the appropriate connection site on the light source. The camera cable is also connected to the camera box on the video cart. The light source, camera, and video monitor are activated and the endoscope is pointed at some object on the field such as surgical gauze. A clear, well-illuminated image of the object should appear on the video monitor. If not, the connections must be rechecked at all levels. During this maneuver the color tone of the camera may be set by activating the white balance on the camera box.

THE OPTICAL CAVITY

Endoscopes function like wide-angle lenses with a very short focal length. When the endoscope is directed toward objects or anatomic structures closer than the focal distance, a blurred image results. A space must therefore be created in which the endoscope can function and which provides adequate room for surgical maneuvering, dissecting, and structure identification. The space is the optical cavity; it provides an open area for clear viewing as well as the necessary space for instrument movement and tissue manipulation. ***Developing and maintaining an optical cavity are essential in the application of any form of surgical endoscopy of the breast.***

In many endoscopic surgical procedures a natural body cavity can provide a ready optical cavity. In endoscopic surgery of the breast, however, these natural body spaces do not exist. Rather they must be created by dissection and maintained throughout the procedure. Four basic breast optical cavities are created during the course of endoscopic breast surgery; these include a *subcutaneous* cavity dissected between the gland and subcutaneous fat, the *intraparenchymal* cavity for removal of masses, a *subglandular* cavity for manipulation of the breast from the deep surface, and a *submuscular* cavity such as is used during transaxillary augmentation. In addition, optical cavities may be created in a supramuscular plane, within the back fat, and submuscularly during endoscopic latissimus dorsi harvest for breast reconstruction. Optical cavities may also involve the layers of the abdominal wall during vascular delay procedures or even the peritoneal cavity during omental harvest.

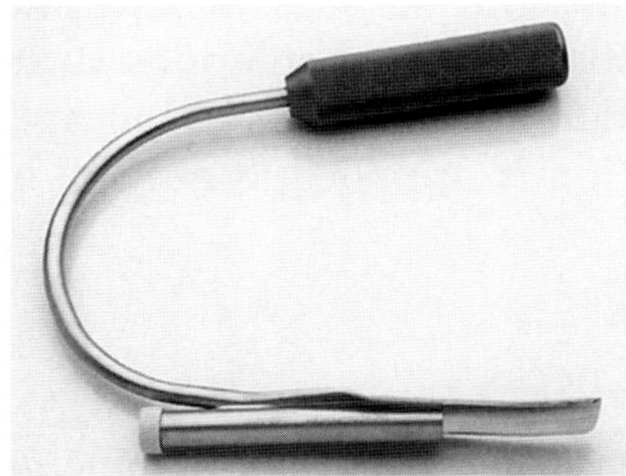

Most endoscopic breast surgery procedures are performed in dissected spaces where the optical cavity must be constantly maintained throughout the course of the operation. The most common method for maintaining the optical cavity during breast surgery is via an endoscopic retractor or endoretractor system, which may be purchased from a variety of manufacturers. The endoretractor consists of a blade that is used to elevate the optical cavity by means of an attached handle. Underneath the blade is a hollow tube or cannula that holds the endoscope in position. The cannula shields the end of the endoscope as it is advanced into the optical cavity. The endoscope can be withdrawn or advanced within the cannula, allowing the relationship of the blade and endoscope to be adjusted for optimal visualization. However, in the normal working position the endoscope is not advanced past the tip of the retractor blade so as to prevent the objective lens from coming in contact with tissues. The endoscope is partially stabilized within the retractor by placing the light cord into its groove on the retractor handle. To firmly stabilize the endoscope, some endoretractors also have a ring that can be tightened at the proximal end of the cannula.

If lens clouding occurs while using the endoscopic retractor, the endoscope and retractor can be removed as assembled, the scope advanced clear of the retractor tip, and the lens cleaned. Alternatively, the scope can be removed from the cannula sheath while the retractor remains positioned within the optical cavity. The endoscope can then be cleaned and reinserted into the endoretractor. Endoscopic retractors do not form an airtight seal with the surrounding soft tissues.

Although insufflation is not frequently used during endoscopic breast surgery, a standard laparoscopic cannula is necessary if insufflation is indicated. This device fits through a small incision, creating an airtight seal between the cannula shaft and soft tissues that prevents the escape of gas. In addition to allowing the endoscope to be placed, the cannulas have ports for the insufflation tubing. Additional cannulas can be positioned to allow the insertion of irrigation, suction, or dissecting instruments.

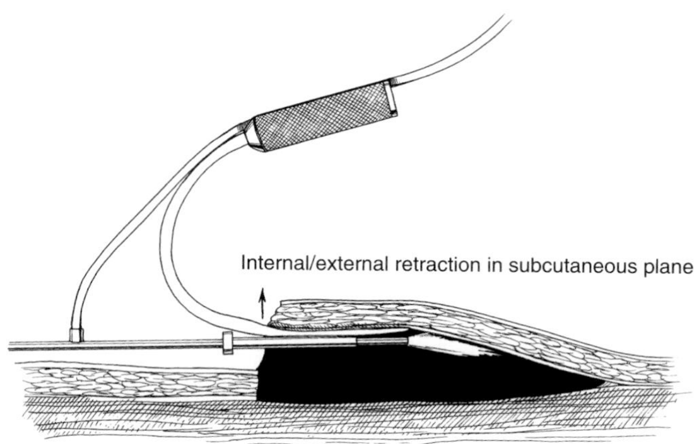

The combined retractor/cannula system allows the surgeon to provide an outward and upward lift that opens the optical cavity. ***A retractor tip positioned at the periphery of the optical cavity places the cavity edges under traction, which facilitates additional dissection to enlarge the cavity.*** Because the cannula and retractor function as a single unit, holding the retractor in place simultaneously positions the endoscope in the appropriate direction.

When the 30-degree endoscope is used, the lift on the retractor tip compensates for the downward-view deflection, and therefore the area of interest is appropriately centered on the monitor. Biofeedback from the retractor position also helps orient the surgeon to the visualized structures and is analogous to the use of the familiar lighted retractor, but rather than peering into a small, suboptimally illuminated hole, the surgeon is able to look at a large, bright magnified image. Furthermore, the retractor/cannula system can easily be pivoted and rotated to allow exposure and dissection of various regions while maintaining the optical cavity for clear visualization. The surgeon is able to control the optical cavity and view with a single (usually nondominant) hand. The other hand is freed for dissection with a variety of instruments.

Special Considerations

PLACEMENT OF ACCESS SITES

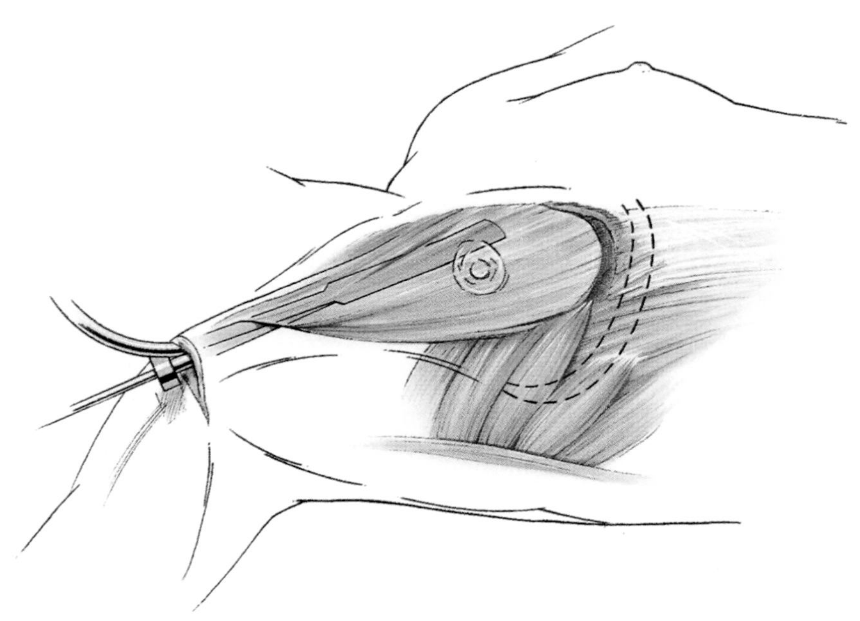

It is desirable to develop a well-defined optical cavity, which on occasion will also serve as an implant or expander cavity. ***To properly develop and access the optical cavity, one or more access incisions for ports must be placed.*** The access incision(s) permits placement of the endoscope and insertion of devices for optical cavity development and instruments for tissue manipulation, hemostasis, smoke evacuation, removal of tissue, and insertion of implantable devices.

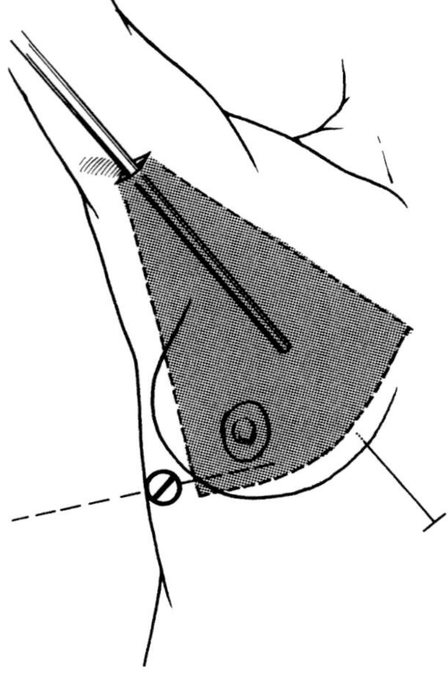

Several factors should be considered in planning the access incision(s). First, since reduction of visible scarring is a primary goal of endoscopic techniques, the incision should be located in relatively hidden sites away from aesthetically sensitive areas. Examples include the use of prominent axillary creases to hide the access incision for augmentation, biopsy, and many other endoscopic breast procedures. A periareolar incision, existing scars, and the inframammary fold are also aesthetically acceptable.

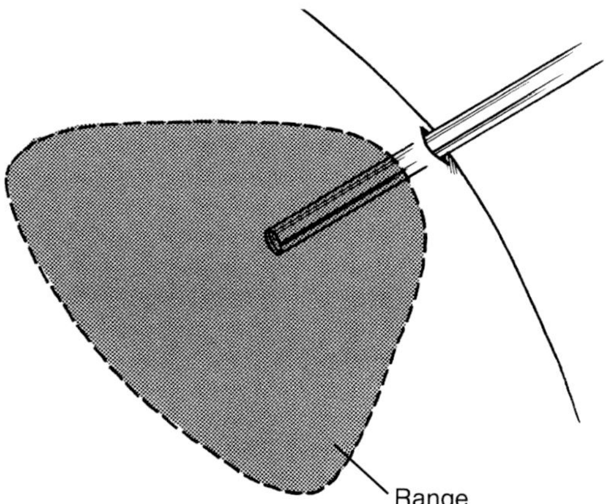

A second consideration is the operating distance, or range, of the endoscope. ***The effective range of the endoscope dictates the distance at which the incision can be placed away from the primary zone of dissection.*** Structures closer than the effective range are dissected using either traditional open methods or blunt blind dissection. Structures distant to the far range of the endoscope must be approached either through additional access incisions or with the assistance of a second, longer endoscope. For example, a standard endoscopic retractor works quite well for transaxillary breast dissection, but it may be too short for complete latissimus dorsi harvest through the same incision.

The location of access incisions is determined on an arc from the center of the proposed optical cavity with a radius equal to the anticipated effective range.

Third, locating the access incision away from the site of expander or implant placement may protect against extrusion or exposure through the access incision. In addition, the length of the access incision is determined by the size and number of instruments to be placed, the dimensions of tissue to be removed, and the size of implants/expanders to be inserted.

The region of the access incision is usually infiltrated with an epinephrine-containing solution to minimize oozing from the skin margins. It may also be used for subcutaneous dissections but is avoided for submuscular dissections.

CONTOUR CONSTRAINTS

The curvature of the chest wall may further impact the effective working range, and this can be partially compensated by using a curved-blade retractor. With a longer endoscope the entire latissimus dorsi can be harvested through a single periareolar incision. Positioning the incision toward the posterior aspect of the axilla further extends the effective range. However, if a large muscle is to be harvested, secondary incisions may be necessary in certain cases.

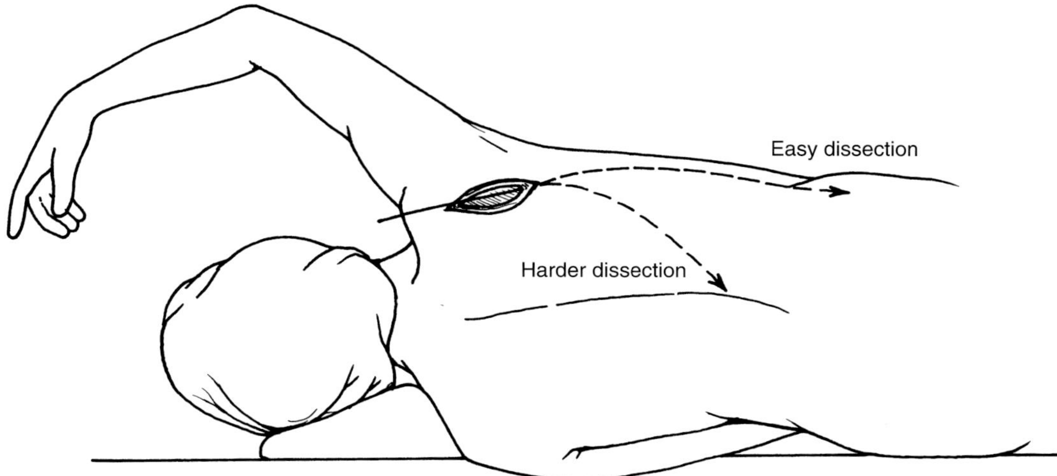

Mobilization of the muscle primarily in a superior to inferior orientation allows a straighter path to be followed, partially avoiding the anterior to posterior curvature. Flexible fiberoptic endoscopes can be used to overcome curvature restrictions; however, poorer light transmission and image clarity are the drawbacks.

CONVERSION TO OPEN DISSECTION

Occasionally the surgeon may choose to complete a portion of the dissection as an open procedure. In this situation incisions for open dissection may function as "free" access sites. Open dissection of the vascular pedicle may be desired for harvesting muscle flaps and mandates an incision in this region. For this reason we use an axillary incision as the first access site for free latissimus dorsi harvest, which allows traditional pedicle isolation under loupe magnification.

INITIAL DISSECTION

The endoscope is in essence nonfunctional until a pocket has been developed. Therefore the initial dissection is performed in an open manner or blindly without the endoscope. For example, to develop a subpectoral pocket the loosely adherent deep muscular surface is elevated bluntly without the need for endoscopic visualization. For fascia lata or latissimus dorsi muscle harvest, several centimeters of fascia/muscle can be exposed with traditional dissection techniques to develop an initial pocket and to define the appropriate tissue plane for dissection. In these cases the dissection planes can subsequently be followed under endoscopic guidance.

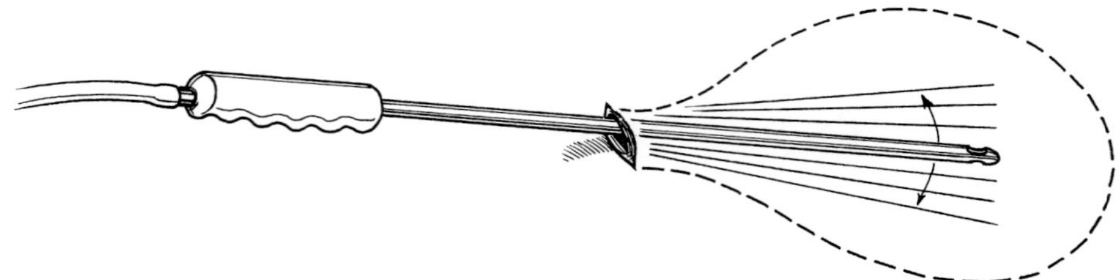

In anatomic regions with adequate subcutaneous tissue we have found that pretunneling or liposuction of the area after infiltration of a wetting solution and blunt elevation prior to insertion of the endoscope may simplify endoscopic dissection. We infiltrate a solution containing 1000 ml of Ringer's lactate, 1 ml of 1:1000 epinephrine, and 25 ml of 1% lidocaine prior to pretunneling. This combination of fluid with vasoconstriction and blunt elevation can markedly reduce bleeding in the optical cavity, and the lidocaine reduces postoperative pain.

Guidelines for Endoscopic Applications in Breast Surgery

Endoscopic Applications in Breast Surgery

Augmentation (transaxillary, inframammary, and periareolar)
Biopsy
Mastectomy (gynecomastia)
Expander placement
Expander inspection
Expander exchange
Implant exchange
Capsulotomy
Complete or partial capsulectomy
Capsulorrhaphy
Latissimus dorsi muscle harvest for implant/expander cover
Autologous latissimus dorsi harvest
Reconstruction of Poland's deformity
TRAM flap harvest
Vascular delay for TRAM flap
Excision of fat necrosis after TRAM flap
Revision of autologous or implant reconstruction
Omentum harvest for breast reconstruction
Chest wall modification (cartilage removal/reshaping)

Breast Augmentation

The endoscope facilitates the development of the subpectoral pocket, specifically the release of the lower pectoralis major muscle, and accurate dissection and control of the position of the inframammary fold. A 2.5 to 3.0 cm axillary incision usually provides adequate access; however, an inframammary incision is also useful. After the subpectoral pocket is created, the endoscope permits direct, clear visualization of the deep surface of the pectoralis major muscle for division. The improved accuracy and predictability represent a major advance for axillary augmentation.

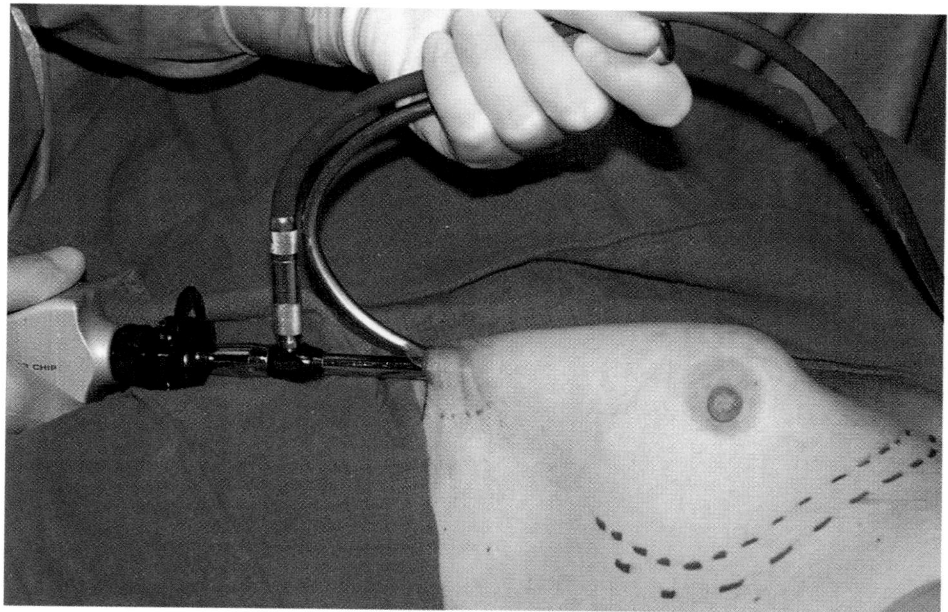

After an upper subpectoral pocket is created using blunt dissection, the lower medial and central pectoralis major muscle origins are divided from their deep surface under direct vision. The remainder of the pocket is dissected, and the breast implant is positioned and inflated with the patient sitting upright on the operating table (see Chapter 6).

Breast Biopsy

The endoscope can permit biopsy of benign breast masses through a distant incision in an aesthetically acceptable position. Infiltration of wetting solution and pretunneling can minimize bleeding. Relatively large fibroadenomas have been removed endoscopically using the axillary approach.

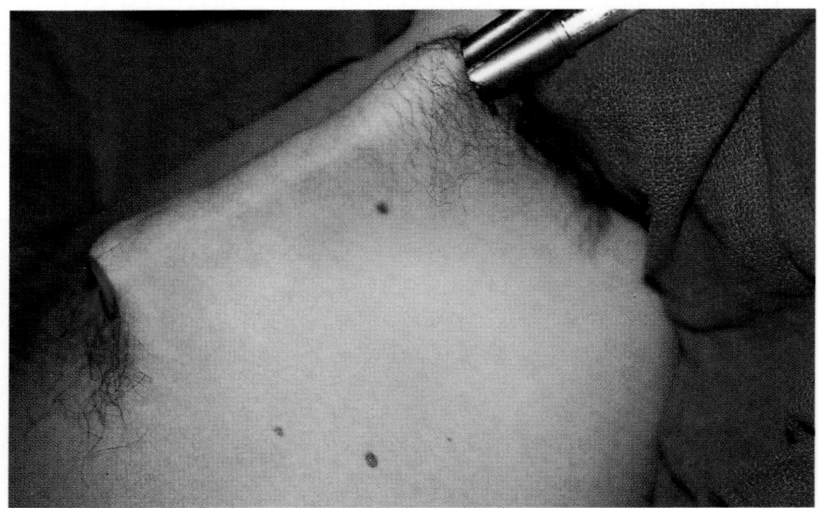

Dissection within the breast through an axillary incision creates an optical cavity that permits localization and visualization of a subareolar mass.

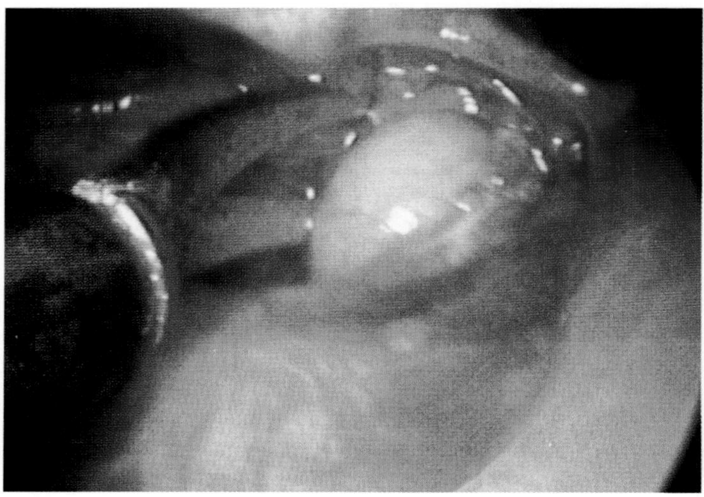

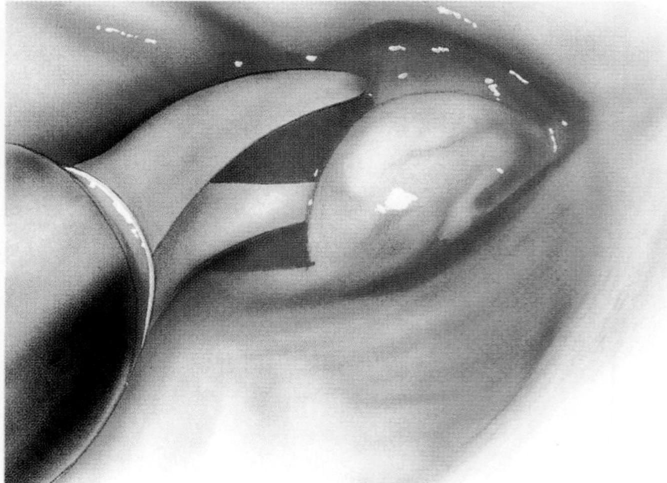

Dissection with the endoscopic Metzenbaum or hook scissors and repeated palpation allow the mass to be exposed and then excised under direct vision. Hemostasis is obtained by direct control with the electrocautery.

Mastectomy (Gynecomastia)

Although the periareolar or inframammary incision is standard for performing mastectomy in patients with gynecomastia, the resulting breast scar may be objectionable to many patients. The mastectomy can be done via an axillary approach under endoscopic visualization. Initially the wetting solution is instilled and pretunneling is performed in the subcutaneous and prepectoral plane. The breast is first lifted from the pectoral and serratus fascia through the axillary incision. It is then dissected from the subcutaneous plane with endoscopic scissors, hemostasis is ensured, and a drain is placed prior to wound closure.

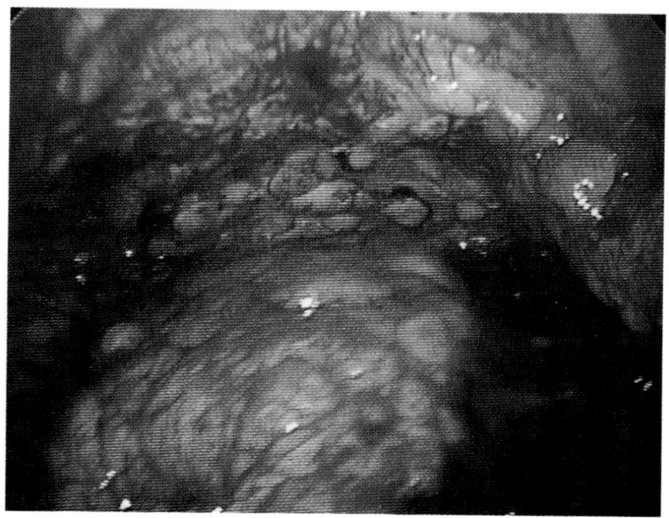

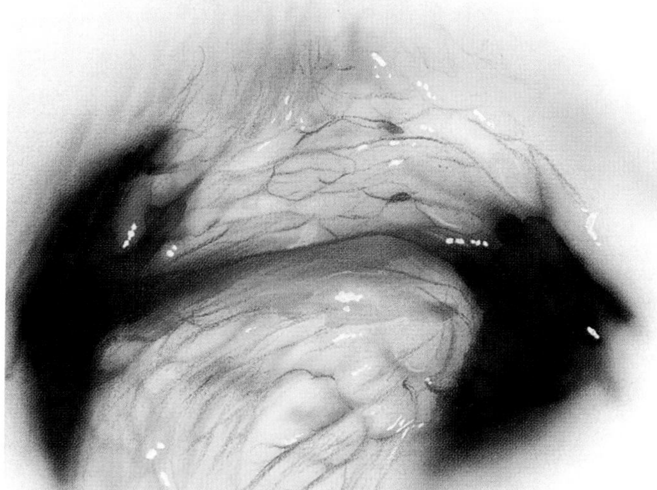

During an axillary mastectomy for gynecomastia the breast specimen is separated from the subglandular plane and the dissection is made in the subcutaneous plane with endoscopic scissors.

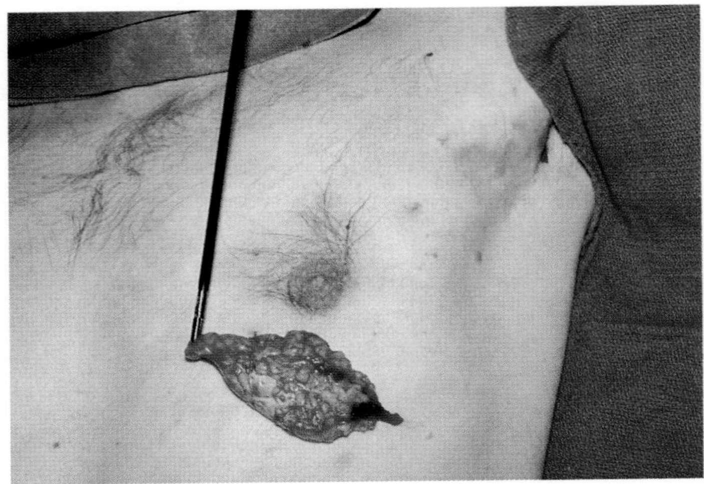

Endoscopic graspers are used to extract the specimen under endoscopic guidance. The endoretractor-mounted endoscope is removed. This provides additional space for withdrawing the specimen from the optical cavity (see Chapter 9).

Expander Placement

The endoscope can facilitate breast expander placement for delayed breast reconstruction through a reduced incision. The technique is similar to axillary subpectoral breast augmentation. The incision is made either in the axilla or lateral portion of the mastectomy scar. After the subpectoral pocket is created, the Agris-Dingman dissector is used for intraoperative dissection, expansion, and definition of the pocket prior to expander placement.

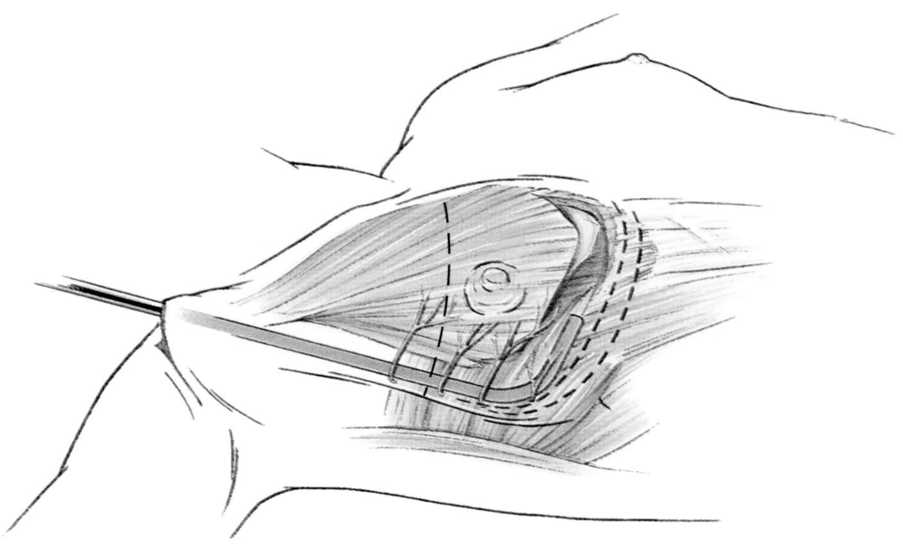

Lateral dissection of the implant pocket is performed bluntly with the Agris-Dingman dissector and the index finger.

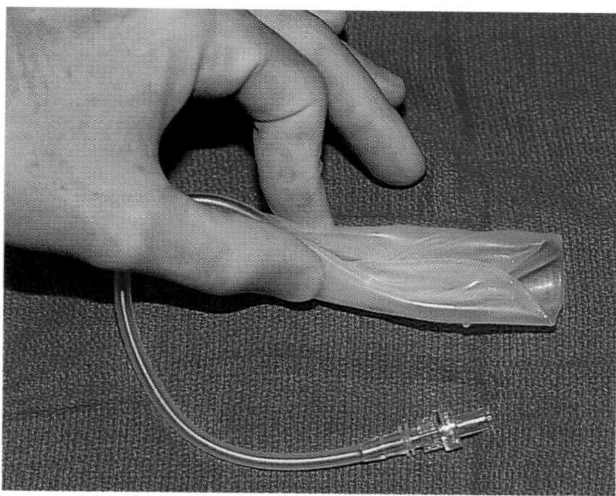

The deflated expander is prepared for insertion by shaping it into a double roll. Narrowing the roll at the end makes insertion easier (see Chapter 13).

Expander Exchange

The endoscope can also provide improved visualization through reduced incisions when exchanging the expander for a permanent implant. If a localized capsulotomy is needed to improve implant position, this can also be done. The expander may need to be deflated so that it can be removed through the short incision. The permanent device is selected, positioned, and inflated.

Implant Exchange

This technique is similar to that used for expander exchange. The endoscope can be useful for localized capsulotomy and shaping of the pocket during the exchange procedure.

Capsulotomy

In some situations the patient may benefit from an open capsulotomy. The endoscope can be introduced through a short incision and a localized capsulotomy performed under direct vision with the insulated electrocautery and blunt instruments. The reduced incision diminishes the chance of wound complications and implant exposure. The capsule provides excellent reflection of light for visualization. An electrocautery is used to make the incision, and a blunt instrument is used to separate the tissues.

Complete or Partial Capsulectomy

Although we have found it difficult to perform a total capsulectomy through a 3 cm endoscopic incision, we have been able to reduce the length of the capsulectomy incision by using the endoscope. It also provides improved visualization and illumination of the cavity to facilitate capsule removal as well as hemostasis.

Latissimus Muscle Harvest for Implant Cover

Breast implants perform better if placed under thick muscular cover. The endoscope is helpful for harvesting the latissimus dorsi muscle through the mastectomy incision and small back access incisions. The muscle is usually transposed for lower implant cover. The pectoralis major is elevated to provide upper breast implant cover. These shorter incisions reduce the postoperative deformity and pain and make this procedure more acceptable to the patient. (See Chapter 14 for a detailed discussion.)

Autologous Latissimus Dorsi Harvest

The latissimus dorsi flap that includes muscle with overlying subcutaneous tissue is useful for partial and total breast reconstruction. A short incision in the axilla, a midback incision, and the mastectomy incision provide access for endoscopic harvest. This more technically challenging procedure is described in Chapter 14.

Reconstruction of Poland's Deformity

The latissimus dorsi transposition is an important component of the treatment of the most extensive deformities such as an obvious infraclavicular flattening and an absent anterior axillary fold. The endoscope can help the reconstructive surgeon harvest the latissimus dorsi muscle through reduced incisions. It also facilitates creation of the anterior pocket for suturing the latissimus dorsi into its new position and for developing a pocket for the breast implant or expander (see Chapter 21).

Vascular Delay of the TRAM Flap

TRAM flap reliability can be enhanced with a vascular delay whereby the superficial inferior epigastric pedicle and the deep inferior epigastric pedicle are divided a few days or weeks before the procedure. The endoscope can be used to approach the deep inferior epigastric pedicle and ligate it without an extended incision. These shorter incisions may be associated with reduced morbidity. (See Chapter 15 for an in-depth discussion of TRAM flap vascular delay.)

Excision of Fat Necrosis After a TRAM Flap

When small nodules of fat necrosis develop in a TRAM flap, many patients want them removed. These areas are often high in the reconstructed breast, and a skin-sparing mastectomy has usually been performed. Before removing the mass, we perform fine-needle aspiration to obtain pathologic confirmation that it is fat necrosis. The mass is approached with the endoscope through the skin-sparing incisions or the axilla. Wetting solution and blunt dissection help create a nonbloody optical cavity through which the mass is removed. We also use the ultrasound device for cavitating and emulsifying these areas of fat necrosis. Tissue samples can be evaluated by the pathologist.

Revision of Autologous Tissue or Implant Reconstruction

An endoscopic approach can be used to remove or revise an autologous tissue reconstruction. It is also useful for adjusting the implant position with capsulotomies under endoscopic visualization if indicated.

Omentum Harvest for Breast Reconstruction

Harvest of the omentum was one of the applications for which endoscopic plastic surgery was conceived. Although the omentum has been used for decades for breast reconstruction, endoscopic harvest of the omentum requires an experienced laparoscopic surgeon and can be challenging if intra-abdominal adhesions are encountered.

Modification of Chest Wall

Some patients have costal cartilage prominences that are aesthetically unattractive. The endoscope can permit visualization of the outer cartilaginous surface and contouring to reduce the deformity. The distant hidden access site makes this procedure more acceptable to the patient.

Caveats

Although specific details of planning and technique will be discussed in subsequent chapters, the following caveats warrant consideration when endoscopic breast surgery is contemplated.

- Insert the retractor before the endoscope. It is generally better to insert the empty retractor into the initial optical space first and then slide the endoscope into the underlying sheath. This prevents smearing the end of the scope against the soft tissues as it is advanced. Before the endoscope tip is advanced free of the sheath, the endoscope is gently lifted to open the optical cavity. The endoscope can then be fully advanced past the sheath tip into the developed space to provide a clear view.
- The endoscope should not be placed directly on the patient's skin or against the drapes. The light sources (especially older models) can generate significant heat, particularly if breaks are present within the light source cord, and potentially cause burns.
- Keep the endoscope warm throughout the procedure to minimize fogging. This is best accomplished by returning the endoscope to the warm fluid bath whenever it is removed from the optical cavity for a significant period of time.
- The initial optical cavity may be best made by blunt dissection, but the surgeon should avoid creating significant bleeding that would compromise the endoscopic view. For example, gentle blunt subpectoral dissection can be used to initiate the development of the subpectoral optical cavity for augmentation, but if too vigorous, it can tear small muscular slips that stain the cavity with blood.
- Because a 30-degree scope is generally used, visualization of the roof of the optical cavity can be difficult. By withdrawing the endoscope and increasing the "toe-in" force applied to the retractor, the roof and upper portion of the dissection zone can be seen more clearly. Pivoting the endoscope at the access incision adjusts the view from side to side.
- In addition, when the endoretractor is used, a "toeing-in" force at the margin of the cavity will place the peripheral tissues under tension and permit easier dissection. Frequently advancing the retractor and adjusting the tip of the endoscope will greatly increase the effectiveness of dissection.

- During enlargement of the cavity the assistant should constantly observe the patient's skin to alert the surgeon if the dissection is becoming too superficial, which could result in skin perforation or burning.
- If a foot pedal is used to activate the cautery, this should always be activated by the surgeon and not by an assistant. Lack of coordination between the surgeon and an assistant in activating the cautery could lead to skin perforation or damage to vital structures.
- If smoke evacuation is insufficient, check the suction-cautery instrument for clogging, which occurs frequently. If this does not facilitate rapid clearance, several other maneuvers can be performed to augment circulation. Depending on the size of the access incision, either a standard plastic Yankauer sucker or a malleable endosuction tip can be placed into the wound. This secondary suction can assist with the outflow factor of cavity circulation. Another way to increase air circulation and thus clearance of the cavity is to promote better inflow. This can be accomplished either by lifting up on the heel of the endoretractor, thus dilating the access incision, or by making the incision slightly longer.
- When dissecting from an axillary incision, it may be efficient to switch the operating hands when switching sides of the patient. For example, a right-handed surgeon generally finds that holding the retractor in the left hand is most comfortable for right breast dissection but that holding the retractor in the right hand works better on the patient's left side.

The endoscope is particularly applicable for aesthetic and reconstructive breast procedures. Many of the operations are facilitated by the enhanced illumination and visualization it provides. Patients are pleased with the shorter incisions and reduced morbidity. Additional developments in equipment and technique should further expand the potential application of endoscopy in breast surgery with the eventual possibility that most breast operations will be able to be performed without the necessity of incisions over the actual breast skin.

REFERENCES

Beer GM, Kompatscher P. Endoscopic plastic surgery: The endoscopic evaluation of implants after breast augmentation. Aesthetic Plast Surg 19:353, 1995.

Bostwick J III, Eaves FF III, Nahai F. Endoscopic Plastic Surgery. St. Louis: Quality Medical Publishing, 1995.

Chajchir A, Benzaquen I, Sagnolo N, Lusicic N. Endoscopic augmentation mammaplasty. Aesthetic Plast Surg 18:377, 1994.

Cho BC, Lee JH, Ramasastry SS, Baik BS. Free latissimus dorsi muscle transfer using endoscopic technique. Ann Plast Surg 38:586, 1997.

Colon GA. Mammoscopy and endoscopic implant and breast tissue evaluation. Clin Plast Surg 22: 697, 1995.

Colon GA, Tancredi F. Mammoscopy: The endoscopy intracapsular evaluation of mammary prosthesis. Plast Reconstr Surg 91:382, 1993.

Dowden RV, Anain S. Endoscopic implant evaluation and capsulotomy. Plast Reconstr Surg 91:283, 1993.

Eaves FF III, Bostwick J III, Nahai F. Instrumentation and setup for endoscopic plastic surgery. Clin Plast Surg 22:591, 1995.

Eaves FF III, Bostwick J III, Nahai F, Murray DR, Styblo TM, Carlson GW. Endoscopic techniques in aesthetic breast surgery. Augmentation, mastectomy, biopsy, capsulotomy, capsulorrhaphy, reduction, mastopexy, and reconstructive techniques. Clin Plast Surg 22:693, 1995.

Eaves FF III, Price CI, Bostwick J III, Nahai F, Jones G, Carlson GW, Culbertson J. Subcutaneous endoscopic plastic surgery using a retractor-mounted endoscopic system. Perspect Plast Surg 7(2):1, 1993.

Faria-Correa MA. Endoscopic abdominoplasty, mastopexy, and breast reduction. Clin Plast Surg 22:723, 1995.

Fine NA, Orgill DP, Pribaz JJ. Early clinical experience in endoscopic-assisted muscle flap harvest. Ann Plast Surg 33:465, 1994.

Friedlander LD, Sundin J, Bakshandeh N. Endoscopic mastectomy and breast reconstruction: Endoscopic breast surgery. Aesthetic Plast Surg 19:27, 1995.

Ho LCY. Endoscopic assisted transaxillary augmentation mammaplasty. Br J Plast Surg 46:332, 1993.

Howard PS, Oslin BD, Moore JR. Endoscopic transaxillary submuscular augmentation mammaplasty with textured saline breast implants. Ann Plast Surg 37:12, 1996.

Kamei Y, Torii S, Hasegawa T, Hishizeki O. Endoscopic omental harvest. Plast Reconstr Surg 102: 2450, 1998.

Karp NS, Bass LS, Kasabian AK, Eidelman Y, Hausman MR. Balloon-assisted endoscopic harvest of the latissimus dorsi muscle. Plast Reconstr Surg 100:1161, 1997.

Kompatscher P. Endoscopic capsulotomy of capsular contracture after breast augmentation: A very challenging therapeutic approach [Letter]. Plast Reconstr Surg 100:1161, 1997.

Masuoka T, Fujikawa M, Yamamoto H, Ohyama T, Inoue Y, Takao T, Hosokawa K. Breast reconstruction after mastectomy without additional scarring: Application of endoscopic latissimus dorsi muscle harvest. Ann Plast Surg 40:123, 1998.

Miller MJ. Minimally invasive techniques of tissue harvest in head and neck reconstruction. Clin Plast Surg 21:149, 1994.

Monticciolo DL, Ross D, Bostwick J III, Eaves FF III, Styblo T. Autologous breast reconstruction with endoscopic latissimus dorsi musculosubcutaneous flaps in patients choosing breast-conserving therapy: Mammographic appearance. Am J Radiol 167:385, 1996.

Narayanan K, Liang MD, Chandra M, Grundfest WS. Experimental endoscopic subcutaneous surgery. J Laparoendosc Surg 2:179, 1992.

Ohyama T, Takada A, Fujikawa M, Hosokawa K. Endoscopic-assisted transaxillary removal of glandular tissue in gynecomastia. Ann Plast Surg 40:62, 1998.

Pitman GH. Liposuction and Aesthetic Surgery. St. Louis: Quality Medical Publishing, 1993.

Price CI, Eaves FF III, Nahai F, Jones G, Bostwick J III. Endoscopic transaxillary subpectoral breast augmentation. Plast Reconstr Surg 94:612, 1994.

Ramirez OM, Daniel RK. Endoscopic-assisted transaxillary submuscular breast augmentation. In Endoscopic Aesthetic Surgery. New York: Springer-Verlag, 1994.

Restifo RJ, Ahmed SS, Rosser J, Zahir K, Zink J, Lalikos JA, Thomson JG. TRAM flap perforator ligation and the delay phenomenon: Development of an endoscopic/laparoscopic delay procedure. Plast Reconstr Surg 101:1503, 1998.

Saltz R. Endoscopic harvest of the omental and jejunal free flaps. Clin Plast Surg 22:747, 1995.

Sasaki GH. Endoscopic, Aesthetic, and Reconstructive Surgery. Philadelphia: Lippincott-Raven, 1996.

Serra JM, Benito JR, Monner J, Zayuelas J, Parraga A. Tissue expansion with endoscopy. Ann Plast Surg 38:101, 1997.

Talamini MA, Gadacz TR. Equipment and instrumentation. In Zucker KA, ed. Surgical Laparoscopy Update. St. Louis: Quality Medical Publishing, 1993, pp 3-84.

Teimourian B, Kroll SS. Subcutaneous endoscopy in suction lipectomy. Plast Reconstr Surg 74:708, 1984.

Van Buskirk ER, Rehnke RD, Montgomery RL, Eubanks S, Ferraro FJ, Levin LS. Endoscopic harvest of the latissimus dorsi muscle using the balloon dissection technique. Plast Reconstr Surg 99: 899, 1997.

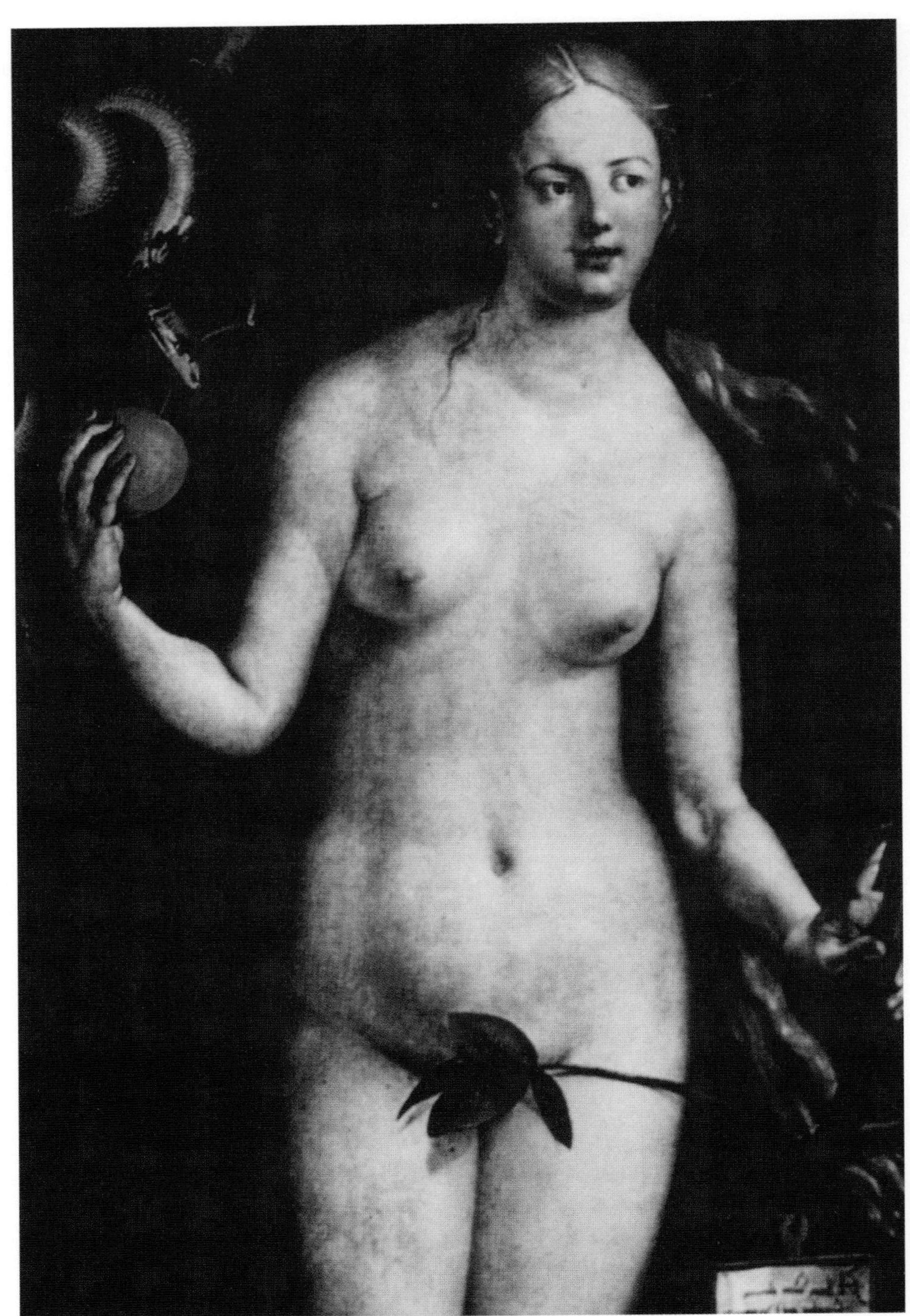

5 Implants and Expanders

Key Topics

Questions About Implants and Expanders

Tissue Response and Surface Bioactivity

Evaluation of Implant and Expander Options

- Smooth Surface vs. Textured Surface
- Round vs. Anatomic Shaped
- Tissue Expander vs. Expander Implant

Selection Criteria

Recommendations

Clinical Applications

- Augmentation Mammaplasty
- Mastopexy-Augmentation
- Breast Reconstruction

Capsular Contracture

- Classification
- Strategies to Decrease Incidence
- Treatment

Observations

Implants and expanders remain essential building blocks in aesthetic and reconstructive breast surgery. Neither controversy nor media attention has served to obviate their value in enhancing breast size, restoring breast shape and contour, and correcting breast and chest wall deformities and asymmetries. As surgeons, we have come to rely on these devices because of the obvious benefits they confer while recognizing the limitations that are associated with any foreign body. Today, in light of public concerns raised about implants, the surgeon needs to be alert to the potential anxieties that may accompany a woman's inquiry about implant surgery. He must be prepared to invest the time to address her questions about these devices, fully apprise her of their potential risks and benefits, and help her to reach an informed decision as to which technique is best for her particular situation and whether implants or expanders play a role in that scenario. The challenge lies in acquiring a working knowledge of the various devices available, in selecting the best implant or expander for each patient's specific problem, in fully educating the patient about these devices and their risks and limitations, in long-term monitoring of patients for problems, and in continuing the quest for the ideal implantable device.

On the surface the choices appear straightforward. Two basic types of implantable devices are available: fixed-volume breast implants and tissue expanders. However, a variety of specialized designs and features serve to increase the options. For instance, the outer envelope is available with smooth or a variety of textured silicone surfaces. Textured silicone appears to help decrease the incidence of capsular contracture in some situations and ensure a softer, more predictably stable breast. Devices have also been designed for variable, incremental, and directional filling of the breast implants and expanders, either intraoperatively or postoperatively, permitting more control over breast volume. Furthermore, the shape of these implants can be modified and anatomic-shaped implants introduced to provide different contours and enhanced projection to meet the individualized needs of patients. These devices are manufactured in a broad range of shapes and sizes. Devices can also be custom designed according to specific physician prescription to provide better contour restoration for individual reconstructive problems than the standard implants.

While choice of shape, size, and surface texture has expanded, options for filling materials have become more limited. Most implants marketed in the United States today are filled with saline solution. Silicone gel–filled implants remain unrestricted in many parts of the world, but they are available on a relatively limited basis in the United States and primarily for breast reconstruction. However, they are being reevaluated by the FDA and may become available again after completion of the clinical studies and FDA evaluation. Other filling materials such as hydrocolloid and purified soybean oil are under investigation, but the long-term safety and efficacy of these fillings has not yet been established and await FDA approval.

The breast surgeon therefore has a panoply of breast implants and expanders for augmentation mammaplasty, mastopexy with augmentation, and breast reconstruction to choose from. Because of the variety of modifications available, it is difficult for any surgeon to gain extensive, long-term experience with every device.*

Surgical Expertise

To avoid the confusion inherent in learning about and using a number of different devices as they become available, some surgeons choose to become familiar with a single device and use it for most augmentation mammaplasties and breast reconstructions. Such conservatism produces few surprises for the surgeon, but it can limit reconstructive versatility, hamper treatment of implant-related complications, and prevent the use of recently introduced devices that may produce a superior result for the patient. Other reconstructive surgeons eagerly embrace the most recently introduced "high-tech" devices for augmentation mammaplasty and breast reconstruction. They change their techniques and devices frequently. The pitfall is obvious; the surgeon may not develop sufficient experience with specific devices and thus his complication rate may increase.

All surgeons using these devices must be aware of the different types of implants and expanders available for breast implantation and have an artistic appreciation and technical understanding of implant form, selection criteria, and principles of implantation. To select the most appropriate implantable device the surgeon must be conversant with clinical data and laboratory studies concerning bioactivity, physical properties, mechanisms of action, capsular contracture, carcinogenicity, toxicology, immunology, and complications.

With that goal in mind this chapter will assess the implantable devices for breast surgery on the market and offer descriptions of many of the currently

*The manufacturers' product information is an important guide for evaluating newer implants and expanders.

available breast implants and tissue expanders. It will also provide key information on educating the patient about implants and expanders and counseling her on risks, benefits, and realistic expectations to promote better doctor/patient communication and to most wisely avoid but also to manage possible risks associated with implant surgery.

This discussion is not intended to be all inclusive; rather the focus is on personal clinical experiences and observations using these devices. It begins with a discussion of the patient education process and the understanding that needs to be established between doctor and patient. Suggestions for addressing frequently posed questions and concerns about implants and expanders are presented. The remainder of the chapter examines the different categories of devices, with attention directed to the specific properties, qualities, and characteristics of each; their advantages and disadvantages; and particular applications and anticipated results. Suggestions are provided for implant selection, placement, and postoperative management. Special attention is devoted to capsular contracture and strategies for avoidance and treatment.

*Patient Education: Frequently Posed Questions About Implants and Expanders**

With all of the coverage that implants have received in the popular media, many women who inquire about implant surgery are also interested in learning more about these devices and their possible sequelae. They often inquire about what they are made of, whether they are harmful, how long they will last, and what potential complications may occur. To supplement information provided in consultation with these patients, I also provide them with a patient education manual that comprehensively addresses questions about implants and expanders. In this way, prospective implant candidates are able to read more about the pros and cons of implant surgery and understand the latest scientific findings about these devices before they decide to proceed with surgery. Most patients appreciate this information and find it reassuring.

Following are questions frequently posed by patients and the answers that I typically use to address them when discussing these devices.

*These questions and answers have been excerpted from Berger K, Bostwick J III. *What Women Want To Know About Breast Implants,* a patient education manual published by Quality Medical Publishing, St. Louis, Mo.

What kinds of breast implants are currently available?

Two basic types of implantable devices are available: fixed-volume implants and implants in which the volume can be altered after implantation (tissue expanders). All of the currently available implants have an outer layer or envelope of silicone elastomer that is in contact with the body tissues.

These implants are usually filled with normal saline solution. Silicone gel–filled implants are also available but on a relatively limited basis in the United States and primarily for reconstructive purposes or for replacement in women with silicone implants.*

Implants and expanders are also available with smooth and textured silicone surfaces. These textured surfaces are used to help reduce the incidence of capsular contracture after implant surgery, to stabilize the devices, and to facilitate tissue expansion. However, textured implants have a thicker elastomer shell and for some patients these textured-surface implants may be more visible and may exhibit a rippled appearance through thin skin. The thicker shell may fold and become more susceptible to fold-flaw problems and potential deflation.

Is silicone safe to use in humans?

The versatility and safety of silicone has long been acknowledged by physicians with years of experience using a variety of silicone products for a broad range of medical applications. Patients, however, are far more circumspect in their opinions and often inquire about the safety of silicone. It helps to provide them with an overview of the many ways that silicone is used.

I explain that silicone is a commonly used substance for various implantable devices and is considered by many to be one of the least reactive biomaterials. Initially introduced for evaluation in medical applications in the 1940s, silicone is used for artificial joints, implantable pumps, shunts, drains, ocular implants, and other devices that require a material that is relatively nonreactive, nonallergenic, and easily tolerated by the body. Implantable silicone devices include pacemakers, hydrocephalus shunts, ocular lens implants, breast implants, penile implants, and testicular implants. Anyone who has ever taken a tablet or capsule has probably ingested silicone, for it is used to coat many capsules to make them more easily swallowed. Silicone is also present in processed foods, in cosmetics, and in many drugs (especially antacids). Silicone is used to lubricate syringes, in intravenous tubing, and in shunts used for chemotherapy. Anyone who has had blood drawn or been

*Silicone implants are being reevaluated by the FDA and may be approved again after all clinical studies are completed as well as the FDA evaluation.

given an injection has had some silicone introduced into his or her body. Many infant pacifiers are made of silicone. If silicone represents a serious chemical hazard to the human body, this should already be apparent because of this chemical's widespread use. Nevertheless, ongoing studies continue to rule out the possibility of currently unrecognized and rare problems. New silicone devices are routinely receiving FDA approval. For example, silicone oil, a product for treating complicated cases of retinal detachment, has received FDA authorization to be marketed.

What problems are associated with implants and how often do they occur?

As with all devices, implants are not without problems. They are subject to local complications such as rupture, possible leakage, deflation, displacement, deformation, and capsular contracture, the latter being the most common problem. They also may interfere with mammograms and cause calcium deposits to accumulate in the capsule tissue that forms around implants. Breast implant surgery may cause changes in breast and nipple sensation. These problems are not life threatening, however, and are usually correctable.

What is capsular contracture? What risks does it pose for women who have implant surgery?

A capsule is firm, fibrous scar tissue that forms around a breast implant. This is a characteristic response of the body to isolate any foreign substance; similar scar formation with collagen deposition can be observed around most other implants regardless of whether they contain silicone, including hip implants, artificial joints, hydrocephalus shunts, heart valves, and pacemakers. For unknown reasons, in some cases the scar tissue capsule may become thick and constrict a soft implant. This phenomenon is referred to as capsular contracture. This condition can make the breast feel harder and firmer than desirable, producing a rounded or spherical breast appearance; sometimes it can also cause pain and rarely it may incite a fluid accumulation or even precipitate implant exposure through thin skin. The severity of this problem varies with each individual. Ideally, the capsular layer surrounding the implant does not thicken, tighten, or contract and affect the shape of the breast. In some women it manifests itself as a slight breast firmness and requires no treatment. Actually, most implants feel somewhat firmer than when first implanted once the initial healing process is over. Many women find this minimal firmness acceptable and are not motivated to undergo further adjustments of their reconstructed or augmented breasts. In more severe cases of capsular contracture, however, a woman may experience significant discomfort and elect to have an operation to release some or all of the scar tissue (capsulotomy) or to remove it (capsulectomy), usually with replacement of the implant. During this secondary operation the surgeon may reposition the implant under the pectoralis major muscle if previously placed over the muscle or he may exchange the implant for one with different surface characteristics after releasing or removing the capsule. The textured-surface implants appear to have a lower incidence of capsular contracture in the subglandular position and when used for tissue expansion. Patients who continue to experience problems after surgical correction may decide to have their implants removed (explanted). After explantation, an aesthetic procedure such as a breast lift (mastopexy) may be necessary to achieve an optimal breast appearance, or rarely the implant is replaced with autologous tissue.

Although capsular contracture may be uncomfortable and produce breast distortion and asymmetry, it is not a health hazard. With the use of textured-surface breast implants in the subglandular position, capsular contracture is estimated to occur in approximately 2% to 4% of cases in some studies and in as many as 4% to 9% in others. Smooth-surface saline implants, while having a higher reported capsular contracture rate in the subglandular position, have a low incidence when placed subpectorally.

What can be done to avoid capsular contracture?

The incidence of capsular contracture is lower when the implant is placed behind the pectoral muscle. Using implants with a textured surface also seems to reduce the likelihood of capsular contracture in the subglandular position. When smooth-surface implants are used, some surgeons recommend breast massage of the implant in the breast pocket in an effort to prevent or reduce the incidence and severity of fibrous capsule formation around the implant. There is no scientific evidence, however, that breast massage is helpful in preventing contracture. Massage is not necessary for implants with a textured surface.

Can calcium deposits be mistaken for calcifications associated with breast cancer?

Sometimes calcium forms in the capsule around the breast implant after it has been implanted for many years. These deposits may increase the hardening; however, they have a characteristic appearance on mammography and can be differentiated from calcifications associated with breast cancer. Breast surgery, including breast reduction, breast lift, and breast reconstruction with a woman's own tissues, can also cause calcifications visible on mammography. Women with calcified capsules should usually have a total capsulectomy when their implants are changed.

What effects will breast implant surgery have on breast sensation?

Women having implant surgery for augmentation may experience changes in breast and nipple-areola sensation. A knowledge of the specific breast nerves and careful blunt dissection to avoid dividing them reduce the possibility of denervation and anesthetic breasts. Although most of these changes are temporary, in some cases they prove permanent. Women having breast reconstruction with or without implants already have diminished sensation because of the nerves severed during the mastectomy.

Will implants or expanders interfere with mammograms?

Both saline-filled and silicone gel–filled implants are radiopaque and can pose some breast imaging problems. Silicone implants are opaque to x-rays; saline implants are less so; therefore breast tissue overlying or underlying the implant may be masked by the implant on the breast films. Women should make sure that they inform the breast imager that a breast implant or expander is present so that well-defined additional tangential and special displacement and compression mammographic views can be taken. Imaging of the parenchyma therefore requires additional views combined with upward displacement of the implant and anterior, forward compression of the breast. Ultrasound, magnetic resonance imaging (MRI), computed tomography (CT), and positron emission tomography (PET) are other techniques for delineating breast implants and defining breast masses. In addition, if the implant is positioned submusculofascially, the gland can be more easily pulled away from the chest wall if spherical contracture develops. The overlying breast parenchyma can become compressed and more dense when capsular contracture develops around a subglandular implant or expander, making it more difficult for an early breast cancer to be seen on a mammogram and inhibiting the early detection of a breast cancer. The spherical shape and the noncompressibility of an implant within a tight capsule can pose imaging problems when only the standard two screening mammographic views are used. But when the submusculofascial position is used, the implant is located behind the breast parenchyma, which can be pushed forward for better visualization; thus breast biopsies and even partial and total mastectomies can be done with the implant left undisturbed in the submusculofascial position. Most oncologic surgeons and breast radiologists now recommend that the breast implant be inserted in the submusculofascial or subpectoral position. Lumpectomy/irradiation for the treatment of small breast cancers is now used in selected women who have had augmentation mammaplasty. The breast implant does not affect the amount of therapeutic radiation that is administered.

It should also be noted, however, that the presence or absence of capsular contracture is more important than implant site in determining the effectiveness of mammography in women with implants. Because a woman with breast implants usually has small thin breasts, breast self-examination and regular physician examination are very effective for detecting small masses and breast cancer.

Will implants or expanders mask or delay the detection of cancer?

Periodically reports appear in the literature concerning the problem of detection of breast cancer in the presence of a breast implant. A breast implant should always be placed behind the breast parenchyma after augmentation or behind subcutaneous fat and any breast remnants after mastectomy. Thus, except in the rarest of circumstances, a breast cancer or recurrence would develop in front of the device.

The position of the implant or expander relative to the musculofascial layer and especially the presence of a spherical capsular contracture also can affect the physical examination as well as breast imaging. Implant folds and palpable edges can mimic a breast lump and may prompt the physician to do a breast biopsy. (These folds have been aspirated with a needle, causing implant deflation.) When a breast biopsy is planned for a patient who has a breast implant, the patient should be examined preoperatively by a plastic surgeon and preparations made to exchange the implant or perform a capsulotomy or other modifications if the mass is related to an implant defect or rupture. Rupture of a silicone gel–filled implant can cause siliconoma if the material extravasates through the capsule into the adjacent breast parenchyma. Patients with an implant in place who are scheduled for a breast biopsy should undergo breast imaging before the procedure to assess implant integrity and to better define the mass. MRI with a special program for the detection of silicone can accurately identify small extracapsular droplets of silicone.

The presence of a breast implant or expander does not alter a woman's risk of breast cancer or change the incidence or course of existing breast cancer. A woman and her physicians should always be vigilant for signs of breast cancer. A yearly examination by a plastic surgeon or a qualified member of the breast management team is recommended. She must look for a developing breast mass through monthly breast self-examination, have regular physician monitoring, and undergo scheduled breast imaging with appropriate views to image the implanted breast under the suggested guidelines. Any changes should be brought to the attention of her plastic surgeon.

Can the implant be rejected by a woman's body?

"Rejection" refers to the allergic or immune response that causes the body to literally reject a foreign substance through an antigen-antibody response. In this sense implants are not rejected. However, capsular contracture can develop, the overlying breast skin may become thinned, infection can develop, or healing may be incomplete, leading to implant exposure and necessitating implant removal. Although these are complications, they are not tantamount to rejection.

Can an implant be removed?

When an implant is not performing as intended or if the woman feels that she would be better off without the implant, it can be removed in an operation called explantation. In most cases explantation can be performed on an outpatient basis. The capsule may also have to be removed in a procedure called capsulectomy, especially if it is thickened, contains calcium, or distorts the breast. Additional aesthetic corrections may be necessary after removal, most frequently a mastopexy, usually with a periareolar or vertical incision.

How long do implants last?

There are no precise figures on the life span of implants at present. We do know that silicone breast implants have been available for use in patients since 1964 and that many of the original devices are still in place. Implants can last from a very short time to many years, depending on the surgical technique used, the patient, and the type of implant. However, just as human and artificial organs can fail and require transplantation, breast implants also may fail or leak and have to be replaced. Breast implants should not be considered "lifetime" devices. A woman who has implant surgery should be followed by her physicians over the long term so her breasts can be monitored for possible problems as a part of her general health regimen.

How strong are implants? Can they be broken during mammography? What factors increase the chance that an implant will rupture?

Although breast implants are manufactured to specific standards requiring that they withstand breast compression as well as multiple and long-term physical stress, these devices are not indestructible. The outer shell of the implant can break if subjected to severe physical trauma such as pressure from a seat belt during a car accident, and certainly from a needle stick. Compression views taken during mammography are calibrated to avoid undue pressure that could rupture or deflate a breast implant.

The chance for rupture or deflation may increase with normal wear and tear and the length of time the device has been implanted. The incidence of rupture increases when the implant develops folds or rippling on the outer surface. Implants with thicker elastomer envelopes can develop more distinct folds and leak at a fold-flaw point. Trauma or injury to the breast also increases the chance of rupture as may closed capsulotomy (a technique to correct capsular contracture in which strong pressure is applied to the breast to break up the scar tissue around the implant). This technique is less frequently used today and is not recommended by the manufacturers.

What happens if a saline-filled implant deflates?

There is a possibility of deflation of saline implants if a leak develops in the implant covering and may require reoperation with implant replacement. When a saline implant begins to leak, the breast typically begins a slow deflation over a period of hours to days. Leaking implants should be exchanged over the next month before development of a capsular contracture, which would complicate the simple replacement process. Currently available saline implants have a relatively low deflation rate reported to range from 1.7% to 5.5% over 5 years.

What happens if a silicone gel–filled implant leaks?

When the cover of a silicone implant is pierced or ruptures, the gel usually remains within the fibrous capsule or membrane that develops naturally around the implant and does not travel to other parts of the body. Significant trauma can cause tears in the surrounding capsule, and the gel can migrate into the breast and possibly beyond the breast to form lumps (granulomas or siliconomas) nearby. Some of this silicone can cause enlarged lymph nodes in the armpit area (lymphadenopathy). When silicone escapes to other parts of the body such as the arm or upper abdomen, removal can be difficult. Gel migration outside the capsule rarely occurs, however, and if it does, the viscosity or thickness of the gel seems to reduce its ability to migrate. Currently magnetic resonance imaging is the most sensitive test for assessing silicone implant integrity or detecting extracapsular silicone.

What is silicone bleed?

Silicone bleed refers to microscopic amounts of silicone fluid that seep through the silicone implant's envelope. Although most of this is trapped within the implant pocket or the surrounding scar tissue, minute amounts of silicone could possibly migrate through the capsule. The majority of implants manufactured after 1985 have a low-bleed elastomer design and more cohesive gel that reduces leakage.

Are implants or expanders toxic or linked to cancer?

The possibility that a mammary implant or expander could increase the risk of breast carcinoma has worried surgeons, patients, basic scientists, and other interested observers since these devices first became available in the early 1950s. Although it is possible for breast cancer to develop in a woman whose breasts have been augmented, no evidence exists in either clinical or research data collected over 35 years to indicate that women with any of the breast implants or expanders available today are at increased risk for breast cancer. In the years that breast implants have been available they have been studied extensively by plastic surgeons, implant manufacturers, scientists, and government regulatory agencies such as the FDA. In all that time no scientific studies have documented an increased risk of breast cancer attributable to implants nor is there any evidence that these devices have adversely affected the course of breast cancer when they are used for breast reconstruction. Large population studies from California, Denmark, Sweden, France, and Canada have all indicated that the incidence of breast cancer in women with silicone breast implants is the same or possibly lower than in women who have not had implants. The FDA's current informed consent document serves to underscore these findings by stating that "there is presently no scientific evidence that links either silicone gel–filled or saline-filled breast implants with cancer." The research from cancer experts and institutions through the world, such as the U.S. National Cancer Institute, the Karolinska Institute in Sweden, the Danish Cancer Registry, the Fred Hutchinson Cancer Research Center, the Institute Gustave Roussy in France, the Alberta Canada Cancer Board, and the U.S. Centers for Disease Control and Prevention, among others, seems to indicate a general consensus that breast implants do not increase a woman's risk of developing breast cancer and that there is no greater incidence of breast cancer among women with implants than in the general population.

Can implants cause connective tissue or autoimmune disease in healthy women?

There have been allegations that implants can cause or exacerbate immune-related or connective tissue disorders (rare disorders such as lupus erythematosus, dermatomyositis, scleroderma, and rheumatoid arthritis in which the body reacts to its own tissue as though it were a foreign material). This possibility has been carefully evaluated by respected immunologists and rheumatologists in numerous national and international scientific studies. The consensus after extensive scientific investigation is that there is no conclusive scientific evidence to indicate that there is an increased incidence of such diseases in patients with breast implants. Although these conditions may exist concurrently, there is no evidence that a silicone implant has caused or contributed to autoimmune disease. Even the FDA's own *Epidemiological Review* published in 1996 concurs that "current research has tended to rule out large increases in risk for connective tissue disease caused by breast implants."

Should women diagnosed with connective tissue diseases or autoimmune diseases have reconstruction with breast implants?

These diseases are rare, and scientific studies are under way to define and better understand these conditions. Because of their unpredictable clinical course, however, if a woman has any of these conditions or a family history of these conditions, she should probably not have either silicone or saline implants. Some rheumatologists recommend that patients with scleroderma minimize trauma of any kind. That includes all cosmetic or elective surgery, not just operations involving implants. The natural history of these conditions is progressive, and if implants are placed the patient naturally questions if this progression will be affected by the implants. Radiation oncologists also do not recommend radiation therapy for these women.

What possible complications can occur with implant surgery?

As with any surgical procedure, there is the potential for complications, including reactions to anesthesia as well as infection, hematoma, bleeding, seroma, delayed wound healing, and capsular contracture with possible implant exposure requiring removal.

How does the incidence of complications from implant surgery compare to that encountered with other common operations such as appendectomy, mastectomy, and hysterectomy?

The rate of complications experienced after breast implantation is comparable to and sometimes lower than the rate of complications from other commonly performed operations. A study by Gabriel et al. published in 1997 in *The New England Journal of Medicine* examined the rate of local complications requiring reoperation in women with breast implants and found that approximately 24% of women studied experienced at least one surgically treated complication over the period of follow-up. According to Dr. Gabriel, "These rates are about the same as the rates reported for breast reconstruction without implants and are comparable to reports from other centers." Patients having breast implant surgery generally have a lower incidence of conditions such as infection, hematoma, pulmonary emboli, and deep vein thrombosis. However, reoperation because of capsular contracture or to achieve a better final breast appearance is necessary in a significant number of cases.

Implants

The silicone breast implant is the prototype for breast implants. After its introduction in 1963 by Cronin and Gerow it was the most frequently used implant for augmentation mammaplasty and for breast reconstruction. Over the years more than 1 million of these devices were implanted and numerous modifications introduced. It proved to be a predictable and safe device for enlarging the breasts and improving the chest wall contour for congenital, developmental, and mastectomy deformities. Inflatable implants were developed to permit breast augmentation without silicone gel, to provide more control of implant volume, and to lower the incidence of capsular contracture. Today, in light of the restricted availability of silicone gel–filled implants, saline inflatable implants have become the standard implants widely used for plastic surgery of the breast. Saline is a safe, biocompatible material, and should a leak or deflation occur, the primary side effect is loss of breast volume.

Although early saline-inflatable implants had unacceptably high deflation rates, sometimes related to improper volume of saline filling and fatigue spots and fold-flaw failures in the elastomers, current devices have proved quite durable with acceptably low deflation rates. When the saline-inflatable implant is used, the manufacturer's recommendations regarding specific volume requirements should be followed meticulously. The volume listed is the recommended minimal volume; infiltration of an additional 10% volume can help avoid folds, ripples, and deflation. If underinflated, folds can develop and surface fatigue from constant motion at these sites can contribute to early implant fold-flaw failure.

TISSUE RESPONSE AND SURFACE BIOACTIVITY

The normal wound healing associated with the smooth-surface breast implant is a well-defined process. An initial acute inflammatory phase during the first few days is followed by fibroplasia. When these devices are implanted, fibroblasts enter the wound and lay down collagen. As the collagen becomes cross-linked, it entirely surrounds the breast implant and a capsule or interface forms around the implant. The capsule characteristically has a low vascularity and a small number of fibroblasts. Myofibroblasts have been found in the capsule and are postulated to contribute to the development of capsular contracture. It is also postulated that a low-grade or subclinical infection, usually caused by *Staphylococcus epidermidis,* normal flora in most women's breasts, is responsible for modifying the healing process and contributing to capsular contracture. These organisms have been shown to adhere to the surface of the breast implant. Topical antibiotics are thought to decrease the incidence of capsular contracture. The firmness of the breast is not related to the thickness or thinness of the capsule surrounding the implant, and bacteria are not always found in the capsular contracture. The infection rate reported in several series of breast augmentation patients averages about 1%. The implant does not need to be removed if an infection develops. Other rare types of infection such as those caused by *Mycobacterium* and other unusual organisms can occur around breast implants, and capsulectomy as well as culture-specific antimicrobials may be necessary.

Implants with textured, bioactive surfaces that bond with host tissue are more likely to provide a stable interface than are inert smooth-surface devices that become separated from the host by a fibrous capsule. When the fibrous capsule tightens or constricts, a firm breast develops. It is for this reason that displacement exercises and postoperative physical therapy using implant motion seem critical to breast softness when smooth-surface implants are used. Because there is no bonding between the implant and tissue, bacterial contamination of the entire surface of a smooth-surface implant is possible.

SELECTION CRITERIA

The base diameter and measurements of the breast implant are important clinical criteria for selecting the proper implant. Manufacturers provide charts and templates of the implant diameters that help in making this determination. The implant diameter must be related to the actual planned breast diameter and is a more important measurement than the volume estimate, which is helpful but of secondary importance. The implant diameter must also be appropriate for the vertical breast dimensions as well as the nipple position. The implant must fit properly and aesthetically behind the breast and have the correct relationship to the inframammary crease, nipple-areola, and supra-areolar area. For example, a wide implant inserted behind a breast with a high inframammary crease and low nipple can produce too much upper breast fullness.

The diameter of the implant should be approximately the same or slightly less than the proposed breast diameter. Implants with a base diameter greater than the base diameter of the breast tend to produce a flattened, broad breast appearance with the implant extending beyond the natural breast limits laterally and superiorly toward the clavicle and axilla. If a patient desires a larger volume, which often means more breast projection than can be obtained with an implant that is the appropriate base diameter for the breast, immediate expansion can be used. ***Wider implants often do not provide significantly more projection despite the added volume.***

Implant options

- Round smooth-surface saline inflatable
- Round textured-surface saline inflatable
- Anatomic-shaped or contoured textured-surface saline inflatable
- Postoperatively adjustable textured-surface saline inflatable

ROUND SMOOTH-SURFACE IMPLANT

Smooth-surface implants have a low incidence of capsular contracture when placed in a subpectoral position. These devices are manufactured solely in round shapes, which, when placed in a generous subpectoral pocket, have some mobility that enables them to respond to gravity and produce a more natural breast appearance. The smooth surface facilitates implant insertion and positioning through reduced incisions associated with endoscopic procedures. Results using these smooth-surface devices have been generally acceptable; however, their performance is compromised by the occurrence of clinically significant capsular contracture when they are placed in a subglandular position for breast augmentation.

SMOOTH-SURFACE IMPLANT SPECIFICATIONS

Round Saline Implant

(Courtesy Mentor Corporation)

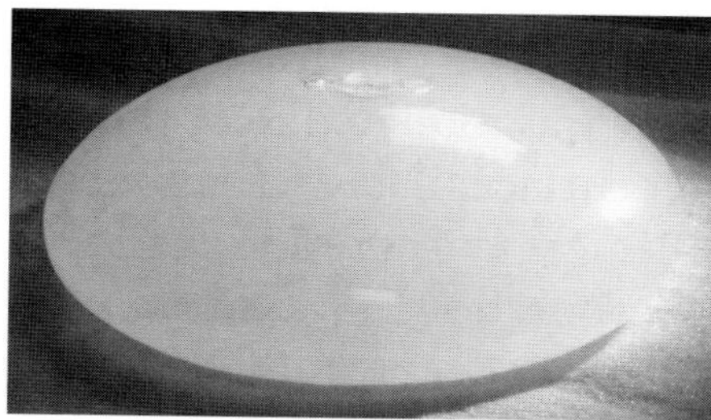

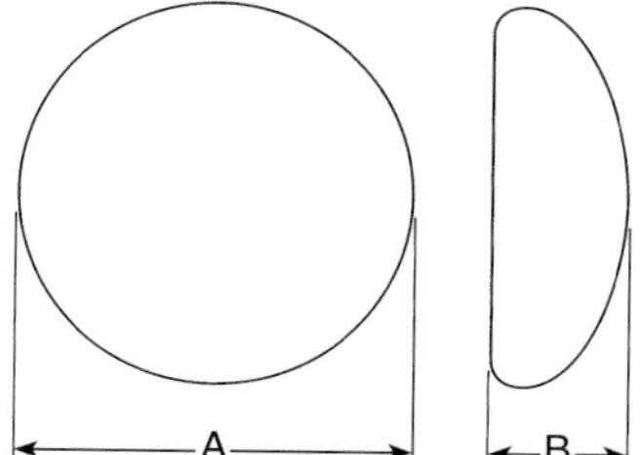

Device Volume (cc)	A Diameter (cm)	B Projection (cm)
125 + 25	9.5	3.0
150 + 25	10.0	3.1
175 + 25	10.6	3.3
200 + 25	11.0	3.4
225 + 25	11.5	3.5
250 + 25	11.9	3.6
275 + 25	12.3	3.7
300 + 25	12.6	3.7
325 + 50	13.0	3.8
350 + 50	13.3	3.9
375 + 50	13.6	4.0
425 + 50	14.2	4.1
475 + 50	14.8	4.2
525 + 50	15.0	4.2
575 + 50	15.0	4.5
625 + 75	15.2	4.6
700 + 75	15.6	4.9

Style 68 Round Saline Implant

(Courtesy McGhan Medical Corporation)

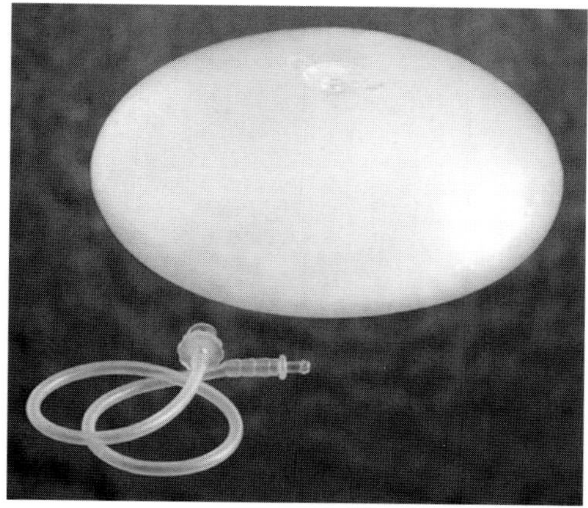

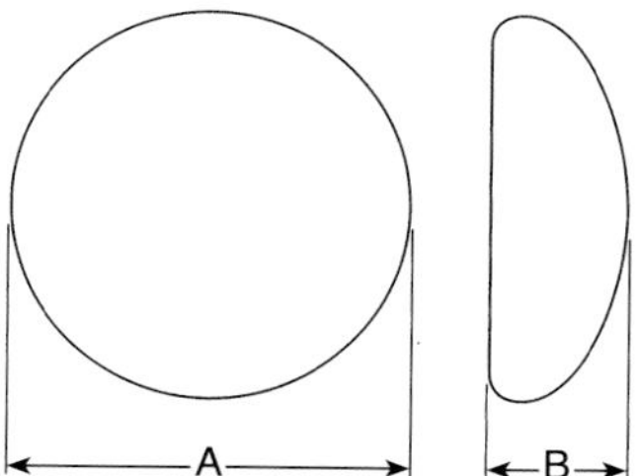

Fill Volume (cc)	A Diameter (cm)	B Projection (cm)
120-150	9.0	3.0
150-180	9.6	3.3
180-210	10.2	3.4
210-240	10.6	3.7
240-270	11.1	3.8
270-300	11.6	3.9
300-330	11.9	4.1
330-360	12.3	4.2
360-390	12.7	4.2
390-420	13.0	4.5
420-450	13.4	4.5
450-480	13.7	4.6
480-510	14.1	4.6
510-540	14.4	4.6
550-600	14.6	4.9
600-650	15.0	5.0
650-700	15.2	5.3
700-750	15.6	5.4
750-800	15.9	5.6
800-850	16.4	5.6

ROUND AND ANATOMIC-SHAPED TEXTURED-SURFACE IMPLANT

Favorable clinical reports on the softness and performance of polyurethane-covered implants, which are no longer available in the United States, combined with studies of the relationship of physical surface properties to implant biologic reactivity led to the development of the textured-surface breast implant in 1987. The outer silicone elastomer was modified to provide a roughened, irregular, textured silicone elastomer surface that externally actually resembles an open-pore foam (McGhan Medical Corporation) or the surface of the polyurethane implant (Mentor Corporation). Studies show that the textured-surface and smooth-surface implants affect wound healing differently. These laboratory studies have also demonstrated that the physical properties of the textured surfaces may promote adherence. Bonding of textured-surface implants to the surrounding tissues may also decrease the potential for pericapsular infection.

These devices are manufactured in round as well as contoured shapes. The outer textured shells on these implants tend to be thicker with significant surface folds that can be visible and palpable when there is thin skin cover overlying them, resulting in noticeable outer ripples and surface irregularities. The implant's uneven surface is less noticeable when there is good skin and subcutaneous tissue or breast parenchyma cover.

TEXTURED-SURFACE IMPLANT SPECIFICATIONS

Siltex Round Saline Implant

(Courtesy Mentor Corporation)

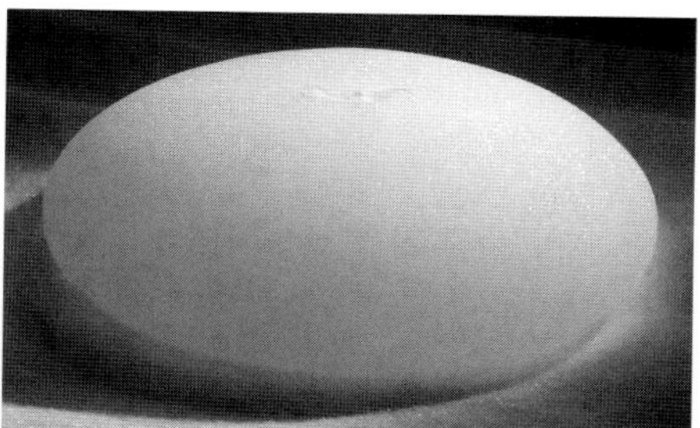

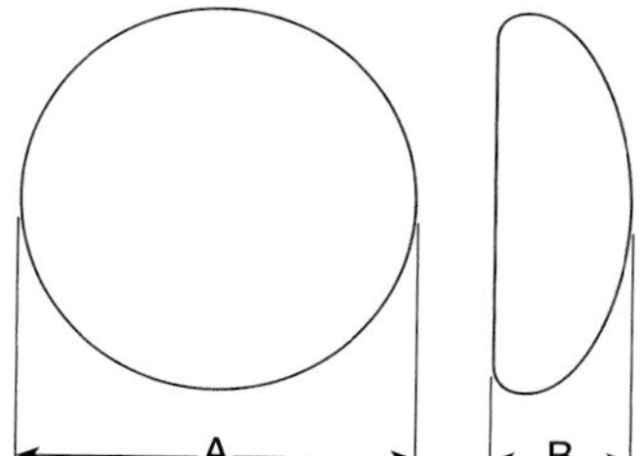

Device Volume (cc)	A Diameter (cm)	B Projection (cm)
125 + 25	9.5	3.0
150 + 25	10.0	3.1
175 + 25	10.6	3.3
200 + 25	11.0	3.4
225 + 25	11.5	3.5
250 + 25	11.9	3.6
275 + 25	12.3	3.7
300 + 25	12.6	3.7
325 + 50	13.0	3.8
350 + 50	13.3	3.9
375 + 50	13.6	4.0
425 + 50	14.2	4.1
475 + 50	14.8	4.2

Style 168 Biocell Round Saline Implant

(Courtesy McGhan Medical Corporation)

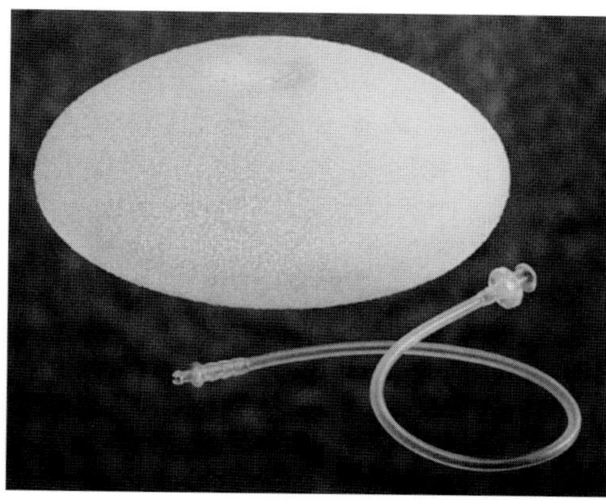

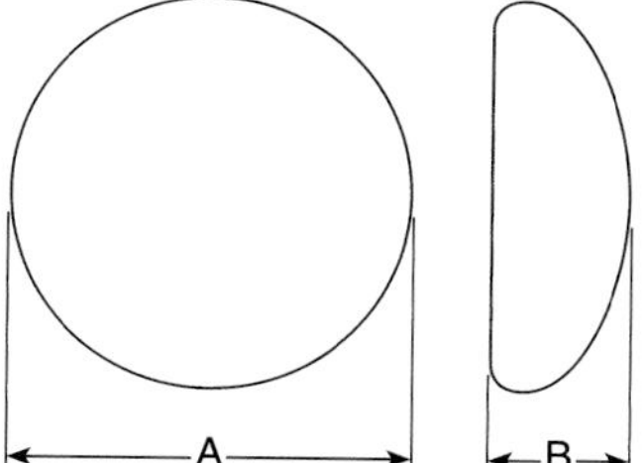

Fill Volume (cc)	A Diameter (cm)	B Projection (cm)
120-150	9.0	3.0
150-180	9.6	3.3
180-210	10.2	3.4
210-240	10.6	3.7
240-270	11.1	3.8
270-300	11.6	3.9
300-330	11.9	4.1
330-360	12.3	4.2
360-390	12.7	4.2
390-420	13.0	4.5
420-450	13.4	4.5
450-480	13.7	4.6
480-510	14.1	4.6
510-540	14.4	4.6
550-600	14.6	4.9
600-650	15.0	5.0
650-700	15.2	5.3
700-750	15.6	5.4
750-800	15.9	5.6
800-850	16.4	5.6

TEXTURED-SURFACE IMPLANT SPECIFICATIONS—cont'd
Styles 363 and 163 BioDIMENSIONAL Anatomic-Shaped Saline Implant for Reconstruction

(Courtesy McGhan Medical Corporation)

Style 363

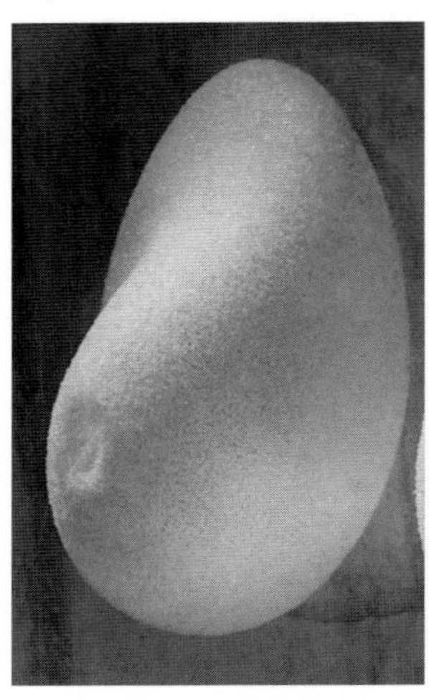

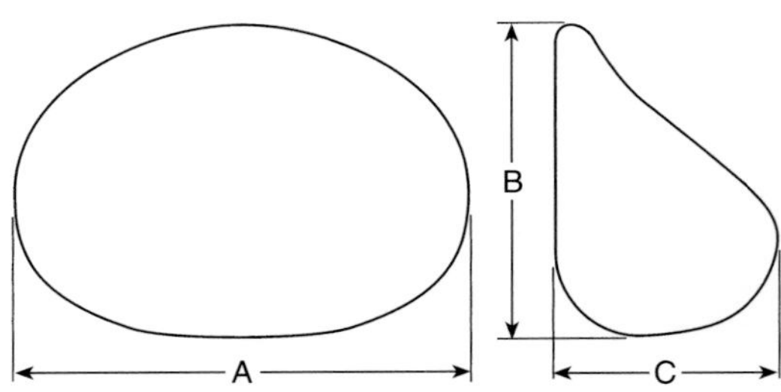

Fill Volume (cc)	A Width (cm)	B Length (cm)	C Projection (cm)
230-240	11.5	9.5	4.4
310-325	12.5	10.5	4.8
390-410	13.5	11.5	5.4
510-535	14.5	12.5	5.8
650-685	15.8	13.5	6.1

Style 163

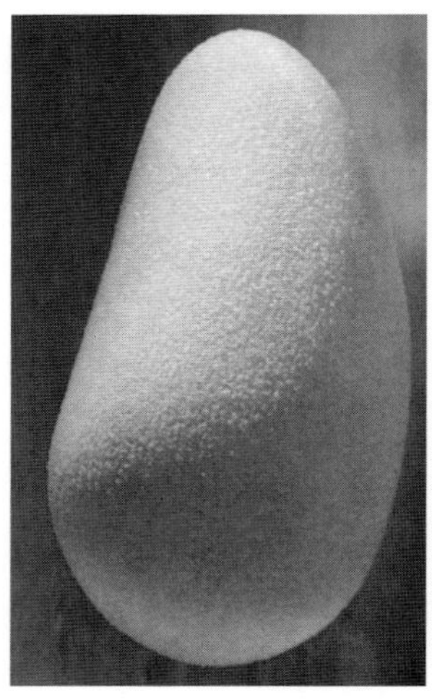

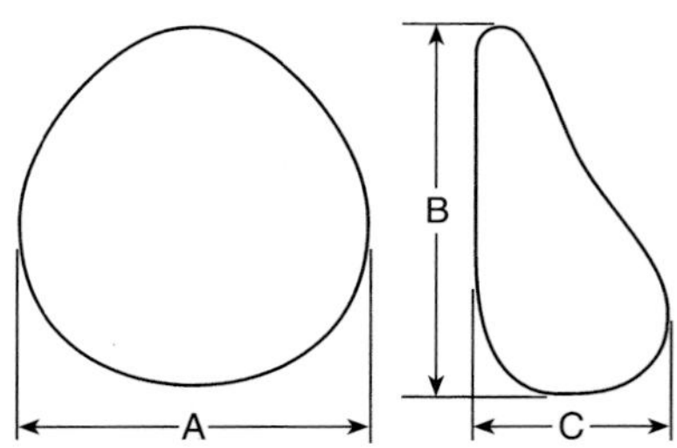

Fill Volume (cc)	A Width (cm)	B Length (cm)	C Projection (cm)
360-380	12.0	12.8	4.9
440-460	12.8	13.6	5.2
530-555	13.5	14.6	5.5
655-690	14.6	15.6	5.8
780-820	15.5	16.5	6.1

Style 468 BioDIMENSIONAL Anatomic-Shaped Saline Implant for Augmentation

(Courtesy McGhan Medical Corporation)

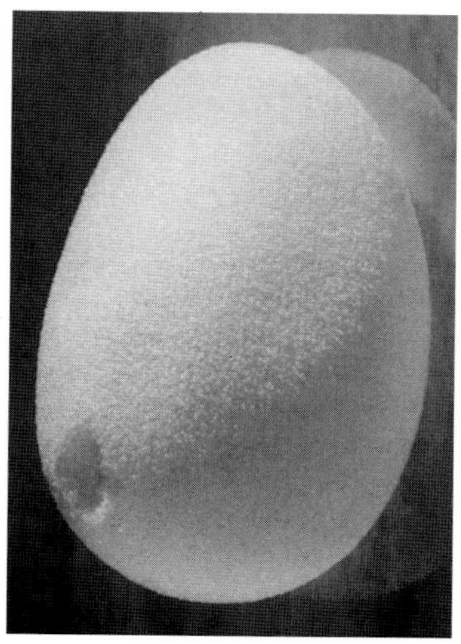

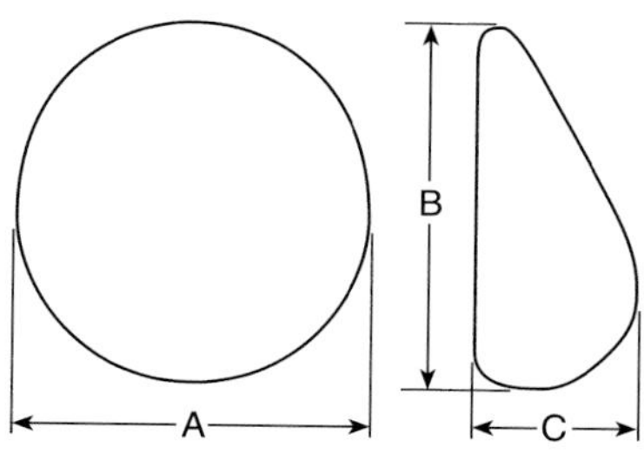

Size (cc)	A Width (cm)	B Height (cm)	C Projection (cm)
195-205	10.0	10.5	4.0
230-240	10.5	11.0	4.2
270-285	11.0	11.5	4.3
300-315	11.5	12.0	4.6
350-370	12.0	12.5	4.8
380-400	12.5	13.0	4.9
450-475	13.0	13.5	5.3
495-520	13.5	14.0	5.5
560-590	14.0	14.5	5.7
620-650	14.5	15.0	5.9

Contour Profile Natural Anatomic-Shaped Saline Implant

(Courtesy Mentor Corporation)

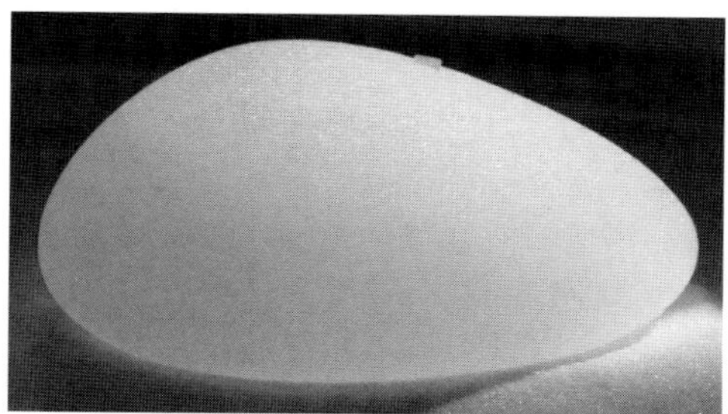

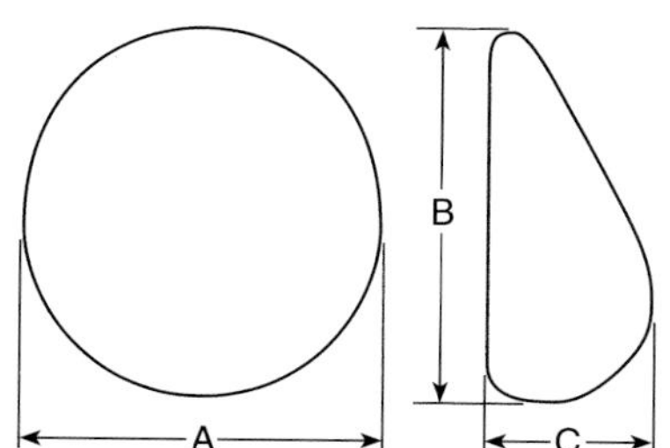

Device Volume (cc)	A Width (cm)	B Height (cm)	C Projection (cm)
175 + 25	10.2	8.5	4.3
225 + 25	11.2	9.4	4.5
275 + 25	12.2	10.3	4.5
350 + 50	13.1	11.0	4.7
425 + 50	13.8	11.6	5.2
525 + 50	14.9	12.5	5.6

POSTOPERATIVELY ADJUSTABLE IMPLANT

A modification of the textured-surface saline implant is the postoperatively adjustable textured-surface implant. It is not a tissue expander; however, it is useful when the breast volume may need to be changed in the postoperative period.

IMPLANT SPECIFICATIONS
Siltex Round Spectrum Saline Implant

(Courtesy Mentor Corporation)

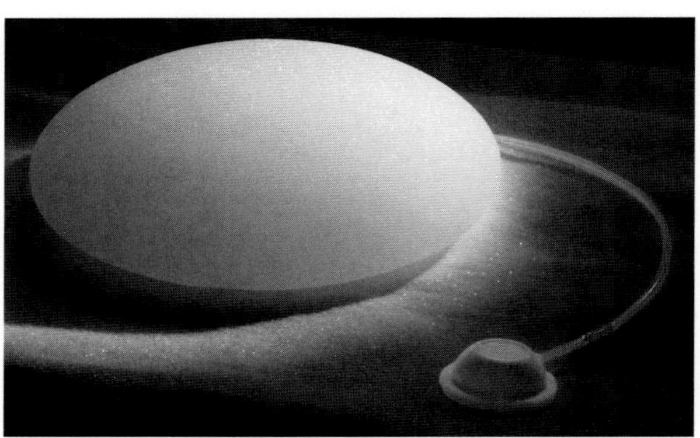

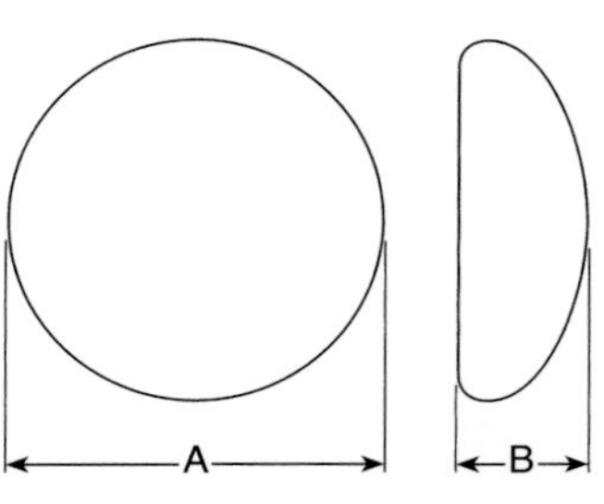

Device Volume (cc)	Temp. Min. Volume (cc)	Minimum Fall: Final Volume (cc)	Minimum Fall: A Diameter (cm)	Minimum Fall: B Projection (cm)	Maximum Fall: Final Volume (cc)	Maximum Fall: A Diameter (cm)	Maximum Fall: B Projection (cm)
125	105	125	9.4	3.0	150	9.2	3.5
175	150	175	10.5	3.1	210	10.4	3.9
225	190	225	11.3	3.3	270	11.1	4.2
275	235	275	12.0	3.6	330	11.4	4.4
325	275	325	12.9	3.7	390	12.6	4.5
375	320	375	13.4	3.9	450	13.1	4.8
425	360	425	14.0	4.2	510	13.6	5.0
475	405	475	14.5	4.5	570	14.2	5.7

RECOMMENDATIONS

The round smooth-surface saline implant has been my device of choice for breast augmentation for the past 8 years. It has a number of advantages. When placed in the subpectoral position, which I use almost exclusively, this device has a very low incidence of capsular contracture. It also has a more natural appearance because the saline fill responds to gravity and assumes a more anatomic shape when the woman is upright. The implant can be filled incrementally to modify the projection, diameter, and volume of the implant. This feature is helpful in treating breast asymmetries or in making small intraoperative contour adjustments. The elastomer shell and valve protect against rupture. The smooth surface is also less palpable than a textured surface and less susceptible to visible folds and ripples.

The round textured-surface implant is preferred for subglandular augmentation if there is good cover because it has a lower incidence of capsular contracture in this position. The implant's uneven surface is less noticeable when there is good skin and subcutaneous tissue or parenchymal cover. Therefore, to minimize potential palpability and ripples and the inherent firmness of the implant, there needs to be 2 cm or more of tissue cover or the implant needs to be placed subpectorally. With thin tissue cover for subglandular augmentation I often choose the smooth-surface implant for a firmer breast, which may be preferable to a very palpable, folded textured-surface implant. Textured-surface implants are also used after capsulectomy when firmness develops after placement of a smooth-surface implant or when there is an increased risk of capsular contracture or an increased risk of infection.

For breast reconstruction I use round smooth-surface implants when there is good muscular cover because they feel more natural and the capsular contracture rate does not seem to be increased. I use textured-surface implants for secondary reconstructions if there is a need for a capsulectomy after placement of a smooth-surface implant. I use very few anatomic-shaped implants because I have found that the round smooth-surface implant performs well and creates a satisfactory breast shape when placed in a well-developed pocket formed by an anatomic-shaped textured-surface expander.

The anatomic-shaped implant is useful to match the opposite breast with significant upper pole flattening and may obviate the need for an opposite breast implant. Anatomic-shaped saline implants are also placed following the use of anatomic-shaped expanders when the shape of the opposite breast requires a specific breast contour. I have noted that the amount of saline required to maintain the proper fill and achieve the appropriate shape after using these anatomic-shaped devices often results in breasts that are firmer than those augmented or reconstructed with round implants. The shaped devices can also rotate, distorting breast shape and obviating the benefit of the anatomic correction.

I prefer the postoperatively adjustable implant for augmentation or reconstruction when there is some breast asymmetry and the patient is young and still experiencing breast growth. However, the value of the somewhat limited adjustability must be weighed against the presence of the retained valve and the need for postoperative injections.

Tissue Expanders

Tissue expansion has been an important component of breast reconstruction since the early 1980s. Before tissue expanders were developed, the tissues were stretched manually when the surgeon created the pocket for the breast implant, expanding the overlying cover and recruiting the surrounding tissues. This expansion approach was modified when serially larger or smaller breast implants were used to replace the initial implant. Radovan introduced the initial tissue expander device for breast surgery. It was greeted with enthusiasm by the surgical community because it provided an alternative to the complex musculocutaneous flaps and the additional scars created by transposition of autologous tissue for breast reconstruction. This first-generation tissue expander was a saline-filled device with a single smooth elastomer shell and a separate fill port. The expander often had a flat backing to maintain the base diameter and for positioning on the chest wall. This thick backing adhered to the chest wall and helped the expander maintain a larger footprint on the chest wall. These expanders had a relatively narrow base in comparison to their volume, with relatively large-volume expanders having a narrower base than the expander implant. These initial expanders often did not have appropriately wide dimensions relative to breast width and vertical requirements, even with volumes of 600 to 800 cc. When these expanders were inflated, they tended to become spherical and their diameters decreased further, leaving an even smaller footprint on the chest wall. The first-generation of smooth-surface expanders permitted limited tissue expansion; frequently a capsulotomy and manual reexpansion of the pocket were necessary at the time the permanent implant was placed when a breast of significant size and projection was reconstructed.

Today's expanders have textured surfaces and are available in a variety of sizes and shapes so that they are able to stretch the skin appropriately to accommodate implants of different sizes and shapes. These devices have the advantage of holding their position better and providing better definition of the inframammary fold than the smooth-surface expanders formerly used. The textured surface allows capsular ingrowth into the device surface, thereby inhibiting migration during the expansion process and capsular contracture formation around the expander, allowing the expansion process to have a direct effect on the overlying skin. The capsule around these expanders resists contracture. Current expanders for breast reconstruction are designed for greater expansion of the inferior half of the device to permit development of a natural breast contour with the appropriate ptosis after implant placement.

Breast reconstruction using expansion is usually a two-staged process: during the first stage a temporary expander is inserted and inflated to stretch the skin appropriately; at a second stage the temporary device is removed and replaced with a permanent implant. Expander implants are also available with remote removable ports. When the desired skin envelope is achieved through expansion, the distant port is removed. This technique avoids the necessity of a second-stage procedure. The tissue expander implant is now also advocated for the occasional patient who requests breast augmentation and has marked asymmetry and breast constriction.

MECHANISM OF ACTION

Several mechanisms are involved in tissue expansion. When the skin is initially stretched or expanded, adjacent skin is also recruited; that is, the adjacent skin is brought onto the circumferential base area of the expander. Additionally, a certain amount of expansion is derived from elasticity and stretch following the actual stretching of the skin and underlying tissues. When the skin is expanded over a long period of time, additional elastic stretching of the skin results. Increased vascularity of the expander capsule and the tissues surrounding the tissue expander is related to the expansion process. Speed, frequency, and volume of the expansion are primary considerations. More rapid expansion before the onset of wound contraction is becoming a more predictable and efficient method. Some thinning of these tissues accompanies expansion, which can subject the implant to increased palpability and even exposure and compromise the aesthetic result. This problem is most often seen in immediate breast reconstruction when the expander is close to the dermis.

BIOACTIVITY

The recruitment characteristics of tissue expansion contribute to its efficacy. The expander brings adjacent skin from the surrounding chest and abdominal area to contribute additional breast projection and shape. The underlying saline compartment results in minimal silicone bleed. Serial saline injections after the procedure, however, do increase the possibility of introducing bacteria and subsequent low-grade or clinical infection that can contribute to capsular contracture and implant exposure. Expanders with a textured silicone surface have a lower propensity for motion and displacement and are helpful for defining the margins of the reconstructed breast, particularly the inframammary fold. These expanders are also softer clinically because of less firm spherical capsular contracture. There is increased bioactivity at the implant-tissue interface; however, there is still an underlying layer of laminated collagen.

SELECTION CRITERIA

The actual preinflation dimensions of the expander, its diameter after it is inflated, and the proposed final permanent implant dimensions are important determinants in selecting the appropriate expander. The width and positioning of the expander are also key. For instance, the diameter of the expander decreases somewhat as it is inflated and overinflated; skin is recruited onto its surface as the inframammary fold is elevated. The textured-surface expander can be positioned at the proposed inframammary fold, and when combined with directional, anatomic expansion, it remains relatively fixed and can give a more desirable shape. Expanders are now selected with the final shape of the breast in mind. When considerable projection is necessary even after directional expansion to match the opposite breast, the choice of the permanent implant should be determined by the need for projection. Using a permanent implant with a moderate or low projection after directional expansion loses the expansion gained.

Expander options

- Temporary textured-surface tissue expanders
    - Contained port and external port
    - Round and anatomic shaped
- Permanent expander implants

ROUND AND ANATOMIC-SHAPED TEMPORARY TISSUE EXPANDER

Temporary textured-surface tissue expanders are available in a wide range of sizes, shapes, and designs. They are produced in round shapes as well as contoured and anatomic shapes. They also are available with two basic types of injection ports: integral ports that are incorporated directly in the shell or remote ports that are connected by a closed tube system.

Anatomic-shaped expanders permit directional expansion. These directional devices are increasing in popularity because they permit selective expansion of tissue and avoid lower breast deficiency when the upper breast is unnecessarily expanded. These directional tissue expanders are designed for use in patients who require additional projection or who have tightness in the future lower breast region. Some of these have modifications of the outer elastomer that permit directional expansion during fill in the lower areas of the expander. This customized textured-surface directional expander with an integral magnetic finder valve is filled percutaneously after locating the fill valve with a magnet. ***Although directional devices are effective, I have also found that in most cases the direction of tissue expansion can be controlled during the initial procedure by the specifics of the dissection.*** More release of the muscle cover is done inferiorly so that more expansion goes in this direction of reduced resistance.

REMOTE AND CONTAINED PORTS

The remote port is designed for placement just under the skin surface so that it can be readily identified by palpation. The integral port is located by direct palpation or with a magnetic finder. A needle is subsequently inserted through the skin into the injection port for infusion of saline solution.

The standard expander with a distant port requires a tunnel between the port site and the expander for the connecting tube. The port is subsequently placed in a subcutaneous position or may be located outside the skin. With a remote port a needle can be inserted into the port to accomplish expansion.

A valve for saline injection is incorporated in the anterior surface of the contained port expander. This valve can usually be palpated through the thin skin after a mastectomy. The manufacturer provides a finder to assist in locating the valve. This valve has advantages over the separate external valve. It does not pose problems with displacement, kinking of the tubing, or separate infection in the valve pocket. The contained port expander does not require removal, and thereby problems of external port displacement and fill-tube failure are avoided. Drawbacks are the possibility of expander deflation with puncture of the device during filling and the palpable valve, which is objectionable to some patients with permanent implants who have thin cover over the expander.

The advantage of the remote port is that it can be positioned away from the tissue expander in an easily identified subcutaneous position. It is usually removed; however, some of the newer "micro" ports can be left in for a longer period of time. Although they are somewhat more difficult to locate and inject, they are more acceptable to the patient.

ROUND AND ANATOMIC-SHAPED TISSUE EXPANDER SPECIFICATIONS

Round Tissue Expander

(Courtesy Mentor Corporation)

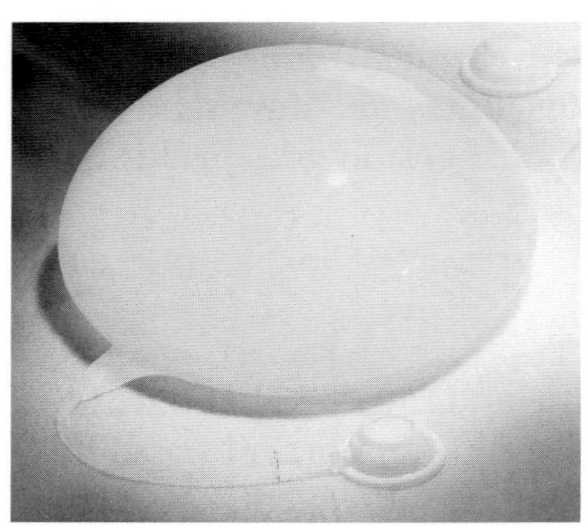

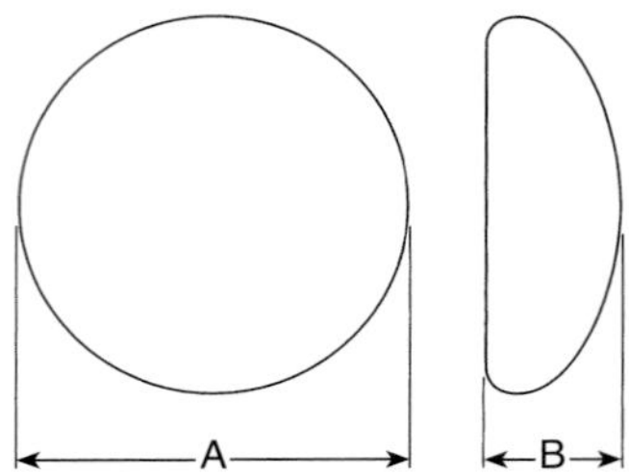

Device Volume (cc)	A Diameter (cm)	B Projection (cm)
400	11.3	5.9
550	13.4	5.8
700	14.6	6.7
850	15.0	7.2
1000	15.5	7.8

Contour Profile Anatomic-Shaped Tissue Expander

(Courtesy Mentor Corporation)

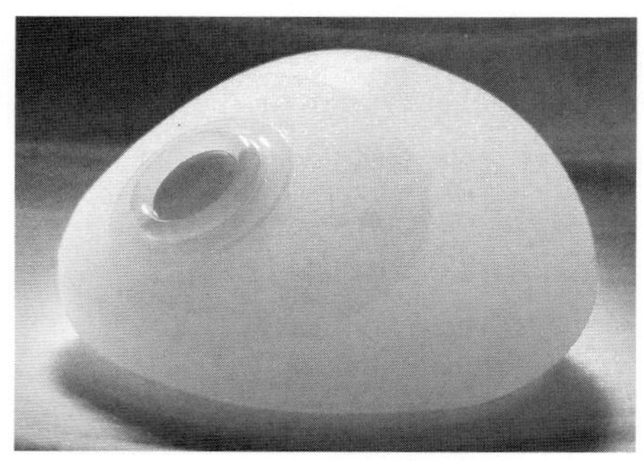

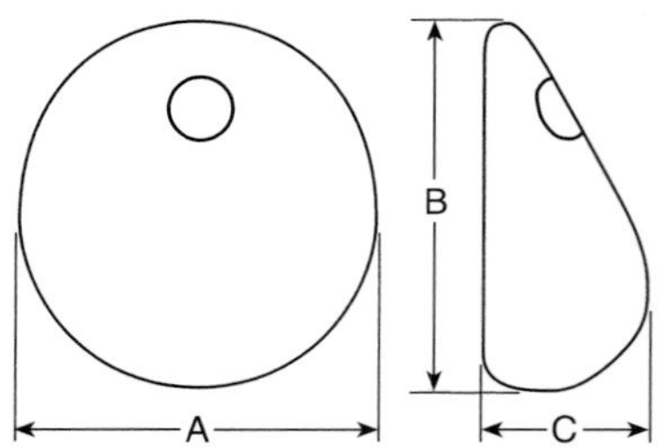

Volume (cc)	A Width (cm)	B Height (cm)	C Projection (cm)
350	11.6	9.9	6.4
450	12.7	10.7	6.8
550	13.7	11.5	7.0
650	14.8	12.5	7.2
800	15.9	13.0	7.7

Styles 131 and 133 Biospan Anatomic-Shaped Tissue Expanders for Reconstruction

(Courtesy McGhan Medical Corporation)

Style 131

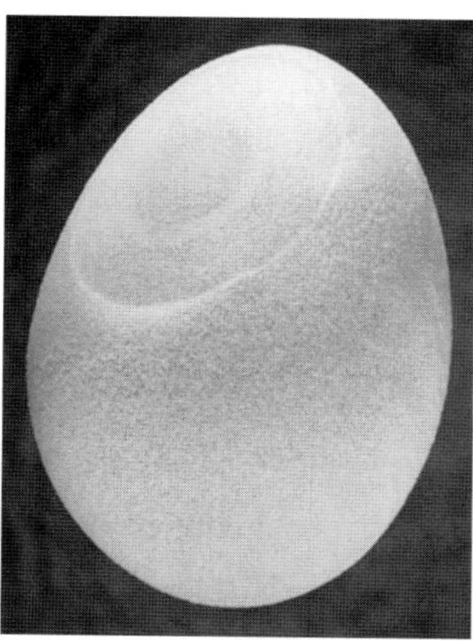

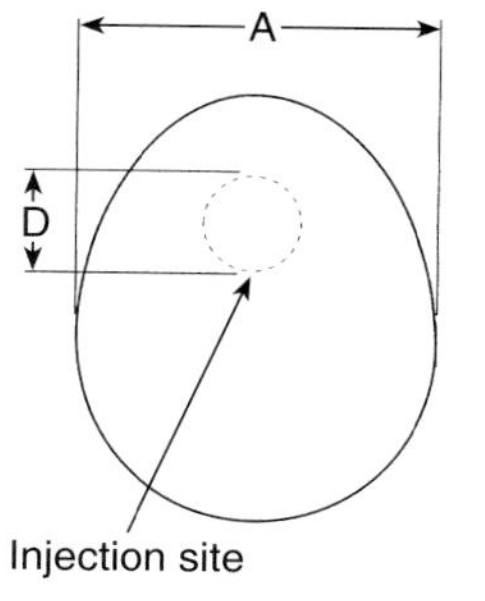

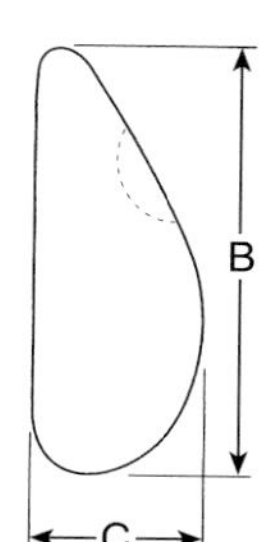

Volume (cc)	A Width (cm)	B Length (cm)	C Projection (cm)	D Injection Site Diameter (cm)
500-600	11.5	14.0	5.0-7.5	2.8
600-800	12.0	14.5	7.0-8.7	2.8
800-900	13.0	15.5	6.5-8.5	2.8

Style 133

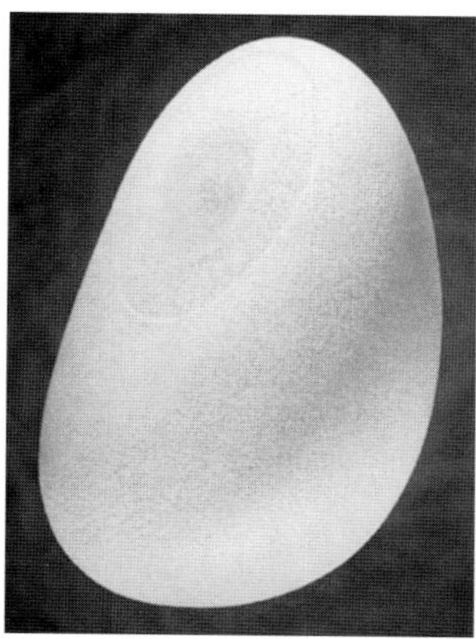

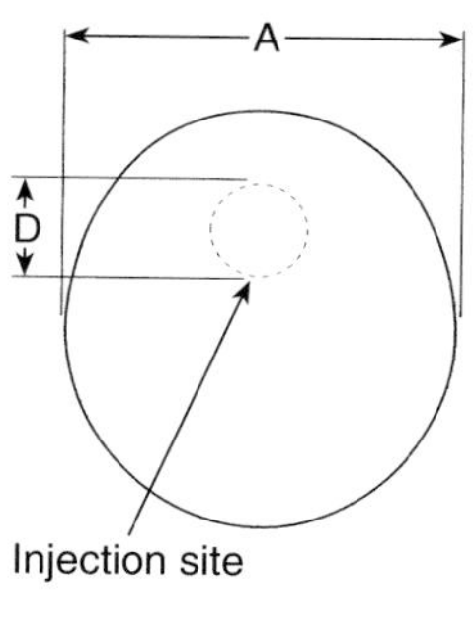

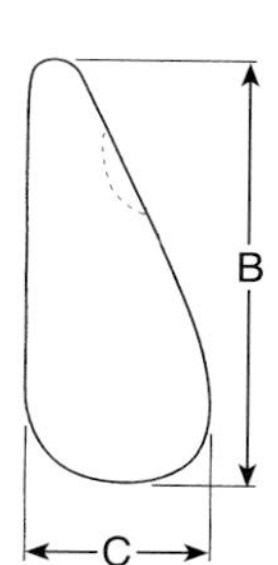

Volume (cc)	A Width (cm)	B Length (cm)	C Projection (cm)	D Injection Site Diameter (cm)
200	10.0	11.0	4.0	2.8
300	11.0	12.0	4.5	2.8
400	12.0	13.0	5.0	2.8
500	13.0	14.0	5.0	2.8
600	14.0	15.0	5.5	2.8
700	15.0	16.0	6.0	2.8
800	16.0	17.0	6.0	2.8

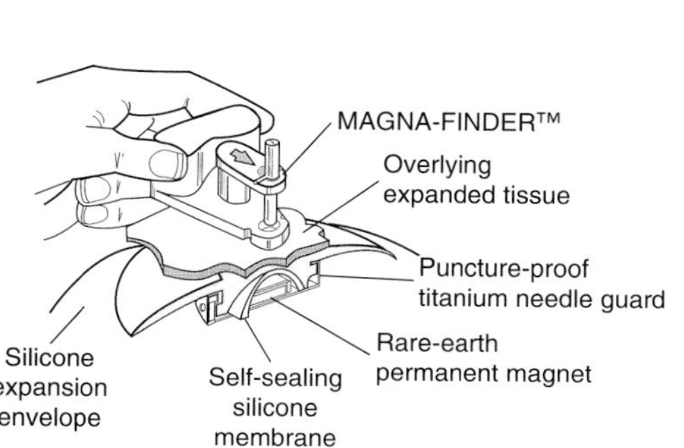

Magna-site locating system

PERMANENT EXPANDER IMPLANTS

The tissue expander implant represents the second generation of expanders. This is essentially a textured-surface double-lumen implant that has a silicone gel contained within its outer lumen and an inner saline-inflatable compartment. This implant has a removable fill tube and two seal valves that can convert it from an expander to a permanent implant. The permanent tissue expander implant is a good expander choice when the device is available and the patient is not resistant to the use of silicone gel. The external port is connected to a fill tube that enters the inflatable pocket through two valves. This device is currently available in the United States for breast reconstruction under FDA-monitored clinical trials.

The device has proved very reliable; current models have had less than a 1% failure rate. The initial low profile of this device permits the expander volume and diameter selected to be more accurately determined—the diameter is about 4 cm wider than the final volume needed. When a wider expander is placed, the device base narrows during expansion and this extra tissue is later recruited for breast reconstruction. The wall of this device is made of low-bleed silicone. The textured surfaces added to these implants have further enhanced the potential for a soft reconstruction; however, the texture is less distinct and there is usually less tissue adherence than with the anatomic-shaped textured saline devices.

EXPANDER IMPLANT SPECIFICATIONS
Siltex Round Becker and Becker 50 Expander Implants

(Courtesy Mentor Corporation)

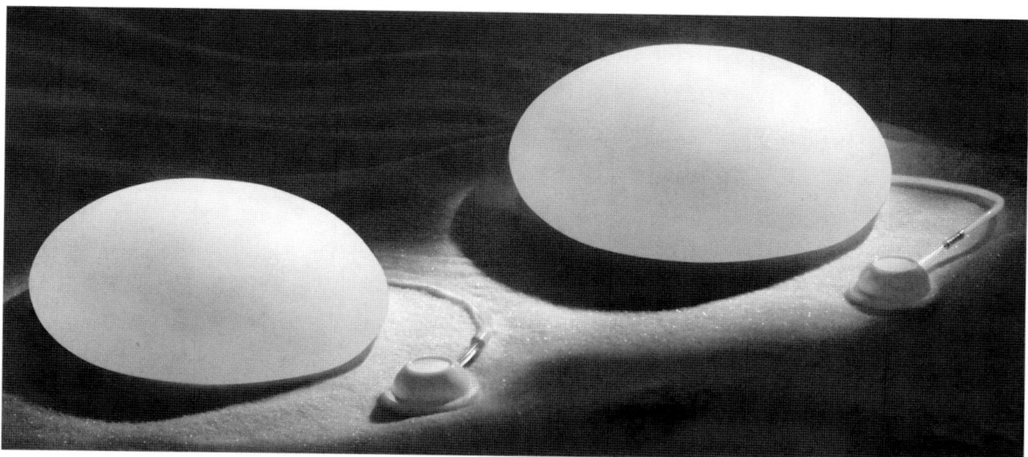

Round Becker Becker 50

Classic Becker: 25% Silicone Gel in Outer Lumen, 75% Saline in Inner Lumen

		Temporary Overexpansion Volumes					
Size (cc)	Gel Volume (cc)	Maximum Saline (cc)	Total Gel-Saline (cc)	Total Saline (cc)	Total Gel-Saline (cc)	A Diameter (cm)	B Projection (cm)
150	40	185	225	85-150	125- 190	10.7	2.4
200	50	250	300	125-200	175- 250	11.6	2.7
250	60	315	375	165-255	225- 315	12.1	3.0
300	75	375	450	200-300	275- 375	12.9	3.0
350	90	435	525	235-350	325- 440	14.1	3.0
400	100	500	600	275-400	375- 500	13.9	3.4
500	125	625	750	350-500	475- 625	14.7	3.7
600	150	750	900	425-600	575- 750	15.6	4.2
700	175	875	1050	500-700	675- 875	16.8	4.3
800	200	1000	1200	575-800	775-1000	17.2	4.6

Becker 50: 50% Silicone Gel in Outer Lumen, 50% Saline in Inner Lumen

Size (cc)	Gel Volume (cc)	Total Saline (cc)	Total Gel-Saline (cc)	A Diameter (cm)	B Projection (cm)
300	150	150-200	300-350	12.9	3.0
400	200	200-300	400-500	13.9	3.4
500	250	250-350	500-600	14.7	3.7
600	300	300-425	600-725	15.6	4.2
700	350	350-500	700-850	16.0	5.0

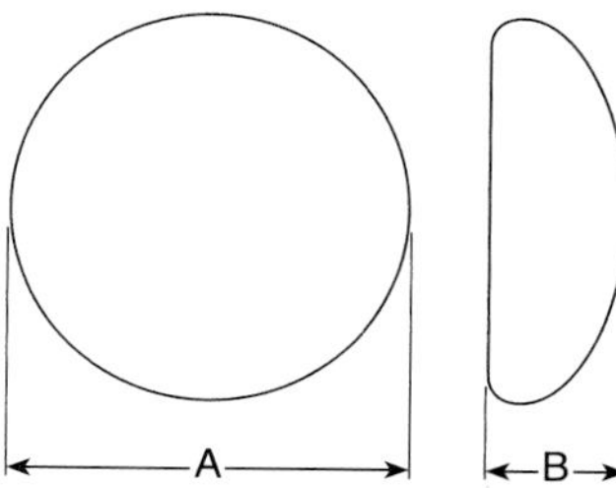

RECOMMENDATIONS

Anatomic or contoured expanders permit selective expansion and are particularly effective in stretching and creating a more projecting lower breast area. I use them almost exclusively because of their versatility. When the reconstructed breast requires additional projection, a temporary expander with an integral valve that has differential expansion capabilities is a good choice. An integral valve is selected when the expander will need to be replaced with a permanent implant. I prefer the tissue expander implant when there is a high probability that the tissues will expand as expected and the proposed reconstructive breast needs a full, rounded appearance. A remote valve, a component of the first-generation expanders, is used for the tissue expander implant.

I usually select the anatomic-shaped saline device for unilateral delayed reconstruction, followed by a permanent implant chosen to give the best breast symmetry. This may be either a round or anatomic-shaped permanent saline implant. I also prefer the anatomic-shaped textured-surface expander for unilateral immediate breast reconstruction when a device replacement is planned.

For bilateral reconstruction, when the shape and symmetry of the breasts are determined almost totally by the implants, the permanent expander implant is a good choice and can avoid the need for a second operation for many women. The patient and surgeon often prefer the flexibility of the expander implant with the retained microport, which enables volume adjustments to be made over the long term.

Specific Clinical Applications

AUGMENTATION MAMMAPLASTY

Both smooth-surface and textured-surface implants are recommended for augmentation mammaplasty. However, I prefer smooth-surface saline implants for this operation. ***They are easier to introduce through the shorter endoscopic-assisted incisions; they are also more easily positioned, and the saline weight can produce the additional lower postoperative breast expansion necessary after an axillary augmentation to get the best final result.*** For the axillary subpectoral approach the smooth-surface saline implant usually performs better than the textured-surface implant. Subglandular textured-surface implants probably have a lower incidence of capsular contracture. When the patient desires a periareolar incision, I prefer to place the implant in the subpectoral or submusculofascial position. When the patient's areola is small, it is easier to insert a smooth-surface saline implant through a smaller periareolar incision than a textured-surface implant. If the areolar diameter is larger and a 5 cm periareolar incision can be made or the periareolar incision can be extended, a textured-surface implant is used when the implant is placed subglandularly.

For axillary subpectoral breast augmentation I use a smooth-surface saline implant. The saline implant can be placed through the reduced incision and inflated when in position.

When patients prefer additional control over their final implant and breast size, the postoperatively adjustable implant for breast augmentation may be considered. The size of the implant selected must have a base diameter to correspond with the final estimated breast volume. The implant is positioned in the subpectoral position (see Chapter 6). The manufacturer provides a small fill port, which is placed near the inframammary incision, and the implant is then expanded to the appropriate volume. Intraoperative expansion may be helpful when the patient requests a significantly larger augmentation. During the postoperative period the expander implant can be adjusted either by additional fill or deflation to obtain the desired size. I prefer to leave the valve in for at least 6 months to 1 year to ensure that the patient is satisfied with the volume. Then the implant fill tube is removed in the office under local anesthesia.

MASTOPEXY-AUGMENTATION

For mastopexy-augmentation I select and position the implant to maximize an attractive, natural breast shape and minimize the potential for capsular contracture. This is particularly important with mastopexy-augmentation because the implant must remain low and behind the breast mass. Any capsular contracture with subsequent elevation of the breast implant will have a double-bubble effect as the breast ptoses over the implant. I use smooth-surface saline subpectoral implants for mastopexy-augmentation with the lower cover provided by the breast parenchyma. I release the lower pectoral muscles up to the fourth intercostal space to ensure that the implant is low enough.

When the patient has minor ptosis (the nipple at the level of but not below the inframammary fold), acceptable contour correction can usually be obtained by placement of an implant of generous volume either subpectorally or in the subglandular space. When the patient has major ptosis (the nipple

IMPLANT AND EXPANDER OPTIONS FOR AUGMENTATION MAMMAPLASTY

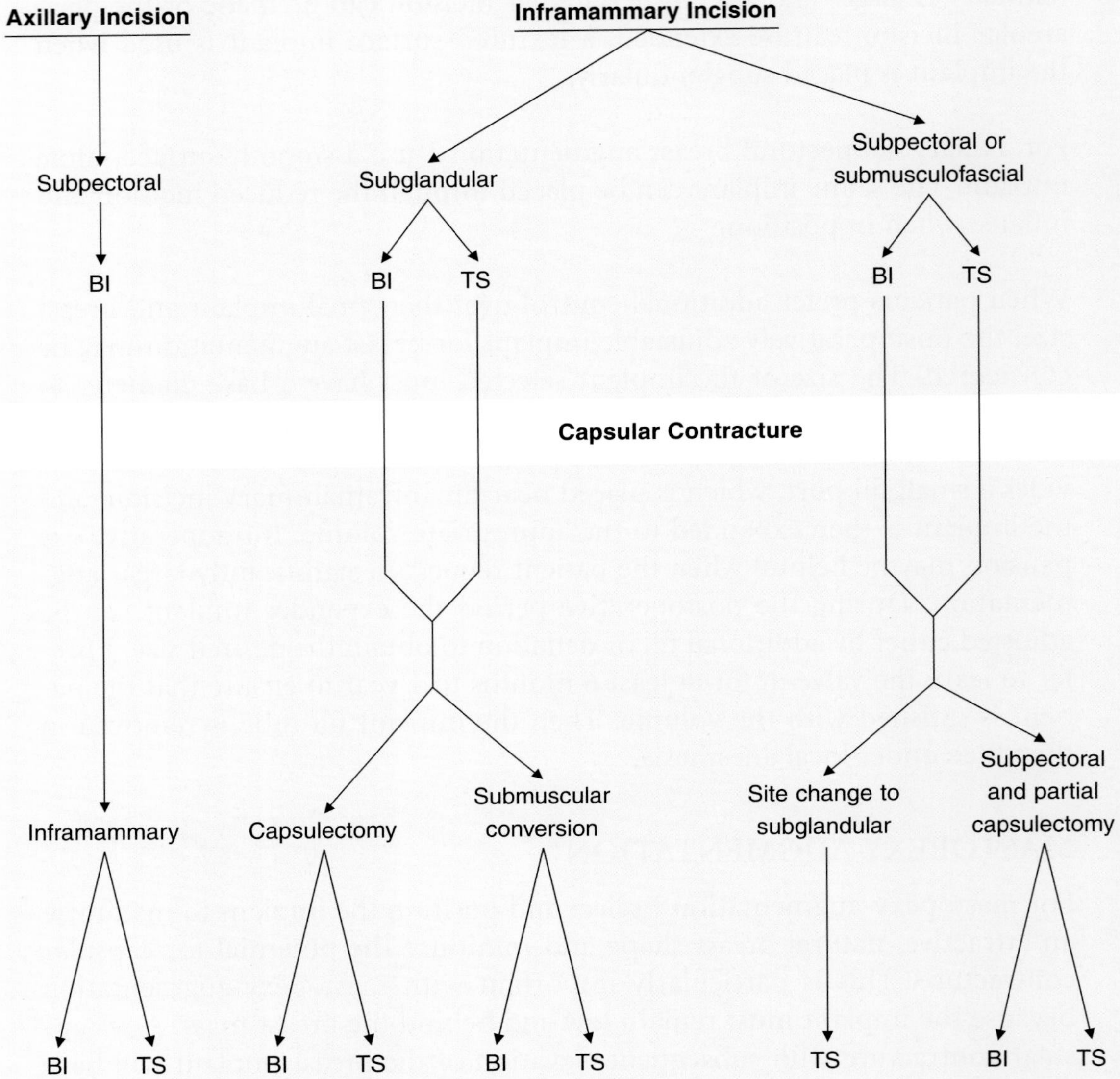

BI = round smooth-surface saline implant; TS = round textured-surface saline implant.

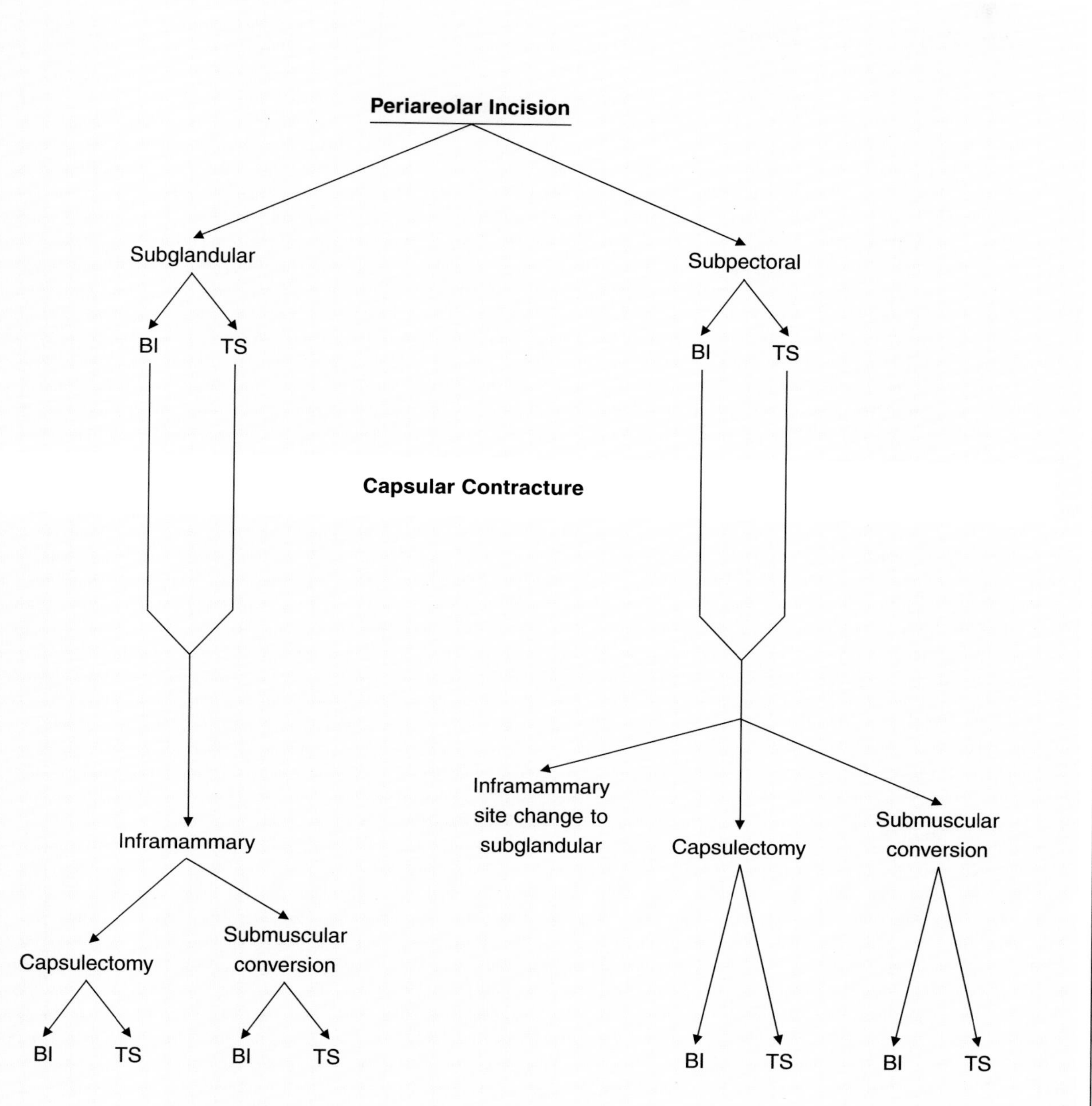
Periareolar Incision
Subglandular
Subpectoral
BI
TS
BI
TS
Capsular Contracture
Inframammary
Inframammary site change to subglandular
Capsulectomy
Submuscular conversion
Capsulectomy
Submuscular conversion
BI
TS
BI
TS
BI
TS
BI
TS

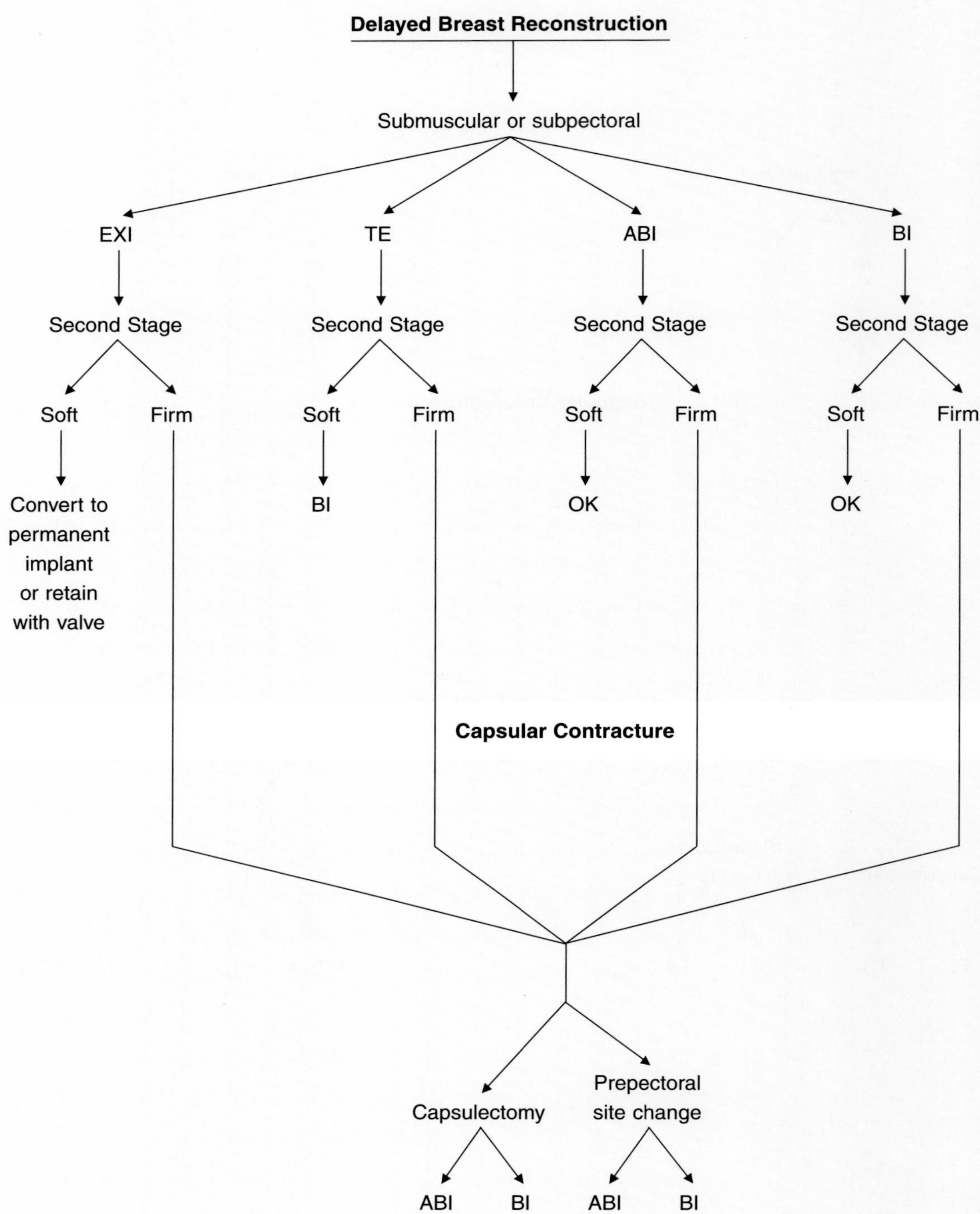

EXI = expander implant; TE = anatomic-shaped textured-surface expander;
ABI = anatomic-shaped breast implant; BI = smooth-surface saline implant.

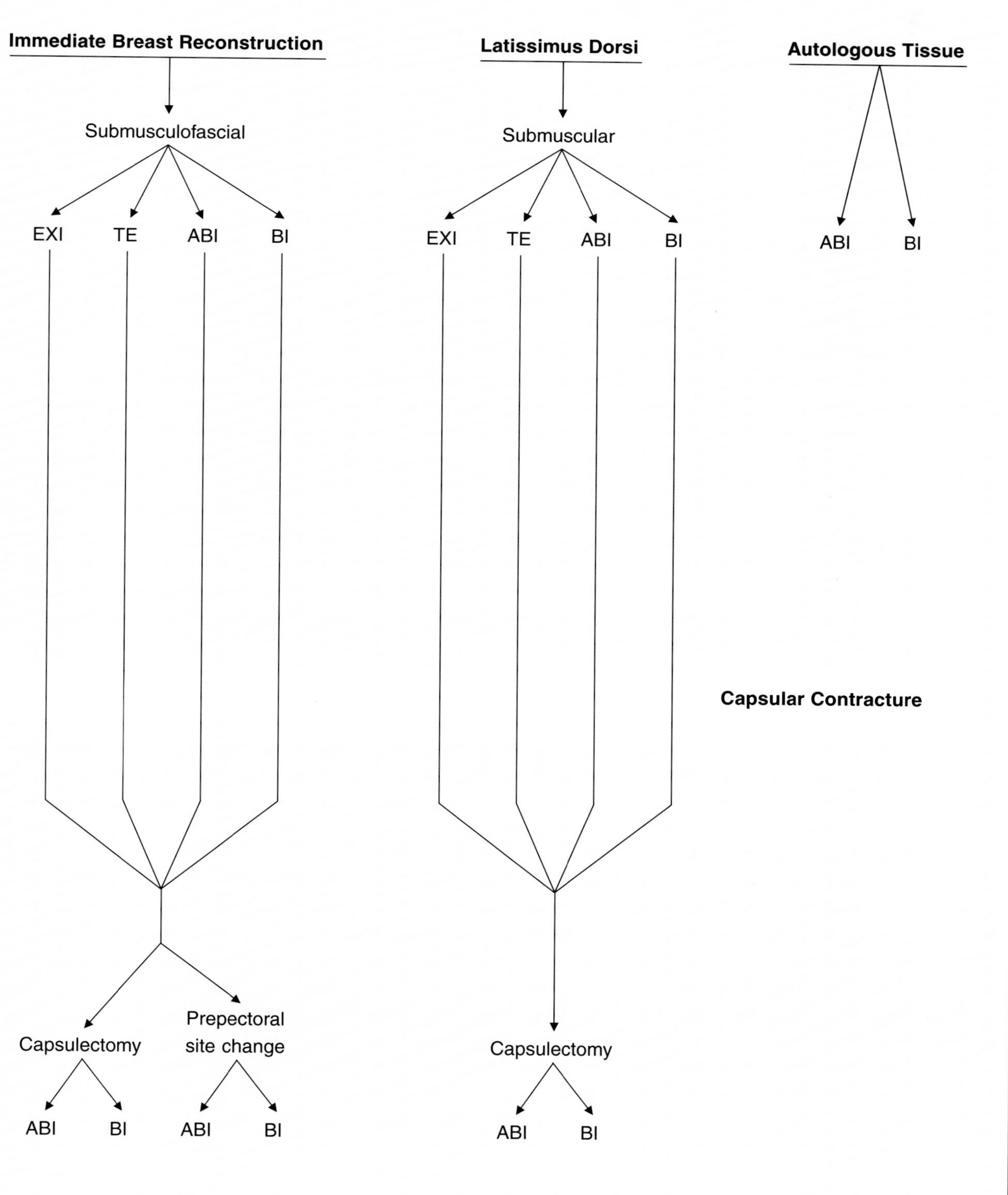
Immediate Breast Reconstruction
Submusculofascial
EXI
TE
ABI
BI
Capsulectomy
Prepectoral site change
ABI
BI
ABI
BI
Latissimus Dorsi
Submuscular
EXI
TE
ABI
BI
Capsulectomy
ABI
BI
Autologous Tissue
ABI
BI
Capsular Contracture

below the inframammary fold), a vertical mastopexy with nipple-areolar elevation will be needed for adequate contour correction. As first popularized by Regnault, the use of a mammary implant as a component for correction of ptosis has the advantage of providing improved supra-areolar contour. An additional advantage is that the increased volume provided by the implant decreases the amount of skin excised and length of incisions necessary for contour and skin correction and nipple elevation. When the breast is narrowed, constricted, and ptotic, I may choose a periareolar mastopexy rather than a vertical mastopexy.

BREAST RECONSTRUCTION

For breast reconstruction I use smooth- and textured-surface implants and round and anatomic-shaped textured-surface expanders. When the tissue expanders need to be replaced, I usually exchange them for smooth-surface implants. If a specific contour must be achieved, I use anatomic-shaped textured-surface implants when there is enough cover to allow these devices to perform appropriately to avoid visible and palpable ripples and folds.

Immediate Reconstruction After Mastectomy With Implant Only

The initial and standard studies of immediate breast reconstruction after total mastectomy and subcutaneous mastectomy involve smooth-surface implants in the submusculofascial position. Noone, Little, and Jarrett reported a low incidence of capsular contracture with smooth-surface implants. When sufficient tissue is present for reconstruction without preliminary expansion after mastectomy, I currently use smooth-surface implants in the submuscular position for immediate reconstruction. If skin flaps are of sufficient thickness and have adequate vascularization, the implant can be placed in the partially submuscular position, which often permits reconstruction of a breast mound with more natural contours and projection than could be obtained with complete submuscular positioning of the implant.

Reconstruction Following Preliminary Tissue Expansion

The anatomic-shaped textured-surface implant can be used as the "permanent" implant following initial expansion with an anatomic-shaped textured-surface expander; the results can be excellent when there is good cover for the device. When the cover is thin and the expander exhibits ripples, I often replace the expander with a submuscular smooth-surface implant. Ideally this technique results in low capsular contracture rates and a more natural-feeling soft reconstruction.

Use of Implants After Flap Surgery

Implants are sometimes necessary after flap surgery, particularly after a latissimus dorsi flap. The latissimus dorsi flap, even when harvested with an overlying layer of subcutaneous tissue, may not have the appropriate volume for breast symmetry. In these situations I usually place a tissue expander beneath the latissimus dorsi flap and under the latissimus dorsi muscle. When there is a thick cover of autologous tissue overlying the implant, I sometimes prefer to use an expander with a remote valve rather than one with an integral valve that may be more difficult to identify and to inflate. This is particularly true in the postoperative period if there is edema of the overlying autologous tissue. After a TRAM flap a woman may request larger breasts, which requires the placement of a breast implant behind the autologous tissue.

Breast Projection

Certain anatomic situations require more projection than can be obtained by simply using a larger volume implant. In these cases anatomic-shaped textured-surface implants can produce a satisfactory result. In the past implants were stacked to create a more projecting breast appearance; however, with the currently available implants this approach is not suitable because they will not adhere together sufficiently to hold their position.

Capsular Contracture

Capsular contracture is manifest as a breast firmness after the placement of a breast implant or expander. The use of postoperative exercises after placement of a smooth-surface breast implant is advised by many plastic surgeons to maximize breast softness. Since some capsule naturally forms about any implanted device, the diagnosis and determination of when the breast implant is "contracted" are clinical decisions. I tell my patients to expect the implants to become firmer over time and that this is a natural occurrence.

HISTOLOGY

Histologically, a contracted capsule may not appear different from a capsule associated with a soft breast, and capsular thickness is not always related to implant softness. Generally, however, contracted capsules are somewhat thicker and demonstrate linear bands of collagen. Sometimes, particularly when associated with earlier models that had a thin elastomer coating, actual foreign body silicone droplets can be seen in the contracted capsule.

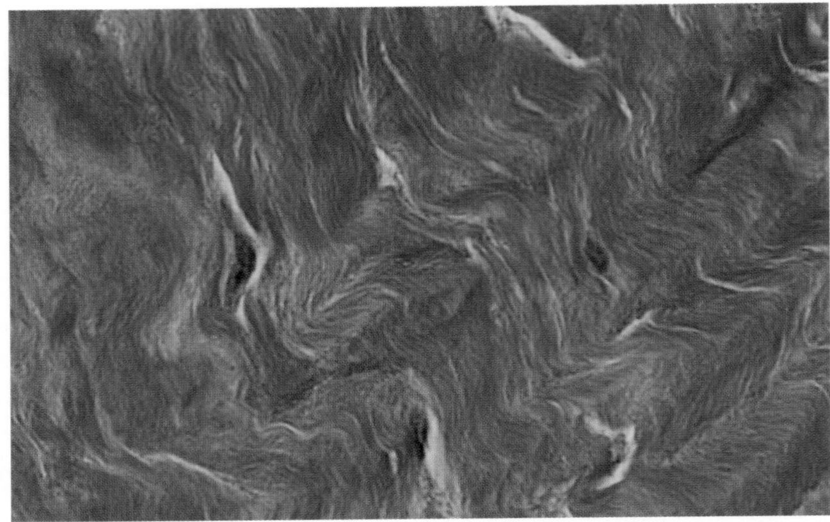

Note the pattern of collagen deposition around this standard smooth-surface implant. The longitudinal deposition of fibers contributes to a concentric, central constricting force.

CLASSIFICATION

The Baker classification presented in 1976 categorizes capsular contracture by degrees:

Grade I	Normally soft and natural appearance
Grade II	A natural appearance despite palpable firmness
Grade III	Firm with visible distortion
Grade IV	Obvious spherical distortion

Most reports on capsular contracture use the Baker classification to rate postoperative results.

Practically speaking, however, the breast is either soft or firm after augmentation mammaplasty. The firmness with the accompanying distortion is either of a degree to be tolerated without an operative procedure or is hard enough to necessitate a specific intervention to improve the softness and appearance of the breasts. At Emory Clinic we use a simpler classification:

Class I	A normal soft breast, fully compressible
Class II	A slightly firm but acceptable breast, minimal resistance to compression
Class III	A firm breast that requires an operative procedure

STRATEGIES TO DECREASE CAPSULAR CONTRACTURE

Implant Type

A lower incidence of capsular contracture has been reported with the saline breast implant and the double-lumen implant than the silicone breast implant containing silicone gel only. This phenomenon has been attributable to lower silicone bleed and the pressure of the saline fill. The introduction of the low-bleed outer shell perhaps lowered the incidence of capsular contracture with the silicone breast implant. The textured-surface silicone breast implant with the low-bleed outer shell has lower capsular contracture rates when placed in the subglandular position than the smooth-surface implant.

Capsular contracture can develop around tissue expanders, particularly the smooth-surface varieties. This is seen most often when there is a low-grade infection. For this reason I prefer to leave tissue expanders in for a longer rather than shorter period of time to determine if a capsular contracture will develop and plan the second-stage strategy. When the breasts are very soft with good contour with the tissue expander in place, particularly if a permanent expander implant is used, the expander implant can be converted to a permanent implant. If a capsular contracture does develop, it should be determined if a low-grade infection is present. The textured-surface expanders are more predictably soft than the smooth-surface expanders and today only textured expanders are available on the market.

Implant Position

Smooth-Surface Implants

The position of the breast implant relative to the breast parenchyma and ducts affects the incidence of capsular contracture. After augmentation mammaplasty with smooth-surface gel breast implants in the subglandular position, capsular contracture has been reported to be as high as 74%. Placing the breast implant in the submuscular position has been reported to significantly reduce the incidence of capsular contracture. With this approach the breast parenchyma and ducts are not divided or elevated off the deep fascia. Most breast ducts contain resident *Staphylococcus epidermidis,* which has been cultured from a high percentage of breast capsules when the breast implant was positioned subglandularly. Perhaps another reason for the enhanced softness of the implant when placed in the submuscular position is the basic contour and firmness of the underlying rib cage. It has been postulated that the overlying muscle compresses and massages the implant over the chest wall and thereby resists the development of a spherical condition. The enhanced overlying tissue thickness when the implant is in the retromuscular position also contributes to less obvious spherical capsular deformity than when the implant is in the subglandular position.

Textured-Surface Implants

One of the primary advantages of the textured-surface implants is that they can be used in the submuscular or subglandular position with minimal difference in the incidence of capsular contracture. Patients with adequate thickness of breast tissue and minimal ptosis are the best candidates for subglandular placement of the implant. Thin patients are usually better served by placement in the submuscular space to provide better cover for the implant; however, if a patient is athletic, she should be told that breast flattening and distortion may occur with flexion and contraction of the overlying pectoralis major muscle. In general implants should not be placed in the complete submuscular space in patients with ptosis. The implant may not descend properly, and the breast tissue can droop over the device, giving a double-bubble appearance. I prefer to release the lower pectoralis major muscle and place the implant under the upper pectoralis major muscle and in the subglandular position in the lower breast.

Most surgeons agree that patients with mammary ptosis and postpartum glandular involution have better aesthetic results when the breast implant is placed in the subglandular position in the lower breast region. However, the high rate of capsular contracture around standard smooth-surface implants placed in the complete subglandular position has led many surgeons to use upper subpectoral placement even in the presence of high-grade ptosis.

TREATMENT

Smooth-Surface Implants

The treatment of capsular contracture following the use of smooth-surface silicone implants using standard techniques of open and closed capsulotomy has failed to control the problem in a predictable manner. Manufacturers do not recommend closed capsulotomy because of the possibility of implant rupture and silicone extrusion.

Capsulectomy

Capsulectomy is usually the best approach in patients with severe subglandular contractures. It is particularly important if there are calcifications or ossifications of the capsule. The procedure can be accomplished with relative ease using a generous inframammary incision and dissection just beyond the outer capsule. The capsule is totally excised and the textured-surface saline implant placed in the freshly dissected, nonscarred pocket if there is good cover; otherwise I use a smooth-surface saline implant. This approach produces a better aesthetic result than transferring the implant to a submuscular pocket from the subglandular space. When there is thin cover, a more limited capsulectomy is sometimes done to avoid increased palpability of the device.

If the techniques described are adhered to, a significant reduction in recurrent capsular contracture can be expected as compared to simple capsulotomy and implant replacement. (See Chapter 6 for clinical descriptions of these techniques.)

Textured-Surface Implants and Expanders

A capsular contracture around a textured-surface implant is usually caused by a low-grade infection, seroma, or lack of implant adherence that occurs when a textured-surface implant is placed in a previous smooth-surface implant pocket. If the implant is in the subpectoral position, I either perform a lower capsulectomy in the area of the breast below the pectoralis major muscle or reposition the implant in a prepectoral position. When good cover is available, prepectoral repositioning is effective. A posterior capsulectomy is not done when the subpectoral implant is on the ribs and intercostal muscles in view of the associated heavy bleeding and proximity of the pleura.

Implant Site Change

Changing the implant site is most often indicated when capsular contracture occurs around submuscular implants. Total capsulectomy may be difficult in this setting, and it is usually technically easier to simply abandon the submuscular pocket and dissect a new subglandular pocket for placement of the implant.

Closing Thoughts

The perfect implantable mammary device remains an elusive goal, and no dramatic breakthrough in terms of new materials is foreseen in the immediate future. At present manufacturers are spending most research funds on "re-proving" the efficacy and safety of current devices, both saline and silicone gel–filled, in keeping with the FDA mandate. For the present surgeons must be content to identify which available devices and variations of surgical technique will produce the best results in the largest number of patients for the longest period of time.

REFERENCES

Ahn CY, Ko CY, Wagar EA, Wong RS, Shaw WW. Clinical significance of intracapsular fluid in patients' breast implants. Ann Plast Surg 35:455, 1995.

Ahn CY, DeBruhl ND, Gorczyca DP, Bassett LW, Shaw WW. Silicone implant rupture diagnosis using computed tomography: A case report and experience with 22 surgically removed implants. Ann Plast Surg 33:624, 1994.

Ahn CY, DeBruhl ND, Gorczyca DP, Shaw WW, Bassett LW. Comparative silicone breast implant evaluation using mammography, sonography, and magnetic resonance imaging: Experience with 59 implants. Plast Reconstr Surg 94:620,1994.

Ahn CY, Shaw WW, Narayanan K, Gorczyca DP, DeBruhl ND, Bassett LW. Residual silicone detection using MRI following previous breast implant removal: Case reports. Aesthetic Plast Surg 19:361, 1995.

Ahn CY, Shaw WW, Narayanan K, Gorczyca DP, Sinha S, DeBruhl ND, Bassett LW. Definitive diagnosis of breast implant rupture using magnetic resonance imaging. Plast Reconstr Surg 92: 681, 1993.

American College of Rheumatology Statement on Silicone Breast Implants. Oct., 1995.

Angell M. Science on Trial: The Clash of Medical Evidence and the Law in the Breast Implant Case. New York: WW Norton, 1996.

Angell M. Do breast implants cause systemic disease? Science in the courtroom. N Engl J Med 330: 1748, 1994.

Angell M. Breast implants—Protection or paternalism? N Engl J Med 326:1695, 1992.

Beekman WH, Scot MG, Taets van Amerongen AH, Hage JJ, Mulder JW. Silicone breast implant bleed and rupture: Clinical diagnosis and predictive value of mammography and ultrasound. Ann Plast Surg 36:345, 1996.

Berg WA, Caskey CI, Hamper UM, Kuhlman JE, Anderson ND, Chang BW, Sheth S, Zerhouni EA. Single- and double-lumen silicone breast implant integrity: Prospective evaluation of MR and US criteria. Radiology 197:45, 1995.

Berg WA, Caskey CI, Hamper UM, Anderson ND, Chang BW, Sheth S, Zerhouni EA, Kuhlman JE. Diagnosing breast implant rupture with MR imaging, US, and mammography. Radiographics 13:1323, 1993.

Berkel H, Birdsell DC, Jenkins H. Breast augmentation: A risk factor for breast cancer? N Engl J Med 326:1649, 1992.

Berrino P, Casabona F, Santi P. Long-term advantages of permanent expandable implants in breast aesthetic surgery. Plast Reconstr Surg 101:1964, 1998.

Bilbey JH, Connell DG. MRI diagnosis of a ruptured breast implant presenting as an infraclavicular mass. Can Assoc Radiol J 44:224, 1993.

Birdsell DC, Jenkins H, Berket H. Breast cancer diagnosis and survival in women with and without breast implants. Plast Reconstr Surg 92:795, 1993.

Bostwick J III. Breast reconstruction following mastectomy. Cancer J Clin 45:289, 1995.

Breast implants—An information update. Rockville, Md.: U.S. Food & Drug Administration, Department of Health & Human Services, July, 1997.

Brink RR. Sequestered fluid and breast implant malposition. Plast Reconstr Surg 98:679, 1996.

Brinton LA, Malone KE, Coates RJ, Schoenberg JB, Swanson CA, Daling JR, Stanford JL. Breast enlargement and reduction: Results from a breast cancer case-control study. Plast Reconstr Surg 97:269, 1996.

Brinton LA, Malone KE, Coates RJ, et al. Breast implants and subsequent breast cancer risk. Am J Epidemiol 141:S85, 1995.

Brody GS, Conway DP, Deapen DM, Fisher J, Hochberg MC, LeRoy EC, Medsger TA Jr, Robson MC, Shons AR, Weisman MH. Consensus statement on the relationship of breast implants to connective-tissue disorders. Plast Reconstr Surg 90:1102, 1992.

Brohim RM, Foresman PA, Hildebrandt PK, Rodeheaver GT. Early tissue reaction to textured breast implant surfaces. Ann Plast Surg 28:354, 1992.

Brown SL, Silverman BG, Berg WA. Rupture of silicone-gel breast implants: Causes, sequelae and diagnosis. Lancet 350:1531, 1997.

Bryant H, Brasher PMA. Breast implants and breast cancer—Reanalysis of a linkage study. N Engl J Med 332:1535, 1995.

Bryant H, Brasher PMA, van de Sande JH, Turc J-M [Alberta Cancer Board]. Review of methods in "Breast augmentation: A risk factor for breast cancer?" N Engl J Med 330:293, 1994.

Burns CJ, Laing TJ, Gillespie BW, Heeringa SG, Alcser KH, Mayes MD, Wasko MC, Cooper BC, Garabrant DH, Schottenfeld MD. The epidemiology of scleroderma among women: Assessment of risk from exposure to silicone and silica. J Rheumatol 23:1904, 1996.

Caffee HH. Vitamin E and capsule contracture. Ann Plast Surg 19:512, 1987.

Caffee HH, Hardt NS, La Torre G. Detection of breast implant rupture with aspiration cytology. Plast Reconstr Surg 95:1145, 1995.

Caskey CI, Berg WA, Anderson ND, Sheth S, Chang BW, Hamper UM. Breast implant rupture: Diagnosis with US. Radiology 190:819,1994.

Cederna PS, Yates WR, Chang P, Cram AE, Ricciardelli EJ. Postmastectomy reconstruction: Comparative analysis of the psychosocial, functional, and cosmetic effects of transverse rectus abdominis musculocutaneous flap versus breast implant reconstruction. Ann Plast Surg 35:458, 1995.

Chandler PJ Jr. An outcome analysis of 100 women after explanation of silicone gel breast implants and connective tissue disease and other rheumatic conditions following breast implants in Denmark. Ann Plast Surg 40:103, 1998.

Chung KC, Wilkins EG, Beil RJ Jr, Helvie MA, Ikeda DM, Oneal RM, Forrest ME, Smith DJ Jr. Diagnosis of silicone gel breast implant rupture by ultrasonography. Plast Reconstr Surg 97:104, 1996.

Cohen BE, Biggs TM, Cronin ED, Collins DR Jr. Assessment and longevity of the silicone gel breast implant. Plast Reconstr Surg 99:1597, 1997.

Coleman EA, Coon SK, Thompson PJ, Lemon SJ, Depuy RS. Impact of silicone implants on the lives of women with breast cancer. Oncol Nurs Forum 22:1493, 1995.

Cook RR, Delongchamp RR, Woodbury M, Perkins LL, Harrison MC. The prevalence of women with breast implants in the United States—1989. J Clin Epidemiol 48:519, 1995.

Council on Scientific Affairs, American Medical Association. Silicone gel breast implants. JAMA 270:2602, 1993.

Cronin TD, Gerow F. Augmentation mammaplasty—A new "natural feel" prosthesis. In Transactions of the Third International Congress of Plastic Surgeons. Amsterdam: Excerpta Medica, 1964.

Deapen DM, Brody GS. Augmentation mammoplasty and breast cancer: A five-year update of the Los Angeles study. J Clin Epidemiol 48:551, 1995.

Deapen DM, Bernstein L, Brody GS. Are breast implants anticarcinogenic? A 14-year follow-up of the Los Angeles study. Plast Reconstr Surg 99:1346, 1997.

Deapen DM, Pike MC, Casagrande JT, Brody GS. The relationship between breast cancer and augmentation mammoplasty: An epidemiologic study. Plast Reconstr Surg 77:361, 1986.

Dempsey WC, Latham WD. Subpectoral implants in augmentation mammaplasty. Plast Reconstr Surg 42:515, 1968.

Destouet JM, Monsees BS, Oser RF, Nemecek JR, Young VL, Pilgram TK. Screening mammography in 350 women with breast implants: Prevalence and findings of implant complications. Am J Roentgenol 159:973, 1992.

Dobke MK, Middleton MS. Clinical impact of breast implant magnetic resonance imaging. Ann Plast Surg 33:241, 1994.

Dowden RV. Detection of gel implant rupture: A clinical test. Plast Reconstr Surg 9:548, 1993.

Duffy FJ Jr, May JW Jr. Tissue expanders and magnetic resonance imaging: The "hot" breast implant. Ann Plast Surg 35:647, 1995.

Duffy MJ, Woods JE. Health risks of failed silicone gel breast implants: A 30-year clinical experience. Plast Reconstr Surg 94:295, 1994.

Elkund GW, Busby RC, Miller SH, et al. Improved imaging of the augmented breast. Am J Roentgenol 151:469, 1988.

Englert HJ, Brooks P. Scleroderma and augmentation mammoplasty—A causal relationship? Aust N Z J Med 24:74, 1994.

Englert HJ, Morris D, March L. Scleroderma and silicone gel breast prostheses—The Sydney study revisited. Aust N Z J Med 26:349, 1996.

Everson LI, Parantainen H, Detlie T, Stillman AE, Olson PN, Landis G, Foshager MC, Cunningham B, Griffiths HJ. Diagnosis of breast implant rupture: Imaging findings and relative efficacies of imaging techniques. Am J Roentgenol 163:57, 1994.

Fee-Fulkerson K, Conaway MR, Winer EP, Fulkerson CC, Rimer BK, Georgiade G. Factors contributing to patient satisfaction with breast reconstruction using silicone gel implants. Plast Reconstr Surg 97:1420, 1996.

Ferguson JH. Silicone breast implants and neurologic disorders—Report of the practice committee of the American Academy of Neurology. Neurology 48:1504, 1997.

Forsberg F, Conant EF, Russell KM, Moore JH Jr. Quantitative ultrasonic diagnosis of silicone breast implant rupture: an in-vitro feasibility study. Ultrasound Med Biol 22:53, 1996.

Forster DW. "False bursae" concept in augmentation mammaplasty. Aesthetic Plast Surg 2:419, 1978.

Frankel SD, Occhipinti KA, Kaufman L, Hunt TK, Kerley SM. MRI of a silicone breast implant surrounded by an enlarging hemorrhagic collection. Plast Reconstr Surg 94:865, 1994.

Friedman RM, Gyimesi I, Robinson JB Jr, Rohrich RJ. Saline made viscous with polyethylene glycol: a new alternate breast implant filler material. Plast Reconstr Surg 98:1208, 1996.

Friis S, McLaughlin JK, Mellemkjaer L, Kjoller KH, Blot WJ, Boice JD Jr, Fraumeni JF Jr, Olsen JH. Breast implants and cancer risk in Denmark. Int J Cancer 71:956, 1997.

Gabriel SE, Woods JE, O'Fallon WM, Beard CM, Kurland LT, Melton LJ III. Complications leading to surgery after breast implantation. N Engl J Med 336:677, 1997.

Gabriel SE, O'Fallon WM, Kurland LT, Beard CM, Woods JE, Melton J III. Risk of connective-tissue diseases and other disorders after breast implantation. N Engl J Med 330:1697, 1994.

Gayou RM. A histological comparison of contracted and noncontracted capsules around silicone breast implants. Plast Reconstr Surg 63:700, 1979.

Giltay EJ, Moens HJB, Riley AH, et al. Silicone breast prostheses and rheumatic symptoms: A retrospective follow-up study. Ann Rheum Dis 53:194, 1994.

Godfrey PM, Godfrey NV. Response of locoregional and systemic symptoms to breast implant replacement with autologous tissues: Experience in 37 consecutive patients. Plast Reconstr Surg 97:110, 1996.

Goldman JA, Greenblatt J, Joines R, White L, Aylward B, Lamm SH. Breast implants, rheumatoid arthritis, and connective tissue diseases in a clinical practice. J Clin Epidemiol 48:571, 1995.

Gorczyca DP, DeBruhl ND, Ahn CY, Hoyt A, Sayre JW, Nudell P, McCombs M, Shaw WW, Bassett LW. Silicone breast implant ruptures in an animal model: Comparison of mammography, MR imaging, US, and CT. Radiology 190:227, 1994.

Gorczyca DP, Schneider E, DeBruhl ND, Foo TK, Ahn CY, Sayre JW, Shaw WW, Bassett LW. Silicone breast implant rupture: Comparison between three-point Dixon and fast spin-echo MR imaging. Am J Roentgenol 162:305, 1994.

Gorczyca DP, Sinha S, Ahn CY, DeBruhl ND, Hayes HK, Gausche VR, Shaw WW, Bassett LW. Silicone breast implants in vivo: MR imaging. Radiology 185:407, 1992.

Greenwald DP, Randolph M, May JW Jr. Mechanical analysis of explanted silicone breast implants. Plast Reconstr Surg 98:269, 1996.

Gumucio CA, Pin P, Young VL, Destouet J, Monsees B, Eichling J. The effect of breast implants on the radiographic detection of microcalcification and soft-tissue masses. Plast Reconstr Surg 84:772, 1989.

Gruber RP, Friedman GD. Periareolar subpectoral augmentation mammaplasty. Plast Reconstr Surg 67:458, 1981

Gruber RP, Jones HW. Review of closed capsulotomy complications. Ann Plast Surg 6:271, 1981.

Gutowski KA, Mesna GT, Cunningham BL. Saline-filled breast implants: A Plastic Surgery Educational Foundation multicenter outcomes study. Plast Reconstr Surg 100:1019, 1997.

Handel N, Silverstein MJ, Gamagami P, Collins A. An in vivo study of the effect of various breast implant filler materials on mammography. Plast Reconstr Surg 91:1057, 1993.

Handel N, Jensen JA, Black Q, Waisman JR, Silverstein MJ. The fate of breast implants: A critical analysis of complications and outcomes. Plast Reconstr Surg 96:1521, 1995.

Handel N, Wellisch D, Silverstein MJ, Jensen JA, Waisman E. Knowledge, concern, and satisfaction among augmentation mammaplasty patients. Ann Plast Surg 30:1, 1993.

Handel N, Silverstein MJ, Jensen JA, Collins A, Zierk K. Comparative experience with smooth and polyurethane breast implants using the Kaplan-Meier method of survival analysis. Plast Reconstr Surg 88:475, 1991.

Hang-Fu L, Marmolya G, Feiglin DH. Liposuction fat-fillant implant for breast augmentation and reconstruction. Aesthetic Plast Surg 19:427, 1995.

Hardt NS, Yu L, LaTorre G, Steinbach B. Complications related to retained breast implant capsules. Plast Reconstr Surg 95:364, 1995.

Hart D. Women and saline breast implant surgery. Plast Surg 15:161, 1995.

Hennekens CH, Lee I-M, Cook NR, et al. Self-reported breast implants and connective-tissue diseases in female health professionals. JAMA 275:616, 1996.

Hochberg MC, Perlmutter DL, Medsger TA Jr, Nguyen K, Steen V, Weisman MH, White B, Wigley FM. Lack of association between augmentation mammoplasty and systemic sclerosis (scleroderma). Arthritis Rheum 39:1125, 1996.

Jarret JR, Cutler RG, Teal DF. Subcutaneous mastectomy in small, large, or ptotic breasts with immediate submuscular placement of implants. Plast Reconstr Surg 62:381, 1978.

Kaiser J. Panel discounts implant disease risk. Science 284:2065, 1999.

Karns ME, Cullison CA, Romano TJ, et al. Breast implants and connective-tissue disease. JAMA 276:100, 1996.

Kessler DA. The basis of the FDA's decision on breast implants. N Engl J Med 326:1713, 1992.

Kessler DA, Merkatz RB, Schapiro R. A call for higher standards for breast implants. JAMA 270: 2607, 1993.

Kulber DA, Mackenzie D, Steiner JH, Glassman H, Hopp D, Hiatt JR, Hoffman L. Monitoring the axilla in patients with silicone gel implants. Ann Plast Surg 35:580, 1995.

Laing TJ, Gillespie BW, Lacey JV Jr, et al. The association between silicone exposure and undifferentiated connective tissue disease among women in Michigan and Ohio. Arthritis Rheum 39: S150, 1996.

Leibman AJ. Imaging of complications of augmentation mammaplasty. Plast Reconstr Surg 93: 1134, 1994.

Leibman AJ, Kossoff MB, Kruse BD. Intraductal extension of silicone from a ruptured breast implant. Plast Reconstr Surg 89:546, 1992.

Levine RA, Collins TL. Definitive diagnosis of breast implant rupture by ultrasonography. Plast Reconstr Surg 87:1126, 1991.

Liston JC, Malata CM, Varma S, Scott M, Sharpe DT. The role of ultrasound imaging in the diagnosis of breast implant rupture: A prospective study. Br J Plast Surg 47:477, 1994.

Little JW III, Goembe EV, Fisher JB. The "living bra" in immediate and delayed reconstruction of the breast following mastectomy for malignant and nonmalignant disease. Plast Reconstr Surg 68:392, 1981.

Mahler D, Hauben DJ. Retromammary versus retropectoral breast augmentation. A comparative study. Ann Plast Surg 8:370, 1982.

Malata CM, Feldberg L, Coleman DJ, Foo IT, Sharpe DT. Textured or smooth implants for breast augmentation? Three-year follow-up of a prospective randomised controlled trial. Br J Plast Surg 50:99, 1997.

Malata CM, Varma S, Scott M, Liston JC, Sharpe DT. Silicone breast implant rupture: common/ serious complication? Med Prog Technol 20:251-260, 1994.

Matti BA, Nicolle FV. A simple technique for removing a silastic gel–filled breast implant through the axillary approach. Br J Plast Surg 42:613, 1989.

McLaughlin JK, Fraumeni JF, Nyren O. Silicone breast implants and risk of cancer? JAMA 273:116, 1995.

McLaughlin JK, Fraumeni JF, Olsen J, Friis S, Mellemkjaer L, Fraumeni JF Jr. Re: Breast implants, cancer, and systemic sclerosis. J Natl Cancer Inst 86:1424, 1994.

Mineyev M, Kramer D, Kaufman L, Carlson J, Frankel S. Measurement of breast implant volume with magnetic resonance imaging. Ann Plast Surg 34:348, 1995.

Moran T. Battle scars. For plastic surgeons, psychological effects linger from silicone breast implant controversy. Tex Med 91:30, 1995.

Nachbar JM, Orrison WW Jr. Validation of quantification of breast implant capsule surface area and volume using magnetic resonance imaging. Ann Plast Surg 27:321, 1991.

Netscher DT, Weizer G, Malone RS, Walker LE, Thornby J, Patten BM. Diagnostic value of clinical examination and various imaging techniques for breast implant rupture as determined in 81 patients having implant removal. South Med J 89:397, 1996.

Netscher DT, Sharma S, Thornby J, Peltier M, Lyos A, Fater M, Mosharrafa A. Aesthetic outcome of breast implant removal in 85 consecutive patients. Plast Reconstr Surg 100:206, 1997.

Noone RB. A review of the possible health implications of silicone breast implants. Cancer 79:1747, 1997.

Noone RB, Frazier TG, Hayward CZ, Skiles MS. Patient acceptance of immediate reconstruction following mastectomy. Plast Reconstr Surg 69:632, 1982.

Park AJ, Chetty U, Watson ACH. Patient satisfaction following insertion of silicone breast implants. Br J Plast Surg 49:515, 1996.

Park AJ, Black RJ, Watson ACH. Silicone gel breast implants, breast cancer and connective tissue disorders. Br J Surg 80:1097, 1993.

Park AJ, Walsh J, Reddy PS, Chetty U, Watson AC. The detection of breast implant rupture using ultrasound. Br J Plast Surg 49:299, 1996.

Park AJ, Chetty U, Watson ACH. Patient satisfaction following insertion of silicone breast implants. Br J Plast Surg 49:515, 1996.

Pay AD, Kenealy J. Breast implant rupture following contralateral mammography. Plast Reconstr Surg 99:1734, 1997.

Peters W, Smith D. Calcification of breast implant capsules: Incidence, diagnosis, and contributing factors. Ann Plast Surg 34:8, 1995.

Peters W, Smith D, Fornasier V, Lugowski S, Ibanez D. An outcome analysis of 100 women after explantation of silicone gel breast implants. Ann Plast Surg 39:1, 1997.

Petit JY, Le MG, Mouriesse H, Rietjens M, Gill P, Contesso G, Lehmann A. Can breast reconstruction with gel-filled silicone implants increase the risk of death and second primary cancer in patients treated by mastectomy for breast cancer? Plast Reconstr Surg 94:115, 1994.

Pickrell KL, Puckett CL, Given KS. Subpectoral augmentation mammaplasty. Plast Reconstr Surg 60:325, 1977.

Radovan C. Tissue expansion in soft-tissue reconstruction. Plast Reconstr Surg 74:482, 1984.

Ransjo U, Asplund OA, Gylbert L, Jurell G. Bacteria in the female breast. Scand J Plast Reconstr Surg 19:87, 1985.

Reed ME. Daubert and the breast implant litigation: How is the judiciary addressing the science? Plast Reconstr Surg 100:1322, 1997.

Regnault P. The hypoplastic and ptotic breast: A combined operation with prosthetic augmentation. Plast Reconstr Surg 37:31, 1966.

Regnault P. Experience with augmentation mammaplasty. In Owsley JQ Jr, Peterson RA, eds. Symposium on Aesthetic Surgery of the Breast. St. Louis: CV Mosby, 1978.

Reynolds HE, Buckwalter KA, Jackson VP, Siwy BK, Alexander SG. Comparison of mammography, sonography, and magnetic resonance imaging in the detection of silicone-gel breast implant rupture. Ann Plast Surg 33:247, 1994.

Rheingold LM, Yoo RP, Courtiss EH. Experience with 326 inflatable breast implants. Plast Reconstr Surg 93:118, 1994.

Rohrich RJ, Beran SJ, Ingram AE Jr, Young VL. Development of alternative breast implant filler material: Criteria and horizons. Plast Reconstr Surg 98:552, 1996.

Romanelli JN. More on breast implants and connective-tissue diseases [Letter]. N Engl J Med 332: 1306, 1995.

Rose NR. The silicone breast implant controversy: The other courtroom. Arthritis Rheum 39:1615, 1996.

Rothkopf DM, Rosen HM. Lactation as a complication of aesthetic breast surgery successfully treated with bromocriptine. Br J Plast Surg 43:373, 1990.

Samuels JB, Rohrich RJ, Weatherall PT, Ho AM, Goldberg KL. Radiographic diagnosis of breast implant rupture: Current status and comparison of techniques. Plast Reconstr Surg 96:865, 1995.

Sanchez-Guerrero J, Liang MH. Silicone breast implants and connective tissue diseases: No association has been convincingly established. Br Med J 309:822, 1994.

Sanchez-Guerrero J, Colditz GA, Karlson EW, Hunter DJ, Speizer FE, Liang MH. Silicone breast implants and the risk of connective-tissue diseases and symptoms. N Engl J Med 332:1666, 1995.

Schnur PL, Weinzweig J, Harris JB, Moyer TP, Petty PM, Nixon D, McConnell JP. Silicone analysis of breast and periprosthetic capsular tissue from patients with saline or silicone gel breast implants. Plast Reconstr Surg 98:798, 1996.

Schusterman MA, Kroll SS, Reece GP, Miller MJ, Ainslee N, Halabi S, Balch CM. Incidence of autoimmune disease in patients after breast reconstruction with silicone gel implants versus autogenous tissue: A preliminary report. Ann Plast Surg 31:1, 1993.

Scott IR, Muller NL, Fitzpatrick DG, Burhenne LJ. Ruptured breast implant: Computed tomographic and mammographic findings. Can Assoc Radiol J 39:152, 1988.

Smahel J. Histology of the capsules causing constrictive fibrosis around breast implants. Br J Plast Surg 30:324,1977.

Strom SS, Baldwin BJ, Sigurdson AJ, Schusterman MA. Cosmetic saline breast implants: A survey of satisfaction, breast-feeding experience, cancer screening, and health. Plast Reconstr Surg 100: 1553, 1997.

Troilius C. Total muscle coverage of a breast implant is possible through the transaxillary approach. Plast Reconstr Surg 95:509, 1995.

Vanderford ML, Smith DH, Olive T. The image of plastic surgeons in news media coverage of the silicone breast implant controversy. Plast Reconstr Surg 96:521, 1995.

Venta LA, Salomon CG, Flisak ME, Venta ER, Izquierdo R, Angelats J. Sonographic signs of breast implant rupture. Am J Roentgenol 166:1413, 1996.

Vinnik CA. Spherical contracture of fibrous capsules around breast implants. Plast Reconstr Surg 58:555, 1976.

Vistnes LM, Ksander GA, Kosek J. Study of encapsulation of silicone rubber implants in animals: A foreign body reaction. Plast Reconstr Surg 62:580, 1978.

Weizer G, Malone RS, Netscher DT, Walker LE, Thornby J. Utility of magnetic resonance imaging and ultrasonography in diagnosing breast implant rupture. Ann Plast Surg 34:352, 1995.

Wells KE, Roberts C, Daniels SM, Hann D, Clement V, Reintgen D, Cox CE. Comparison of psychological symptoms of women requesting removal of breast implants with those of breast cancer patients and healthy controls. Plast Reconstr Surg 99:680, 1997.

Wigley FM, Miller R, Hochberg MC, et al. Augmentation mammoplasty in patients with systemic sclerosis: Data from the Baltimore scleroderma research center and Pittsburgh scleroderma data bank. Arthritis Rheum 35:S46, 1992.

Williams HJ, Weisman MH, Berry CC. Breast implants in patients with undifferentiated connective tissue disease. Arthritis Rheum 40:437, 1997.

Wolfe F. Silicone breast implants and the risk of fibromyalgia and rheumatoid arthritis. Arthritis Rheum 38:S265, 1995.

Wong O. A critical assessment of the relationship between silicone breast implants and connective tissue diseases. Regulatory Toxicol Pharmacol 23:74, 1996.

Woods JE, Arnold PE. Fiction obscures the facts of breast implants. The Wall Street Journal, April 7, 1992.

Young VL, Hertl MC, Murray PR, Lambros VS. *Paecilomyces variotii* contamination in the lumen of a saline-filled breast implant. Plast Reconstr Surg 96:1430, 1995.

Young VL, Diehl GJ, Eichling J, Monsees BS, Destouet J. The relative radiolucencies of breast implant filler materials. Plast Reconstr Surg 9:1066, 1993.

Young VL, Bartell T, Destouet JM, Monsees B, Logan SE. Calcification of breast implant capsule. South Med J 82:1171, 1989.

Young VL, Lund H, Ueda K, Pidgeon L, Schorr MW, Kreeger J. Bleed of and biologic response to triglyceride filler used in radiolucent breast implants. Plast Reconstr Surg 97:1179, 1996.

PART II

Aesthetic Breast Surgery

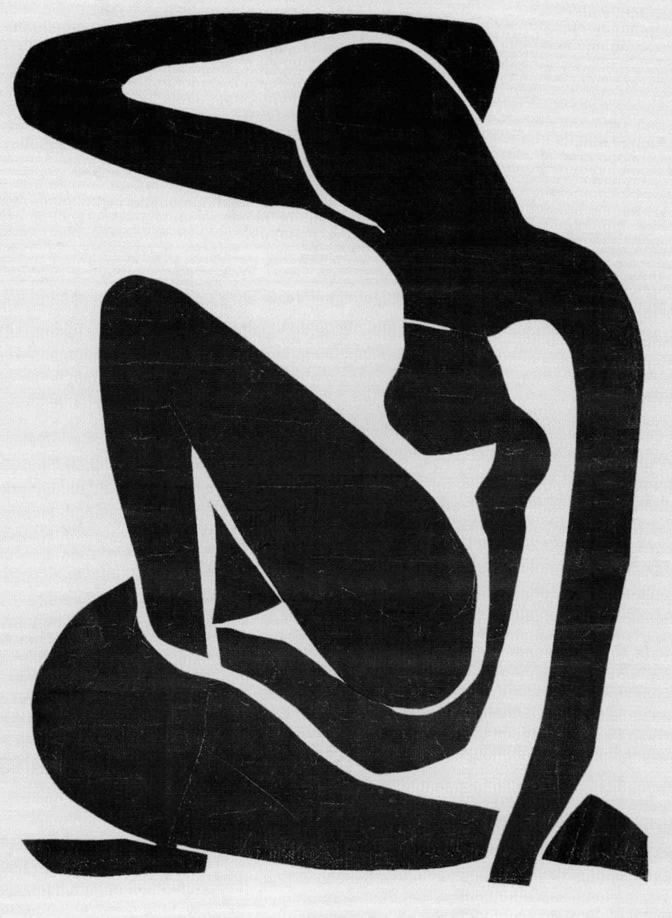

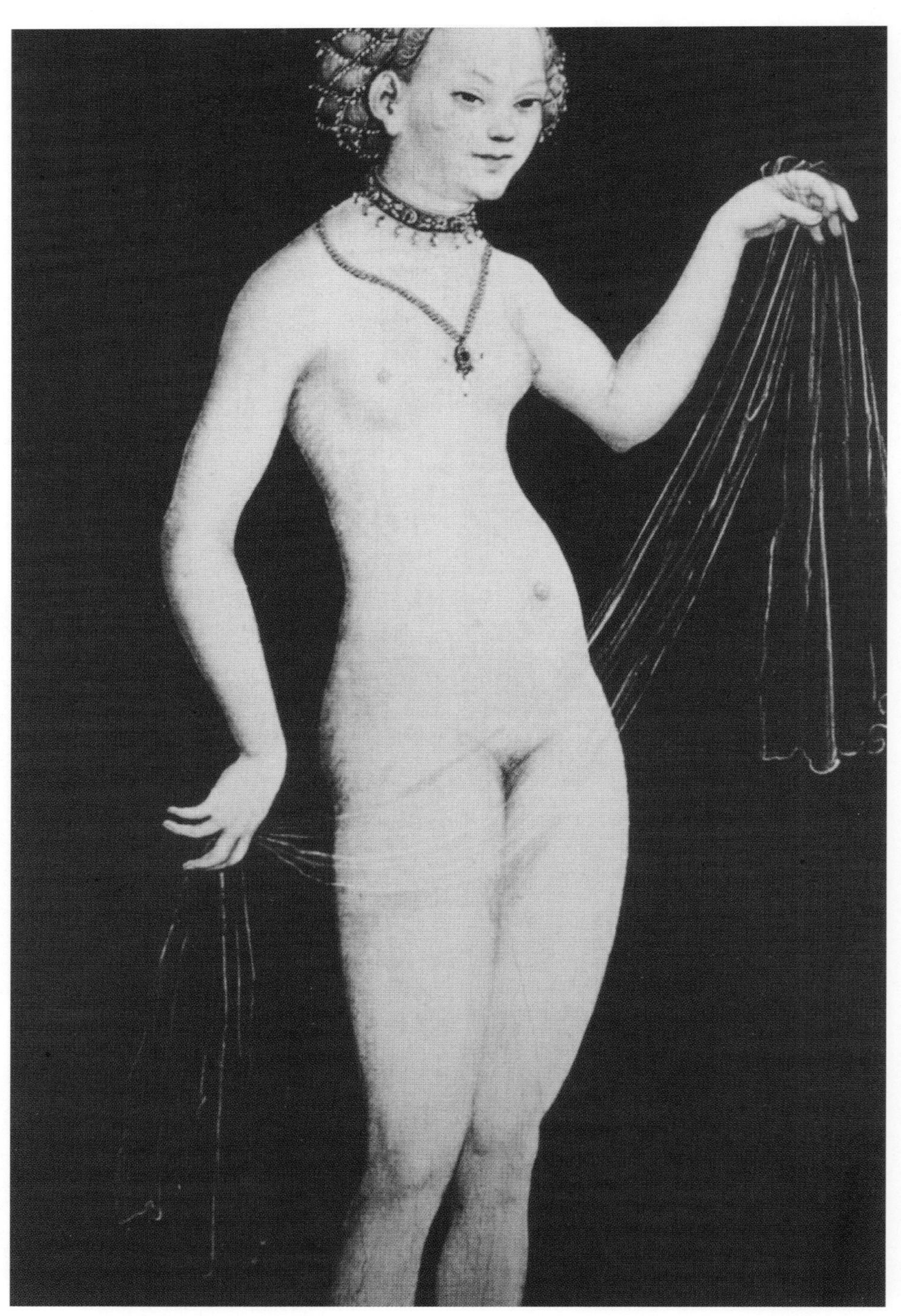

6 *Augmentation Mammaplasty*

Key Topics

Selecting an Implant

- Smooth and Textured Surface
  - Round and Anatomic Shaped

Implant Placement

- Subpectoral
- Subglandular

Incision Placement

Axillary Augmentation

- Standard and Endoscopic Approaches

Inframammary Augmentation

- Standard and Endoscopic Approaches

Periareolar Augmentation

- Standard Approach

Intraoperative Expansion

Augmentation With Tissue Expansion

Augmentation With Abdominal Liposuction or Abdominoplasty

Capsular Contracture

Complications

Long-Term Results

Observations

Each year over 100,000 women in the United States elect to have breast augmentation, an operation noted for its high level of patient acceptance despite ongoing questions and recent controversy over the safety and efficacy of breast implants. Although the popularity of this operation declined after the Food and Drug Administration restricted access to silicone gel–filled implants in the early 1990s, the results of clinical trials and numerous scientific studies now available have provided considerably more information about these devices and their associated risks and benefits. Studies by respected scientists have indicated that implants do not pose a serious health hazard, are not linked to connective tissue disease, and do not increase the risk of breast cancer. In its informed consent document the FDA has concurred with these conclusions. As the controversy has subsided, the demand for implant surgery has increased. Women again feel comfortable requesting this surgical option both for aesthetic and reconstructive purposes. The renewed popularity of augmentation mammaplasty, however, is very different from that which prevailed before the FDA moratorium when implant surgery was greeted with almost unquestioning enthusiasm and acceptance. Although silicone gel–filled implants have not proved the villains they were branded to be, not everyone is aware that they have been cleared of many of the charges leveled against them. Therefore it is only natural that many patients still have lingering concerns about implant surgery and worry about potential problems or complications with these devices. Surgeons also approach implants and implant surgery with more caution and reticence in view of the litigation and media attention that these devices attracted.

Those of us experienced in breast augmentation techniques have long ago abandoned any false notions that augmentation or any implant surgery for that matter is routine as once believed. Creating a long-lasting, soft, and natural augmented breast continues to challenge the surgeon's skill and ingenuity. I now usually insert implants subpectorally, believing that this extra layer helps protect the implant by placing an anatomic layer between the implant and the breast with its bacterial content. This muscle cover appears to minimize the occurrence of capsular contracture. Radiologists say that subpectoral implant placement also facilitates the interpretation of mammograms. During the past few years my approach has been to place saline-filled implants in the subpectoral position. Intraoperative tissue expansion techniques have also given us more versatility in performing augmentation procedures, optimizing prospects for producing breasts of a size that will meet with patient satisfaction.

Endoscopic augmentation mammaplasty has infused a new dynamic into the practice of aesthetic breast surgery, offering patients improved results as a consequence of better visualization, more controlled dissections, shorter incisions, better control of bleeding, and enhanced definition for dissection in the medial cleavage area. Accurate control of the inframammary crease has permitted a broader range of candidates for this procedure. Endoscopic techniques have also improved the predictability of postoperative results.

Patient Assessment and Selection

Women requesting breast augmentation appear to place considerable emphasis on their physical appearance, and they often experience feelings of decreased femininity because of their small breasts. Most women with hypoplastic breasts seeking breast augmentation relate that their feelings of breast inadequacy go back to their teenage years; however, for a variety of reasons, some economic, most patients requesting breast augmentation are in their twenties and thirties. If the patient is self-motivated ("I'm doing this for me" or "I've always wanted larger breasts"), then breast augmentation is associated with a high level of patient satisfaction once the patient's aesthetic concerns and expectations are addressed and an appropriate breast augmentation carried out.

Women requesting breast augmentation today are usually aware of the breast implant controversy, but it does not dissuade them from proceeding with this operation because they feel the advantages of implants outweigh the disadvantages. However, this does not suggest that they do not have questions and concerns about these devices; the bad publicity that implants received has had a definite impact. Women may be more skittish and nervous about this procedure and less accepting of complications and problems. Consequently, it is more important than ever for women considering breast augmentation to be carefully and fully informed of the pros and cons of these devices and of the details of this operation, including possible long-term effects on monitoring and breast cancer surveillance.

PATIENT PROFILES
Women in Their Twenties

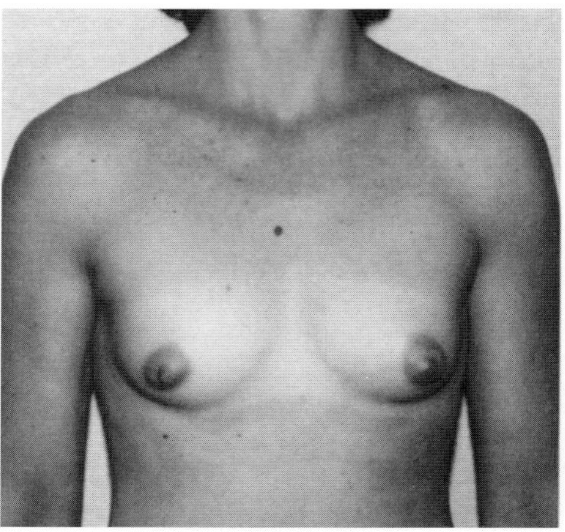
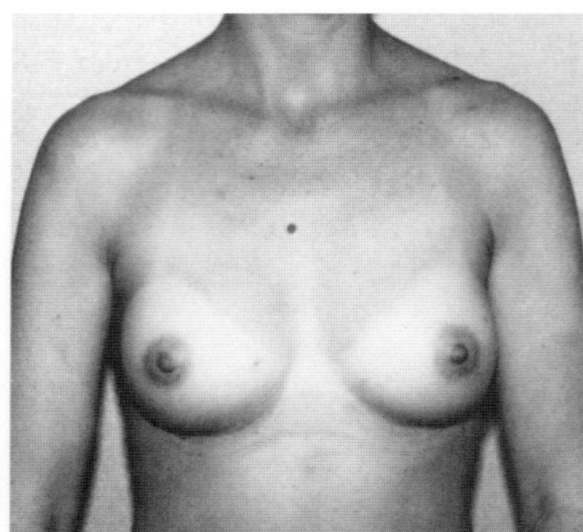

Younger women requesting augmentation are usually nulliparous and are often unmarried. They tend to be thin, muscular, and athletic and often exhibit a striking degree of breast hypoplasia. Highly motivated to have the procedure, they also tend to be very conscious of scar placement and have high expectations for an attractive result. These patients are good candidates, but the details of the operation, potential complications, and anticipated results must be fully disclosed and carefully explained to avoid future disappointment.

Women 25 to 45 Years of Age

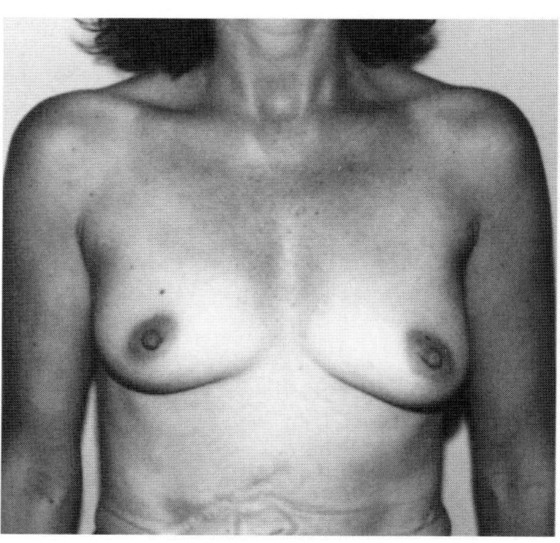
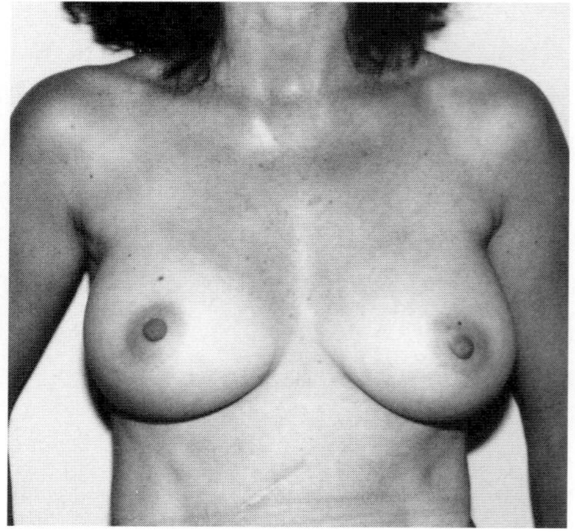

A somewhat older group seeks breast augmentation because of underlying breast hypoplasia, often accentuated by postpartum involution. Frequently they have considered this procedure for several years, tend to be well informed about it, often know a friend or relative who has had the procedure, and have more reasonable expectations as to what can be accomplished. Many liked the increased breast size they experienced during pregnancy and lactation. They look at their now involuted breasts, upper pole flattening, and early glandular ptosis with disappointment. Because they are somewhat older, they express more concerns about the oncologic implications of this procedure and its effect on breast imaging and oncologic surveillance.

Some women in this age group are interested in breast augmentation to offset the emotional impact of a defeminizing procedure such as tubal ligation or hysterectomy. These women are usually pleased with the results of surgery.

Women With Hidden Agendas

Not all women requesting this operation are acting independently nor are they motivated solely by a desire to have larger breasts. It is important for the surgeon to discover the patient's outside influences and hidden motivators before a decision is made for augmentation mammaplasty. These motivations may seem important to the woman at the time; however, she and the surgeon may regret the decision for surgery later. Most plastic surgeons who perform augmentation mammaplasty are familiar with the woman who requests the procedure because she is having marital difficulties; she feels that her husband prefers women with larger breasts and she would be more attractive to him if she made herself more voluptuous.

Some women request breast augmentation to boost general deep-seated feelings of inferiority and unworthiness out of proportion to the typical insecurity exhibited by those with small breasts. These women hope that by enlarging their breasts they will become more popular and admired. When these expectations are not met after augmentation mammaplasty and the insecurities persist, they will be dissatisfied and may even request larger implants that are inappropriate for their body habitus. Sometimes patients with this motivation will focus on the operation as the cause of their unhappiness, feeling that some small deficiency in the operation, a minor asymmetry, volume discrepancy, or nipple malposition, is the root of the problem. These women are frequent visitors to the surgeon's office, voicing vague complaints and requesting reoperation.

Still other women request this procedure in the mistaken belief that it will enhance their careers. Although a number of models and actresses have had breast implants, the procedure itself certainly does not guarantee stardom. Augmentation mammaplasty only produces larger breasts; it does not and cannot produce a major transformation in the person's lifestyle or social situation.

Concerns of Patient and Surgeon

BREAST SIZE

For patients requesting breast augmentation, concerns about breast appearance and size are paramount. The surgeon must first get an idea of how the patient perceives her current breast size and question her about how she wants to look after the operation. Meeting her expectations for breast size and shape is the single most important consideration in ensuring a satisfied patient after the operation. Frequently the patient will answer cautiously, "A little larger" or "Not too much, but I do want to get my money's worth!" It must be remembered, however, that the patient is in your office because she desires larger breasts. The surgeon must be sure that her hesitation does not reflect modesty about revealing her true desire for breast size but portrays her real feelings about the amount of enlargement she desires. Many women seem embarrassed to tell the surgeon that they truly want very large breasts, yet they will immediately express their disappointment if they feel they are not large enough postoperatively. In response to patient desires I have gradually increased the average-sized implant for augmentation from a range of 180 to 250 cc to 200 to 400 cc and select the implant based on the diameter of the planned breast size.

SCARS

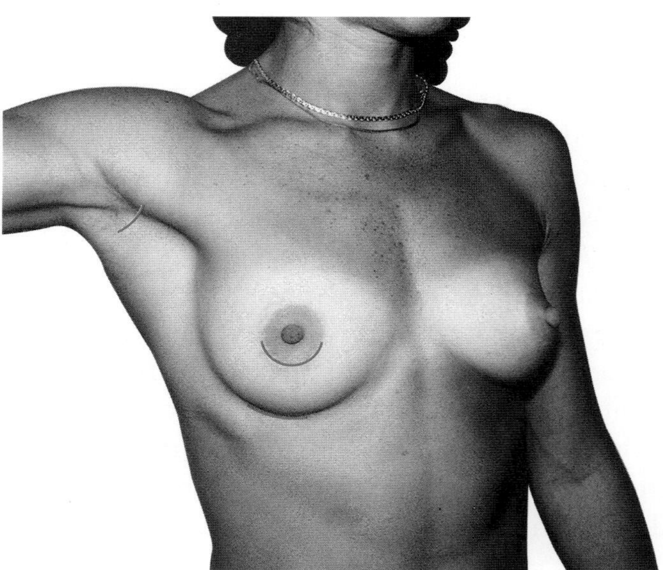

Next to breast size and soft, natural-feeling breasts, the length and placement of scars concern the augmentation patient. She wants to avoid the visible or obvious scars that are the telltale signs that she has had this operation. ***I prefer to place scars away from the breast in the axilla or in the inframammary crease where they are less noticeable and avoid significant dissection of the breast parenchyma that is associated with periareolar scars.***

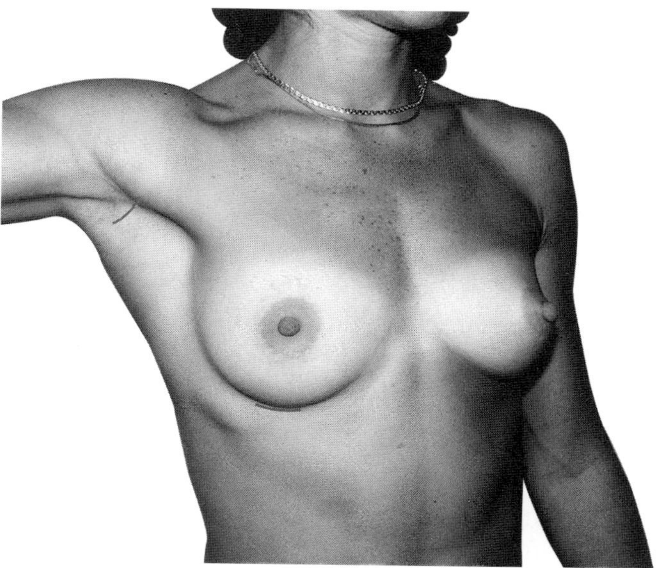

Endoscopic techniques can be used to perform axillary and inframammary breast augmentation with better visualization, shorter scars, more precise dissection, and improved accuracy of implant placement. When axillary incisions are planned, I inform the patient that I may need to make an additional inframammary incision if I encounter unusual bleeding or later if asymmetry or capsular contracture develops. In practice this has occurred in less than 1% of my patients. ***The axillary incision usually heals primarily without scar hypertrophy.*** In patients with a suggestion of hypertrophic healing of previous incisions I avoid the inframammary crease scar since it seems more prone to this type of problem than the axillary or periareolar scar. When the areolar diameter is satisfactory or a small repositioning of the nipple-areola is necessary, the periareolar approach can provide an effective solution to this problem. However, I generally advise women against a central breast incision that requires some division and incision of breast tissue and can leave a visible areolar scar. In addition, incisions through breast parenchyma probably increase the possibility of contamination with *Staphylococcus epidermidis* that colonizes the duct systems of most breasts.

ONCOLOGIC CONSIDERATIONS

Cancer concerns of the augmentation mammaplasty patient focus primarily on the safety of implants for breast enlargement and whether implants can mask a cancer or interfere with imaging for cancer surveillance. Is this operation safe? Will it cause cancer? Will it mask early signs of breast cancer? are frequent questions that need to be addressed. I explain to patients that silicone is not carcinogenic in humans and has not been associated with an increased incidence of breast cancer. A woman's risk of developing breast cancer is not affected by breast implants. Multiple epidemiologic studies have failed to show an increase in breast cancer after breast augmentation, that breast cancer diagnosis and treatment are delayed because of implants, or that survival is compromised (see Chapter 5).

Implant positioning can affect both tumor detection and management. It can also influence healing, the incidence of capsular contracture, and the quality and natural appearance of the result. This topic must be discussed with the patient. I explain that most radiologists and general surgeons are more confident about evaluation and surgical biopsy of a breast mass when the implant is in the subpectoral position. Since the implant is placed behind breast tissue, any breast mass will be in front of the breast implant. Breast imaging techniques (mammography and sonography) generally allow better breast visualization when the implant is underneath the muscle. Radiopaque implants can still pose imaging problems, however, and the patient's doctors and the radiologist should be informed that a woman's breasts have been augmented so that the radiologist can make adjustments in the views taken and use special diagnostic views developed for imaging breast implant patients. He will include additional displacement views to adequately visualize the breast parenchyma and include the "squeeze" technique to pull and project the breast parenchyma beyond the breast implant. In the event that a tumor is detected, stereotactic, ultrasound-guided, or open biopsy or lumpectomy and radiation therapy can usually be done with the implant in place, particularly if it is in a subpectoral position. Immediate breast reconstruction can also be performed after total mastectomy in patients who have had breast augmentation. Sometimes the implant can be preserved or exchanged for a larger one at the time of the mastectomy.

SENSATION

Although some patients inquire about the effect of surgery on breast sensation, this does not appear to be a major consideration for most individuals. I explain that breast and nipple sensation is usually not permanently affected because the breast nerves are stretched but not divided. If sensation is decreased, it usually returns in a few weeks or months; however, paresthesias and dysesthesias may accompany the return of sensation. ***The relative size and diameter of the breast implant appear to be directly proportional to decreased sensation.*** When a large, wide pocket is developed for placement of a particularly large breast implant or sharp dissection is used, more patients report decreased sensation. Breast sensation is more at risk during secondary operations that divide the capsule surrounding the breast implant and extend or enlarge the implant pocket, during which the sensory nerves may be injured.

PREGNANCY AND LACTATION

Many patients seek breast augmentation after their childbearing years. Often these women liked their breast size while they were lactating and were disappointed when their breasts once again shrank to their smaller, more ptotic prelactation size. Breast augmentation can restore their breasts to a fullness they experienced during lactation or before their initial pregnancy. Younger patients, however, frequently request breast augmentation before pregnancy and ask about the safety, timing, and effect of this procedure on their breasts, on a future pregnancy, and on their ability to lactate. ***The potential for lactation is not impaired by breast implants, especially when incisions within the breast parenchyma are avoided and when the implants are positioned behind the breasts and usually also behind the pectoral muscle layer.*** I recommend that a woman wait at least 6 months after lactation before having breast augmentation. This ensures that lactation has subsided and that the breasts have decreased to a stable size and shape. If a lactating breast is augmented, milk can accumulate in the implant pocket from breast ducts divided during the operation. I also suggest that a patient wait at least 6 months after breast augmentation to get pregnant. This delay provides a suitable interval for wound healing. It is also important to ensure the patient is not pregnant at the time of breast augmentation, largely because of the adverse effects of anesthesia and medications on the developing fetus. An accurate menstrual history should be taken and specific questions asked about a possible pregnancy. When there is any doubt, a pregnancy test is done or the procedure delayed.

Breast augmentation does not interfere with lactation or breast-feeding. A number of my patients have successfully breast-fed their infants after augmentation mammaplasty. It is difficult to predict breast appearance following pregnancy, lactation, and breast-feeding. Although most patients' breasts return to their prepregnancy appearance, others may show marked changes after pregnancy, especially if there has been considerable breast enlargement or weight change resulting in poor skin elasticity, striae, and stretched Cooper's ligaments.

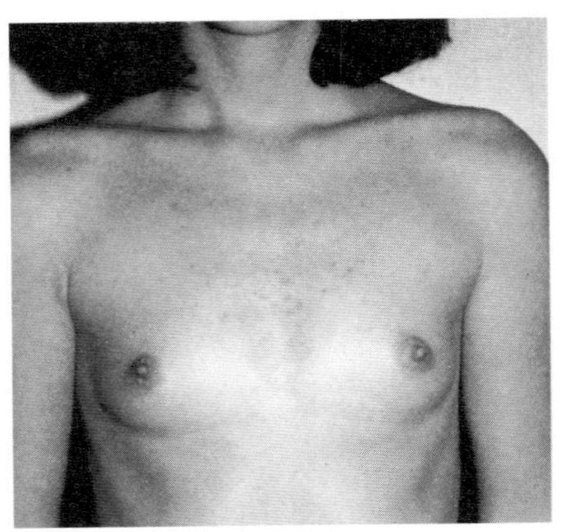
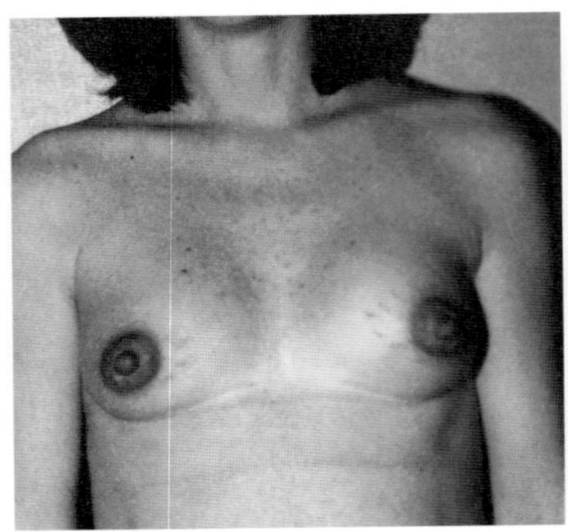
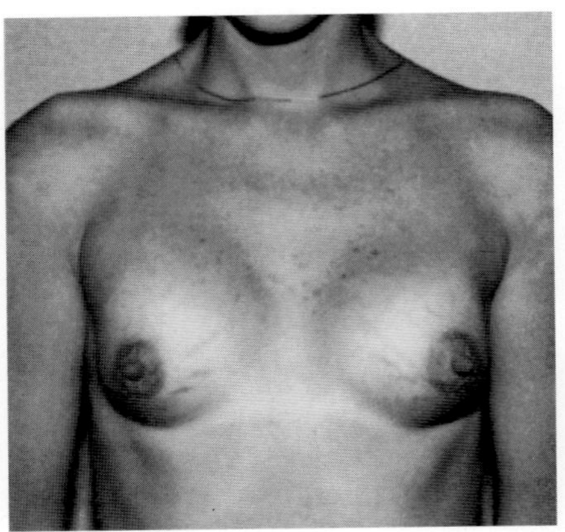

This breast augmentation patient is shown before the initial procedure, at 8 months' gestation, and 4 months postpartum. She breast-fed her infant for 3 months.

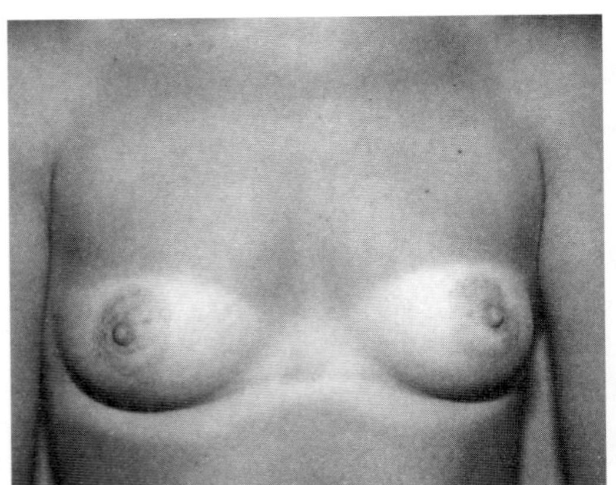
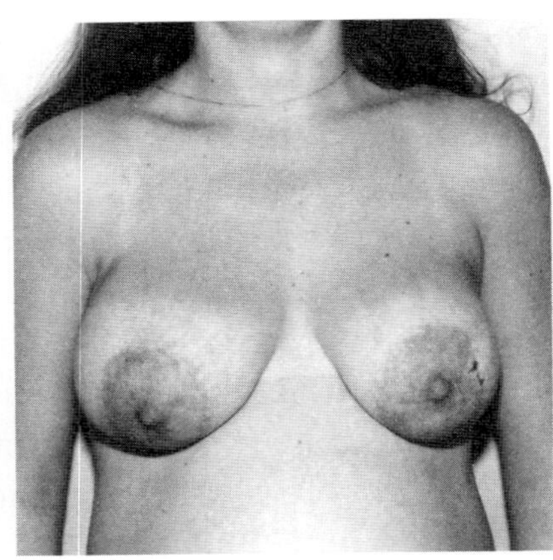
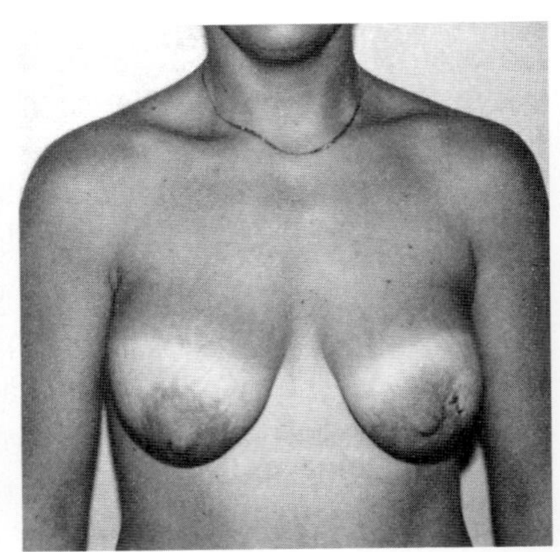

This patient had breast augmentation with subglandular periareolar breast implants. She is shown prior to the initial procedure, at 7 months' gestation, and 4 months following a 6-month period of nursing. She experienced significant breast enlargement during pregnancy, which later resulted in ptosis. Although this patient is displeased with her current breast appearance, she has declined any additional procedures until she completes childbearing.

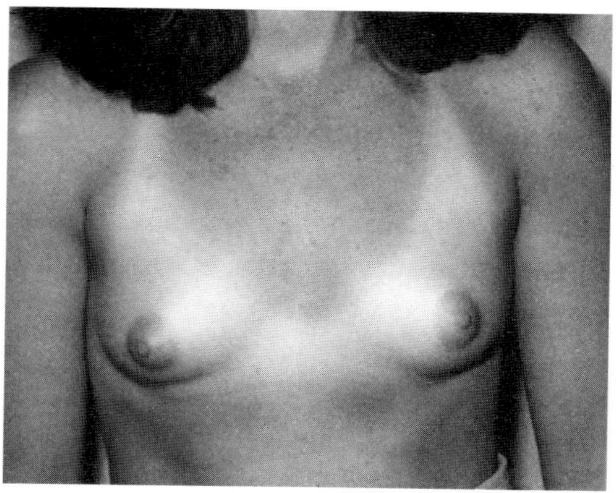

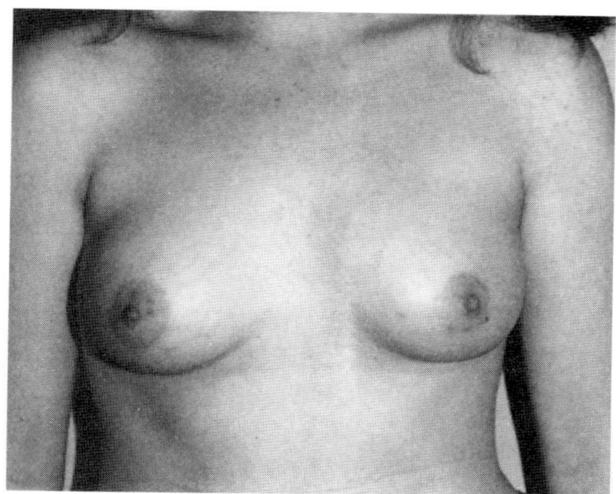

This patient is shown before and 5 years after breast augmentation. She became pregnant 3 years following augmentation and breast-fed her infant for 6 months. Her breast appearance remained basically unchanged, as is ordinarily the case in this situation.

SYMMETRY

Most breasts exhibit some asymmetry. ***An underlying chest wall asymmetry or scoliosis can affect breast appearance and projection.*** As with most conditions, however, asymmetry must be looked for specifically. You can be assured that the patient will examine her breasts frequently and in detail for any differences after the operation, fully expecting aesthetic breast surgery to have resulted in perfectly balanced breasts. Any deviation is therefore a cause for concern. That is why it is important to alert her to any asymmetries that exist before the operation and explain that efforts will be made to improve them as much as possible, but it would be unrealistic to expect a perfectly symmetric result. ***If a woman is unaware of preexisting breast asymmetries, she will not be prepared for the expected asymmetry after the operation.*** She will assume that the distortion has been caused by the operation and should have been resolved or avoided by the surgeon.

Planning

DETERMINING BREAST VOLUME

The patient's concept of her ideal breast size strongly influences the ultimate decision as to breast volume. I always ask the patient about her assessment of present breast size and have her explain the enlargement desired. Some patients bring in padded brassieres or pictures to indicate a breast volume that is more to their liking. The amount of padding in the patient's brassiere provides additional clues to the breast size she feels comfortable with. Sometimes I place a breast implant in the patient's brassiere to help determine the size and appearance she desires. Other patients have even made a point of coming for consultation when they are lactating and their breasts are full to demonstrate the size that they want their breasts to be after augmentation.

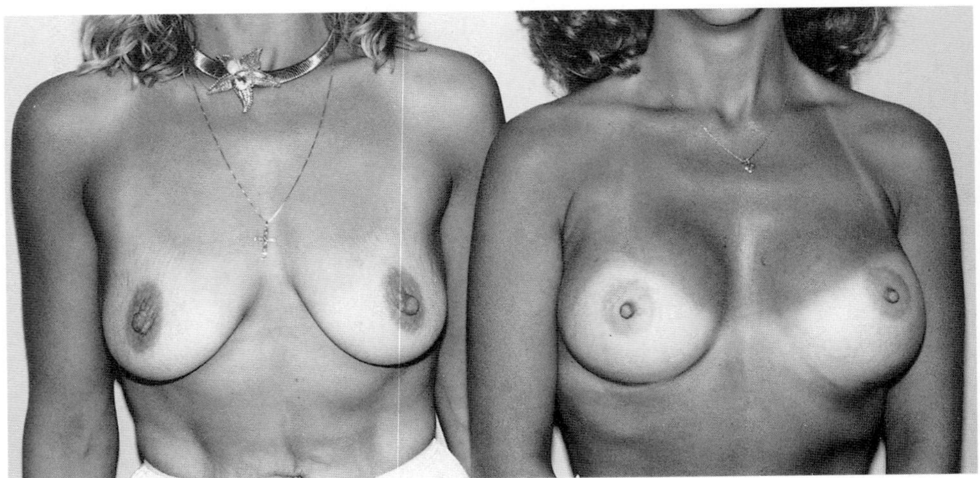

The patient on the left even brought her sister (right), who had previously had a breast augmentation with 360 cc implants, to the consultation to demonstrate the appearance and volume she desired for her own augmentation. Although this was helpful in indicating her desired breast volume, it also provided an opportunity to point out she had some glandular ptosis and her breasts would not look exactly like her sister's.

Still others bring in pictures of themselves with larger breasts during pregnancy or lactation or of other women who have breasts of the desired size. These photographs are helpful in giving me an idea of what the patient expects. Most patients request enlargement to a "normal" size rather than large breasts; however, over the years this "normal" size seems to have increased. The patient must be put at ease during this discussion so that she does not feel embarrassed to state her real expectations concerning the operation and the surgeon can get a better idea of what she really wants.

Digital imaging can facilitate this communication process when trying to determine the appropriate breast size. By using an imaging system, the surgeon can demonstrate the various size increases and the resulting impact these will have on body proportions. No guarantees are implied, but she gets a better idea of possible changes and how they will look. This is an effective tool for helping her to understand the various options she has to select from and for ruling out those that will not be appropriate because they will produce breasts that are too small, too large, or aesthetically unacceptable. It is also an effective adjunct to the informed consent and risk management process. Once a size has been agreed upon, it is documented in the medical record and a copy of the image attached for future reference.

If a digital imaging system is not available, a simple and effective approach is to ask the woman to bring in photographs that illustrate women whose breast size approximates the size that she desires. These pictures can help the surgeon clarify patient expectations and also serve as a means of identifying unrealistic goals that will ultimately lead to patient disappointment.

SELECTING AN IMPLANT

Increases in breast volume are planned in relationship to the patient's expectations and desires; her original breast dimensions, projection, and volume; her chest wall circumference and chest wall symmetry; and her body proportions. I find that the breast and implant diameter is the most important determinant of the implant size and volume selected. Women with larger chest circumferences and wider breasts naturally require wider and larger volume implants. Brassiere sizes also help make a general estimate of volume changes. Patients with smaller breasts of approximately 100 to 150 cc are generally pleased with enlargements that at least double or triple breast size to approximately 300 to 400 cc; their breasts will appear larger and fuller with 180 to 300 cc implants. Less proportional enlargement can be expected from a 200 cc implant in a patient who begins with a larger breast volume, especially if she has a wide chest and breast. If a woman has breasts of 300 cc, she will require implants of 300 to 400 cc or larger to at least double her breast volume. Because patients with larger, wider breasts initially need more volume to make a significant difference in appearance, they frequently are not as satisfied with the results of breast enlargement as women with smaller breasts. The larger volume breast implants have relatively less projection per volume unit; therefore breasts augmented with these devices will be larger but will not demonstrate a similar increase in projection. Part of the problem is inherent in the design of the implant, which frequently minimizes the effect of breast projection. ***As implants get larger, most of the volume is added to the periphery as the diameter of the implant is increased, with relatively less increase in anterior projection.*** Women with large, wide chests and small, tight breasts who require large-diameter and large-volume implants despite intraoperative expansion have tight, flattened breasts in the early postoperative period that will soften and project to a greater degree after a few weeks have elapsed and some constriction of the breast implant capsule develops.

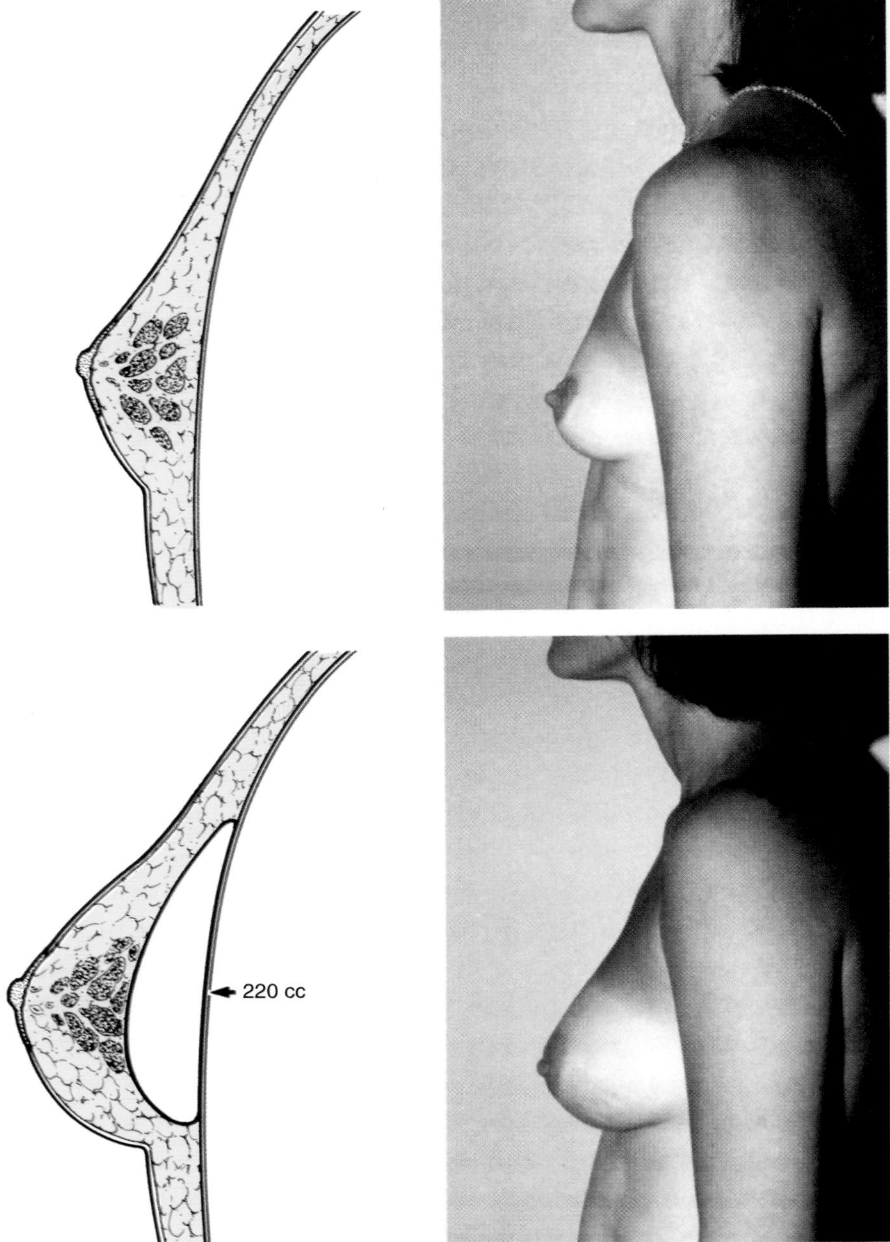

Volume requirements become even more extreme and the results less satisfying for overweight patients. Although a 220 cc implant will provide good contour improvement for a thin patient, this same implant will not provide adequate contour enhancement for an obese patient.

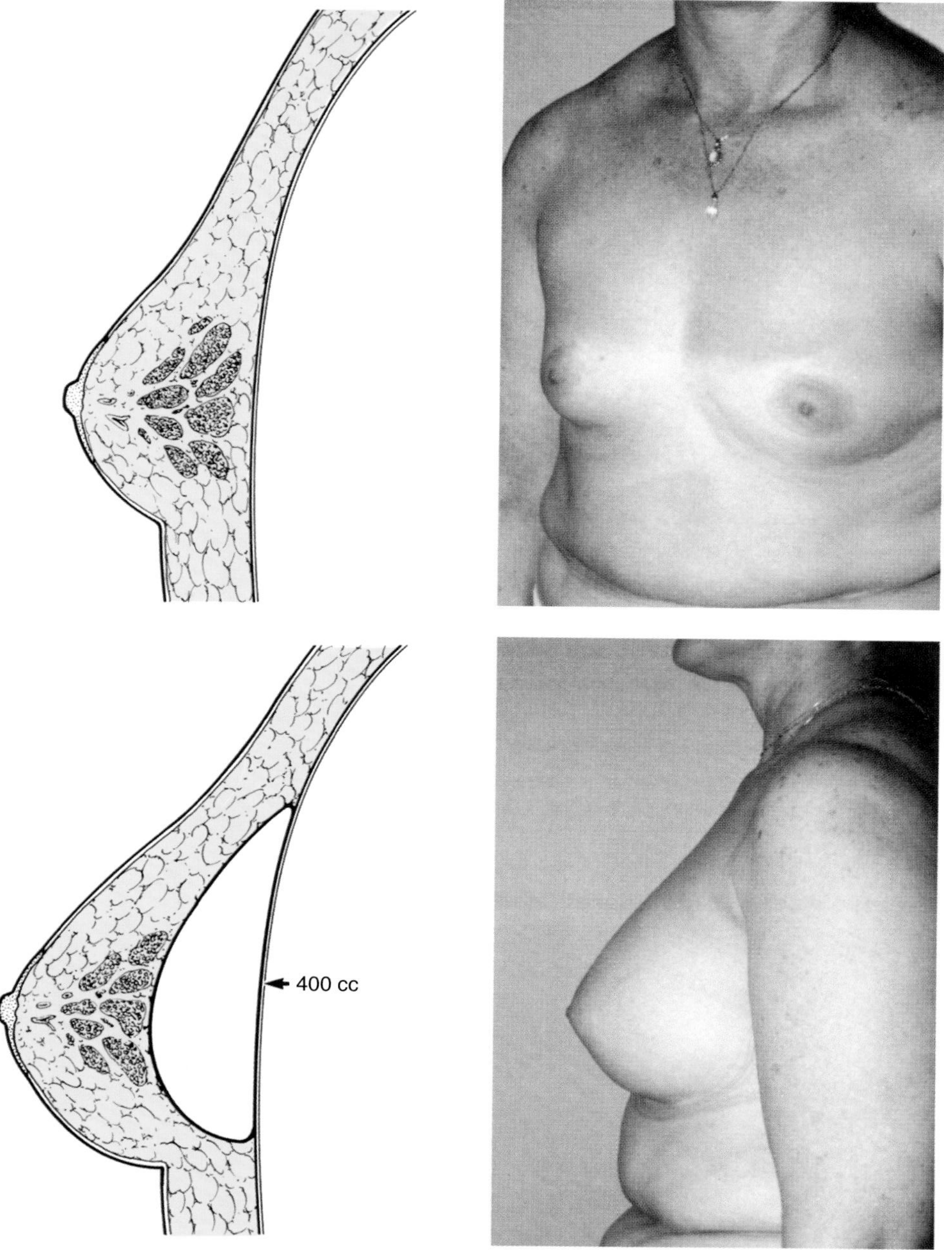

In patients with larger breasts and obese patients with relatively small breasts a thicker subcutaneous tissue layer and an epigastric prominence reduce breast projection and diminish the attractiveness of their breasts after enlargement. In some cases the thickness of the subcutaneous tissue of the upper abdomen and upper chest wall can be equal to the projection of a small breast implant. These women need larger implants to provide a suitable breast appearance. For example, a patient with thicker subcutaneous tissue will require a 400 cc implant to obtain a contour improvement comparable to that obtained with a 200 cc implant in a slender woman.

Breast augmentation can either ameliorate or exacerbate problems of asymmetry. ***When there is a marked difference in breast volume, adding more volume reduces the percentage of difference between the breasts to provide a more balanced breast appearance.*** If one breast is twice the size of the other, for example, with a volume of 200 and 100 cc, respectively, both breasts will appear more balanced if a 300 cc implant is added to each breast, thereby achieving respective volumes of 500 and 400 cc—a much lower percentage of disparity. When implants of different width and volume are used, the asymmetry can be reduced even further, but true symmetry is unlikely. The different volumes and diameters can become even more noticeable over time. ***Therefore I try to use implants of the same dimensions when the asymmetry is not extreme.***

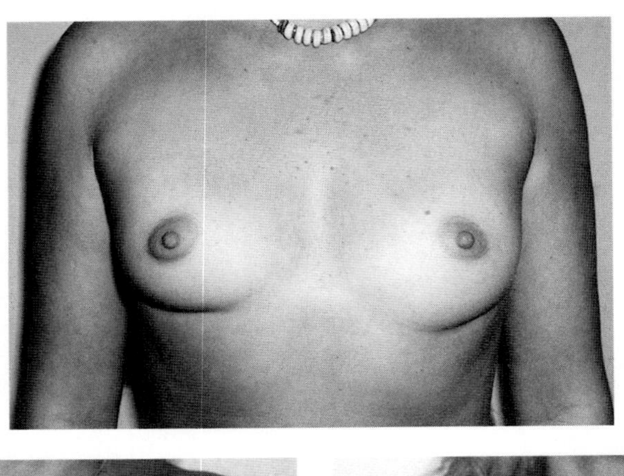

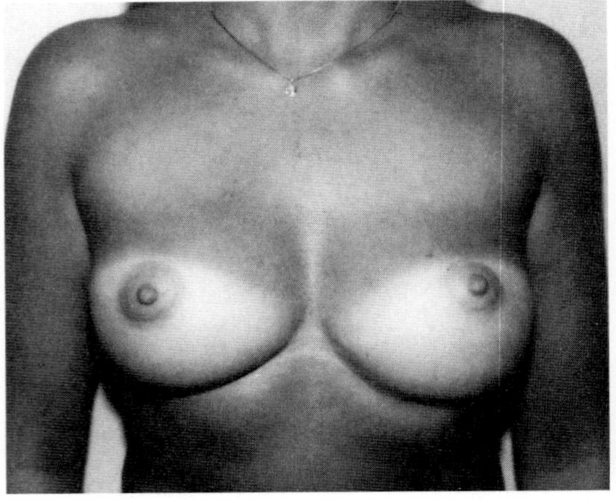

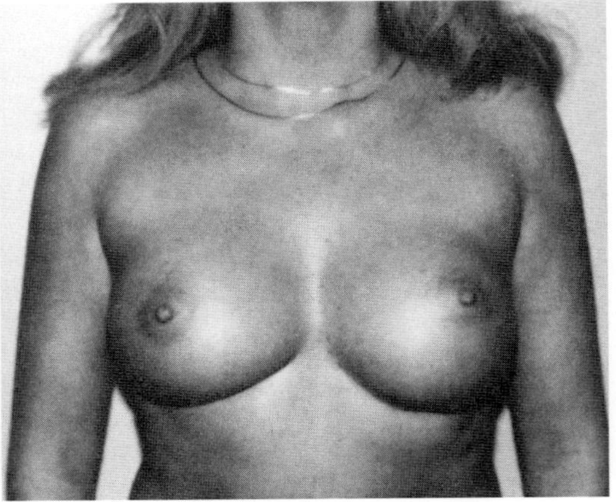

When there is a difference in the vertical position of the breasts (especially when the inframammary folds are at different levels) and they project vertically and obliquely in different directions, the proper placement of breast implants can make the breasts appear more asymmetric. This patient had breast hypoplasia with asymmetry of the inframammary crease, breast, and nipple-areola. The asymmetry persisted after augmentation mammaplasty with 360 cc implants and actually increased with time. She is seen 3 and 6 years postoperatively.

Nulliparous women with small breasts and tight skin may be limited in the volume and width of implant that they can accommodate compared with women whose tissues have been stretched by pregnancy and lactation. Small-breasted patients are generally delighted with the improvements in breast projection and contour produced by smaller implants. Intraoperative tissue expansion techniques also provide these women with an effective method for aesthetically achieving increased breast volume with augmentation mammaplasty. Applying the same basic principles evident in the stretched skin of pregnant women, intraoperative expansion stretches the breast pocket and allows these women to accommodate a larger size implant than otherwise physically possible. This principle also applies to patients in whom pregnancy and the natural process of expansion have led to larger breasts that resulted in greater skin elasticity, thus permitting a larger implant to be used if they request breast enlargement.

Increasing breast implant volume can require an implant base that is too large to produce a natural-appearing breast. ***The implant selected should not be so large that it extends beyond the natural limits of the breast.*** When this occurs, the breast implant extends too far laterally and impinges on arm motion. It also will extend too low and too high and appear unnaturally full. If it extends too far medially, symmastia may develop.

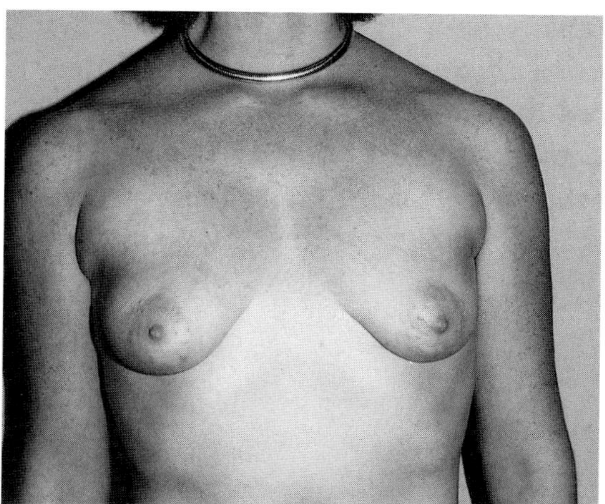

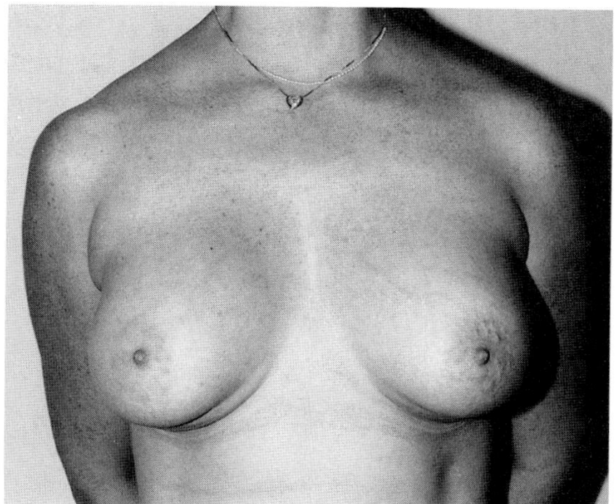

This patient was insistent in her request for “maximal” breast enlargement. Breast augmentation with 495 cc implants exceeded her natural breast limits and extended below the inframammary crease, increasing upper pole fullness and lateral breast fullness. Postoperatively she acknowledged that her breasts were too large and that they restricted her activities. She was unwilling, however, to have any additional procedures, particularly replacement with smaller implants.

The projection and diameter of the implant are also important considerations. ***The implant diameter must fit within the limits of the enlarged breast for the patient's chest wall dimensions.*** Larger implants can extend beyond the natural landmarks that delineate breast position and result in a lowering of the inframammary fold. They may also extend too far laterally under the arm to the midline over the sternum and project unnaturally in the upper pole of the breast.

STANDARD ("OPEN") VS. ENDOSCOPIC APPROACH

Most patients seeking breast augmentation are candidates for an endoscopic procedure either through an axillary or an inframammary incision. An endoscopic technique permits acceptable breast enlargement through reduced incisions, allows the inframammary crease to be more accurately controlled and lowered, and provides greater improvement of mild degrees of ptosis and breast constriction. The endoscope can also be helpful during capsulotomy and capsulectomy to ensure a reduced incision and to increase illumination and provide magnification. ***Patients with moderate or more marked ptosis and those with significant breast constriction are not as well suited to the endoscopic transaxillary approach.*** Patients with severe ptosis who desire enlargement require mastopexy. Although the implants may still be placed endoscopically, the nipple-areolae will need to be repositioned through standard open incisions. Patients with existing scars (either inframammary or periareolar) generally undergo augmentation through these scars. If the patient is having a secondary procedure involving a significant capsulotomy or capsulectomy, this should be performed through a standard open incision. If significant bleeding is encountered during an endoscopic procedure, the operation may have to be converted to a standard open approach. The results of endoscopic augmentation depend in part on the placement of the incision and the surgeon's familiarity and experience with endoscopic techniques.

INCISION PLACEMENT: AXILLARY, INFRAMAMMARY, AND PERIAREOLAR

I commonly use axillary and inframammary incisions for breast augmentation. ***I usually limit the periareolar incision to patients who have made a specific request for this approach or when an areolar approach is needed for other breast corrections.*** All of these approaches can be performed endoscopically; however, the axillary or inframammary approach is preferable.

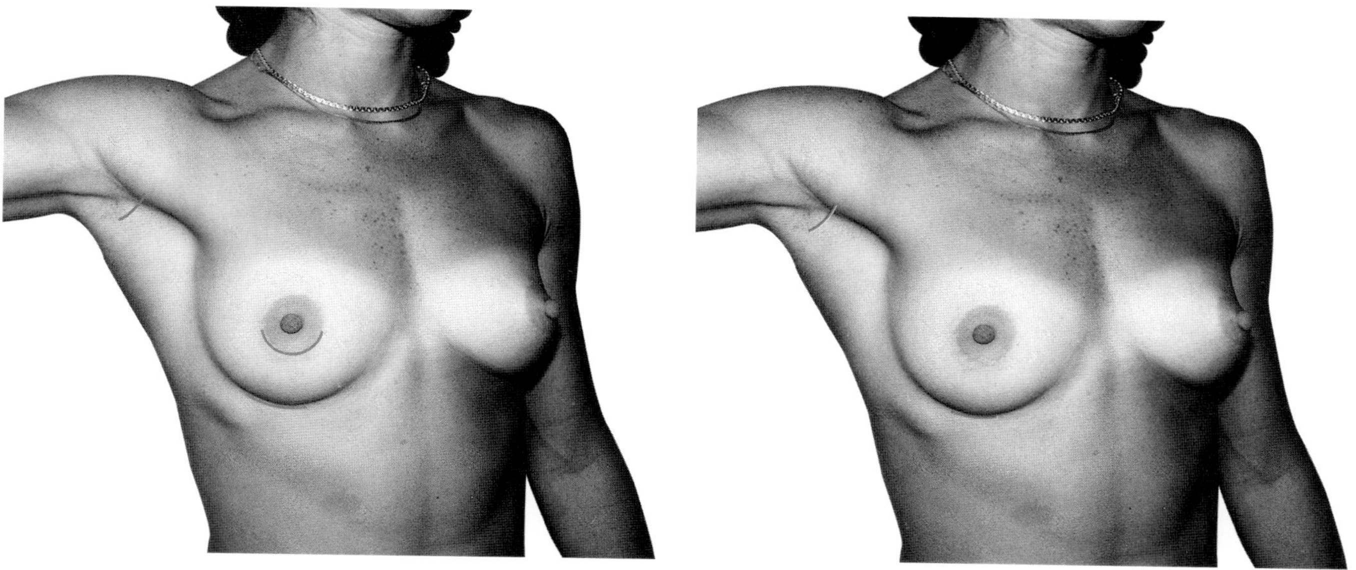

Standard incisions

Endoscopic incisions

The position of the incision for augmentation mammaplasty is critical to the success of the operation and must be individualized. No one incision works best for all women. The preferences and experiences of the surgeon and the preferences of the patient must be considered. Although the patient may have a friend who had a particularly successful augmentation mammaplasty with an incision in one position, the same incision placement may not be ideal for her. The type and size of breast implant to be used also influence the choice of incision position for prefilled implants. The saline implant is particularly compatible with the shorter length scars permitted by endoscopic breast augmentation.

The axillary incision is placed transversely in a natural skin line deep and high within the axilla. Many patients prefer the transaxillary approach because it creates no breast scar, a stigma of breast augmentation. Because hypertrophic scarring is unusual in this area, the transaxillary approach is especially appealing for patients with a history of this problem. At one time visualization of the entire breast pocket was difficult, if not impossible, through this incision, and the lowest dissection of the breast during the axillary approach had to be made blindly using long blunt instruments to create the proper pocket. The introduction and refinement of endoscopic surgery has transformed this operation into one that allows excellent visualization and precision for placement of either subglandular or submuscular breast implants. I prefer subpectoral placement for the reasons discussed previously. In this approach the pectoralis major muscle is divided inferomedially and the pocket dissected appropriately downward to ensure the best implant position. ***With the endoscopic axillary approach, special care is necessary to create symmetric pockets that are dissected low enough to provide a natural breast contour.*** Revision of a breast implant after axillary augmentation often requires another incision, usually inframammary or possibly periareolar; however, surgeons experienced with endoscopic plastic surgery techniques can often make these revisions through the preexisting axillary scar.

I prefer the axillary incision for women with breast hypoplasia who have an absent or poorly defined inframammary fold. I also suggest it for nulliparous women who want an incision that avoids a breast scar. When other scars indicate a patient's propensity for scar hypertrophy, this incision is also a consideration because scar hypertrophy within the region of the axillary hair growth is unusual. Athletic patients or others who object to axillary incisions that are visible when the arms are raised may prefer an alternate approach.

The axillary approach must be undertaken with special care because of the proximity of the intercostobrachial nerve and the underlying axillary fat pad. Injury to this nerve can cause distressing pain, anesthesias, and paresthesias of the upper inner arm.

The inframammary approach provides direct access to the retromammary area and the subpectoral layer without the need for significant incisions in breast parenchyma. This direct approach allows creation of a precise implant pocket. The inframammary crease and breast shadows conceal the scars created by this incision; these scars tend to fade and flatten with time and are usually barely perceptible after erythema subsides, scar maturation occurs, and a few years have elapsed. The use of the endoscope and saline implants permits this incision to be reduced to 2 to 3 cm in length and provides improved visualization for release of the lower medial pectoralis major muscle.

Women who have well-defined inframammary folds, who heal well with no previous evidence of or tendency for hypertrophic scarring, and who have some mild glandular ptosis are the best candidates for the inframammary fold incision, as are women who do not want an axillary scar or women who are active in sports such as tennis requiring considerable arm elevation. These women often opt for an incision that can be covered by a brassiere. This approach is also used frequently when operative adjustments need to be made in the lower breast area; these reoperations are more easily performed through the inframammary incision.

The periareolar approach usually creates inconspicuous scars and places the incision directly over the area of surgical concern. Appropriate for patients with an areolar diameter greater than 35 mm, this incision allows the lower half of the areolar circumference to be 4.5 cm. Breasts with a thin layer of breast parenchyma are also suitable for this incision because less breast tissue must be divided when the retromammary area is approached. ***If the periareolar incisions extend onto normal breast skin, unattractive scars can result. To avoid this problem it is important that the periareolar incision be made just at the margin of the areola and the breast skin.*** If it extends onto the normal breast skin, there is an increased probability of a hypertrophic wide, visible scar. If the incision is made within the areola, it can heal with a white line, which is particularly noticeable on the pigmented areola. I use this approach when the inframammary fold is not well defined and direct operative intervention is necessary in the lower breast or areola, such as in patients with constricted or tubular breasts. In these situations I do not use an endoscopic technique but rely on a standard open approach.

To gain access to the retromammary and retropectoral space some breast parenchyma and ducts must be divided when this approach is used; as a result, scarring and cysts can develop that may complicate breast examination, making biopsy necessary for definitive diagnosis. It is also important to remember that breast parenchyma is frequently colonized by bacteria, most often *Staphylococcus epidermidis;* therefore division of breast ducts and parenchyma during augmentation may also contribute to capsular contracture by increasing the risk of bacterial contamination and low-grade infection or reaction about the implant, especially if it is positioned subglandularly (see Chapter 5).

IMPLANT POSITION

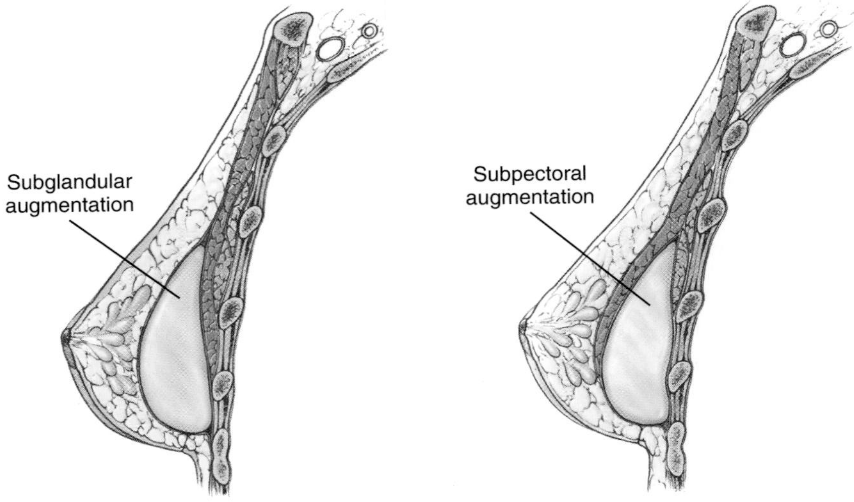

Proper implant position in relationship to the breast and to the musculofascial layer contributes to the long-term success and appearance of augmentation mammaplasty. ***In my experience, subpectoral implant placement of saline breast implants generally results in fewer problems with capsular contracture and produces softer, more natural breasts. Certain strategies are necessary to minimize contraction and distortion of the overlying muscle, especially release of the inferior and inferomedial pectoralis major muscle.*** The medial dissection also improves cleavage.

Sometimes, however, subglandular placement may be appropriate to minimize the elevated appearance of an implant, for patients with fuller ptotic breasts that provide good cover for the implant, and for bodybuilders or athletes who want to avoid muscle contractions that could possibly distort their implants.

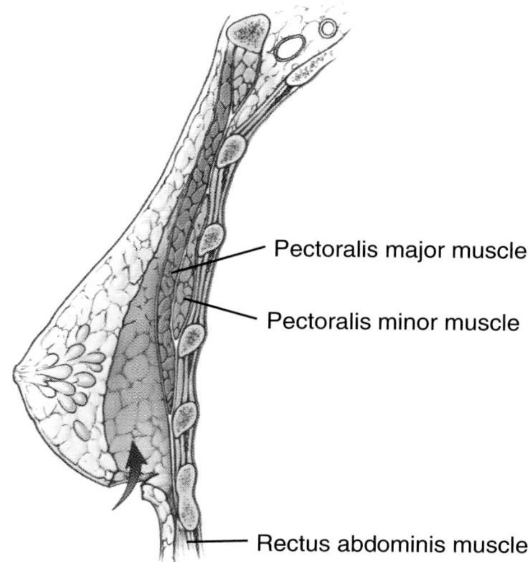

When subglandular placement is planned, the breast is elevated above the musculofascial layer with blunt dissection. Complete hemostasis between the superficial and deep fascia is essential. Fiberoptic lights and a headlight or endoscope are helpful not only for visualization to ensure hemostasis but for sharp dissection as necessary with the electrocautery. This approach is again becoming more popular since the softness obtained with textured-surface implants is similar in either the subglandular or subpectoral position.

In my experience, hematomas occur more frequently with subglandular augmentation than with the submuscular approach, and I am careful to check and recheck for hemostasis. It is also more difficult to identify the anterolateral intercostal neurovascular bundles with the subglandular approach; every effort is made to preserve them. Blunt finger dissection permits the best opportunity for avoiding injury to these nerves.

AUGMENTATION MAMMAPLASTY WORKSHEET

PATIENT DATA
Name: ______
Age: ______ Height: ______ Weight: ______
Married: ______ Single: ______
Nulliparous: ______ Pregnancies: ______
Children: ______ Nursing: ______

ONCOLOGIC INFORMATION
Family history of breast CA: ______
Prev. breast cancer: ______
Prev. breast surg.: ______
Mastodynia: ______
Fibrocystic chg.: ______
Breast disease: ______
Mammogram: ______
Masses: R ______ L ______
Biopsies: R ______ L ______

MEDICAL INFORMATION
Systemic disease: ______
Diabetes: ______
Bleeding problems: ______
Allergies: ______
Medications: ______
Smoking (pk-yr): ______
Alcohol/wk: ______
Other: ______

PHYSICAL EXAMINATION
Chest wall:
Pectus defor.: ______ Scoliosis: ______
Asymmetries: R ______ L ______
Constriction: R ______ L ______
Tubular: R ______ L ______
Striae: R ______ L ______
Breast scars: ______
Neurologic exam:
Normal: ______ Problem: ______

INFORMED CONSENT
Verbal explan.: ______ Signed form: ______
Bleed sheet: ______ Preop. mamm.: ______
FDA info.: ______ Mfg. info.: ______

EXPECTATIONS ______

SPECIFIC DESIRES
To achieve: ______
To avoid: ______

SYMPTOMS ______

MEASUREMENTS AND PLAN 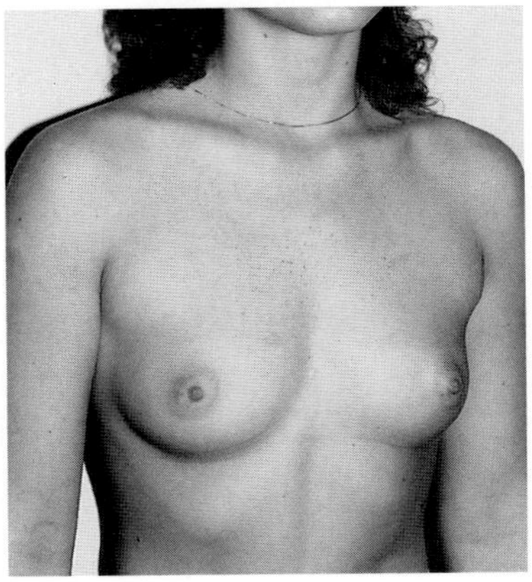
Chest circum.: ______
Bra size: ______
Breast width:
R ____ cm L ____ cm
N → infr. cr.:
R ____ cm L ____ cm
SN → N:
R ____ cm L ____ cm
Vol.: R ______
L ______

Other: ______

PLANNED AUGMENTATION
R ______ cc L ______ cc
Type of implant: Smooth ______ Textured ______

TECHNIQUE
Endoscopic: ______
Subpectoral:
Incision: Inframam. ______ Periareol. ______ Axillary ______
Subglandular:
Incision: Inframam. ______ Periareol. ______
Mastopexy: R ______ L ______

IMPRESSIONS AND NOTES ______

PLAN ______

SURGICAL OPTIONS FOR BREAST AUGMENTATION

AXILLARY APPROACH

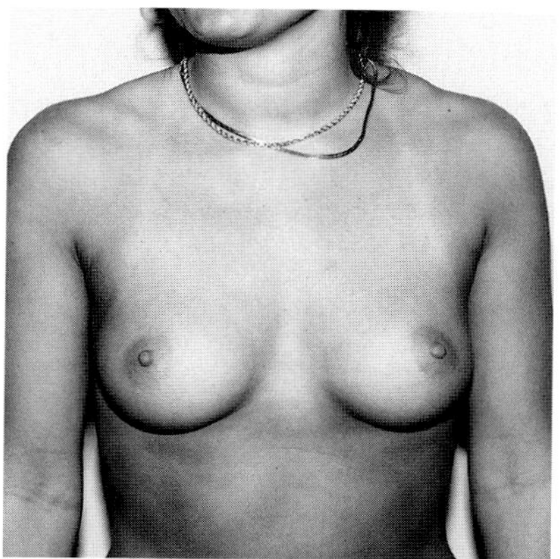

Age: Younger
Skin quality: Elastic
Breast size: Small (no ptosis)
Implant: Smooth-surface saline

PERIAREOLAR APPROACH

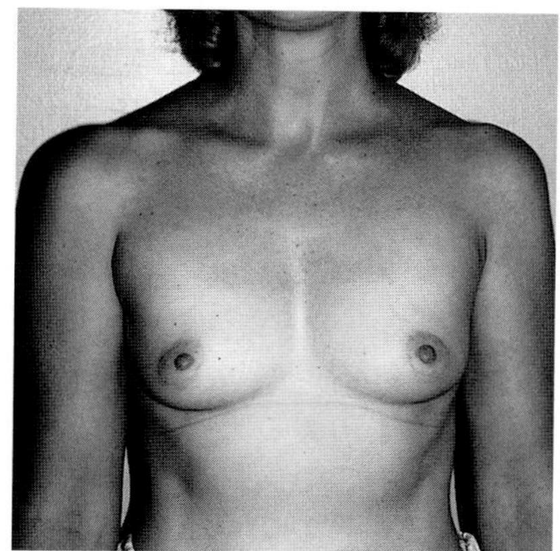

Age: Older
Skin quality: Any
Breast size: Any
Nipple-areola: Large
Implant: Smooth- or textured-surface saline

INFRAMAMMARY APPROACH

Small Breast

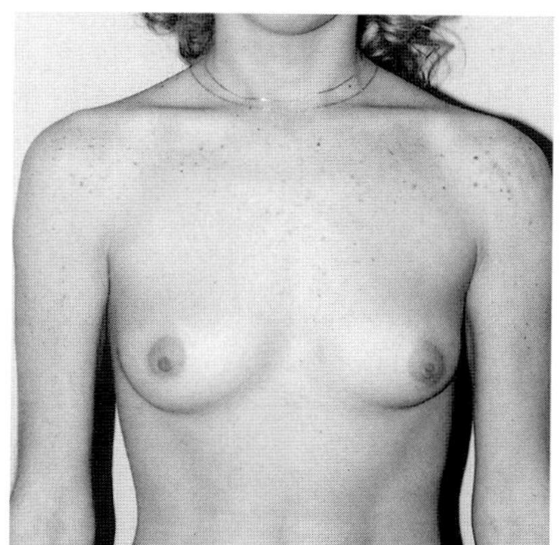

Age: Any
Skin quality: Any
Implant: Smooth- or textured-surface saline

Minimal Ptosis

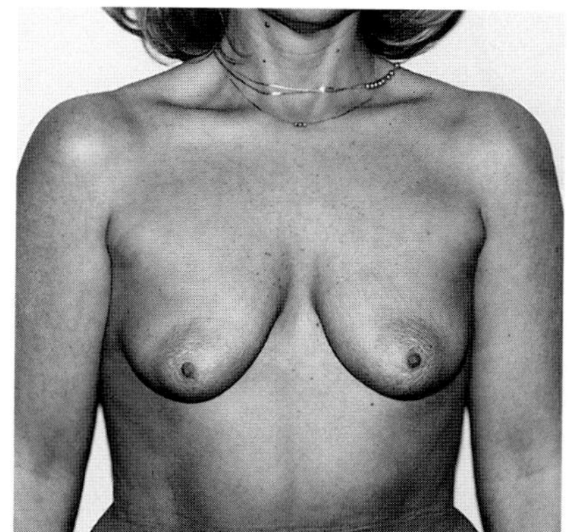

Age: Older
Skin quality: Inelastic
Implant: Smooth- or textured-surface saline

Constricted

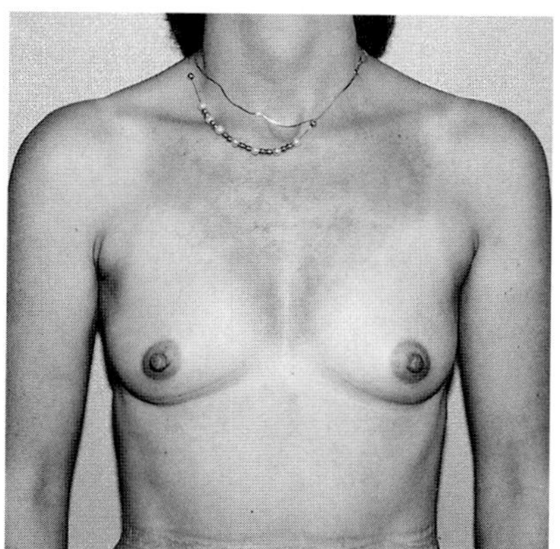

Age: Younger
Skin quality: Tight
Implant: Smooth- or textured-surface saline

Surgical Approach: Matching the Technique to the Problem

The selection of a specific technique for breast augmentation depends on a number of variables: the age of the patient, skin quality, the presence of ptosis, and the present and projected breast size. Elements of breast constriction and inframammary fold elevation must also be noted and decisions made concerning the type of breast implant, the surgical incision and approach (whether endoscopic or standard open), and the placement of implants above or below the musculofascial level. ***For most patients I favor round smooth-surface saline implants with anterior fill valves.*** Smooth-surface saline implants can create an element of postoperative expansion by their mobility and the increased weight of saline solution relative to silicone gel. Textured-surface implants may decrease capsular contracture in the subglandular position; however, if coverage is thin, they can be more palpable and have ripples, visible irregularities, and an unnatural feel. In the subpectoral position the capsular contracture rate is low with both smooth- and textured-surface saline implants. Oncologic concerns for postoperative management and monitoring of the breast for masses generally favor the subpectoral approach. ***Mammography usually visualizes more breast parenchyma and the implants are protected from any diagnostic procedures by the subpectoral layer.***

Options for breast implants

Design
- Saline inflatable

Surface
- Smooth
- Textured

Shape
- Round
- Anatomic shaped

Options for approach
- Standard
- Endoscopic

Options for incisions
- Axillary
- Inframammary
- Periareolar

Options for implant position
- Submusculofascial or subpectoral
- Subglandular

Thin, small-breasted patients with minimal overlying fatty tissue seem more prone to development of capsular contracture around subglandular smooth-surface implants. Especially in these patients as well as in most patients I prefer subpectoral smooth-surface saline implants. When these patients decide to have an axillary incision, I use an endoscopic technique to place subpectoral saline implants. Patients with larger areolae and early breast ptosis are candidates for a periareolar incision. The saline implant placed in the subpectoral position above and the subglandular position below is more likely to produce breast softness and will not limit the postoperative fullness of the breast. Patients with a well-defined inframammary crease and moderate breast volume are good candidates for inframammary incisions. Endoscopic techniques can also enhance and facilitate inframammary breast augmentation. I generally prefer the subpectoral to the subglandular approach because the implants seem to remain softer in that position. It is also the preferred positioning for breast cancer surveillance. When a smooth-surface saline implant is selected, a large subpectoral pocket permits the implant to remain mobile and soft without visible or palpable rippling or folds in the upper breast region.

Although I generally prefer subpectoral placement of breast implants, there are times when it is advisable to place breast implants in the subglandular position. ***When there is considerable breast ptosis and satisfactory upper breast thickness, subglandular implant placement can be useful for minimizing the elevated appearance of an implant that is positioned too high.*** I generally prefer the upper pole of the breast implant to lie beneath the pectoralis major muscle to minimize the chance that it will be visible and palpable through thin skin and breast parenchyma, particularly when textured-surface implants are being used that may show rippling. The subglandular approach is also considered for patients with fuller ptotic breasts that provide good potential cover for the implant or for patients who are active bodybuilders and want to avoid any distortion of the breast implant by muscular contractions. I usually prefer a textured-surface breast implant in such situations because of the higher incidence of capsular contracture that I have seen with smooth-surface implants in the subglandular position. However, when there is extremely thin breast parenchyma and skin, irregularities and ripples of the subglandular implant will be palpable and visible. When a smooth-surface implant is selected, postoperative displacement exercises and perioperative and local antibiotics lessen the incidence of capsular contracture. I use the smooth-surface implant, however, if there is thin skin or the cover is thinned secondary to capsular contracture and a reoperation is needed.

For the most part, my patients have not been as pleased with textured-surface saline implants regardless of their placement above or below the muscle. The thicker shell is often palpable and ripples are more visible. They usually do not feel as natural. Patients sometimes comment that they have a "plastic" feel. These problems are also seen with anatomic-shaped textured-surface saline implants. When they are underfilled, they are softer but readily ripple and do not give the desired anatomic correction; when they are overfilled to create the desired anatomic shape, they feel firmer than round smooth-surface saline implants. In my experience, patient satisfaction with these anatomic-shaped devices for breast augmentation has been somewhat disappointing.

MARKINGS

Preoperative markings are made with the patient sitting upright or standing with her arms comfortably to her side. Plans to achieve breast symmetry are determined before the markings are made and incorporated into the plan; the markings must include the necessary adjustments and allowances made for optimal balance. The size and diameter of the breast implants to be inserted are also determined; the extent of the markings is related to these measurements and the defined dimensions for the breast implant pocket. ***When there is uncertainty about implant size, inflatable sizers should be available to aid the surgeon in determining the best implant size.***

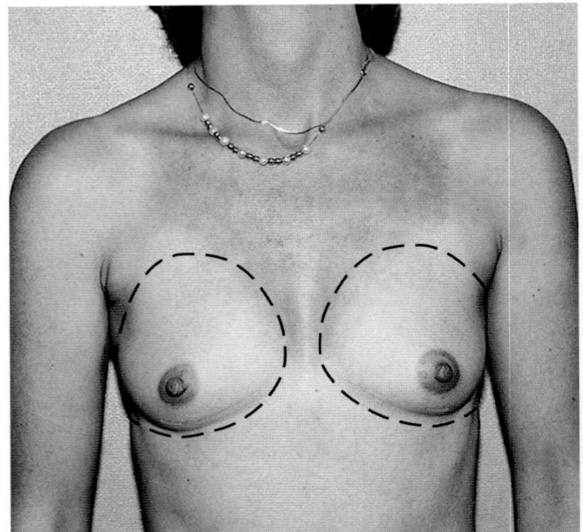

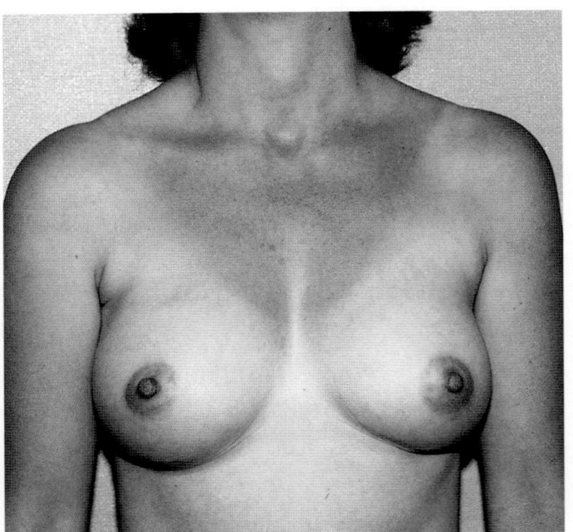

The limits of the implant pocket and the limits of dissection are marked above, usually to the second rib; laterally to the midaxillary line or to the lateral extent of the proposed breast after augmentation; and medially to the most medial extent of the pectoralis major origins but not to the midline.

Symmastia is difficult to treat and must be avoided to ensure enhanced symmetry. The lower inframammary crease dissection line is defined next. When the breast is small with an areolar-inframammary crease distance of less than 5 cm or when there is some breast constriction, the inframammary crease must be lowered to 5 to 6 cm below the areola and the pocket dissected downward. ***A high or constricted inframammary fold must not be allowed to define the new location of the inframammary fold.*** It must be disregarded and the surgeon must control and define the new crease to accommodate the breast implant dimensions. When the inframammary crease is positioned normally, particularly if a patient has been pregnant or has had breast implants, the pocket of dissection is located at the crease. As a rule, the equator or center of the implant should not be above the nipple level or the breast implant will be too high and the breasts will appear too full above and relatively deficient below. The inframammary crease is adjusted accordingly. ***In determining the implant diameter and crease level the radius of the implant should be equal to or slightly larger than the nipple to inframammary fold measurement on the breast base and chest wall (not over the breast).***

Markings of the lower breast pocket are individualized, depending on the inframammary fold position and level. When there is some constriction of the breasts or a high fold, a new fold must be made consistent with the new breast implant volume and position. When the fold is to be redefined and repositioned, the lower portion of the breast implant is placed in a subglandular deep subcutaneous position rather than beneath the deep fascia. ***It is sometimes necessary to release lower breast parenchyma and structures of the inframammary fold radially to permit expansion and widening to minimize the lower breast constriction in tubular breasts.***

When the subglandular implant position is chosen, markings are the same as for subpectoral breast augmentation except the pocket is dissected toward the clavicle a few centimeters higher than with the subpectoral approach. This approach avoids the necessity of lifting the submusculofascial layer and detaching the pectoralis major muscle, obviates any muscle contraction over the implant, and provides maximal projection without overlying muscular restriction. Textured-surface implants perform better with a lower rate of capsular contracture than smooth implants in the subglandular position; however, these can be more visible and palpable if there is not good cover.

AXILLARY APPROACH

Because blunt dissection away from the actual implant pocket is used for the axillary approach, patience and skill are required; it is also more difficult to create a symmetric pocket. Time spent checking and adjusting to ensure that the pockets are symmetric and sufficiently low is well invested to avoid later asymmetries and patient dissatisfaction. ***Unless the pocket dissection is made lower than the inframammary fold, the breast implant will often be too high.*** I find that it is easier for the anesthesiologist to secure the upper sterile drape close to the table and to have the entire arm and arm board covered with sterile drapes. This permits me to stand above the arm board and have direct access for the blunt submusculofascial dissection and to view the implant placement from above.

ENDOSCOPIC SUBPECTORAL AXILLARY AUGMENTATION

Endoscopic transaxillary augmentation provides the same benefits as the standard open transaxillary augmentation, including short, inconspicuous incisions away from the central breast area, ready access for submuscular implant placement, possibly improved preservation of breast sensibility, and avoidance of parenchymal breast dissection, which may reduce the incidence of infection and postoperative scarring and fibrosis. The incorporation of endoscopic techniques for transaxillary augmentation avoids the inherent shortcomings of the open procedure. The standard open procedure with little direct visibility of the lower operative field is converted to one in which the subpectoral space can be clearly visualized, which also shortens the length of the axillary incision. Endoscopic techniques can help reduce the scar from 4 to 5 cm to an average of 2.5 to 3.0 cm. Furthermore, the muscle and fascia to be divided are at right angles to the endoscopic view, making the axillary approach particularly well suited to endoscopic techniques. Control of the inframammary crease is greatly enhanced by accurate division of the pectoralis major muscle origins and prepectoral fascia under direct vision. Because the muscle is divided with the electrocautery, bleeding is avoided or minimized, and when it occurs, hemostasis is readily achieved with direct coagulation of the vessel. Although difficult to quantitate objectively, postoperative pain may be reduced by eliminating most of the blunt dissection. Control of the subpectoral cavity is maintained by careful dissection of the pocket under endoscopic visualization. Clear visualization of the subpectoral pocket permits cavity revision, implant exchange, or capsulotomy through the same incision if necessary.

Operating Room Setup and Patient Positioning

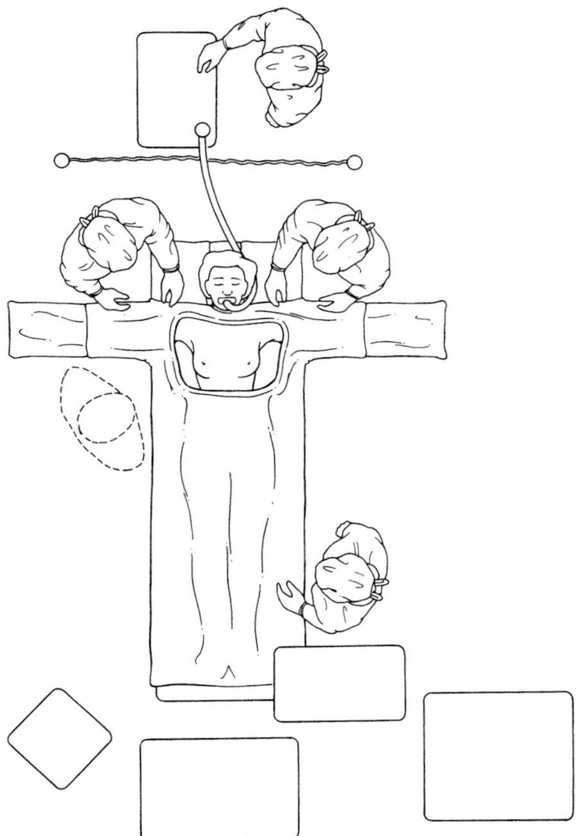

When using the endoretractor, the most comfortable position for the surgeon is one that provides a direct view of the endoscope and the monitor in a straight line. ***For transaxillary endoscopic procedures this alignment is most effectively accomplished with the surgeon positioned above the patient's extended arm and shoulder and the video monitor positioned at the foot of the operating table.*** Although this positioning does not provide ideal alignment, the monitor will not have to be repositioned as the surgeon moves to the opposite side of the table. The light source, video cable, cautery cord, and suction tubing are brought up from the foot of the operating table and also will not require repositioning. To provide adequate space for the surgeon the operating table is moved approximately 2 feet away from the anesthesia cart.

The patient is placed on the operating table in a supine position and secured with her arms abducted. After anesthesia is induced, the patient's arms are carefully positioned and secured to the arm boards at 90 degrees of abduction with soft roll padding. The patient must be positioned so as to allow the table to be adjusted to a full upright (sitting) position for optimal pocket and implant evaluation and adjustment at the end of the operation. Standard padding precautions at pressure points are observed. The incision site is infiltrated with 1% lidocaine with 1:100,000 epinephrine, and the entire anterior chest and axilla from the clavicles to the costal margin are then prepped and draped. The drapes are adjusted so that the surgeon can stand above either arm without being contaminated by the anesthesia equipment.

Surgical plan

- Axillary approach
- Subpectoral dissection of implant pocket
- Endoscopic release of medial and inferior pectoralis muscle fibers
- Development of symmetric subpectoral pockets
- Placement of round smooth-surface saline implants

Markings

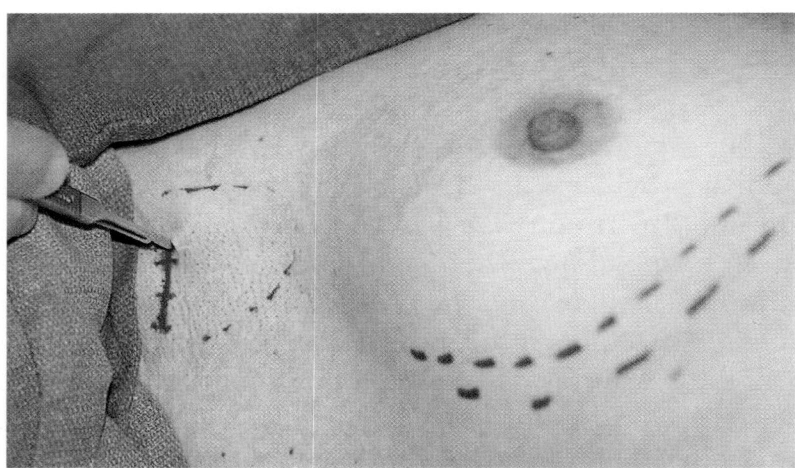

A prominent transverse axillary crease is marked for the access incision. Because of the reach afforded by the endoscope and endoscopic instrumentation, this line can be placed at essentially any point within the axilla; however, I generally place it high in the axillary apex. ***The endoscopic axillary incision can be as short as 1.5 cm (measured at 2 cm on stretch), but the procedure is easier to perform if the incision is 2.5 to 3.0 cm.*** Endoscopic dissection is possible with incision lengths of less than 1.5 cm, but it is difficult to insert the implants, especially those with textured surfaces. When inserting devices are developed (and approved by implant manufacturers), perhaps this length can be reduced even further. ***However, the primary benefit of endoscopic transaxillary augmentation is control of the dissection, which should not be sacrificed for a reduction of incision length.***

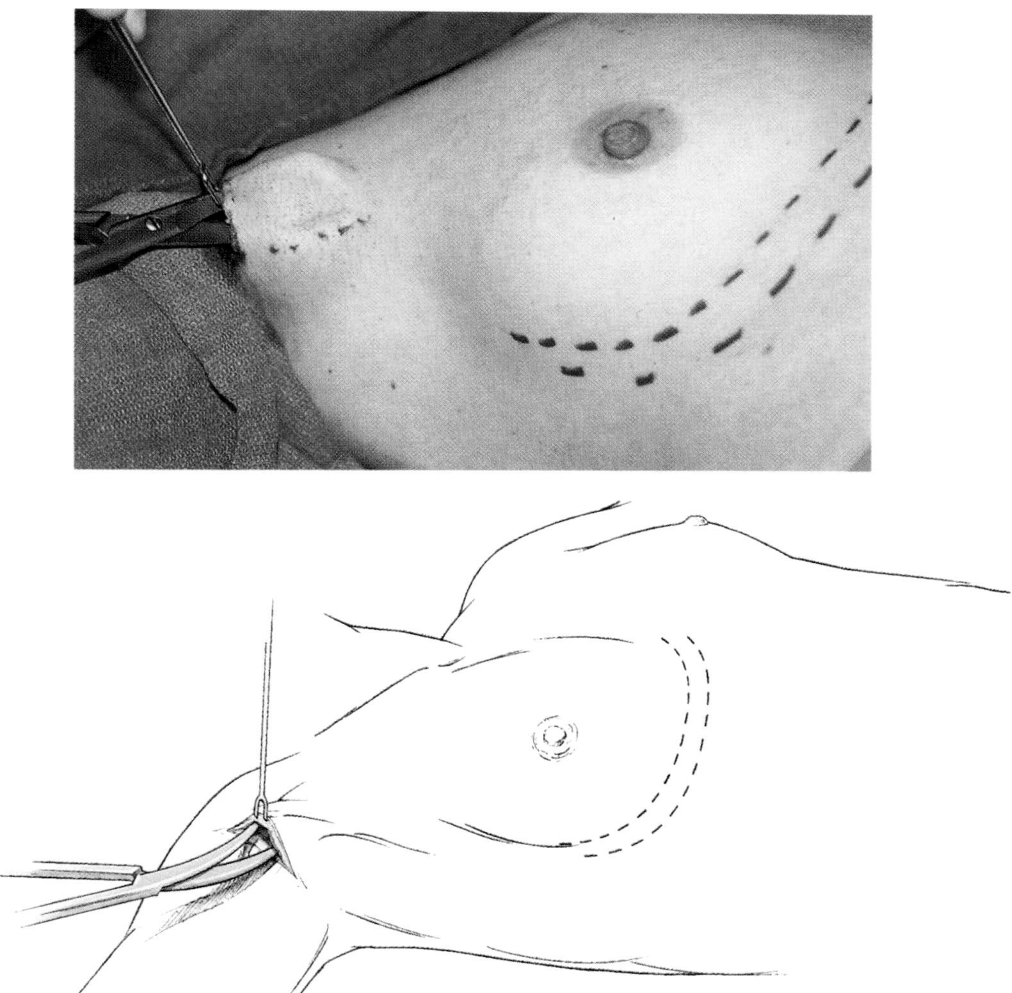

The incision and initial subpectoral pocket dissection are facilitated if the surgeon stands above the patient's extended arm. The axillary skin is placed under tension with the nondominant hand, and the incision is made as marked through the skin only. The anterior edge of the incision is then elevated with sharp double hooks. Spreading scissors dissection creates a tunnel directly medial to the thick anterior axillary fold marking the pectoral muscle. ***Elevating the anterior skin margin and maintaining this dissection in a superficial plane minimize the risk of injury to the intercostobrachial nerve.***

The subcutaneous tissue underlying the incision tends to restrict instrument insertion and mobility unless opened widely. This is accomplished by sharp division of the tissue immediately underneath the ends of the incision and blunt creation of the subcutaneous tunnel to the lateral pectoral border with the scissors.

Development of the Subpectoral Space

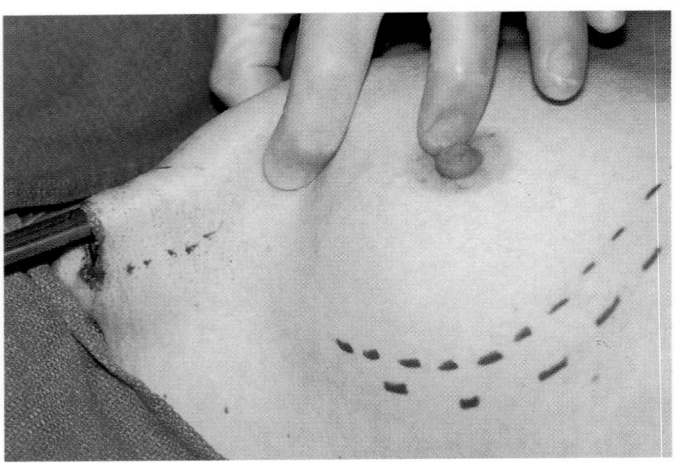

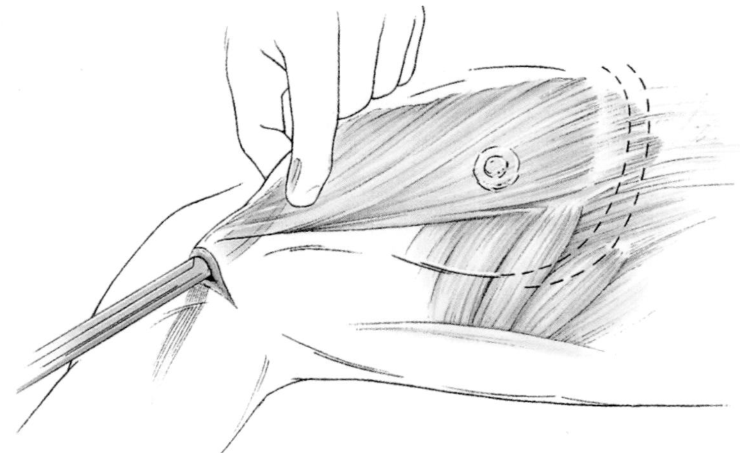

Blunt scissors are placed with the tips closed against the lateral pectoral border and slid posteriorly underneath the muscle. Resistance to advancement of the scissors indicates the lateral pectoral fascia is encountered. This resistance is overcome by firm pressure, and the scissors tips are guided into the subpectoral space. Spreading the tip to the side will enlarge the opening in the lateral pectoral fascia.

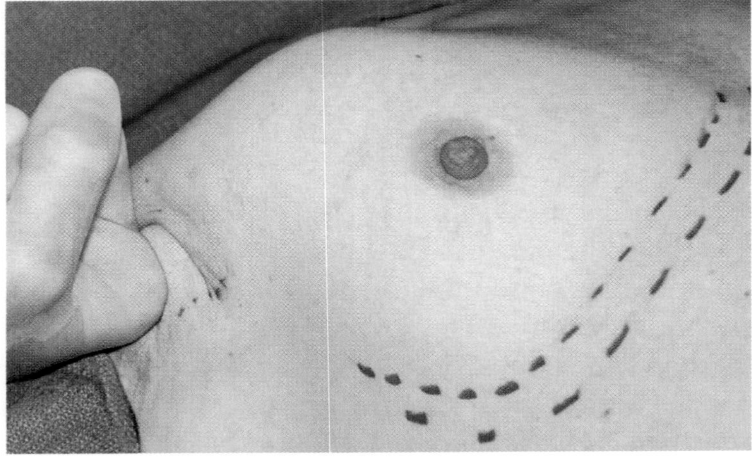

After the incision is extended down to the subpectoral space, the index finger is used to begin the dissection of the subpectoral space; the index finger is gently swept between the upper portions of the pectoralis major muscle.

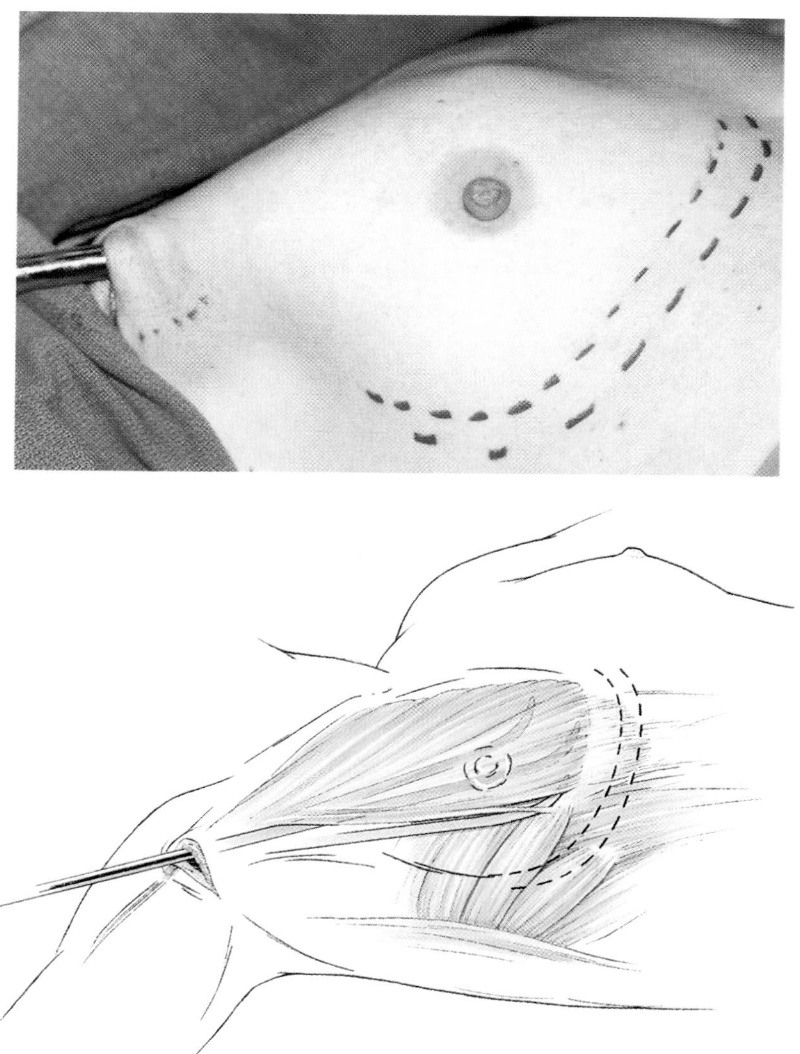

A 36 Fr urethral dilator is placed through this opening into the subpectoral space. ***To facilitate placement of instruments the urethral dilator is used to sweep the superolateral pocket laterally.*** The skin incision then lies at the apex of the optical cavity. A gentle sweeping motion within this subpectoral space divides any loose areolar tissue separating the posterior surface of the pectoralis major from the chest wall inferiorly and pectoralis minor fibers superiorly. A vigorous sweeping motion of the entire space is avoided because this creates bleeding that obscures the endoscopic view. Before the endoscopic approach was developed I used blunt division of the pectoralis major muscle from the chest wall with the Agris-Dingman breast dissectors. However, pectoral muscle fibers are shown to be intact after blunt dissection when viewed endoscopically. The modest bleeding that ensued made visualization for division of these fibers more difficult. In addition, it appears that vigorous dissection may lead to increased postoperative bruising.

Insertion of the Endoretractor

While the skin incision and initial pocket dissection are being completed by the surgeon, the scrub nurse removes the 20 cm long, 10 mm diameter 30-degree endoscope from the warm fluid bath. Alternatively, an antifogging solution may be applied to the endoscope at this time. The endocamera is connected to the endoscope, and if a fixating pin is present on the camera coupler, it is tightened to prevent camera rotation. The light cord is attached, and the camera is white balanced using a clean laparotomy sponge as a reference. The video image is inspected simultaneously, and any initial problems with fogging or blurring are addressed prior to insertion of the scope into the endoretractor.

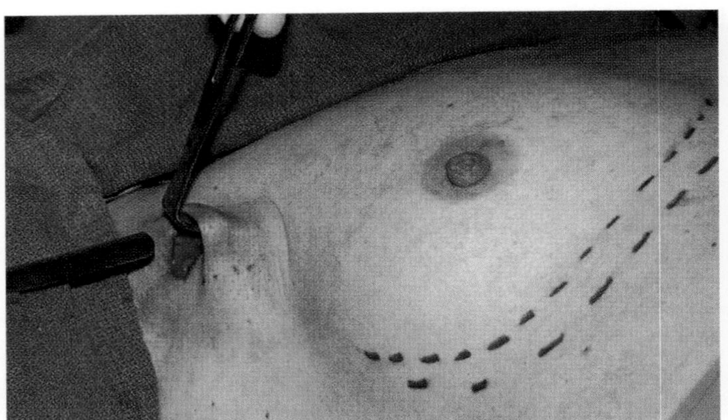

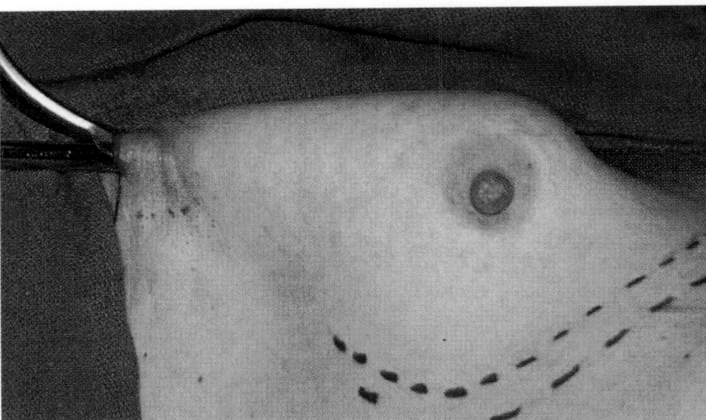

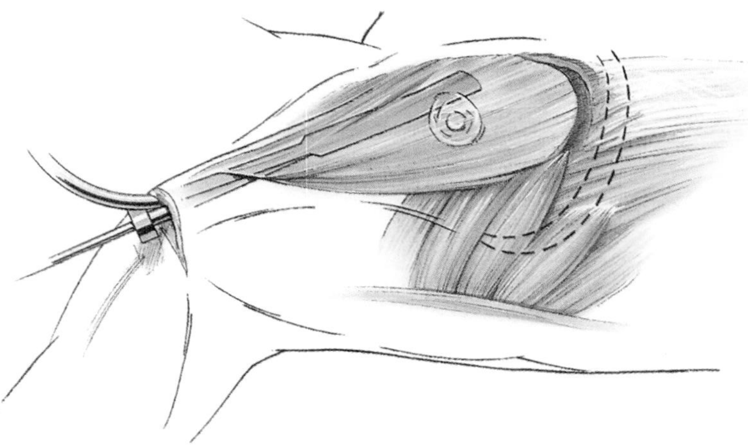

The surgeon then moves to a position above the patient's extended arm. The endoretractor is slid through the incision and into the subpectoral space. The endoscope is inserted into the end of the holding sheath. As the endoscope is slid farther into the sheath, the image is followed on the video screen. If any fluid is present in the sheath, the endoscope can be rotated 90 to 180 degrees to prevent fluid from accumulating on the lens. For the same reason, the endoretractor is lifted off the chest wall before the end of the endoscope emerges from the end of the tubing. The light cord is inserted into its retaining slot on the retractor handle. While maintaining the lift, the endoretractor is advanced or withdrawn and pivoted from a medial to a lateral position to adjust the endoscopic view and inspect the subpectoral space. The focus ring on the camera is adjusted as necessary to obtain a clear view.

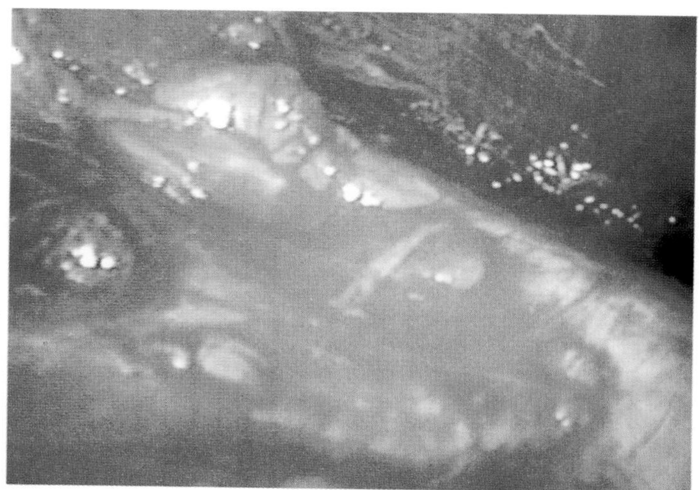

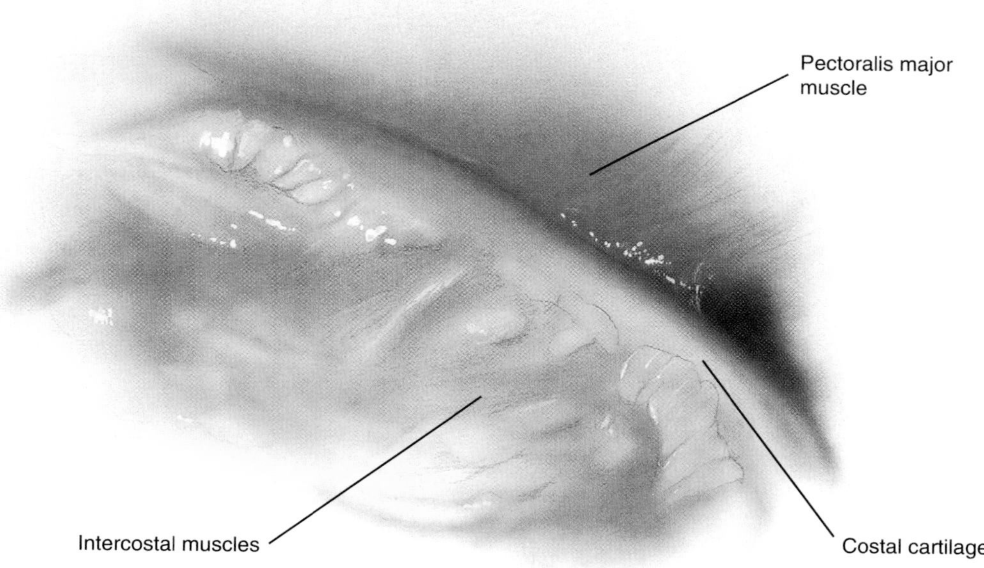

The costal cartilage and intercostal muscle are visible on the inferior aspect of the video monitor. The fibers of the pectoralis major can be seen clearly. In the medial and superomedial views the fibers are seen to course anteriorly and cephalad; inferiorly the fibers course more directly toward the endoscope. ***Pressing a finger along the breast allows the surgeon to correlate the internal structures and the external markings.***

Medial and Inferior Pocket Dissection

The cautery cord and suction tubing are connected to the suction-cautery unit chosen. Depending on the individual cautery unit, cutting off the connector on the suction tubing may provide a better fit. The suction-cautery unit is inserted into the optical cavity underneath the endoretractor. Turning the suction-cautery upward allows the tip of the cautery to slide along the groove between the blade and sheath of the retractor. This helps prevent the cautery tip from catching on the tissue as it is inserted. The cautery is advanced until it comes into view on the video monitor.

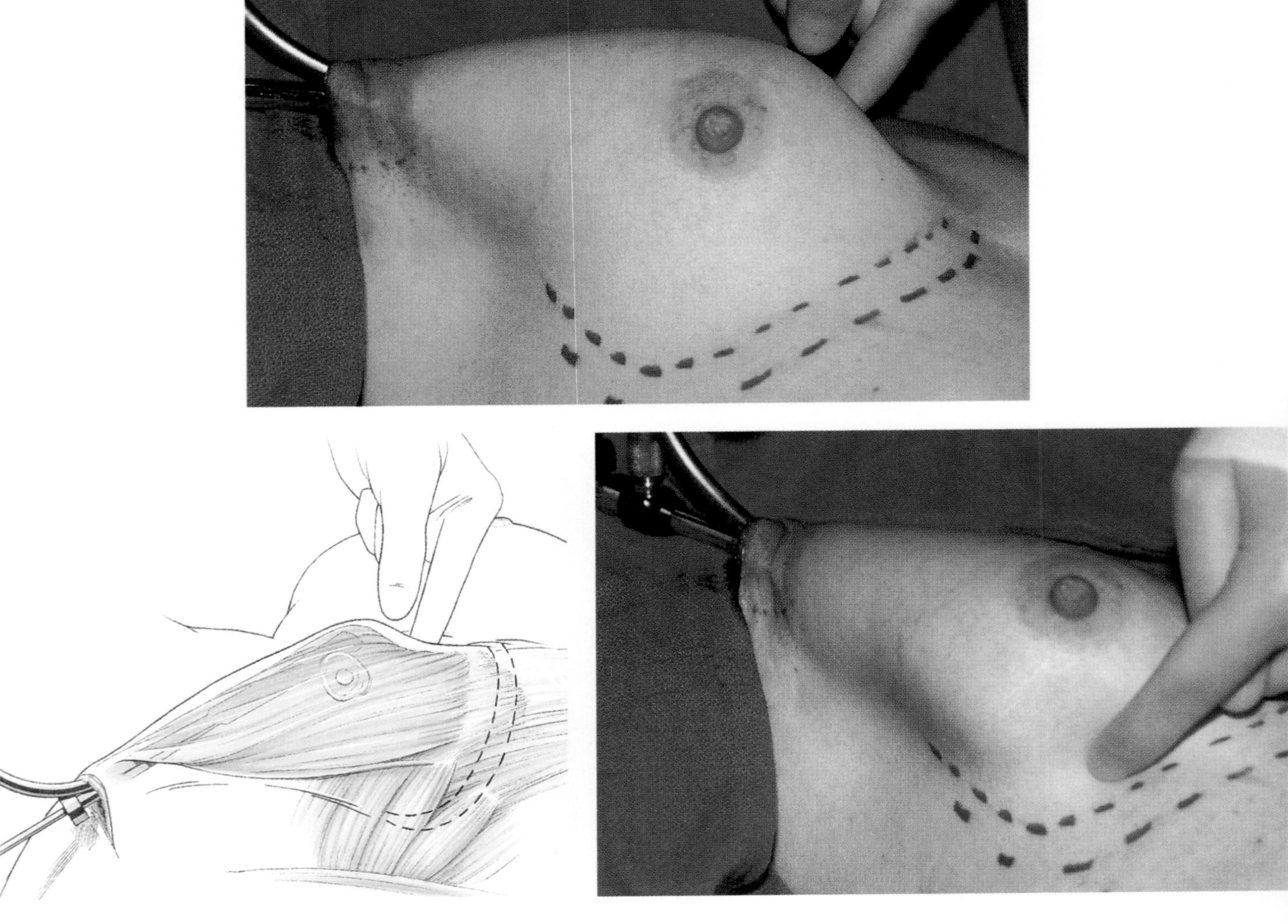

The pectoralis major muscle must be divided from the level of the nipple medially to the lateral extent of the pectoralis major muscle origins. These limits must be defined internally, either by indenting the breast externally while viewing the monitor or by indenting the pectoralis major internally with the cautery tip while viewing the breast directly. When this method is chosen, it is imperative that the cautery tip *not* be activated to avoid burning the breast skin. These points can be marked with the cautery on the muscle fibers if desired.

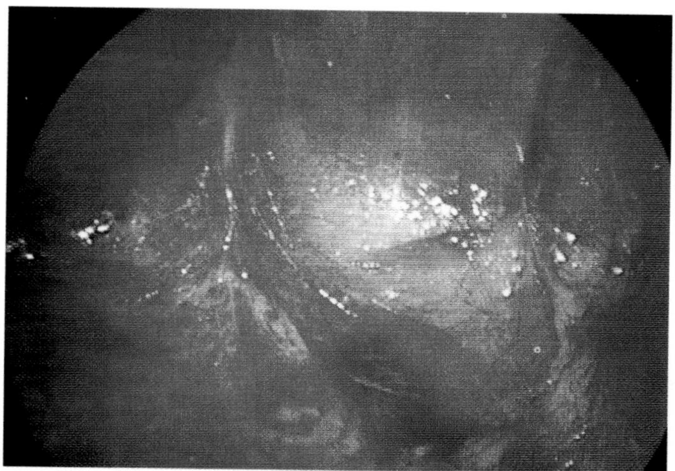

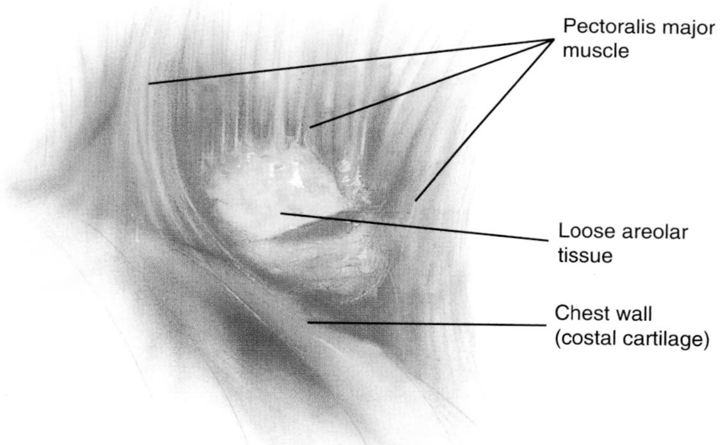

With the endoretractor and 10 mm endoscope in position to visualize the lower medial undersurface of the pectoralis major, the juncture of the muscle origins and the chest wall and ribs is identified.

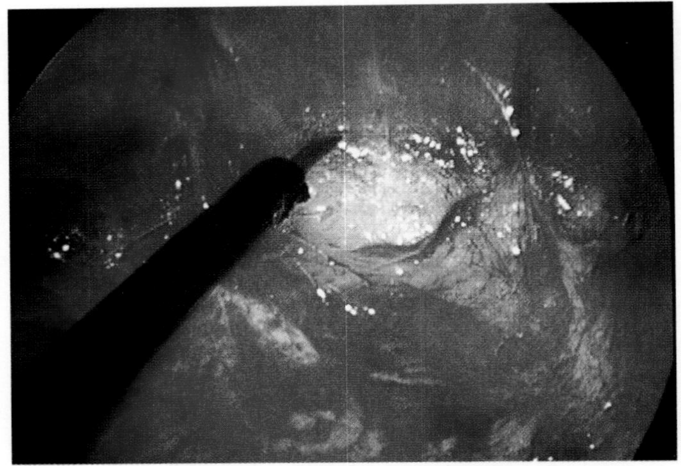

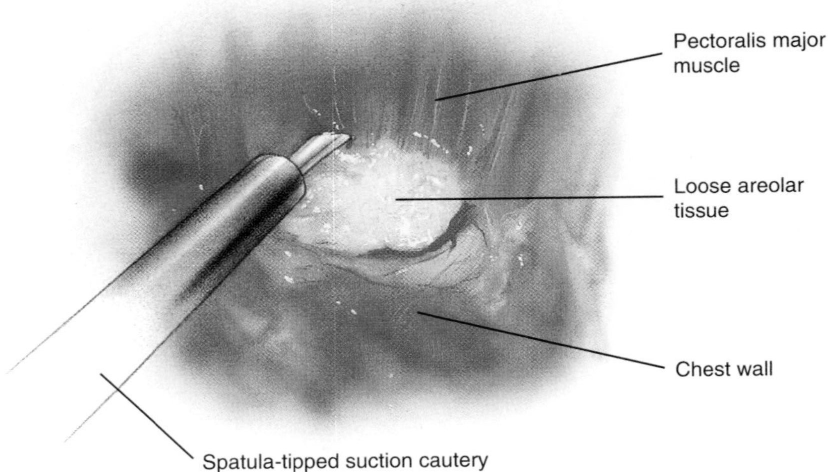

With the undersurface of the pectoralis major clearly visualized, a line of division of the pectoralis major is planned from the level of the areola extending inferiorly and laterally to the lateral extent of the muscle. ***The pectoralis major muscle line of division is made approximately 0.5 to 1.0 cm above the chest wall.*** This position prevents retraction of any divided mammary perforators out of view. The muscle is divided over a broad front and at such a pace that no deep muscle cuts are made initially. This allows identification of the vessels for coagulation prior to division. If they are divided, this is immediately evident in the field and can be controlled either with the electrocautery spatula or an insulated grasper. A deep cut in the muscle can divide a vessel that retracts and is not readily visible without increasing the exposure by dividing additional muscle.

In most patients the muscle is divided at a point approximately 10 mm off the chest wall, leaving a small cuff of muscle. The cuff of tissue seems to prevent the medial perforating vessels from withdrawing beneath the surface of the chest wall, and if bleeding occurs subsequently, it is easier to visualize and control with the cautery. However, in very thin patients that line of division may be palpable or visible, at least in the early postoperative period, and in these patients the pectoralis muscle origin is divided closer to the chest wall. The muscle is divided through the muscle fibers and the thin, lighter prepectoral fascia until the yellow subcutaneous fat is seen.

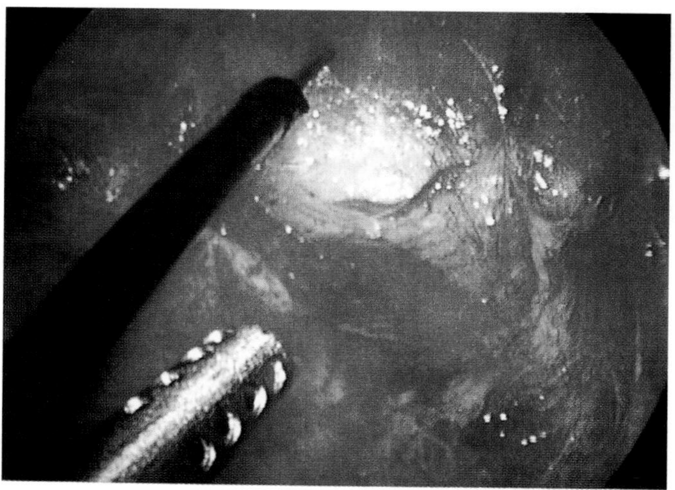

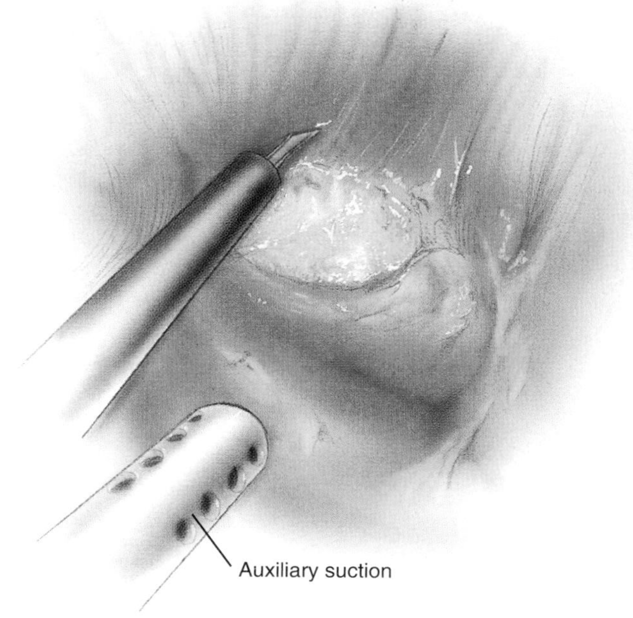

On occasion more smoke is produced during muscle division than can be cleared through the narrow suction-cautery channel. If this occurs, an auxiliary suction device placed through the access incision expedites clearance and permits a clear field of view. Newer retractor models will incorporate suction channels.

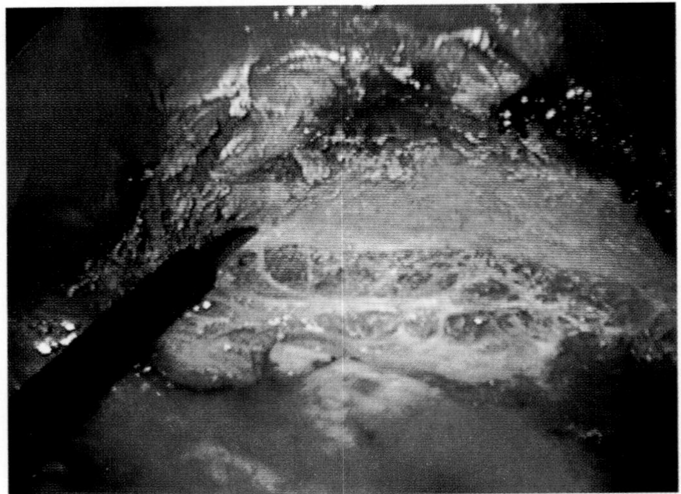

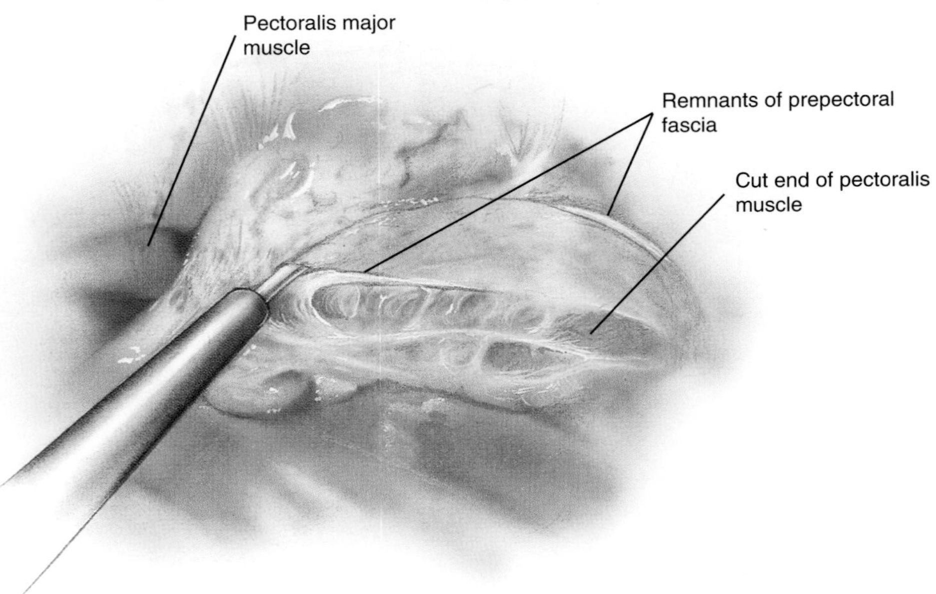

After the pectoral muscle is divided, the superficial pectoral fascia is identified and divided. This will reveal the yellow subcutaneous fat. At this point the surgeon checks to make sure that the muscle division extends from the level of the areola around laterally to the full extent of the pectoralis major muscle. The dissection is then extended inferiorly to the level of the proposed future inframammary fold. Although this could be done with the electrocautery and endoscope, I use the Agris-Dingman dissector for this next step because of the thin skin in this region and the successful results achieved with blunt dissection.

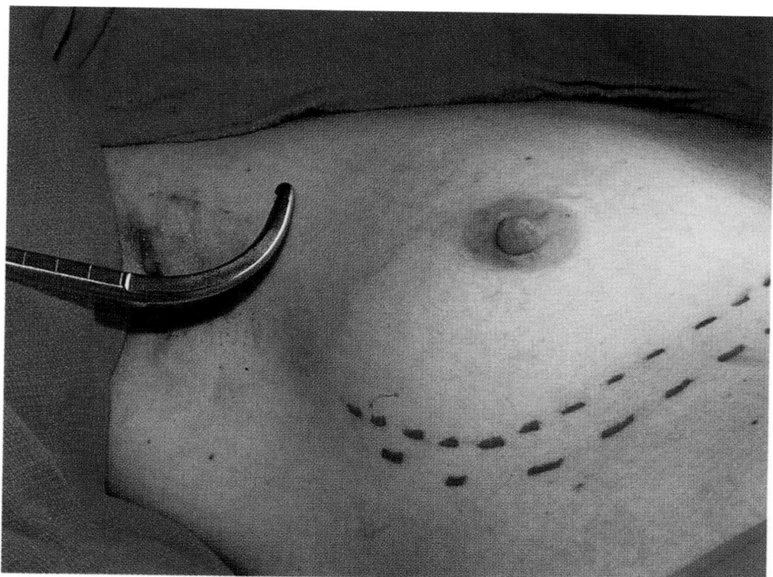

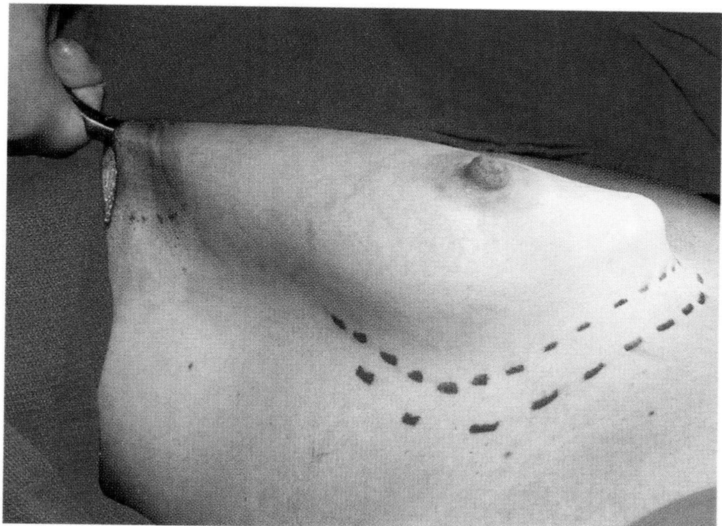

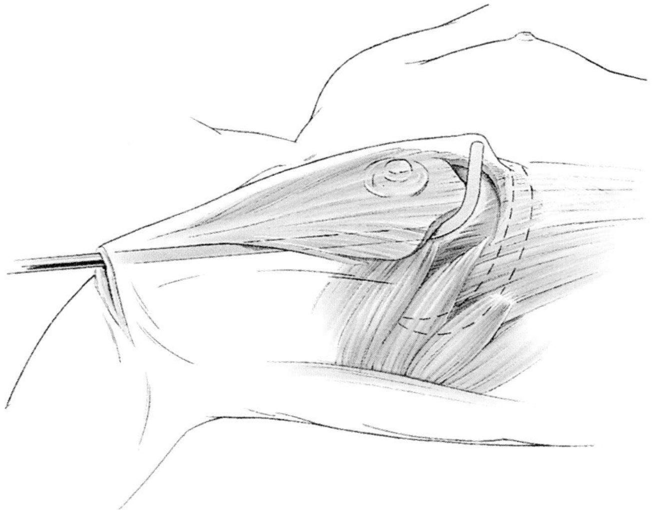

The Agris-Dingman dissector is placed through the incision, and with a sweeping motion, blunt dissection proceeds inferiorly down toward the future inframammary fold. This sweeping motion is effective and prevents the dissection of small irregular pockets in this region. ***The Agris-Dingman dissector is also used to lift upward on the pectoralis major muscle. This creates a generous lower pocket for implant placement by further separating the muscle from the new inframammary fold.*** Separation of the muscle inferiorly and medially allows the pectoralis major to drape less tightly over the implant and results in less muscle contraction and distortion of the implant by the pectoral muscle.

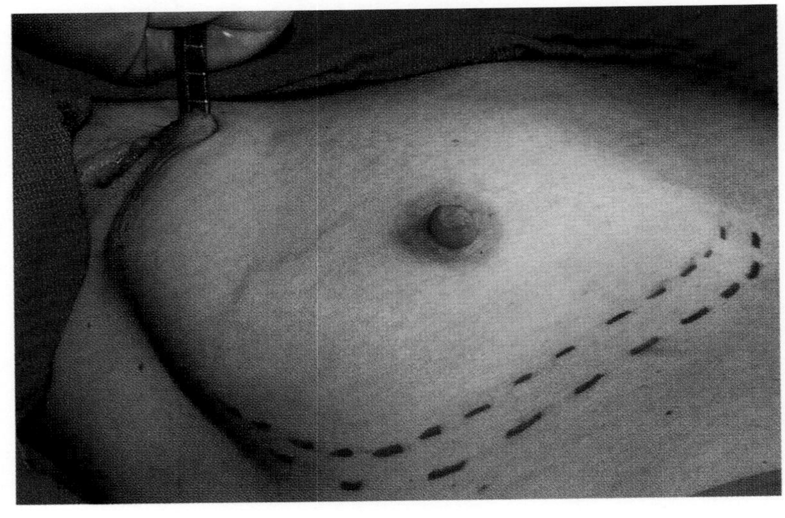

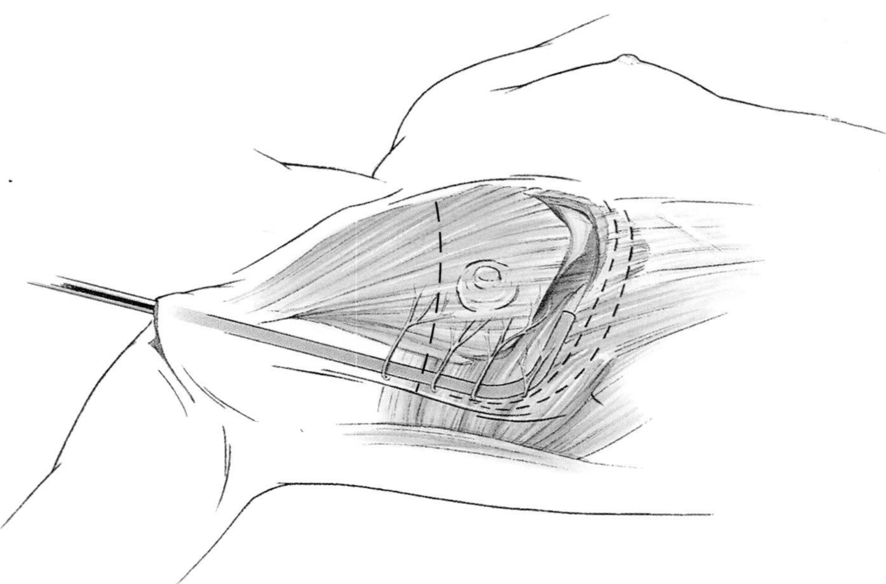

The lateral dissection of the implant pocket is carried out bluntly with the Agris-Dingman dissector as well as with the index finger. Blunt dissection avoids sharp division of the anterolateral sensory nerves and seems to minimize sensory changes after breast augmentation.

Implant Preparation, Insertion, and Inflation

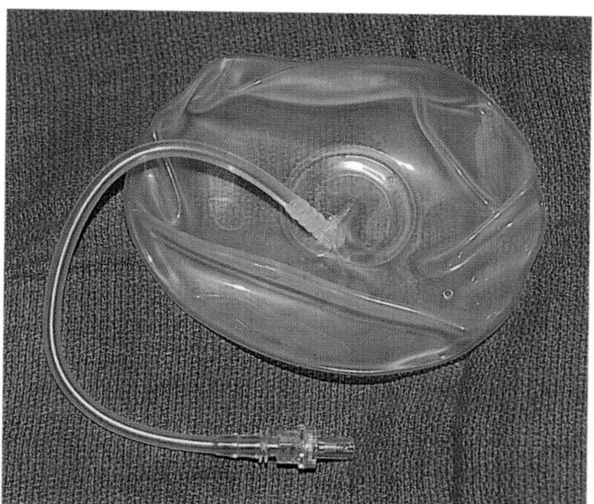

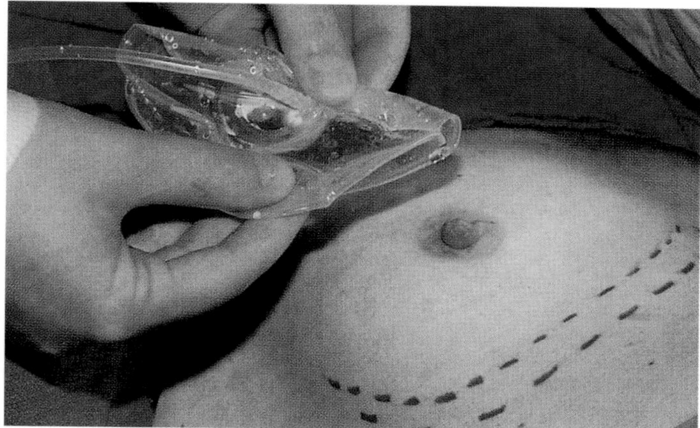

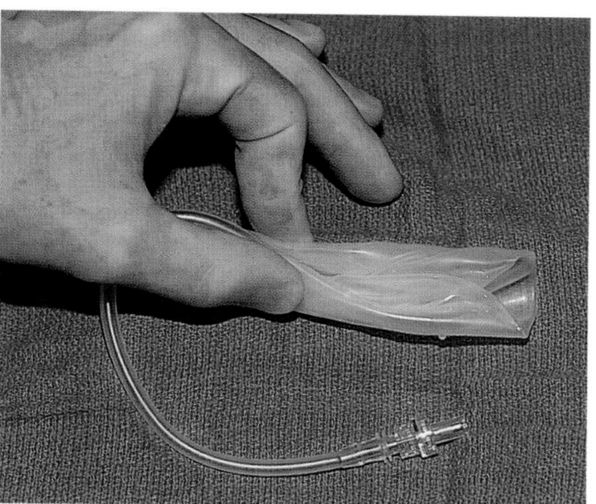

Both right and left implant pockets are developed symmetrically before the implant is inserted. The implants are removed from their containers, fill tubing valves are placed on the ends of the tubing, and a small volume of saline solution is instilled to help remove any residual air. The deflated implant is then prepared for insertion by shaping it into a double roll. If an anterior fill valve device is used, the rolls are folded anteriorly; if a posterior valve is used, the rolls are folded posteriorly. Narrowing the rolls at the ends makes insertion easier.

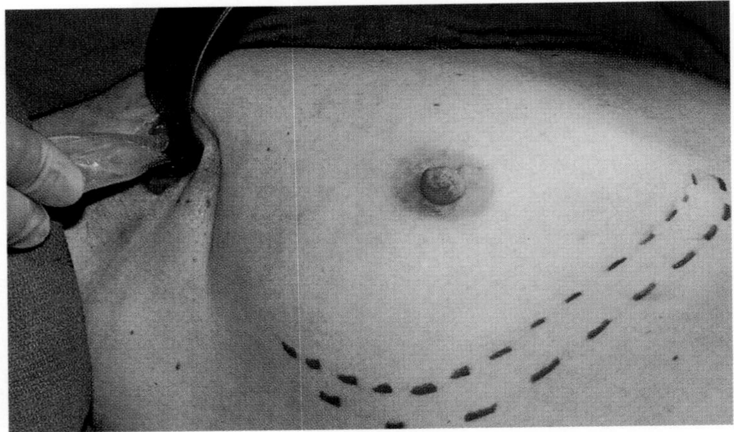

An Army-Navy or small Deaver retractor is placed through the axillary incision with the blade underneath the lateral edge of the pectoralis major in preparation for implant insertion. The surgeon's gloves are wiped with antibiotic irrigation solution as is the patient's axillary skin. I try to avoid contact of the implant with the patient's skin. The rolled implant is then inserted into the cavity with the fill tubing extending from the anterior valve out through the incision. Once the implant is within the superior aspect of the pocket, the retractor is removed and the surgeon positions the implant downward using his fingers.

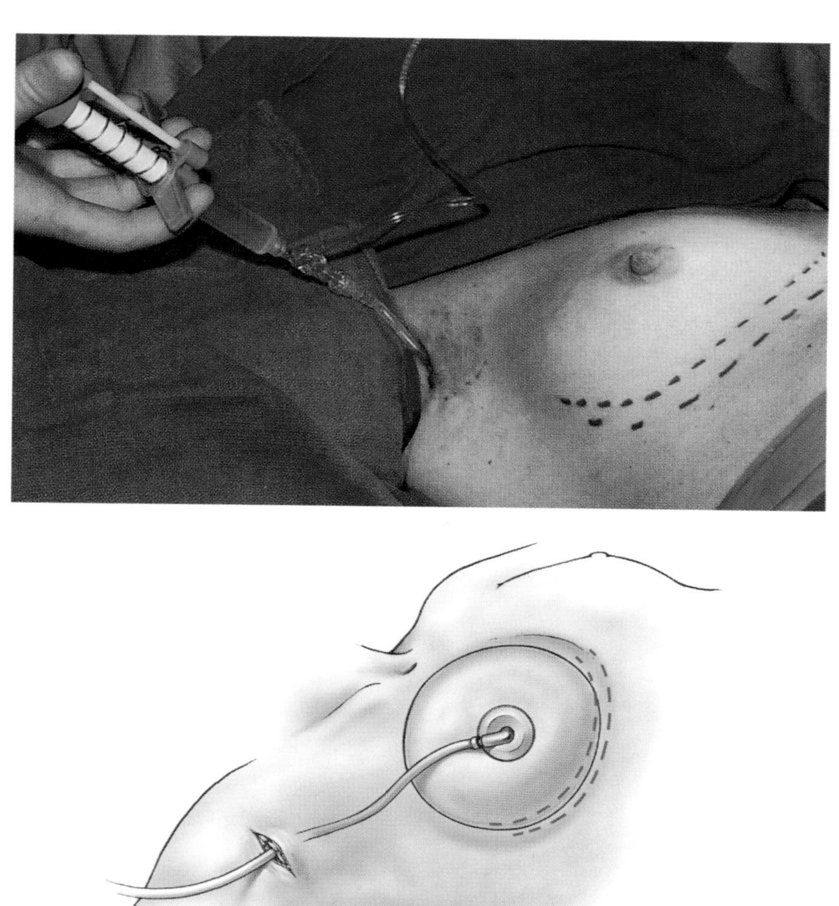

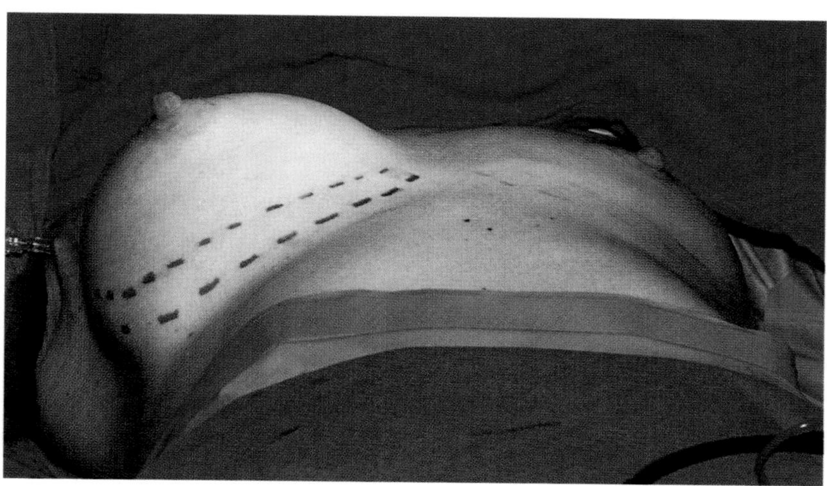

The implant is partially inflated with saline solution, after which the position of the valve is confirmed digitally and the implant seated properly against the inferior aspect of the pocket. The implant may now be filled to the appropriate volume. The opposite implant is prepared and inserted in a similar fashion.

Final Adjustments and Closure

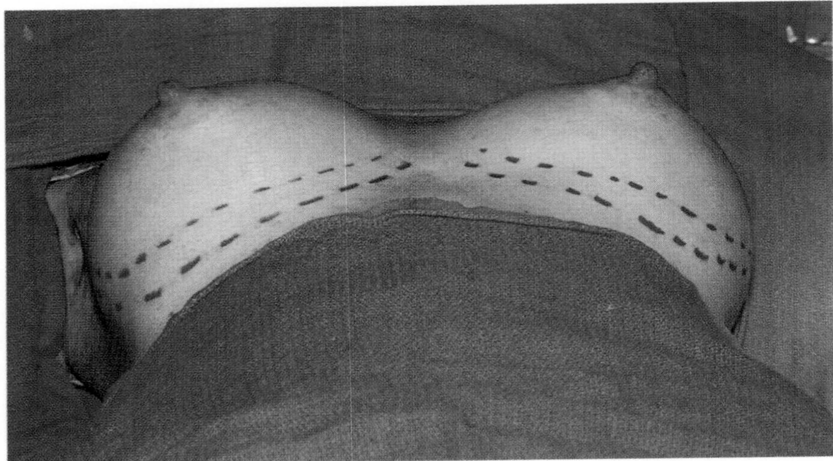

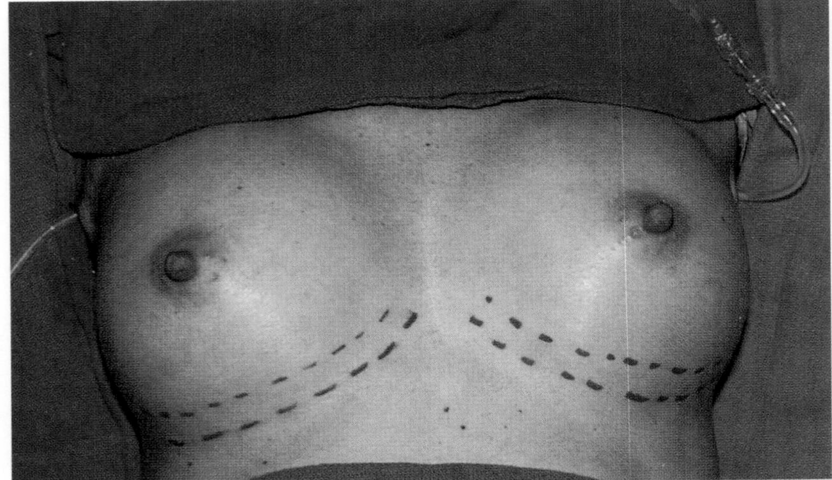

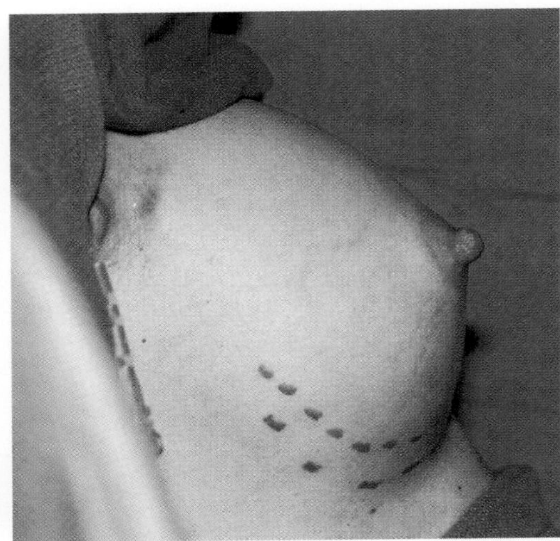

The back of the operating table is now adjusted to place the patient in an upright sitting position. The breast appearance is then evaluated for symmetry, implant position, appropriate volume, and irregularities along the inframammary crease. Implant volume adjustments are made as necessary. Occasionally it is necessary to displace an implant downward digitally, which is not difficult because of the generous pocket dissection.

Occasionally one inframammary fold remains too high or, more commonly, there is a slight fold irregularity. When this occurs, the large, smooth urethral dilator may be carefully placed behind the implant and pressure used to dissect the crease. If the implant is relatively tight within the cavity, 50 to 100 ml of fluid is removed to allow the urethral dilator to be placed behind the implant easily. Pressure on the upper pole of the breast accentuates these irregularities and allows fine adjustment of the crease. After all adjustments are completed, the patient is returned to a supine position for wound closure.

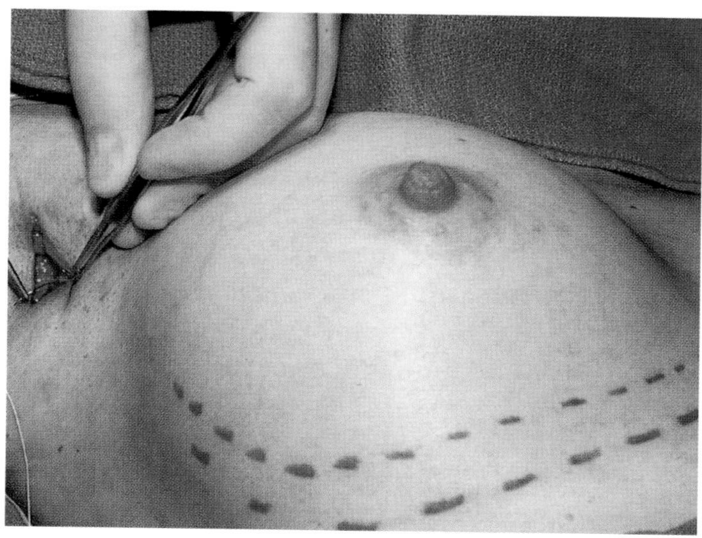

The wound is closed in layers using absorbable suture material. The subcutaneous tissue is reapproximated with two or three 3-0 interrupted absorbable sutures. Deep dermal and intracuticular layers are then closed with a continuous 4-0 running absorbable suture.

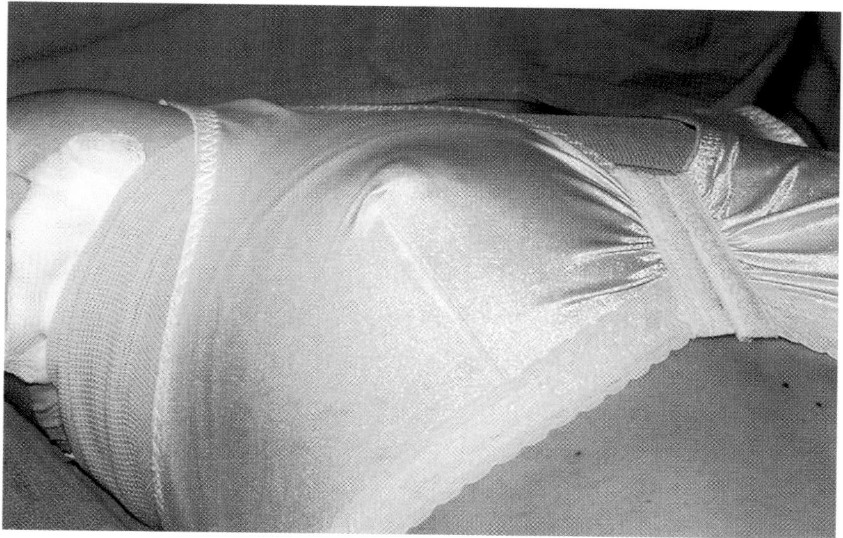

The wounds are cleaned and sterile tapes applied parallel to the incisions. A tube top is positioned over the breasts to provide gentle support without lift. A loose brassiere is used to prevent any upward displacement of the implants. Alternatively, an elastic wrap may be placed over the superior aspect of the breasts during the early postoperative period as shown above.

Results

This healthy 28-year-old woman was concerned that her breasts were disproportionately small; they were also asymmetric, her right breast being somewhat smaller than the left. She wore a size 34A bra but did not fill it. She was particularly embarrassed in a swimsuit and in athletic clothing. Two of her friends who had breast augmentation were pleased with the improvement they had and suggested that she consider having her breasts enlarged. She was fully aware of the breast implant controversy but was not concerned about possible risks and felt comfortable with having her breasts augmented with saline implants. She had thought about breast augmentation for many years and felt that this was a good time in her life to have the operation. She requested a procedure that left no visible breast scars if at all possible. Physical examination revealed a healthy woman 5 feet 6 inches tall and weighing 128 pounds. Mild asymmetry was noted on breast examination. The left breast was estimated at 250 gm and the right breast at 225 gm.

An axillary approach using an endoscopic technique was chosen for this patient because it provided a short, hidden axillary incision while producing the desired breast enhancement. The implant was placed in the subpectoral position to ensure adequate cover and to reduce the risk of capsular contracture. Even though she still has some asymmetry, her enlarged breasts make the asymmetry less noticeable. The breasts are soft and acceptably mobile. The axillary scar is fading. The implants are not palpable and there were no complications following the operation. She is proud of the way she looks and feels that this operation has not only met her expectations but also provided a substantial boost to her self-esteem.

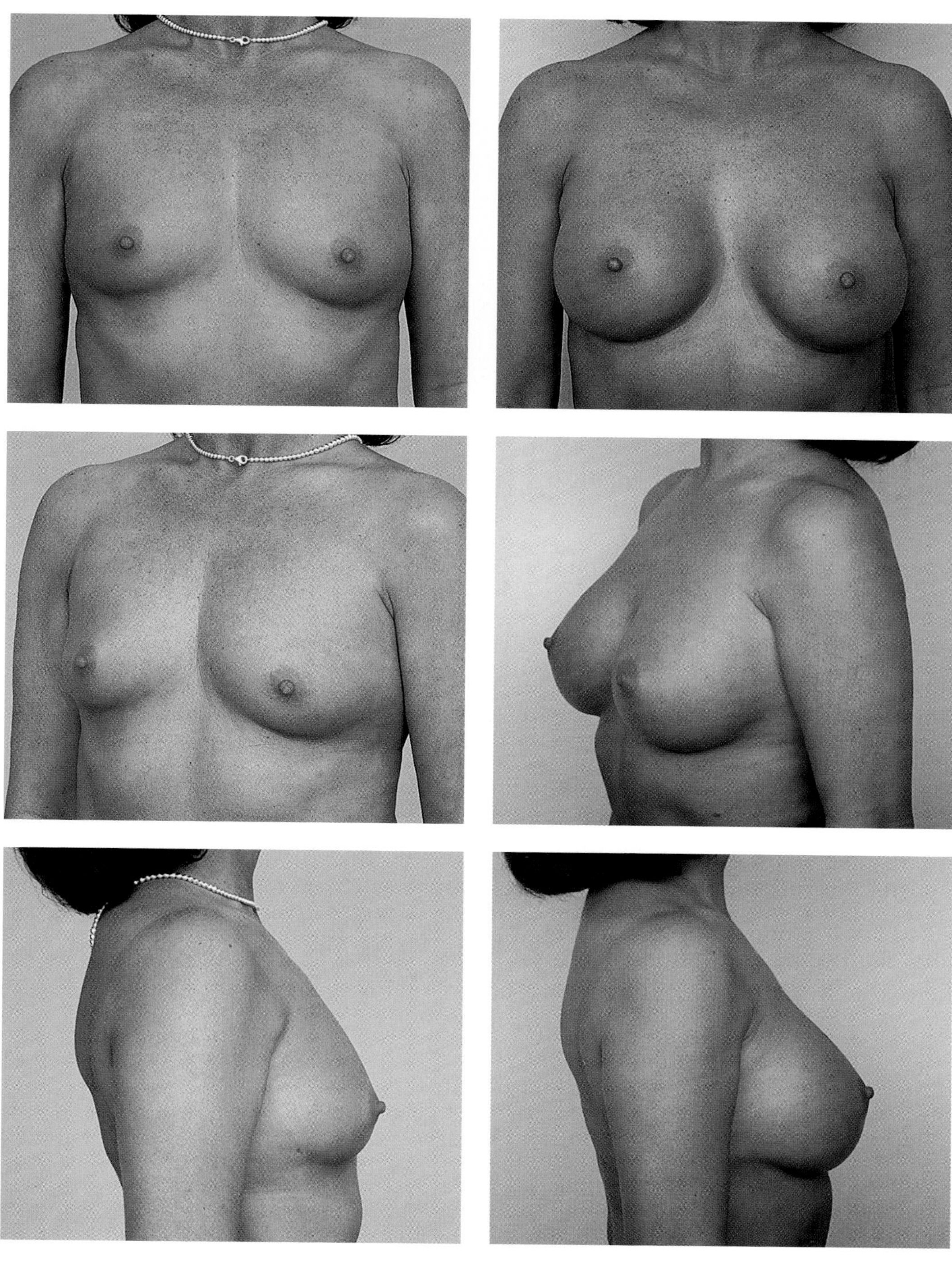

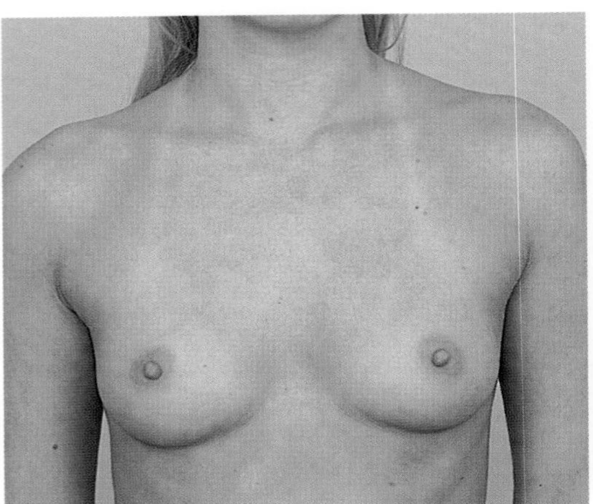

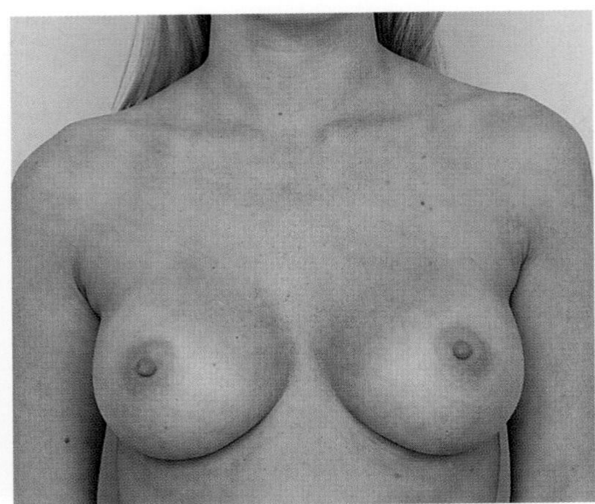

This athletic 22-year-old woman is 5 feet 2 inches tall, weighs 110 pounds, and has a chest circumference of 34 inches. She requested breast augmentation because she felt that her breasts were disproportionately small for her body type. She had some idea what to expect since her mother had breast augmentation 25 years previously and was pleased with her results. She wanted to avoid breast scars and requested an axillary approach for implant placement. Bilateral 300 cc smooth-surface saline implants were placed in the subpectoral position. Good release of the pectoralis major muscle was accomplished inferiorly as well as inferomedially. After insertion the implants were inflated to 320 cc. She healed with no complications. She is shown 2 years following subpectoral axillary breast augmentation. The axillary scars are barely noticeable, her breasts are soft, and the patient is satisfied with her enhanced body contour.

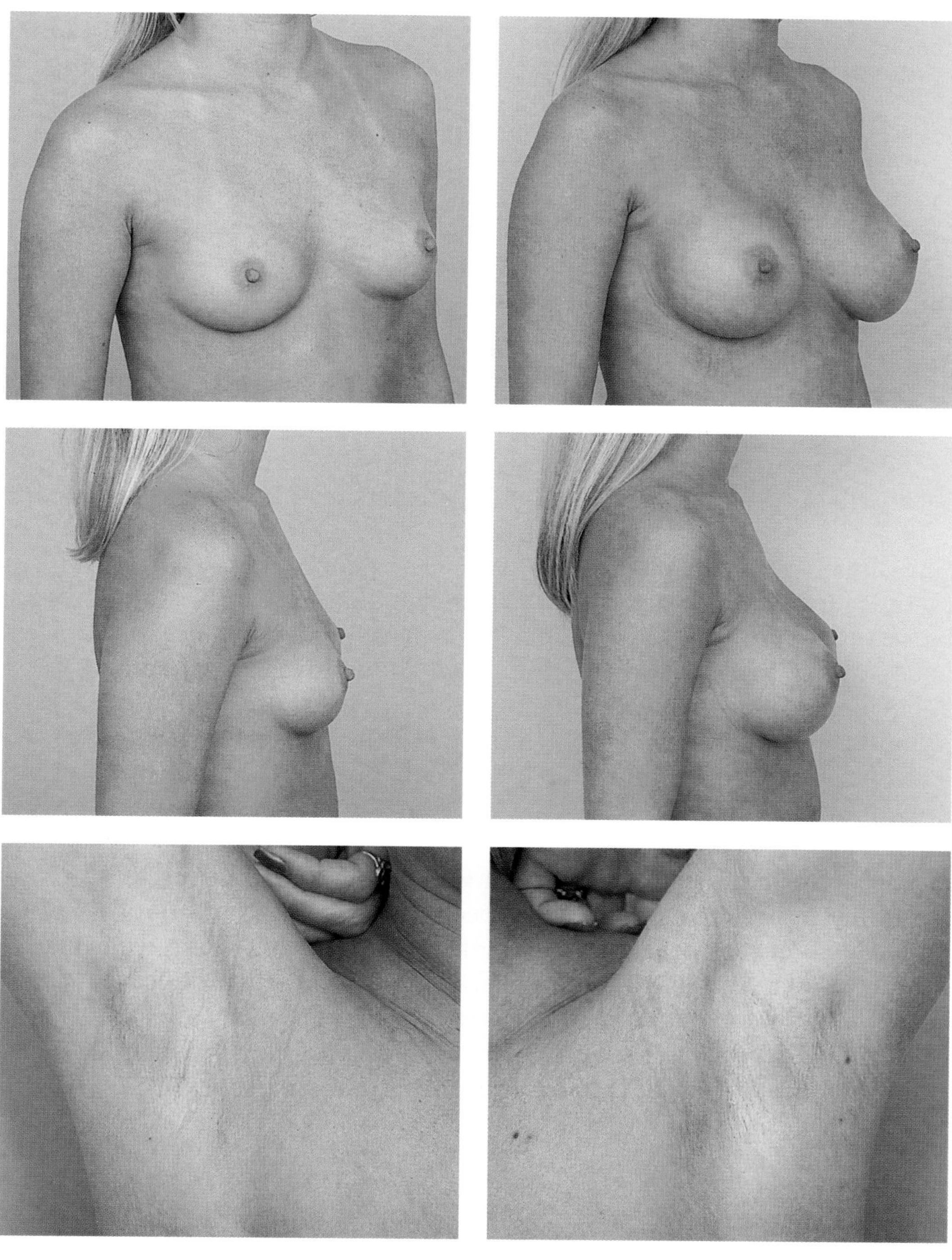

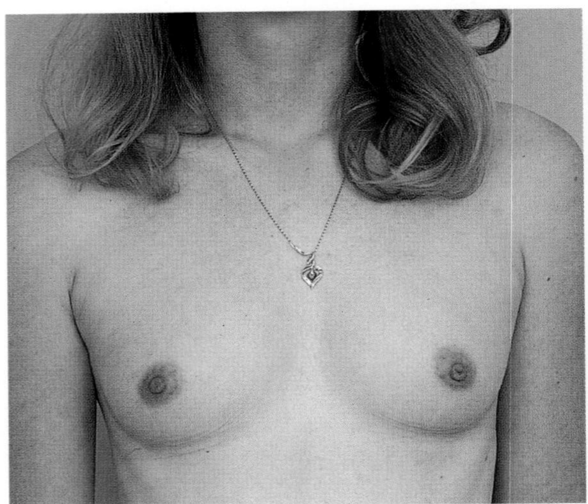

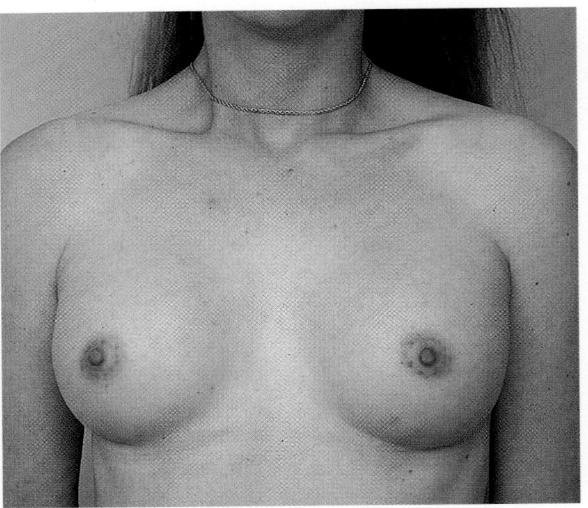

This athletic 24-year-old woman is 5 feet 5 inches tall and weighs 110 pounds. She wore a size 34A bra, which she did not fill. She wanted larger breasts to improve her appearance, to achieve greater balance, and to feel better about herself. She was informed about breast augmentation and about breast implants and did not object to their use. Her breasts were found to be mildly asymmetric, with the right breast slightly larger than the left. She had poor definition of the inframammary fold, but the pectoral muscle was well developed.

An endoscopic axillary augmentation was planned. After release of the pectoral muscle and creation of the subpectoral pocket, 275 cc smooth-surface saline implants were inserted and inflated to 300 cc. These were placed through axillary incisions in a subpectoral position with endoscopic assistance. After augmentation her breasts were soft and the implants mildly palpable in the lower breast region. There were no postoperative complications and the axillary scar faded after 1 year until it was scarcely noticeable.

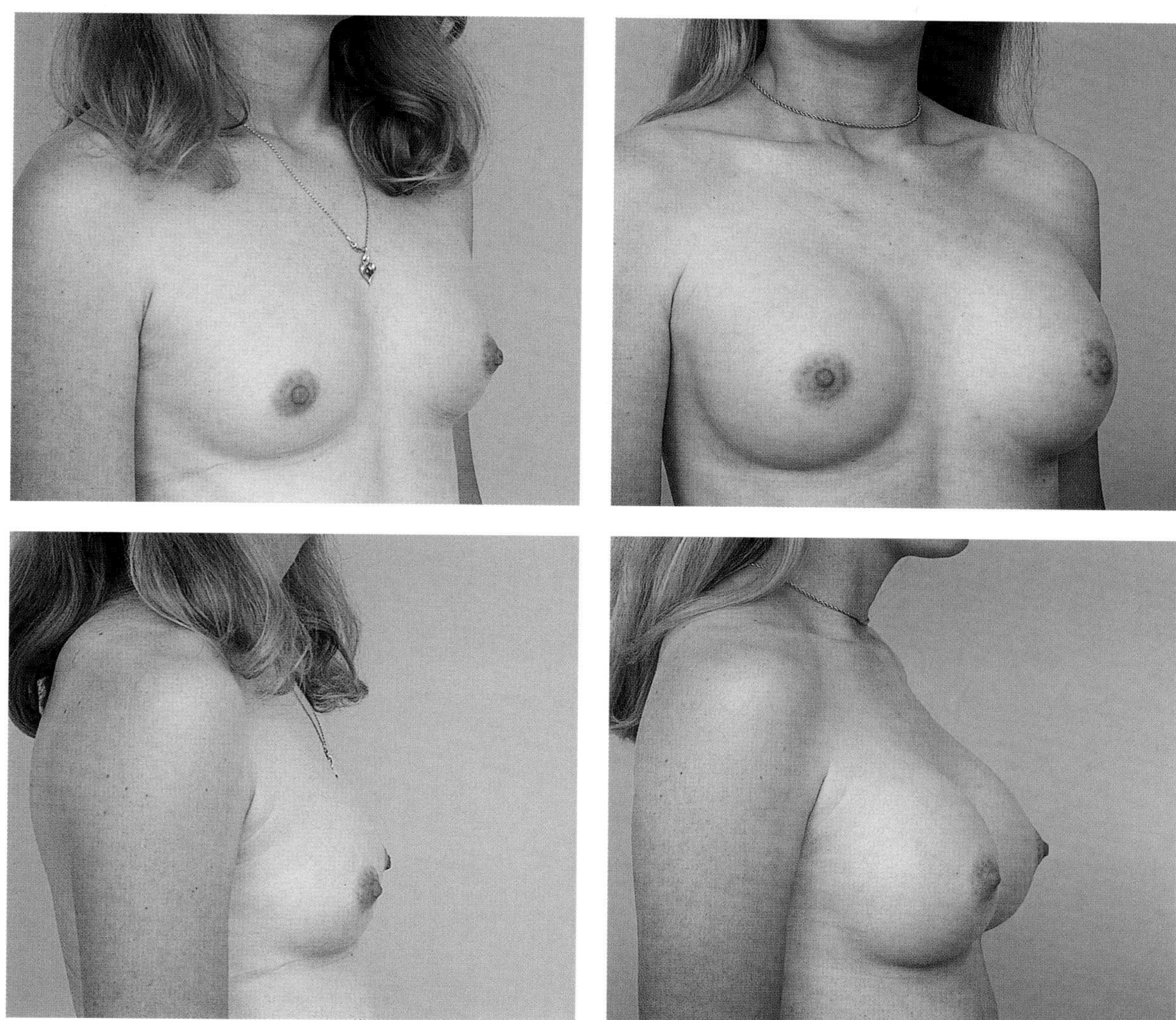

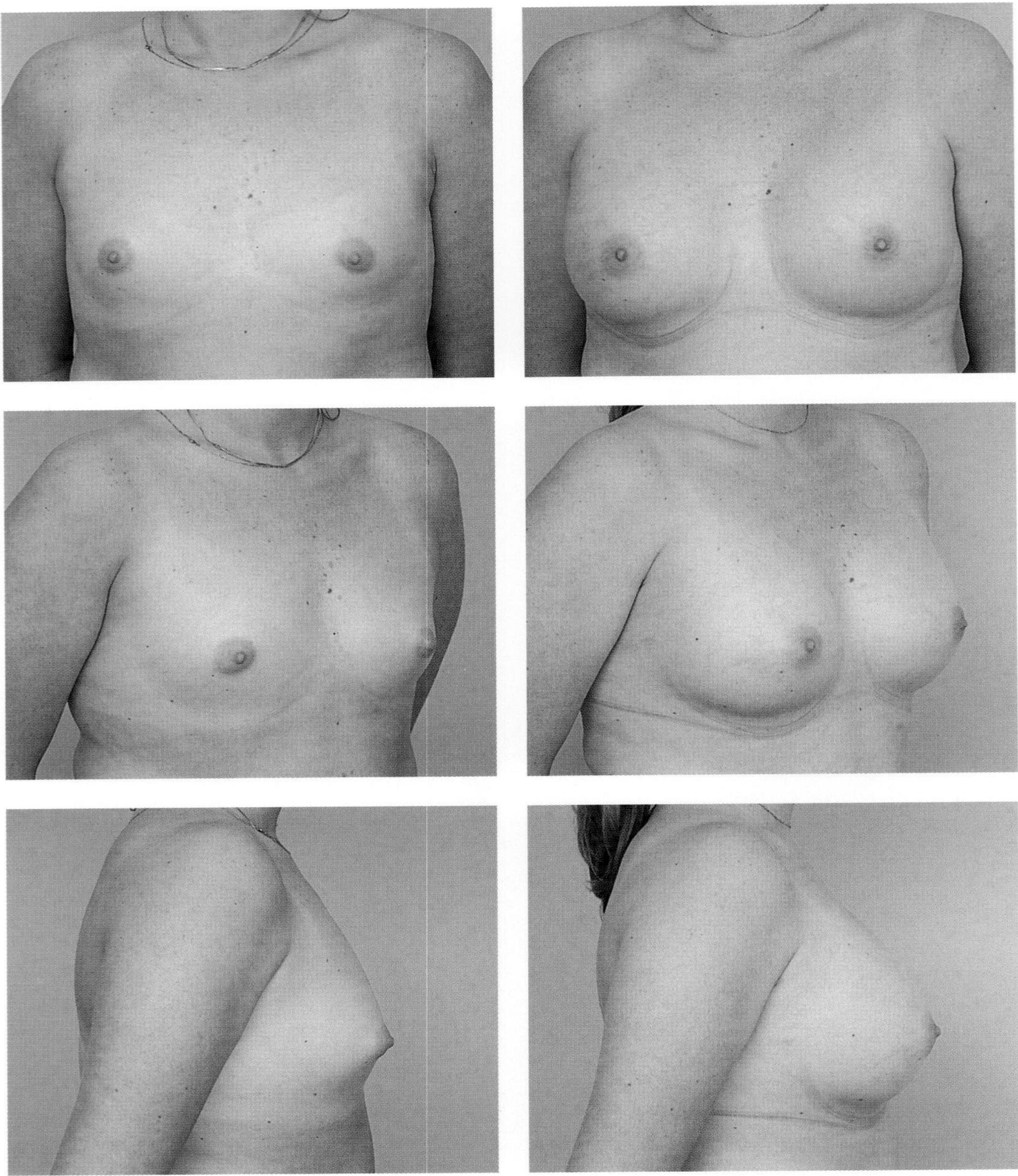

This healthy 28-year-old woman is 5 feet 4 inches tall and weighs 140 pounds. There was minimal breast development and she felt that her breasts were too small for her body habitus. Exercise had not enlarged her breasts. No breast abnormalities were found on mammograms or on physical examination. She requested an endoscopic axillary breast augmentation, which was performed using a general anesthetic. Bilateral 325 cc smooth-surface saline implants were inserted and inflated to a volume of 340 cc. One year later she is pleased with the improvement and her breasts are soft and acceptably symmetric. Satisfactory coverage over the lower aspect of the implants prevented them from being palpable.

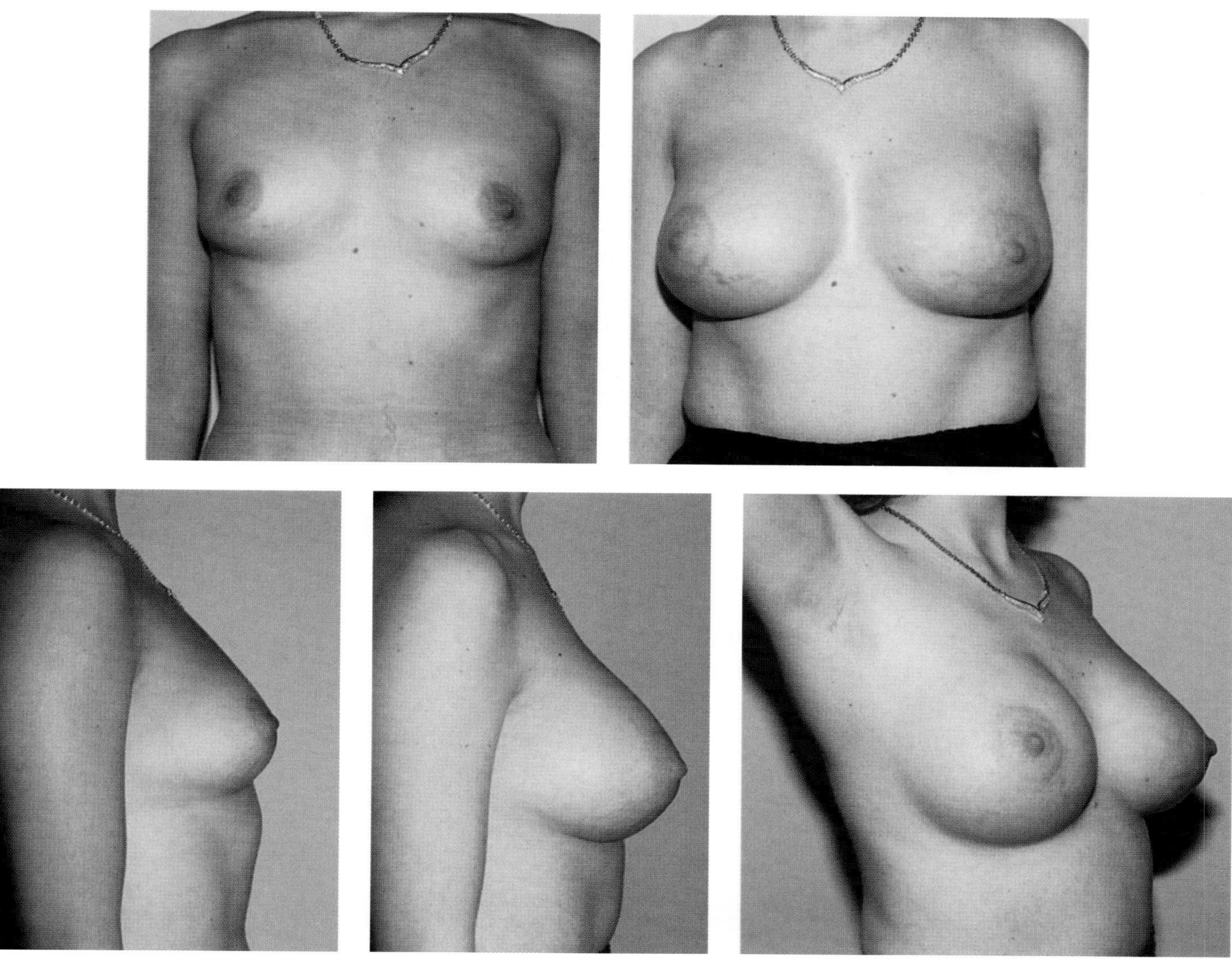

This 26-year-old nulliparous woman requested breast augmentation that would produce a very full look. Her broad chest and wide breast base required a large implant diameter. She underwent endoscopic subpectoral transaxillary augmentation with 425 cc saline implants. Six months postoperatively she has achieved the fullness she desired, and the mild preoperative asymmetry of the inframammary folds has been corrected. Her axillary scar is scarcely noticeable.

STANDARD SUBPECTORAL AXILLARY AUGMENTATION

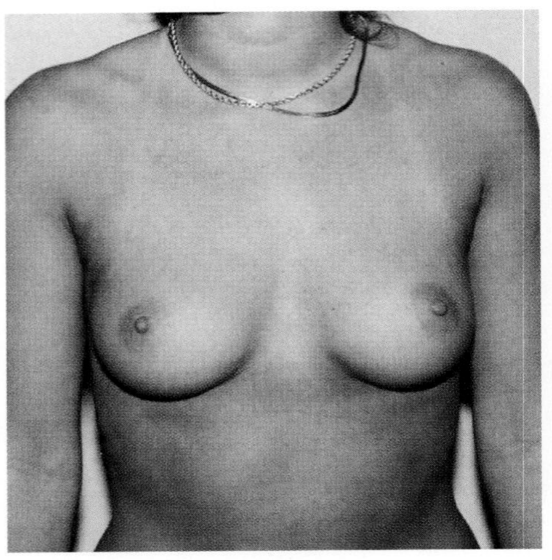

This nulliparous 19-year-old-woman requested breast augmentation that would leave no visible breast scars. Endoscopic techniques had not been introduced at that time. Thus an axillary approach was chosen and the incision was made in the transverse lines of the axilla.

Surgical plan

- Axillary approach
- Subpectoral dissection of implant pocket
- Release of medial and inferior pectoralis fibers
- Development of symmetric subpectoral pockets
- Placement of round smooth-surface saline implants

Markings and Technique

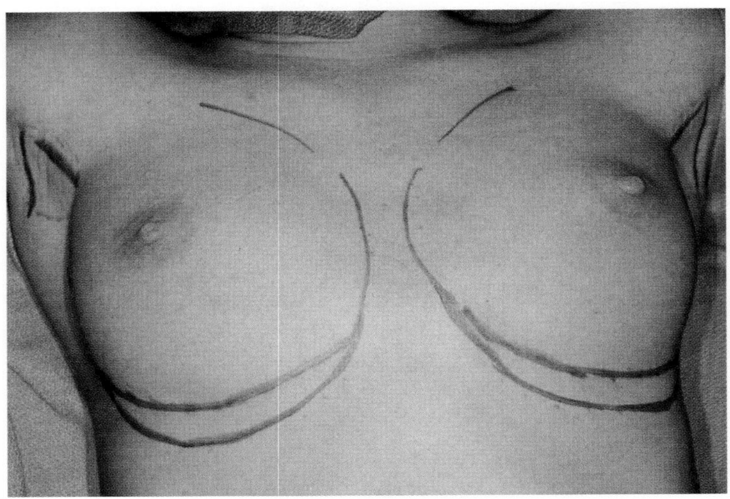

Preoperative markings delineate the extent of dissection of the subpectoral pocket. ***The lower marks for dissection of the pocket are placed 1.5 to 2.0 cm below the proposed inframammary crease.*** The underlying axillary contents contain major vessels and nerves, and the fat pad also contains the intercostobrachial nerve.

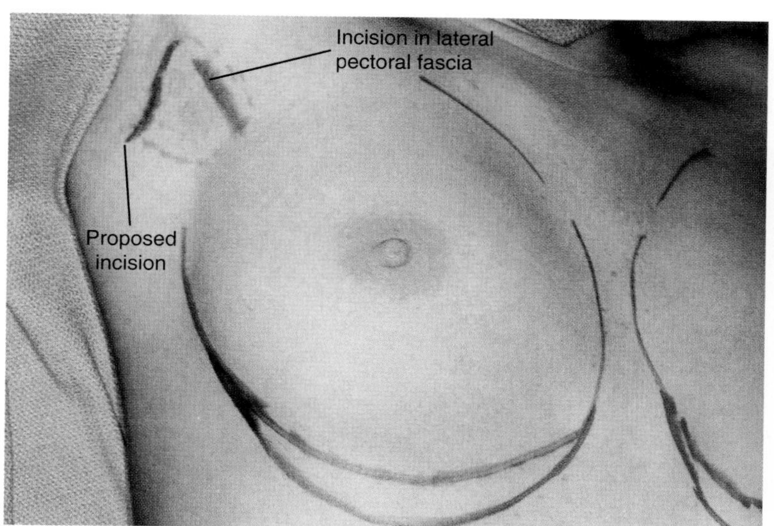

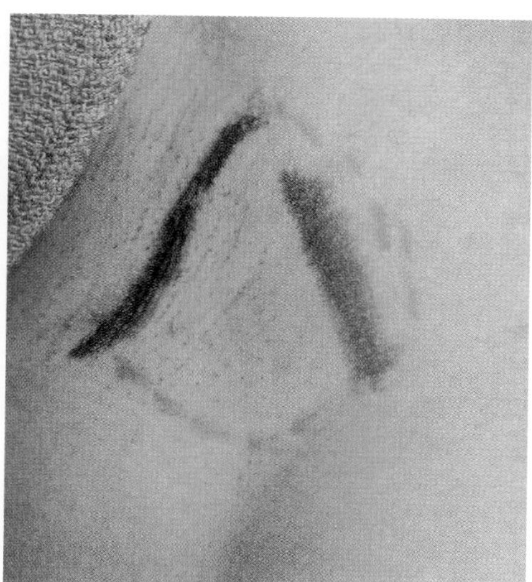

The axillary incision is marked in a transverse direction in a crease in the depth of the axilla. It is approximately 3.5 to 4.0 cm long and is planned within the axillary hair pattern. A second line is marked parallel to the upper lateral border of the pectoralis major muscle. This will be the point of entry for the submusculofascial dissection.

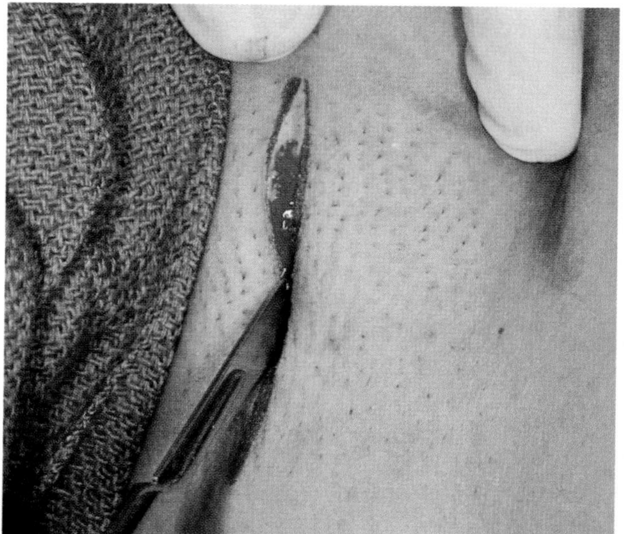

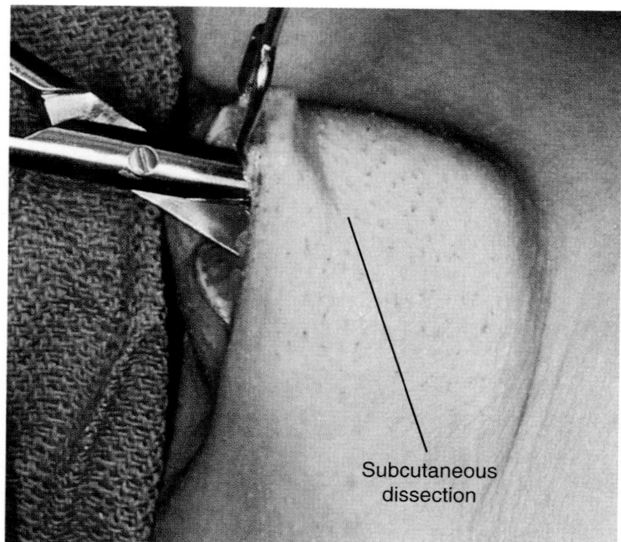

After the incision is made in the axillary skin, the dissection is carried out superficially (subcutaneously) until the lateral border of the pectoralis major muscle is approached.

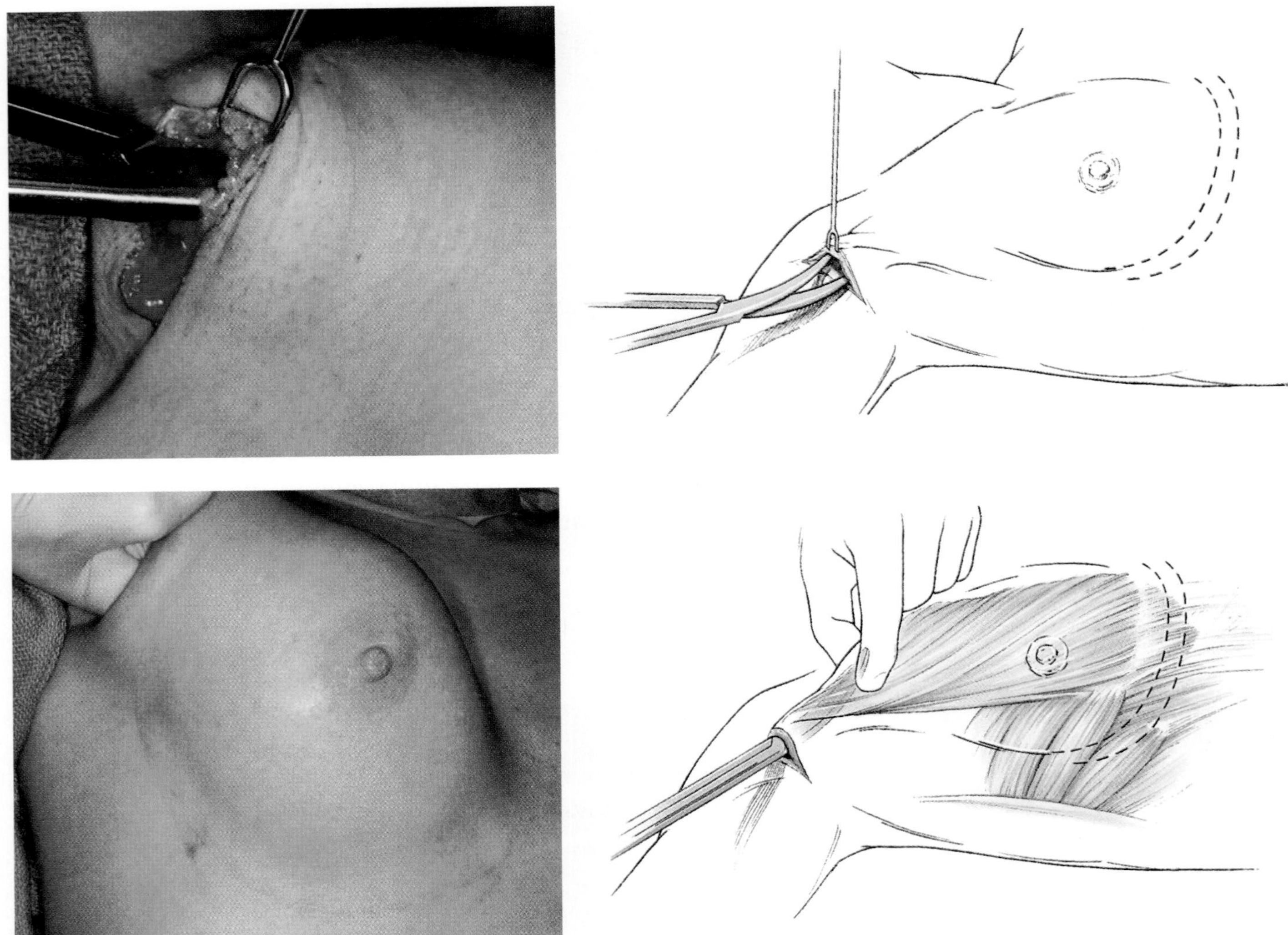

The lateral fascia over the pectoralis major muscle is divided, and the subpectoral space is entered laterally by going under the upper portion of the pectoralis major muscle. ***The dissection underneath the pectoralis major muscle should be made continuously; if undue bleeding is encountered, the surgeon is probably in a deeper plane beneath the pectoralis minor muscle and the dissection plane must be corrected.***

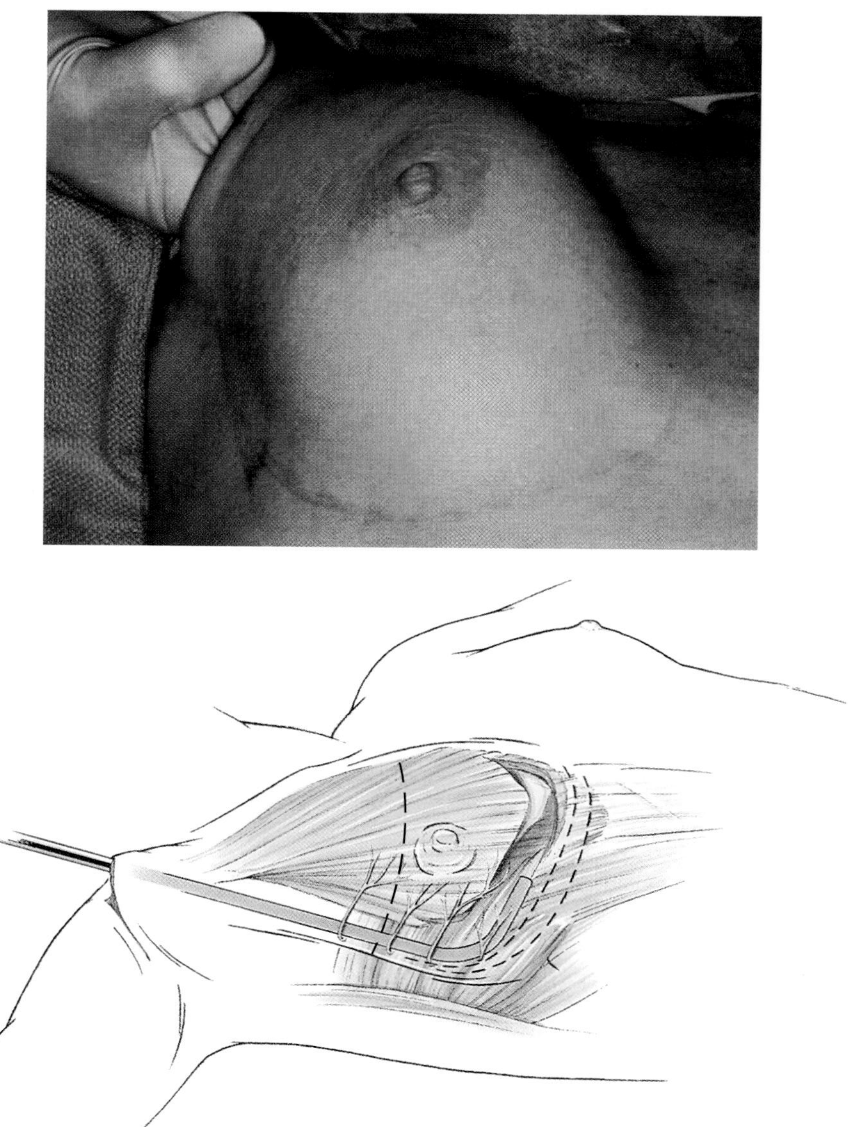

Blunt finger dissection beneath the pectoralis major muscle extends as far laterally and inferiorly as possible. The colored area indicates the extent of blunt finger dissection. The remainder of the dissection must be accomplished using blunt dissecting instruments.

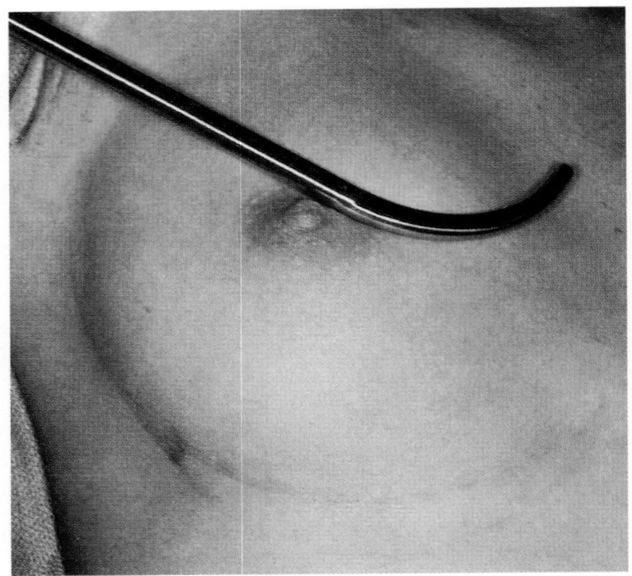

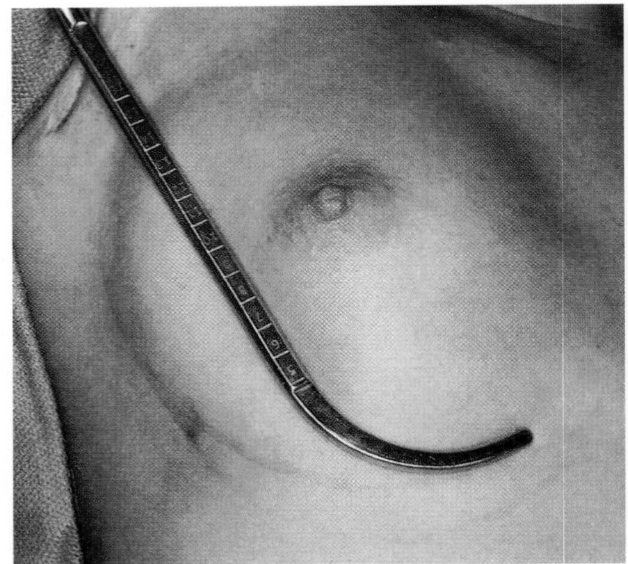

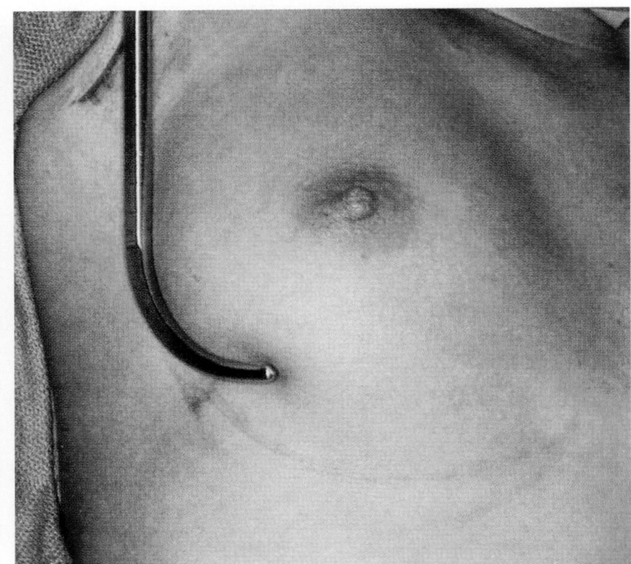

I use a pair of Agris-Dingman axillary dissectors or a large urethral sound (size 36 Fr) to detach the pectoral muscle bluntly from the sternum and from its lower costal origins. The position, orientation, and extent of dissection with the subpectoral dissectors are indicated above. ***The lower pectoralis major fibers must be divided with the dissector to create a sufficiently low and medial pocket.***

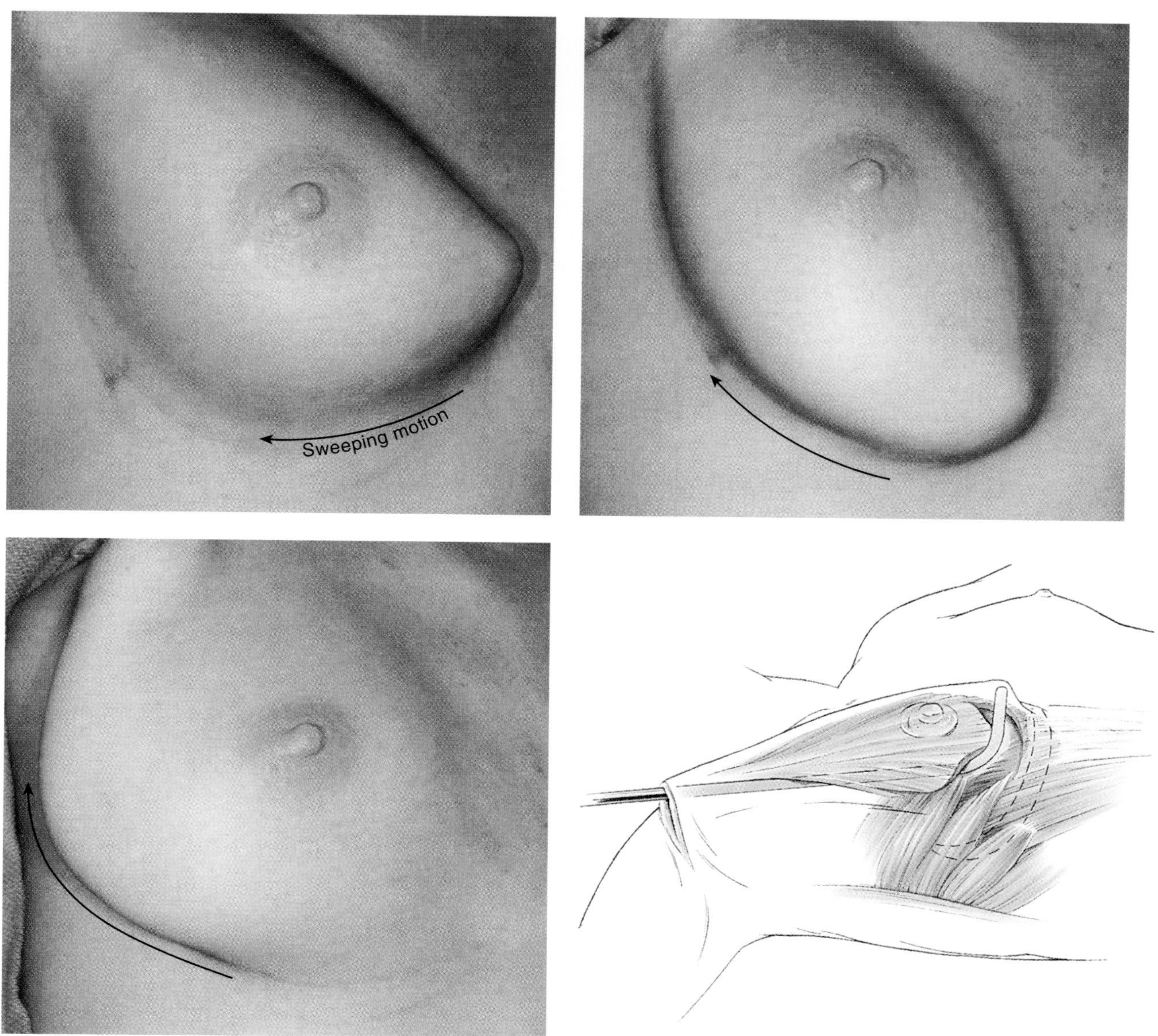

The blunt elevation then proceeds inferomedially to laterally; it extends to the limits of the inferior dissection marked preoperatively over the fascia of the upper rectus abdominis, external oblique, and lateral serratus anterior.

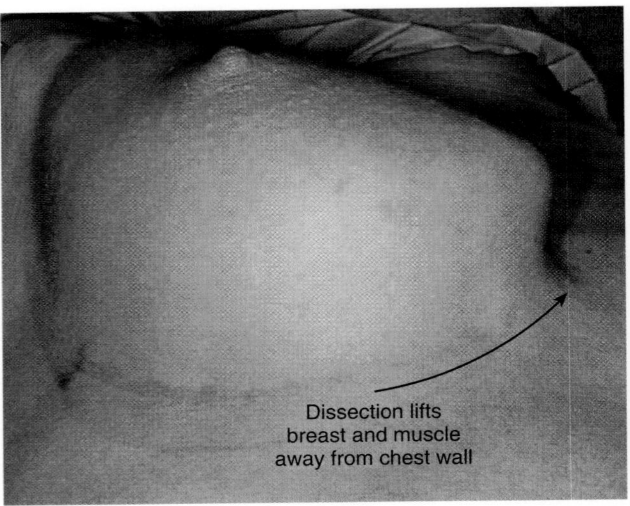

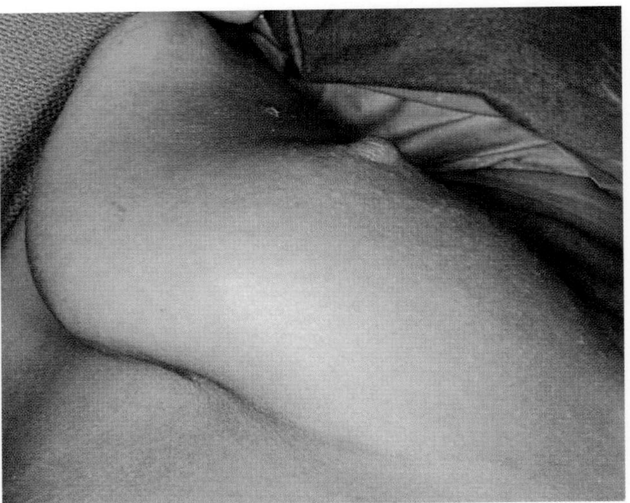

This dissection is more effective when the dissector is moved both in the direction of the periphery of the proposed pocket and in a rotating motion away from the chest wall to stretch and expand the tissues outward and allow them to accommodate the implant.

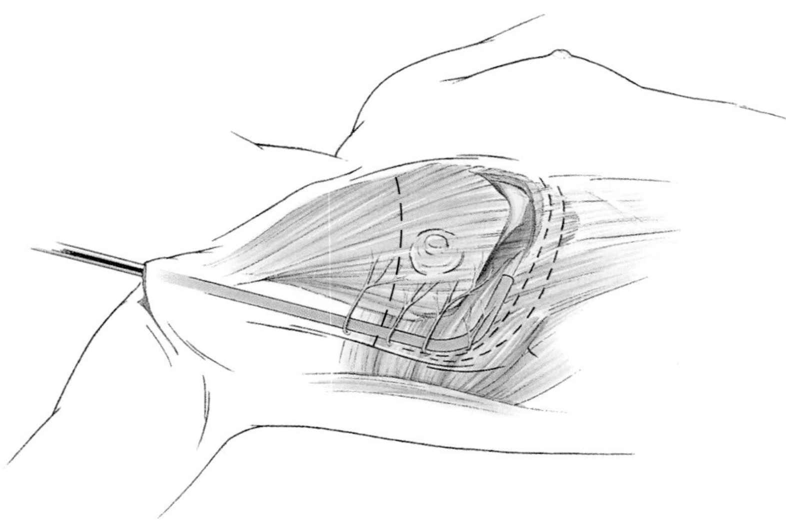

The extent of the instrument dissection is indicated. Anatomic dissections have demonstrated that the dissector breaks through the lower pectoralis major margin and that the inferolateral portion of the pocket is subglandular and superficial to the musculofascial layer.

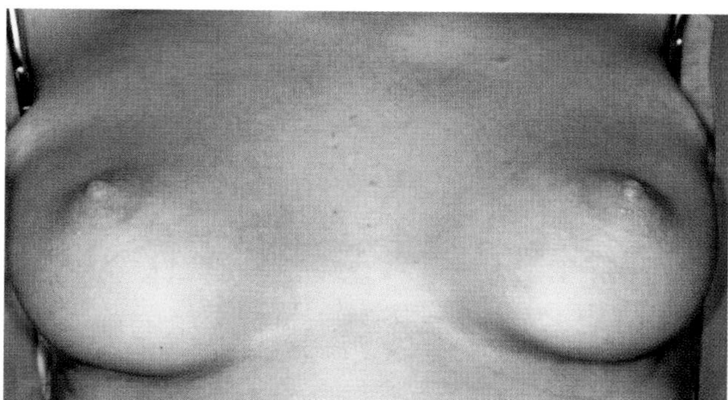

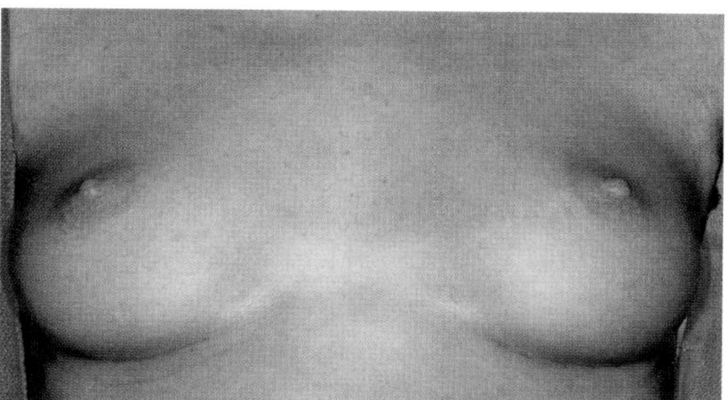

The dissected implant pockets should be examined carefully with the dissectors to ensure that they are symmetric and that they extend smoothly to the desired inferior level.

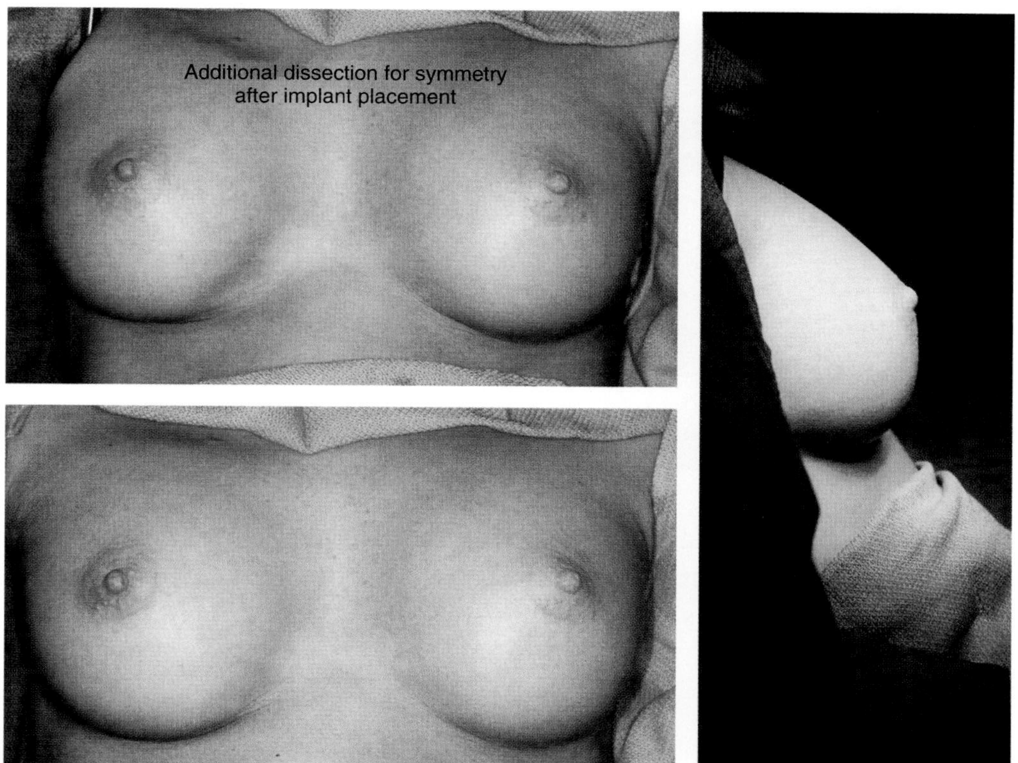

A 320 cc breast implant is then positioned through the axillary incision under the elevated pectoralis major muscle. ***The pockets should be checked for symmetry several times before placement of the implants and again after implant placement.*** At this time the symmetry and the position of the patient's breasts should be observed while she is both sitting and supine. The upright position, however, is most important in determining adequate future symmetry.

When the implants appear too high, the inferior pocket dissection is reevaluated and revised to ensure that the patient's breasts are symmetric and low enough before final closure. ***An appearance of too much upper pole fullness can result from inadequate lower and lateral dissection; this dissection also needs to be extended when larger silicone breast implants are used.*** Additional dissection and adjustment using the blunt dissectors can be made after implant placement with the patient sitting upright. Postoperative external pressure will not adequately lower breast implants that are too high—they must be positioned correctly before the operation is concluded to ensure a symmetric result.

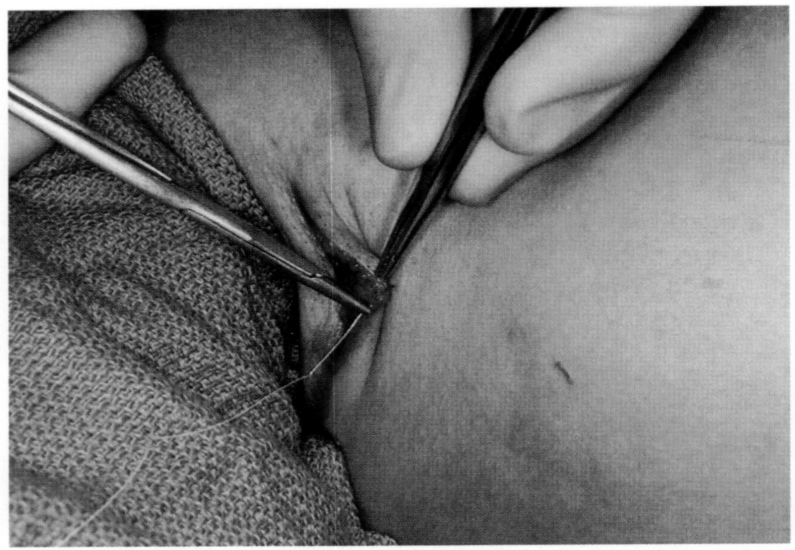

Final closure is done in layers by suturing the lateral pectoral fascia and axillary incision; an intracuticular suture is used for the final closure. The axillary incision usually heals inconspicuously.

Results

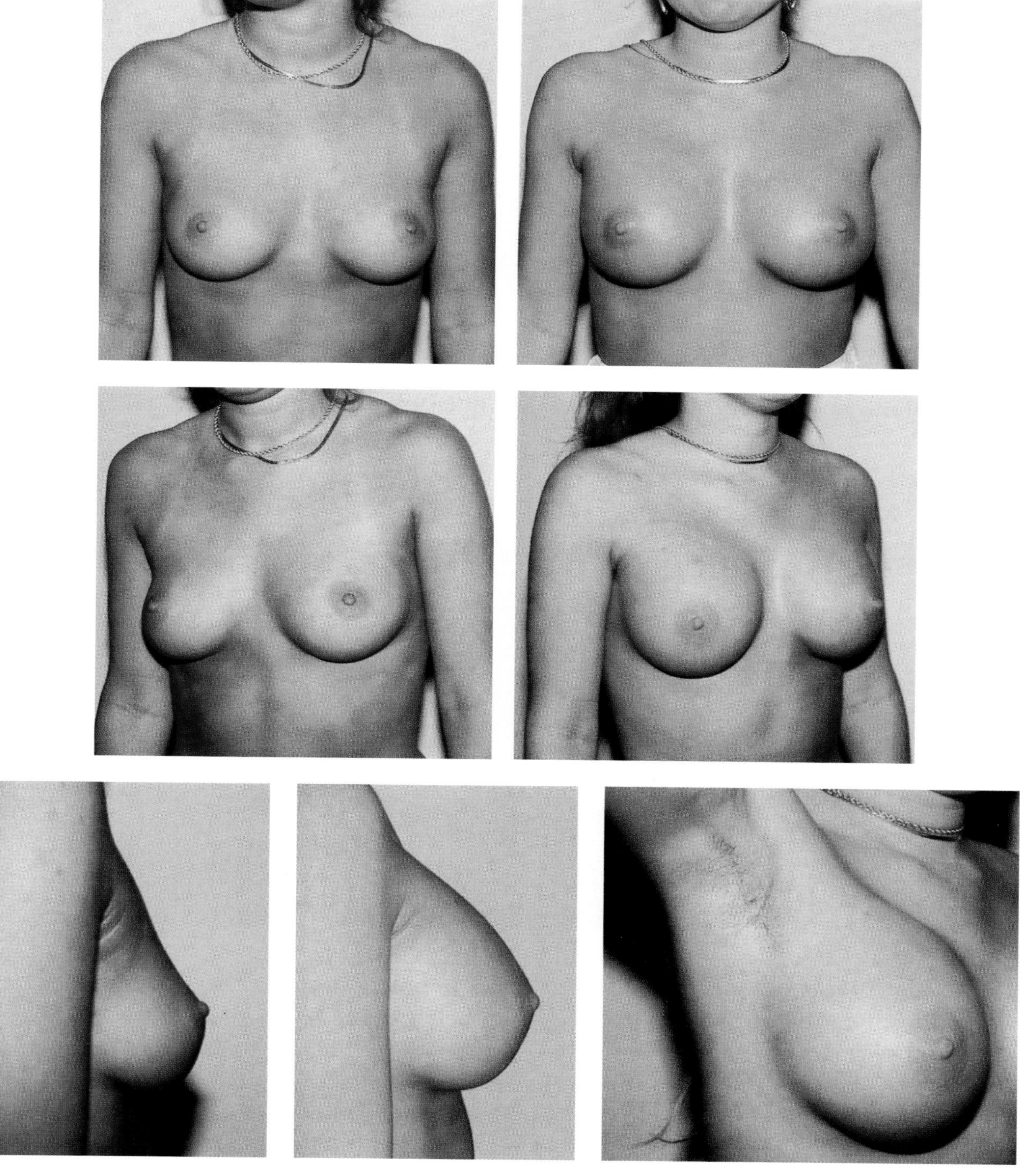

This patient depicted in the preceding operative sequence is pleased with her larger breast size. Three months following axillary breast augmentation her breasts are naturally soft and symmetry has been preserved. The axillary scar, although still erythematous, is in a satisfactory position and is inconspicuous. The implants should settle further during the first year.

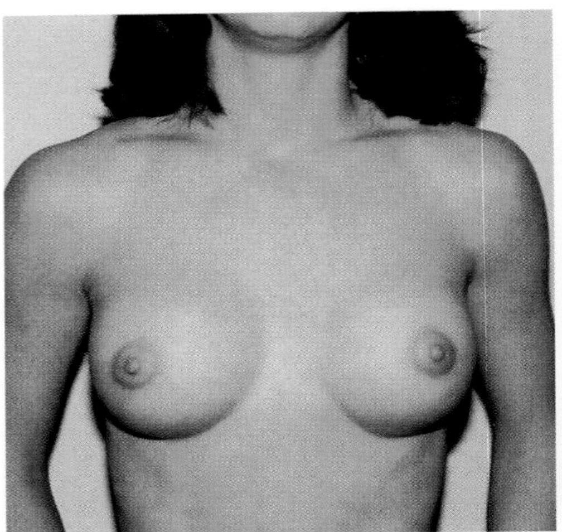
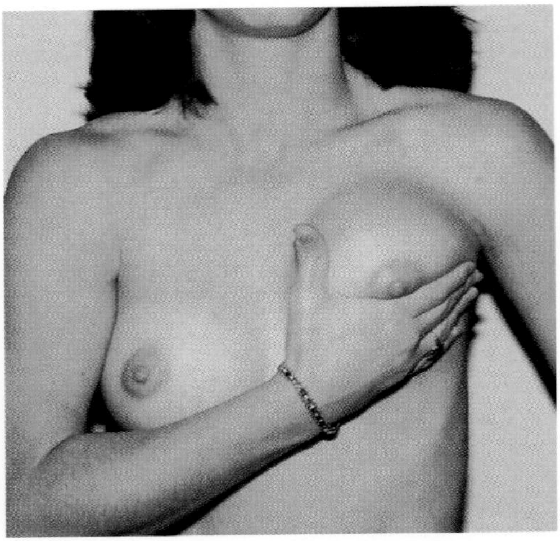

The patient is instructed in upward displacement implant exercises to be done twice daily beginning several days after axillary augmentation.

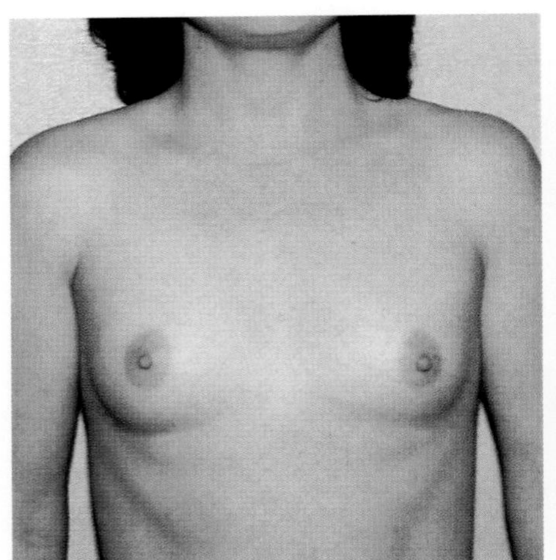
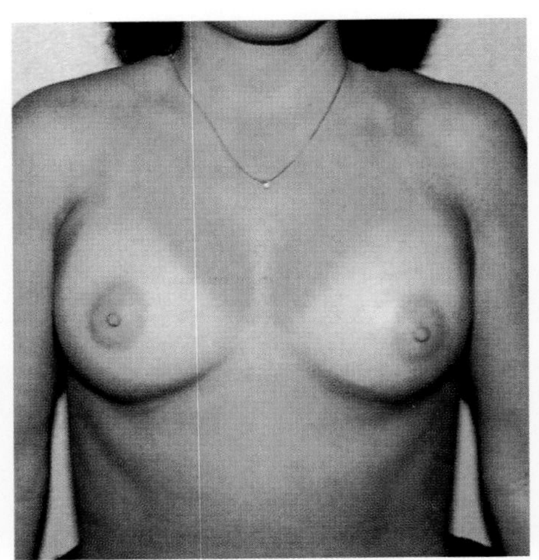
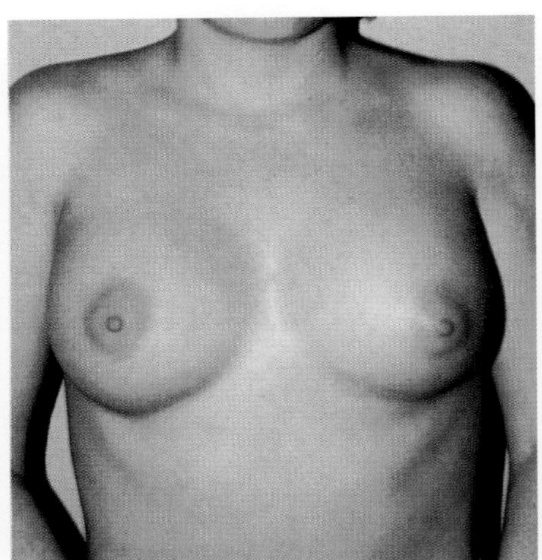

This 20-year-old patient requested breast augmentation via the axillary approach since she did not want scars on her breasts. Augmentation was accomplished with 360 cc smooth implants positioned via the axillary incision. She is shown 6 months postoperatively. One year following breast augmentation the implants have settled further, giving a more natural-appearing result.

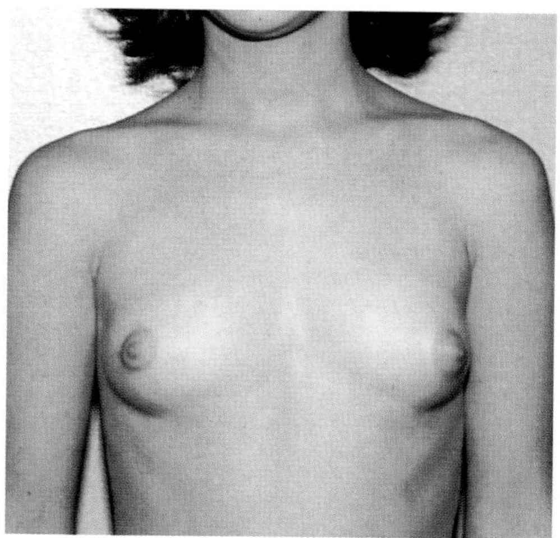
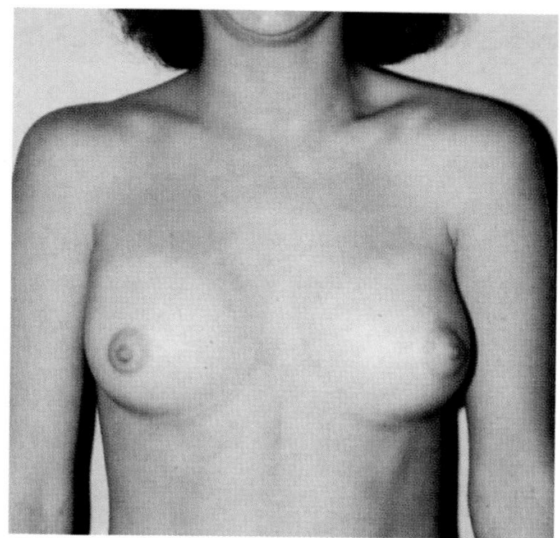

This 18-year-old model was interested in breast augmentation mammaplasty via axillary incisions. She had some preoperative breast asymmetry with a lateral inclination of the left nipple-areola. One year following augmentation she is satisfied with her soft breasts despite some increase in the preoperative asymmetry.

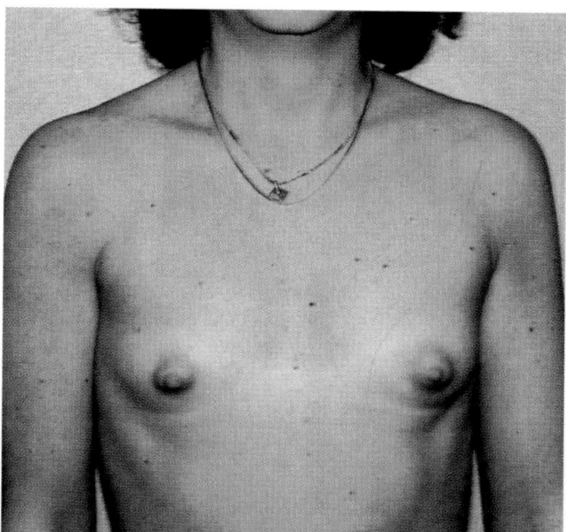
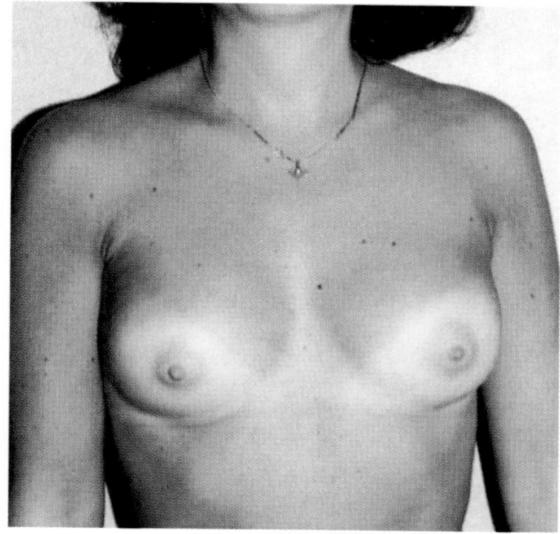

This 25-year-old patient had hypoplastic, somewhat constricted breasts. She requested breast augmentation via the axillary approach. The breasts remain soft 8 months following breast augmentation; however, the constriction and the lower breast deficiency have persisted. It is my experience that the axillary approach does not achieve optimal results in constricted breasts and breasts with a deficiency in the lower pole. For these patients a periareolar approach is a better choice to more accurately define a new lower crease and to expand the lower breast parenchyma.

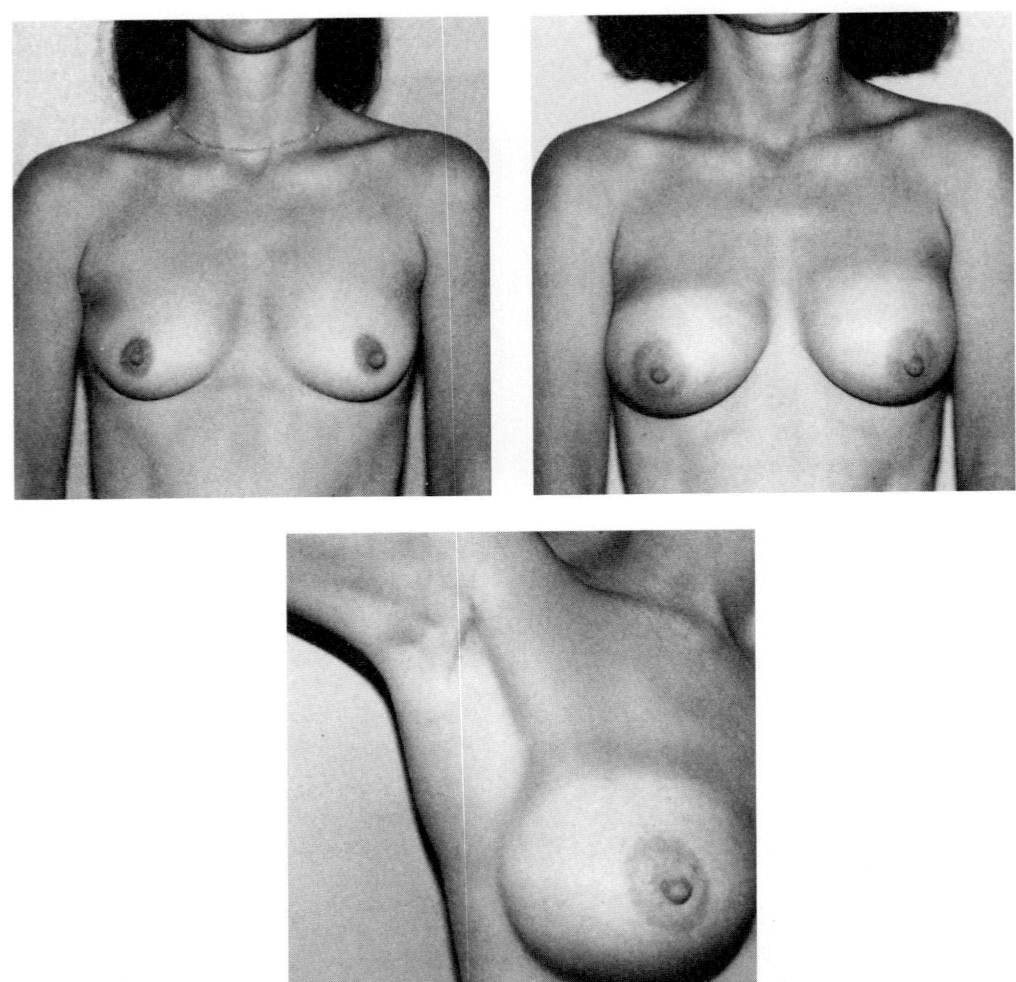

This 28-year-old patient had mild pseudoptosis with involution of her breasts after two pregnancies. She requested an axillary incision. She is shown 8 months following breast augmentation with 320 cc double-lumen implants. The axillary incision has remained somewhat erythematous; however, its position in the axilla is satisfactory.

SUBGLANDULAR AXILLARY AUGMENTATION

In my experience, the subglandular axillary approach with smooth-surface implants results in a higher incidence of capsular contracture and makes it more difficult to obtain symmetry. Textured-surface implants tend to be associated with a lower capsular contracture rate. Open capsulotomy with this approach often requires a second inframammary or periareolar incision for correction. The use of the endoscopic technique permits more accurate subglandular dissection; however, because of concerns about monitoring, imaging, and coverage and the increased likelihood of implant palpability with textured-surface implants, I prefer the subpectoral axillary approach using smooth-surface implants rather than the subglandular approach.

INFRAMAMMARY APPROACH

The inframammary incision is a more direct approach for breast augmentation. It allows direct access to and visualization of the lower breast region and the subpectoral position by dissecting around the lower pole of the breast and up to the lateral margin of the pectoralis major muscle. The subpectoral pocket is then dissected bluntly up to the level of the second rib using either finger dissection or a urethral sound. The initial dissection is made bluntly to preserve the intercostal nerves that provide sensation to the breast and nipple-areolar region. ***For proper medial and inferior positioning of the implant through the inframammary fold, the lower medial and inferior pectoral muscle is released.*** Muscle pull over the implant is reduced by releasing the lowest medial insertions. Although this procedure can be done with a lighted retractor and blunt dissection, the use of the endoscope provides excellent visualization for complete division of the pectoral muscle and permits good control for accurate creation of the breast pocket and positioning of the breast implant to enhance breast symmetry. ***The inframammary incision is usually placed in the crease or slightly above the crease; with the use of the endoscope the scar can often be shortened to 2.5 to 3.0 cm in length.*** The incision generally heals with minimal scarring; however, it can become hypertrophic and require pressure with silicone sheeting.

Patients with minimal to moderate ptosis and a well-defined inframammary crease are candidates for augmentation through an inframammary approach, as are women with a constricted breast and a well-defined crease. Women who want to avoid an axillary scar, however small, are therefore candidates for subpectoral inframammary endoscopic breast augmentation. The inframammary approach is also preferred for women who require intraoperative expansion or expansion of the breast parenchyma because of constriction.

STANDARD SUBPECTORAL INFRAMAMMARY AUGMENTATION

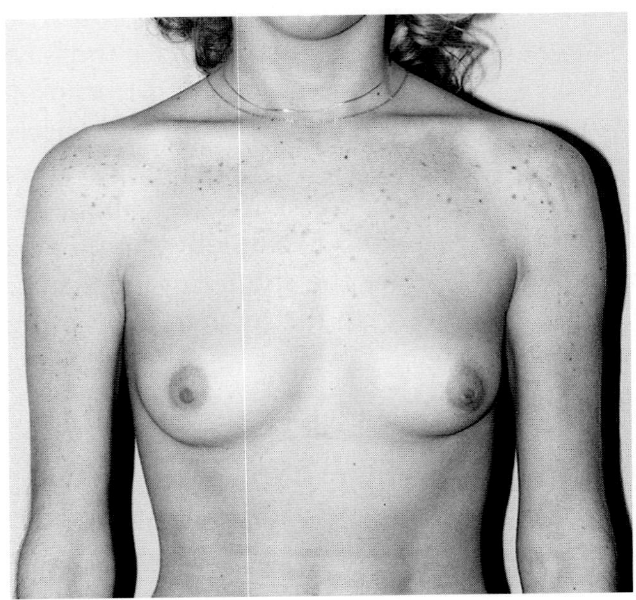

Breast hypoplasia with mild breast asymmetry prompted this woman to request breast augmentation.

Patient Positioning

When inframammary augmentation is planned, patient positioning is an important consideration. The patient must be positioned symmetrically on the operating table. Otherwise the entire procedure can be prolonged by efforts to obtain a symmetric result on an asymmetrically positioned patient. The anesthesiologist and nursing staff should be told that the patient will need to sit up on the operating table before the procedure begins. The anesthesiologist will need to prepare the patient to sit up by securing her arms to the arm boards so that they will not slip off and downward when she is sitting up. Airway control will also be necessary when sitting the patient up; an endotracheal tube is preferable to a mask. I have found it best to sit the patient up by first putting the operating table in the Trendelenburg position at approximately 20 degrees. This helps to prevent the patient from slipping downward when the head of the bed is elevated. The head of the bed is then raised until the patient is in the sitting position. Simply flexing the operating table will not get the patient to the sitting position.

Surgical plan

- Inframammary incisions 3 cm long
- Subpectoral dissection of implant pocket
- Release of pectoralis major muscle inferiorly and medially
- Preservation of lateral sensory nerve pedicles
- Placement of round smooth-surface saline implants

Markings and Technique

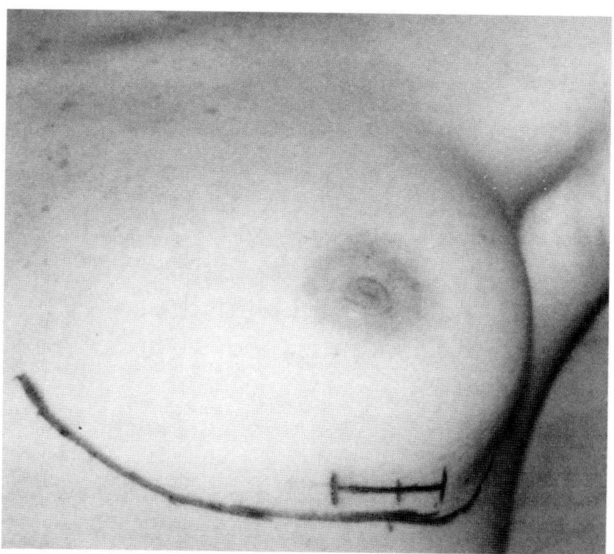

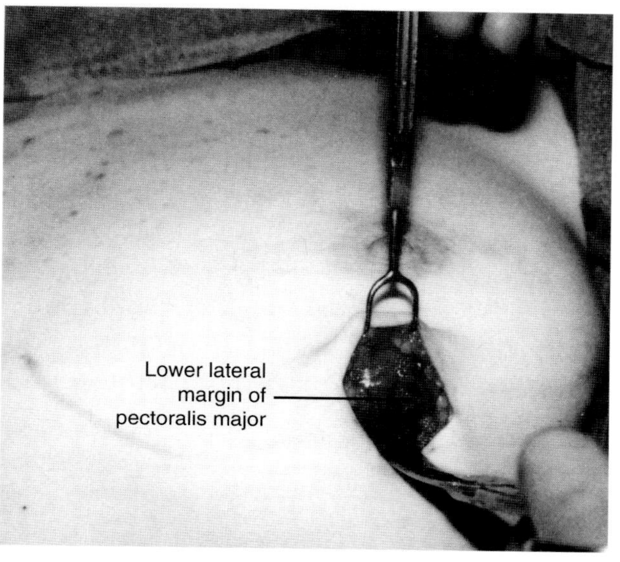

The position of the inframammary fold incisions is usually marked in or slightly above the crease. When the crease is positioned normally, the incision is placed in the crease. When the crease needs to be lowered, I determine how much and mark the inframammary fold incision accordingly. ***I believe it is better to have the scar a bit above the inframammary fold than below since it is less likely to be visible when the patient is upright or wearing bathing attire.*** Care is taken to ensure that these incisions are symmetrically placed. They should be 4 to 5 cm long, depending on the implant size, beginning in the nipple line and extending laterally. ***When the incisions are placed too far medially, they are visible when the women is supine, and there is a greater chance that they will heal with a hypertrophic scar. The incisions, however, should not extend laterally or they will be noticeable from the side when the woman is standing.*** An incision is made and deepened around the lower pole of the breast up to the lower margin of the pectoralis major muscle.

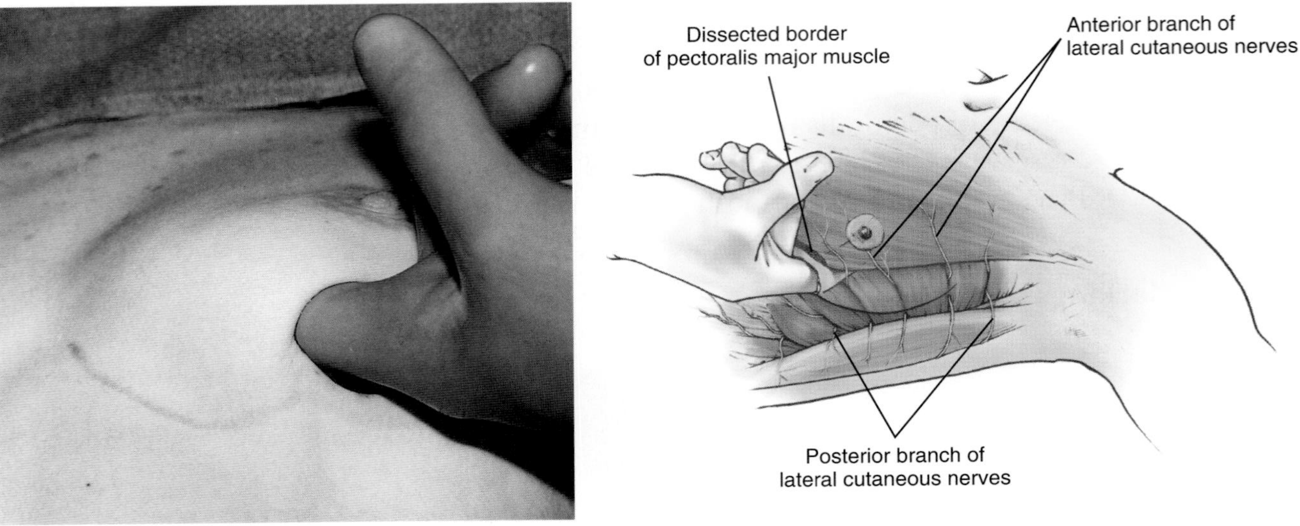

Blunt dissection is used to elevate the pectoralis major muscle from the chest wall and to detach it medially from the level of the nipple downward to include its lowest fibers of origin. This dissection is possible with blunt dissection; however, sharp dissection medially using the electrocautery may be necessary with a lighted retractor to improve visualization.

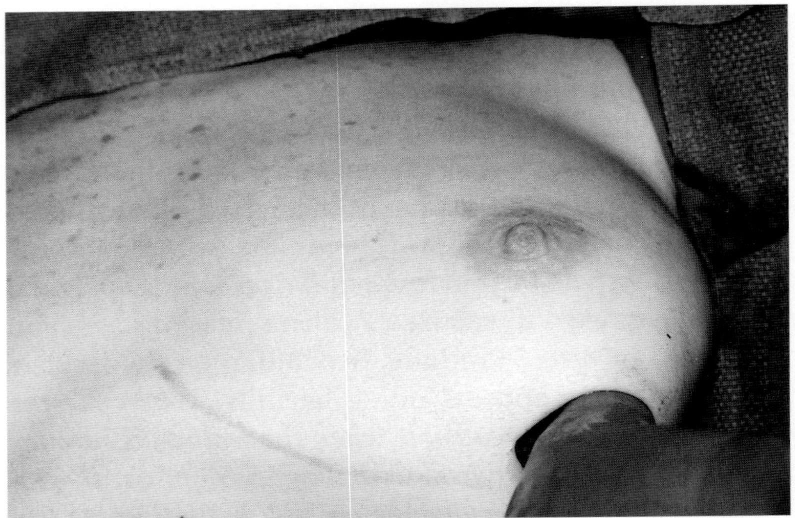

The submusculofascial dissection is then extended laterally beneath the serratus anterior fascia. ***Anterolateral neurovascular bundles are identified with the dissecting finger and are stretched but preserved.*** The dissection is carried out around them to obtain a pocket of the proper dimensions.

At this point the dissection has extended from the inframammary incision around the lower margin of the pectoralis major muscle. This muscle has been elevated and detached medially and beneath the breast to the upper limits of the preoperative markings. When the surgeon's fingers will not extend to the limits of the markings, a blunt dissector such as a Agris-Dingman axillary dissector or a large urethral sound can be used.

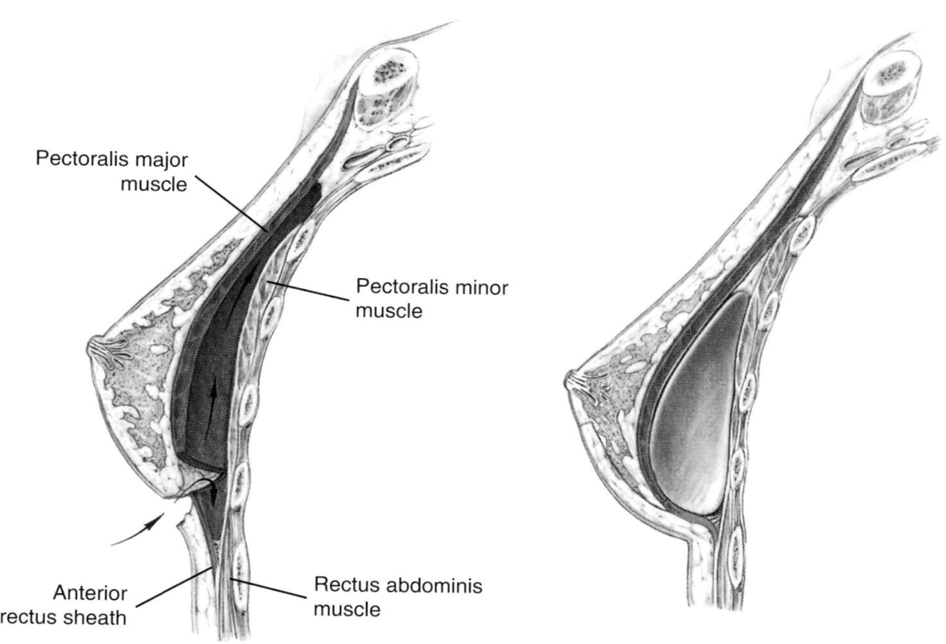

The submusculofascial dissection then proceeds from beneath the pectoralis major muscle toward the lateral limits marked for the implant pocket, usually the line between the midaxillary and anterior axillary line. Blunt finger dissection is continued over the ribs beneath the serratus anterior fascia. It also elevates some of the muscle fibers of the serratus anterior digitations along with the fascia. Blunt finger dissection in this anterolateral area readily identifies the segmental neurovascular bundles coming through the serratus anterior muscle digitations at the juncture of the medial extent of the serratus anterior muscle and the lateral pectoralis major muscle. These neurovascular bundles are freed by digital dissection above, below, and around them and extending laterally to the margins of the pocket. These nerves are resilient, and when necessary, they can be stretched to accommodate placement of a relatively large implant. ***Because the fourth intercostal neurovascular bundle contains the primary sensory innervation of the nipple-areola, its preservation is particularly important.*** If the fifth and sixth inferolateral intercostal branch nerves are divided, the patient will experience some hypesthesia below the nipple-areola area.

The lower outer dissection of the pocket lifts the serratus fascia along with the adjacent external oblique fascia. Again, blunt dissection is used to decrease bleeding and the risk of hematoma. When larger implants are used, this lower outer dissection is important to permit correct implant positioning. During the 5 to 10 minutes it takes to ensure hemostasis, the 250 cc breast implant is prepared and the breast pocket irrigated. Any bleeding usually occurs in the subcutaneous tissue or in breast tissue that has been sharply divided. No specific bleeding points usually remain and drains are not necessary. ***In view of the low incidence of hematoma, I do not use drains for breast augmentation because of the associated risk of infection.***

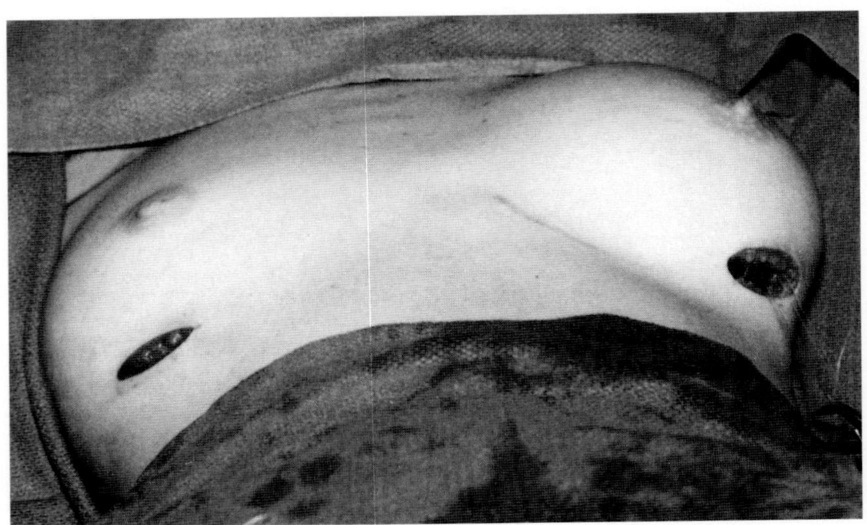

Since absolute symmetry of the dissected pockets is essential, they must be checked carefully for precise balance before placing the implant. I do this by placing the dissecting fingers of both hands in each breast pocket and comparing the pockets to the preoperative marking and to each other. Sterilized implant sizers can be helpful in determining proper implant selection. After the pockets are checked for symmetry, preplaced sutures are positioned at the depths of the incision in the deep subcutaneous tissue.

The first breast implant is inserted and positioned. The implants should be inserted while retracting the breast pocket. Avoid sharp instruments that could damage the implant. The breasts are checked for symmetry with the patient positioned upright on the operating table. ***Many postoperative difficulties and disappointments are averted if the patient's breasts and implants are positioned symmetrically before closure.*** The surgeon can be in for some disconcerting surprises if he waits to view the patient upright in the postoperative period rather than on the operating table.

If there is a problem with balance, the implant pockets can be dissected further to obtain ideal symmetry while the implants are still in place. Optimal symmetry must be achieved before wound closure. Postoperative changes cannot be relied on to improve symmetry. The breasts will not miraculously smooth out and become symmetric in the postoperative period.

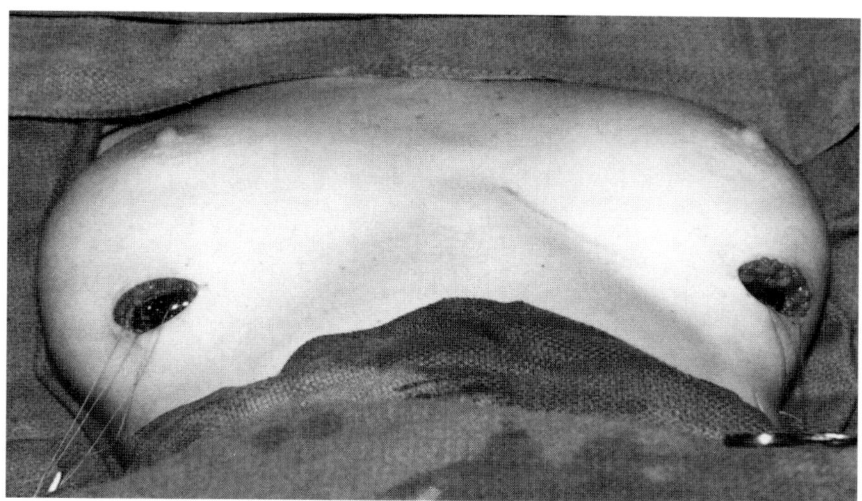

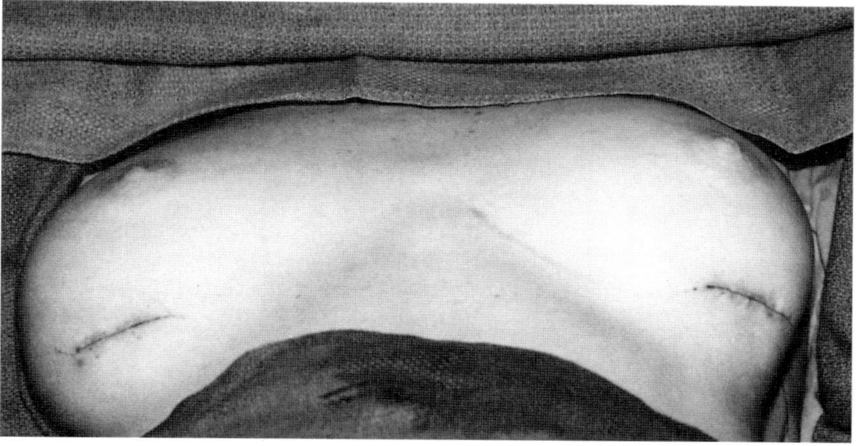

After both implants are positioned, the patient is checked for symmetry in both the upright and supine positions. The incision is then closed in three layers, the last being an intracuticular pullout suture. Steri-Strips are placed along the direction of the incisions. The patient is placed in a brassiere and gauze is positioned at the inframammary crease.

Results

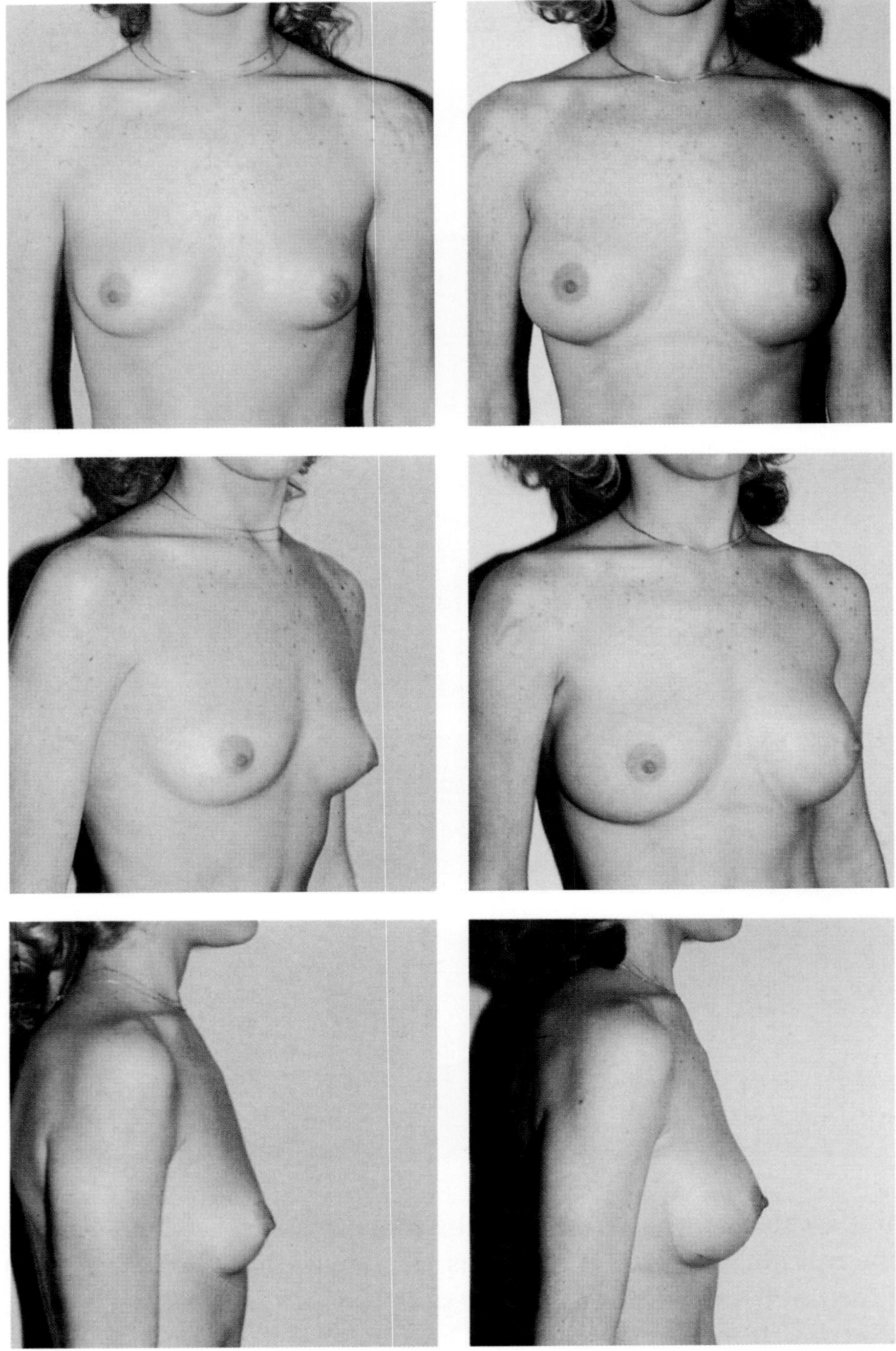

The patient is shown 6 months following breast augmentation with smooth-surface implants. She is pleased with the degree of breast enlargement, and her breasts have remained soft, even though some asymmetry is still noticeable.

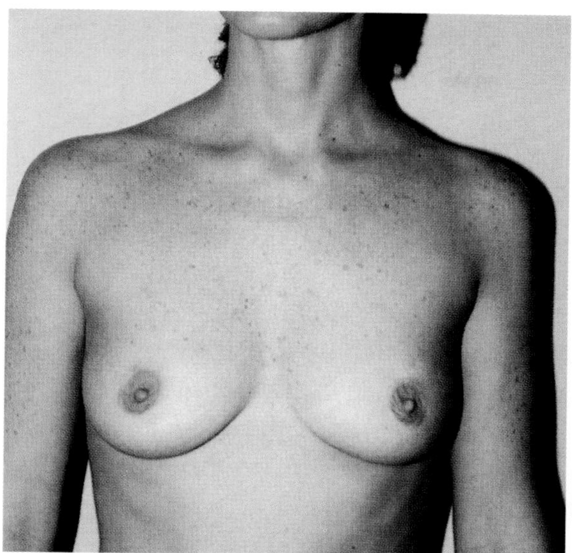

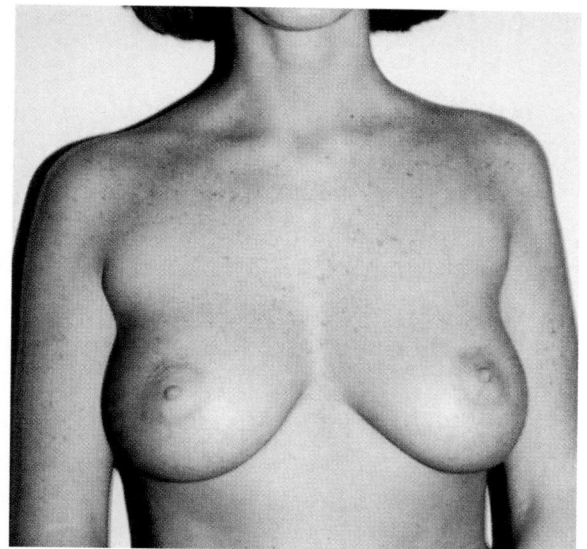

This 26-year-old woman has had one pregnancy; breast involution occurred after breast-feeding. Her breasts were quite large during lactation, and she wanted to restore this appearance. A subpectoral inframammary breast augmentation was performed using 360 cc breast implants. The patient is shown 1 year following the operation. Her breasts are soft, but the weight of the implants has caused some ptosis.

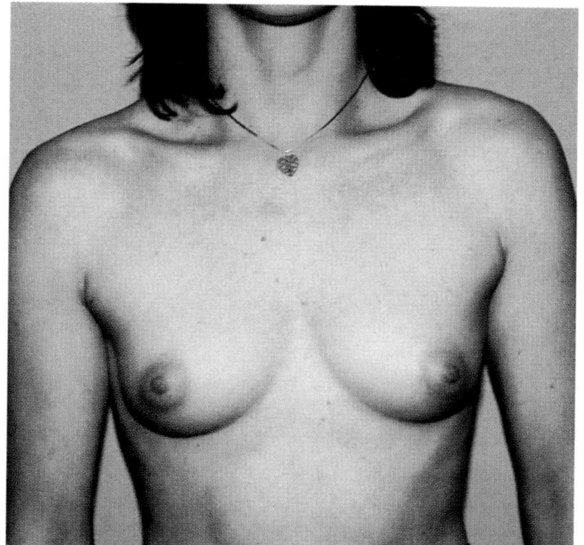

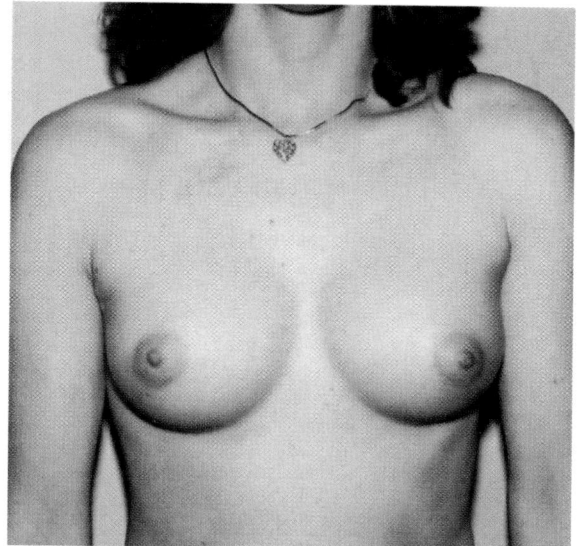

This 23-year-old patient requested moderate enlargement; 220 cc implants were placed in the submusculofascial position using an inframammary approach. She is shown 6 months following this operation. Her breasts have remained soft.

ENDOSCOPIC SUBPECTORAL INFRAMAMMARY AUGMENTATION

Advantages of the endoscopic inframammary approach are the same as those previously cited for the open approach: easy access to the subpectoral space, clear visualization, accurate lower pectoral muscle release under direct vision, and shorter incisions. With the use of endoscopic techniques, inframammary incisions can be reduced from 4 or 5 cm to 2.5 to 3.0 cm while enhancing the surgeon's visualization of the pocket. Visualization is somewhat more difficult than with the transaxillary approach in which the area to be visualized is in direct line with the endoscopic view. ***The endoscope is used primarily for division of the lower medial and inferior pectoralis major muscle origins and can also be used as an adjunct to the inframammary approach to visualize the pocket and control bleeding.***

Although our experience with endoscopic correction of the constricted breast is more limited, endoscopically guided scoring of the inferior pole combined with tissue expansion promises to be an effective approach to the correction of this deformity. Patients with severe ptosis who desire enlargement will require mastopexy through open incisions; for these women the implants can still be placed endoscopically through an inframammary incision, but the nipple will need to be repositioned using an open approach.

Surgical plan

- Inframammary incisions 3 cm long
- Subpectoral dissection of implant pockets
- Endoscopic visualization and direct division of pectoralis major fibers inferiorly and medially
- Preservation of lateral sensory nerve pedicles
- Placement of round smooth-surface saline implants

Operating Room Setup and Patient Positioning

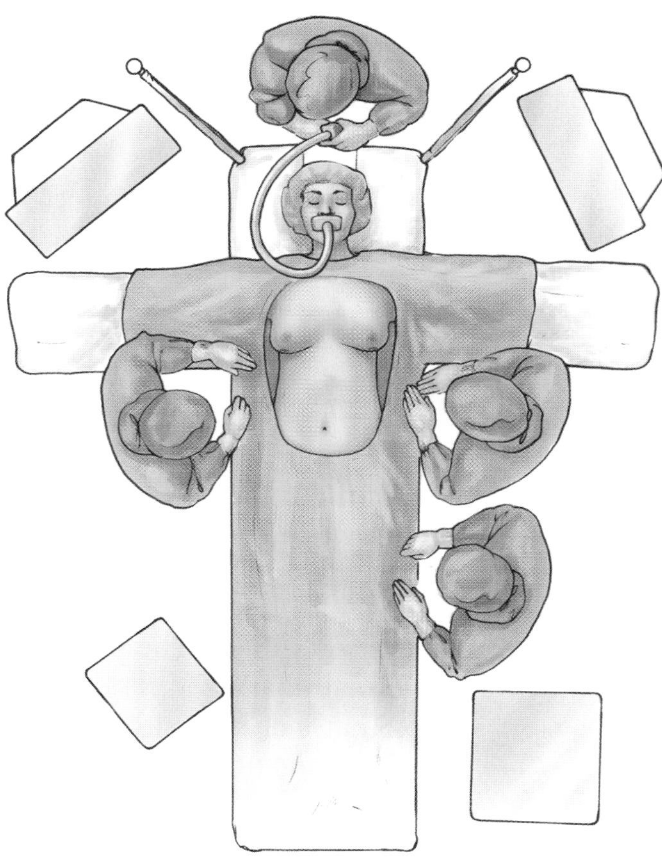

Endoscopic breast augmentation via the inframammary approach is facilitated by the use of two monitors. Alternatively, a single monitor can be moved from side to side. ***The monitor should be in the surgeon's direct line of vision and in line with the operative site.*** This means that when the surgeon is operating on the right breast the monitor should be above his left shoulder.

Markings and Technique

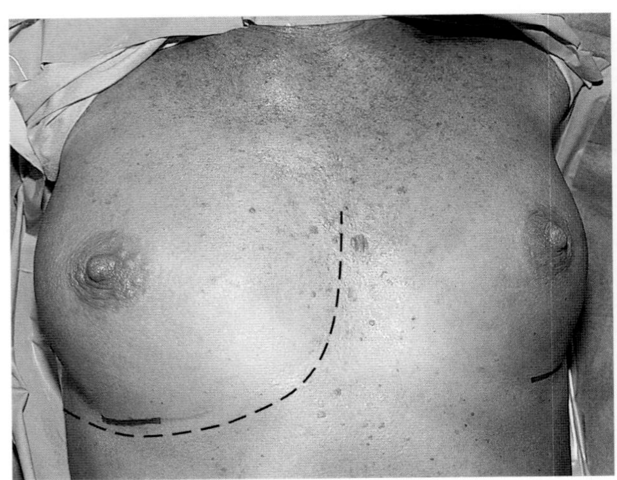

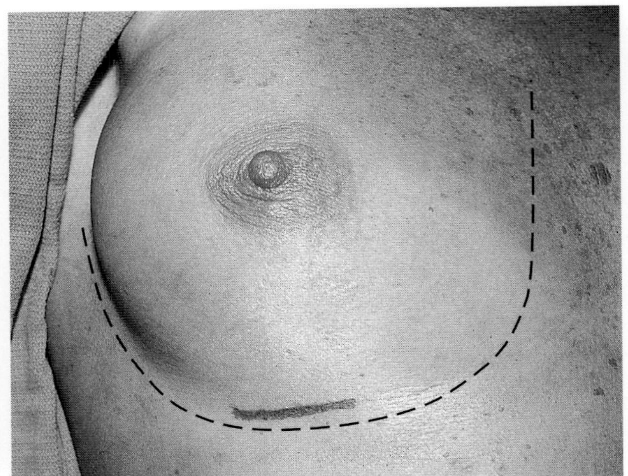

The patient is shown on the operating table after the existing and future inframammary folds were marked while she was in the upright position. Markings for breast augmentation via the inframammary approach include the pocket to be dissected both medially and laterally. The diameter of the implant is determined from this measurement. The present inframammary fold is marked and the future inframammary fold is determined. The extent of the inframammary fold approximates or is slightly longer than the radius of the breast implant. ***I prefer to begin the inframammary incision lateral to the medial areolar border in the breast line approximately 5 mm above the future inframammary fold and extend it laterally approximately 2.5 to 3.0 cm in length.***

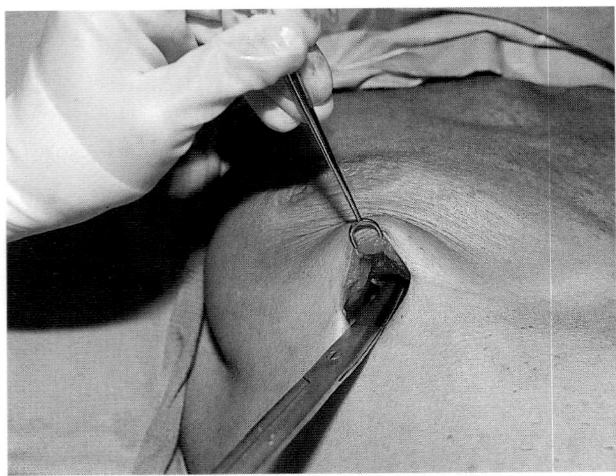

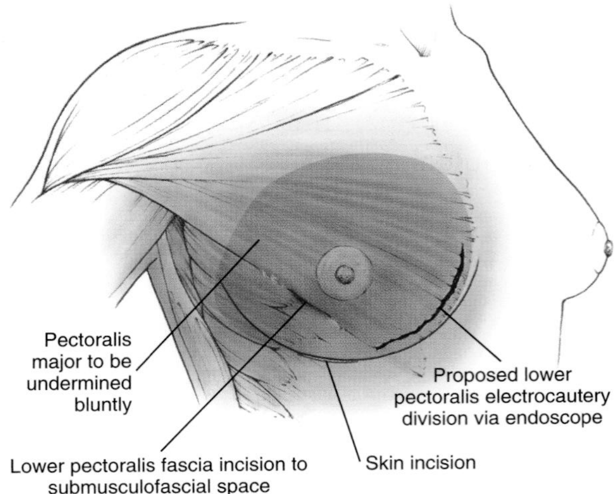

The skin incision is deepened and the dissection extends around the lower pole of the breast parenchyma and on the premuscular fascia up to the lower edge of the pectoralis major.

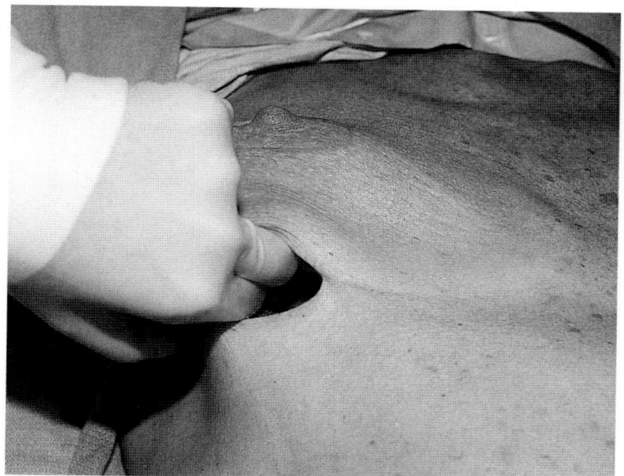

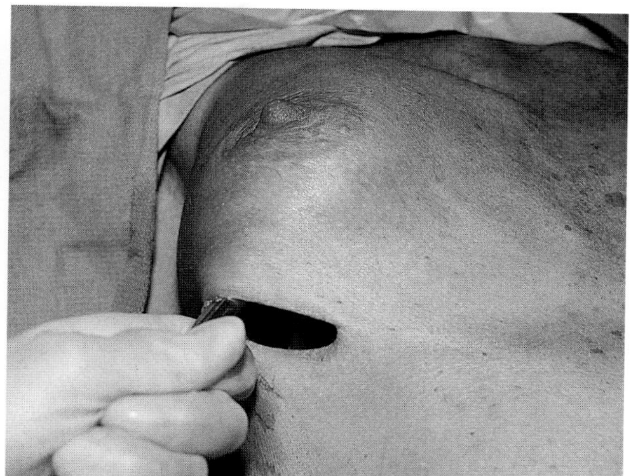

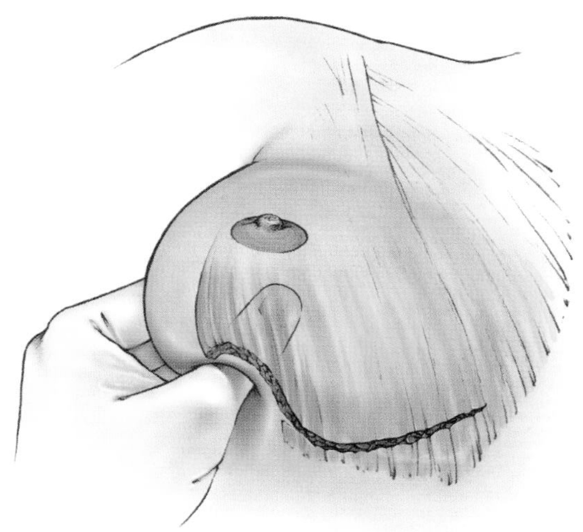

Blunt dissection is used to elevate the pectoralis major muscle from the chest wall. The lateral and superior dissections are also performed bluntly to avoid injury to the nerves in this region.

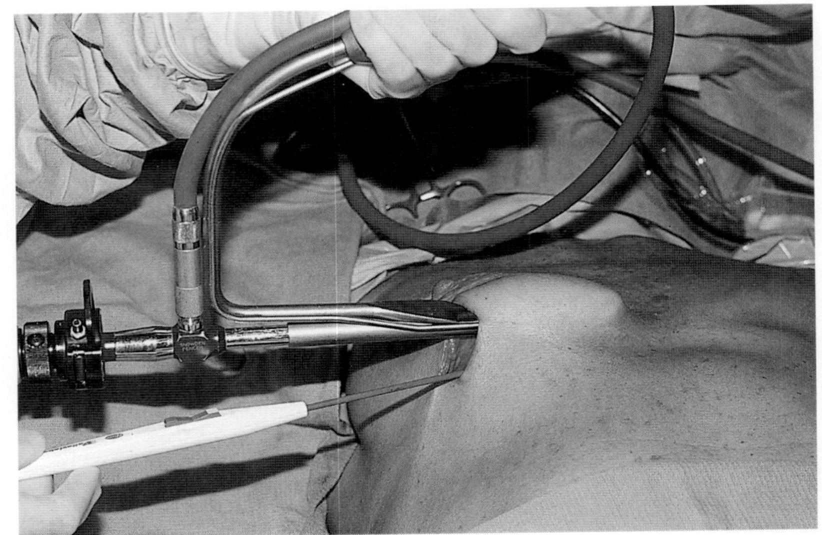

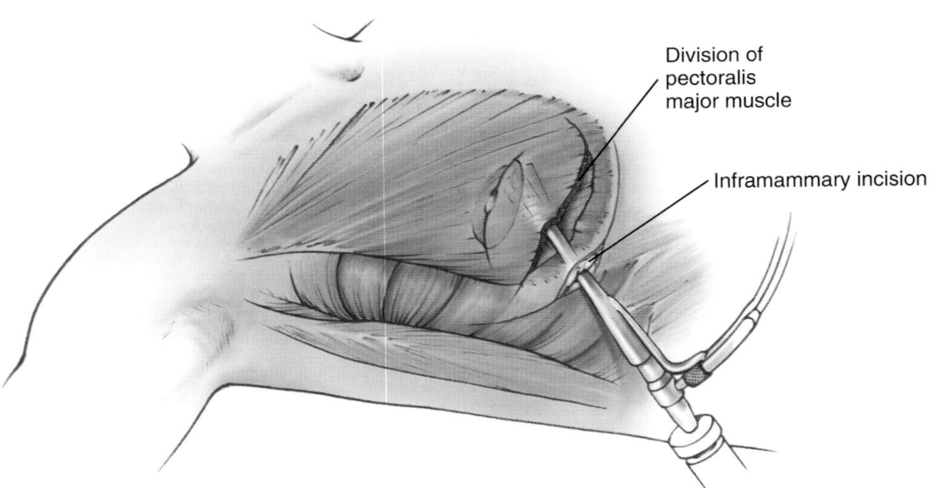

The endoscopic retractor with a 10 mm endoscope is placed through the incision to visualize the pectoral and costal origins of the pectoralis major. These muscle origins are divided with the insulated cautery 1 cm above the chest wall from the level of the nipple inferiorly and laterally; all of the lower medial origins of the pectoralis major are thus divided as described previously. The dissection extends the pocket to the proposed inframammary fold. The subpectoral pocket is then checked for hemostasis, proper dimensions, and extent of dissection. The pocket is lifted anteriorly to ensure that there will be adequate implant projection.

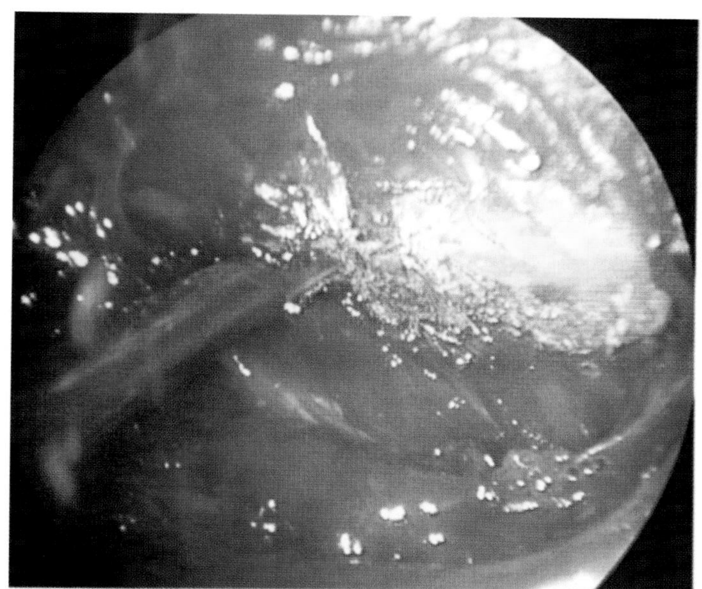

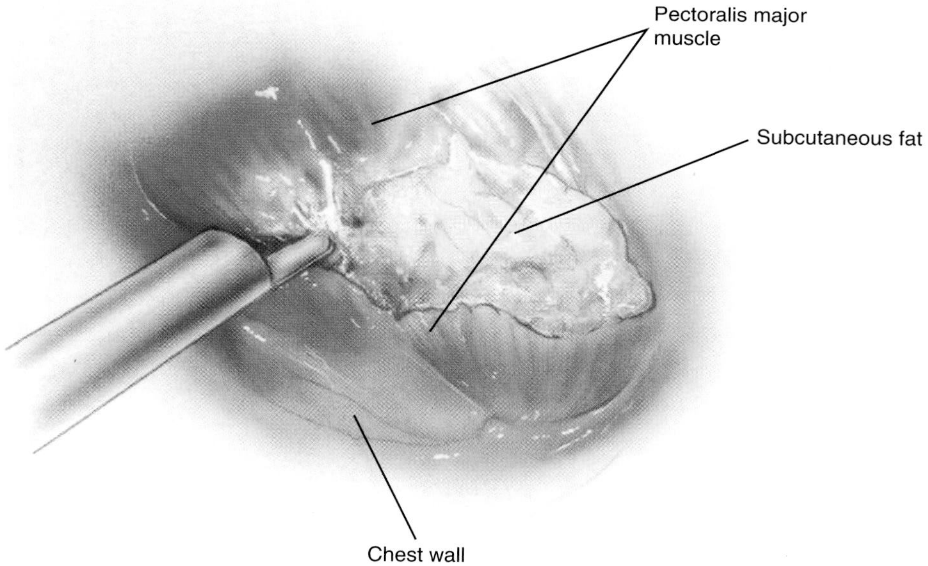
Pectoralis major muscle
Subcutaneous fat
Chest wall

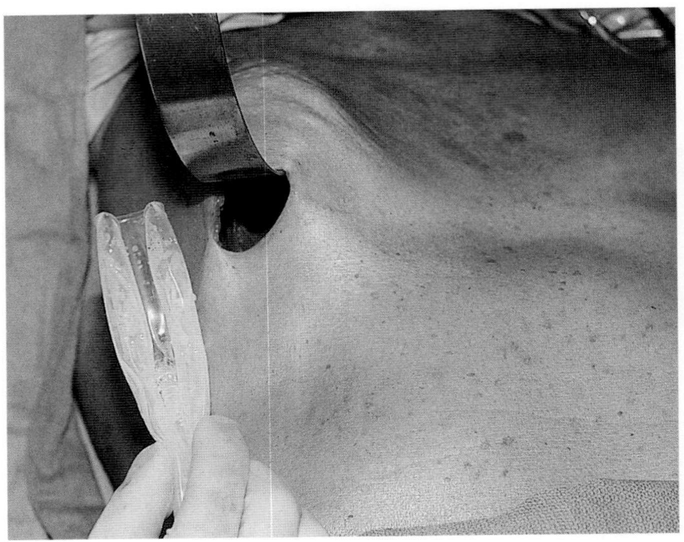

The implant is folded and positioned in the subpectoral space with the patient in the sitting position.

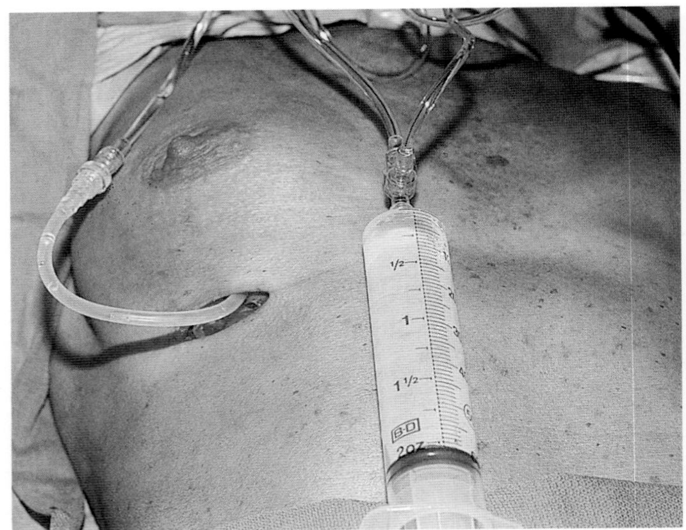

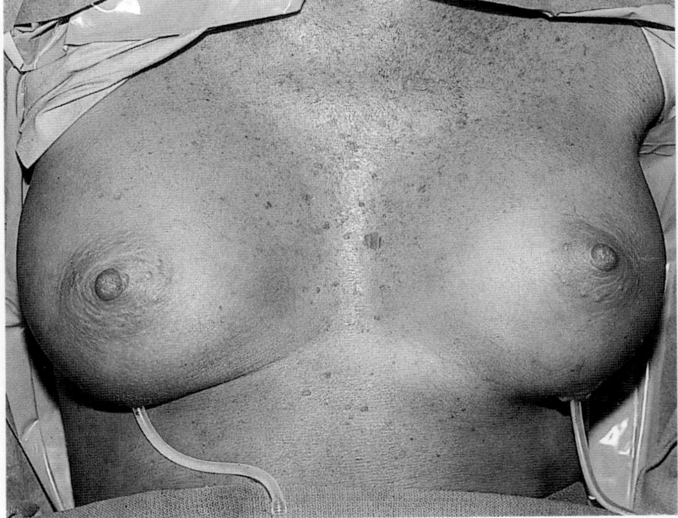

Saline solution is used for inflation to obtain the desired appearance. The patient is checked for symmetry while still in the sitting position, and any final adjustments are made in the implant pocket or implant position and volume. The incisions are closed with three continuous horizontal layers of absorbable sutures. Steri-Strips are applied to the wound.

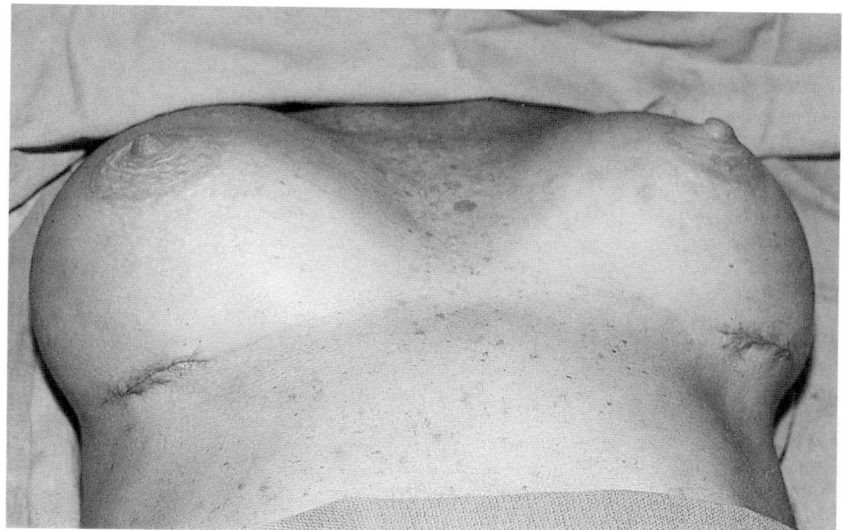

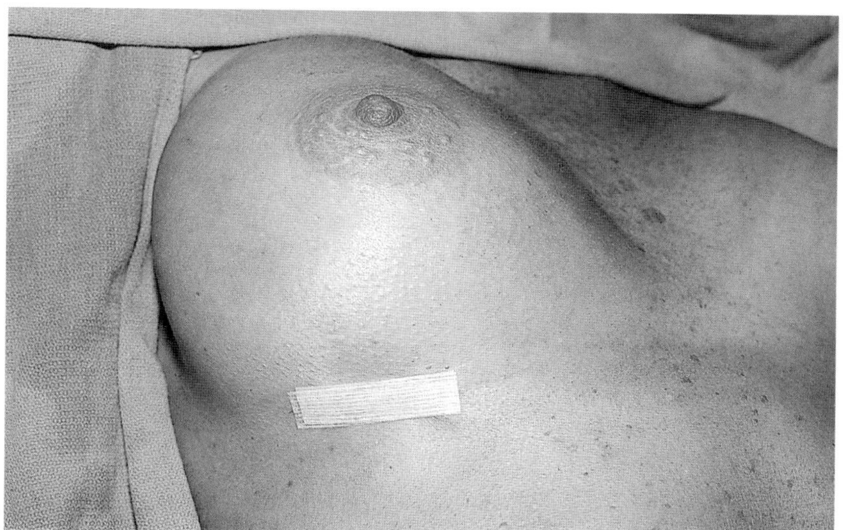

This three-layer closure gives excellent approximation of the tissue at the wound margins and provides the final layer that everts the skin. Tightening the continuous suture will shorten the incision somewhat. A Steri-Strip is placed over the incision and left in place until the first postoperative visit in 1 to 2 weeks. The patient is placed in a loose-fitting brassiere or a tube top. Since it is important that the breast implant not be elevated, I request that the patient not wear a bra so that the implant can settle to an appropriate level.

Results

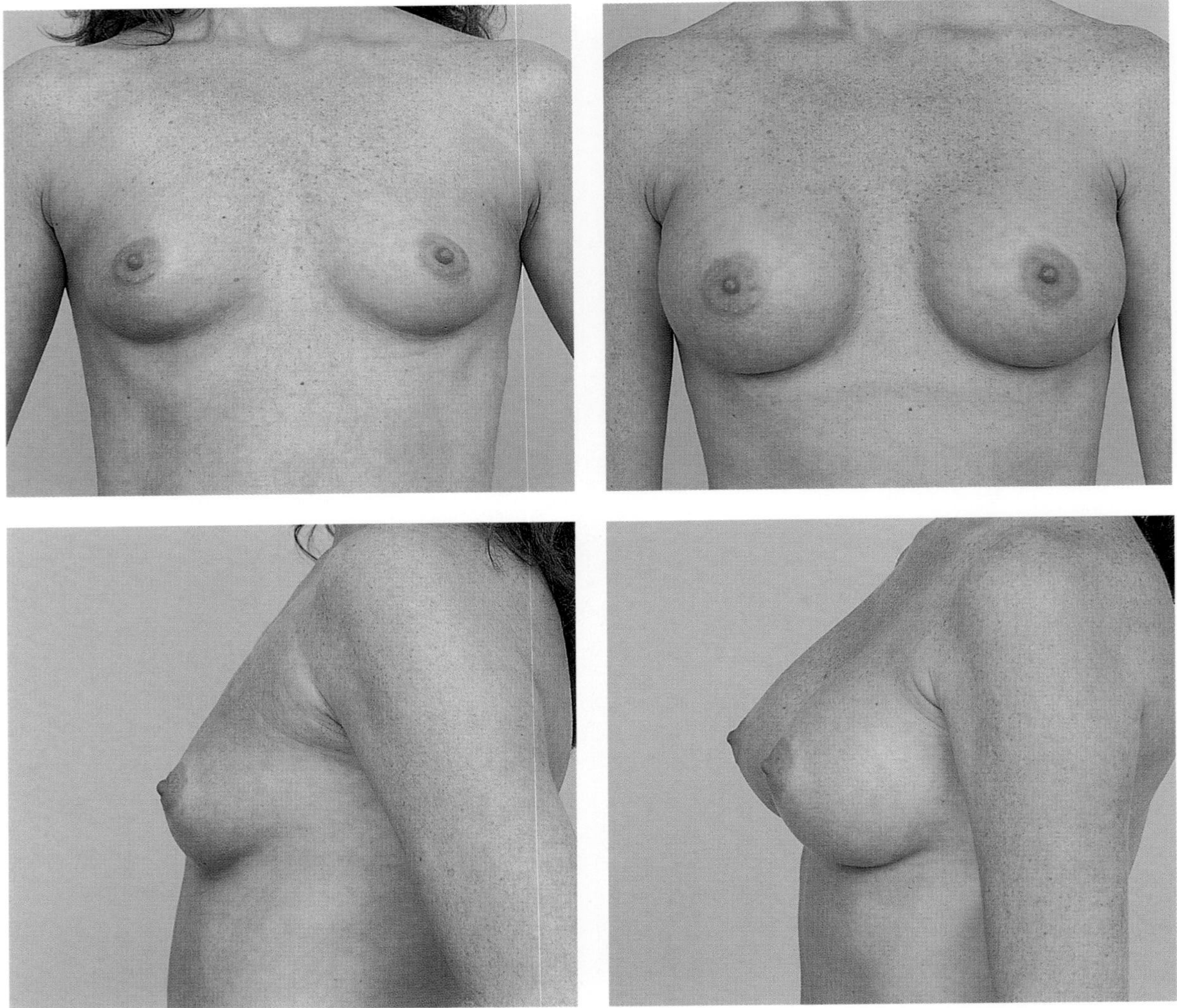

This 30-year-old woman had two children ages 6 and 3. She breast-fed them when they were infants and was pleased with the breast fullness that she noted during lactation. However, when she stopped lactating, her breasts became even smaller than they had been before her initial pregnancy. She requested breast augmentation to a size similar to when she was lactating. Physical examination revealed small, mobile breasts with no observable masses. She had a well-defined inframammary fold.

An inframammary approach was selected with subpectoral placement of 300 cc smooth-surface saline implants that were then inflated to 325 cc. Six months after the operation she was pleased with the improvement in breast size, shape and fullness. Her breasts are soft without capsular contracture and the implants are not palpable.

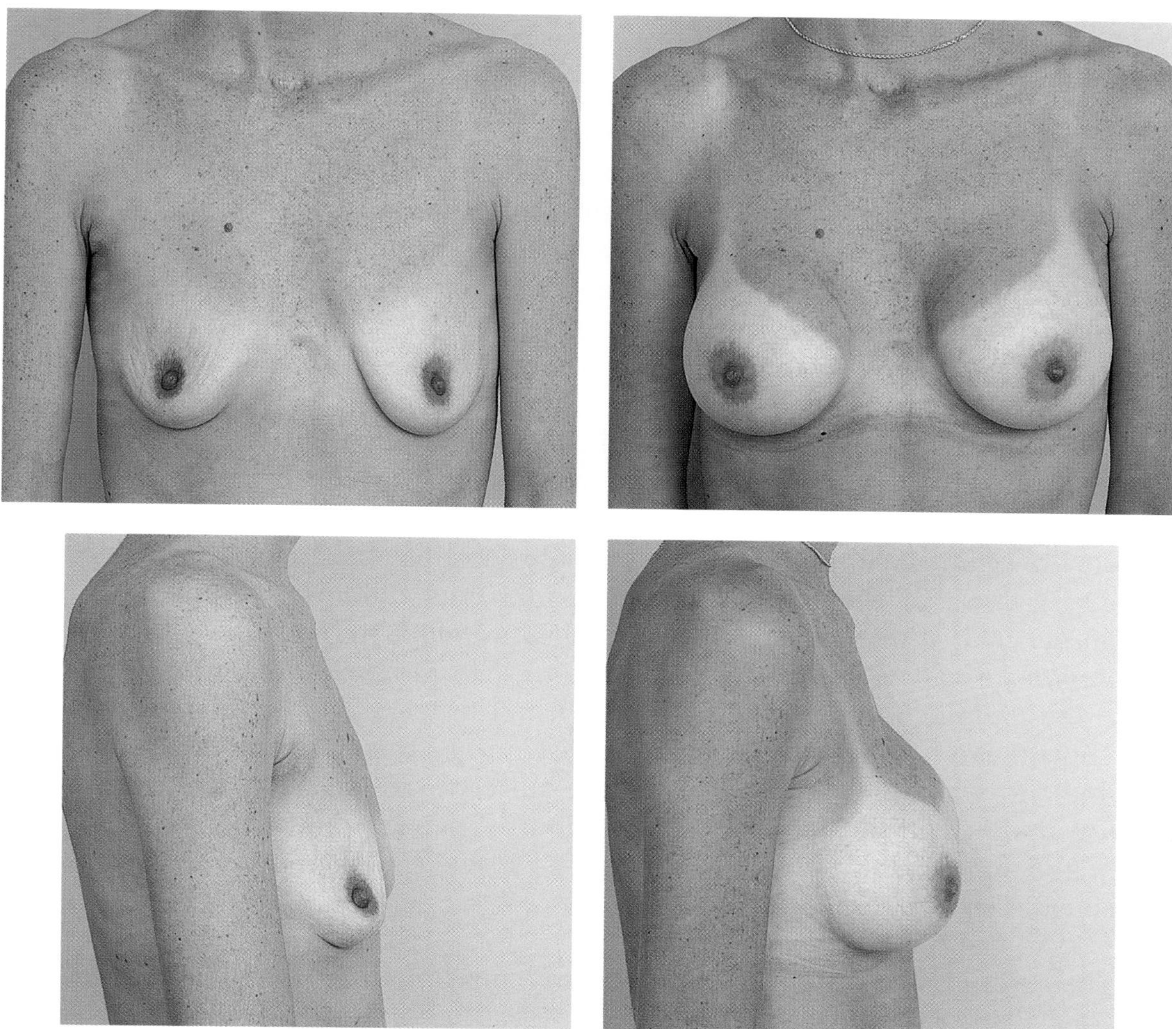

This 32-year-old woman noted a marked breast involution following each of her three pregnancies. She did not breast-feed. She had marked breast engorgement during the perinatal period and liked the size of her breasts before they became involuted and developed a ptotic appearance. She requested breast augmentation. An inframammary approach was selected and 325 cc smooth-surface saline implants were placed in subpectoral pockets. The pectoralis major muscle was released up to the level of the areola. The pectoralis major muscle release and the implants both contributed to an improved breast shape and a diminution of the ptosis. She is delighted with the improvement in the appearance of her chest and breast. Her breast implants are soft and malleable.

SUBGLANDULAR INFRAMAMMARY AUGMENTATION

Implants were placed subglandularly almost exclusively for nearly 15 years after their introduction in the 1960s. When there is satisfactory healing and good cover for the implants, the patient can expect a fine result with this approach. However, the overall capsular contracture rate has been higher for saline as well as silicone implants when they are placed in the subglandular position. The subglandular contracture rate appears to be influenced by the type of implant selected. ***Textured-surface implants perform better in the subglandular position with a lower incidence of capsular formation.*** Because these implants are somewhat firmer and have a thicker shell, it is important that sufficient tissue cover be present to minimize the possibility of palpability and rippling of the implant.

This approach is very similar to the subpectoral inframammary approach in that the incision begins at the inframammary fold, but the dissection is limited to the top of the fascia of the pectoralis major muscle; the pocket is created over the pectoralis major muscle, the serratus anterior fascia, and the upper fascia of the external oblique and rectus abdominis muscles. ***The pocket created should allow minimal implant mobility. The textured-surface implant performs better if it is incorporated in the surrounding tissue and is less mobile.*** A larger implant pocket is necessary when a smooth-surface implant is placed rather than a textured one because the smooth-surface implant, which does not adhere to the adjacent tissues, performs better if it is mobile and the pocket is kept spacious. When the implant remains soft in the subglandular position, the overall result can be natural and quite acceptable.

The subglandular approach is particularly appropriate for the woman with good tissue cover or one who desires a redraping of the breast over the implant to correct some mild ptosis. The approach is also suitable for a woman who does not want her pectoralis muscle disturbed and does not want to risk possible changes in the pectoralis major muscle.

The breast is elevated above the musculofascial layer with blunt dissection. Blunt dissection is used as much as possible to minimize bleeding. Complete hemostasis between the superficial and deep fascia is essential. In my experience, hematomas occur more frequently with subglandular augmentation than with submuscular augmentation, and I carefully check and recheck for hemostasis when using this approach.

The endoscope or fiberoptic lights and a headlight are helpful not only for visualization to check hemostasis, but also for sharp dissection as necessary with the electrocautery. ***It is also more difficult to identify the anterolateral intercostal neurovascular bundles with the subglandular approach; every effort is made to preserve them.*** Blunt finger dissection permits the best opportunity for identifying them and thereby avoiding injury to the nerves. After adequate hemostasis is ensured and symmetry is ascertained, the breast implant is inserted and symmetry checked with the patient sitting upright on the operating table.

Result

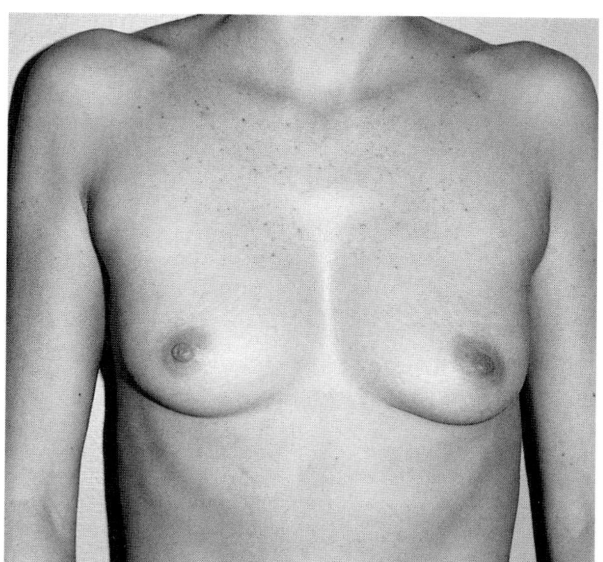

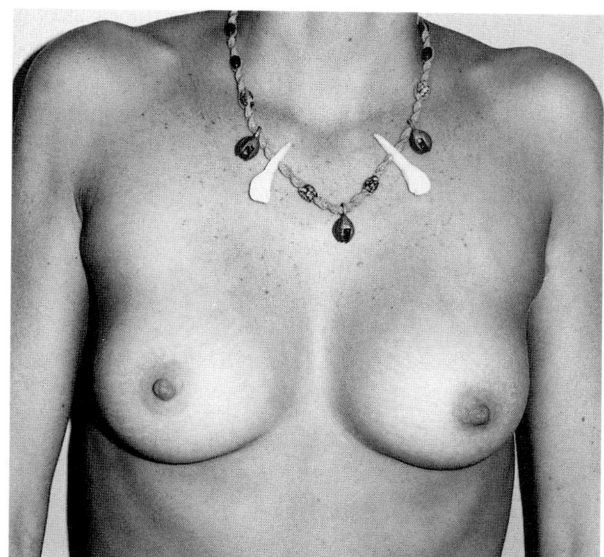

This 25-year-old patient had breast augmentation via a subglandular inframammary approach with 220 cc smooth implants. Two years later she remains satisfied with the result despite some palpable firmness of the left breast. She has refused additional procedures to improve this condition.

PERIAREOLAR APPROACH

The periareolar approach for breast augmentation places the incision directly over the area of dissection. To approach the subpectoral space the dissection can go either directly through the breast parenchyma or down toward the inframammary fold, around the lower pole of the breast, and then up to the pectoralis major muscle. Either of these routes requires some division of breast parenchyma, and most breast ducts contain bacteria, usually *Staphylococcus epidermidis,* increasing the risk of infection. I generally prefer an axillary or inframammary approach to avoid incisions through the breast parenchyma and possible infection. However, some women prefer this approach and it is helpful when adjustments of breast parenchyma must be made. The lower periareolar incision generally heals with a minimally visible scar.

The periareolar approach is particularly helpful when the areola is of moderate to large diameter. I select this approach for the patient with some breast constriction without good inframammary fold definition. It releases and widens the lower breast parenchyma, thereby widening the lower constricted breast and providing better contour when the tissue is redraped over the breast implant.

STANDARD SUBPECTORAL PERIAREOLAR AUGMENTATION

Surgical plan

- Lower periareolar incision
- Subcutaneous dissection toward inframammary fold
- Blunt division of breast parenchyma and subpectoral pocket with direct release of inferior and medial pectoralis major fibers
- Development of symmetric subpectoral pockets with lateral blunt dissection to preserve sensory pedicles
- Placement of round smooth-surface saline implants

Markings and Technique

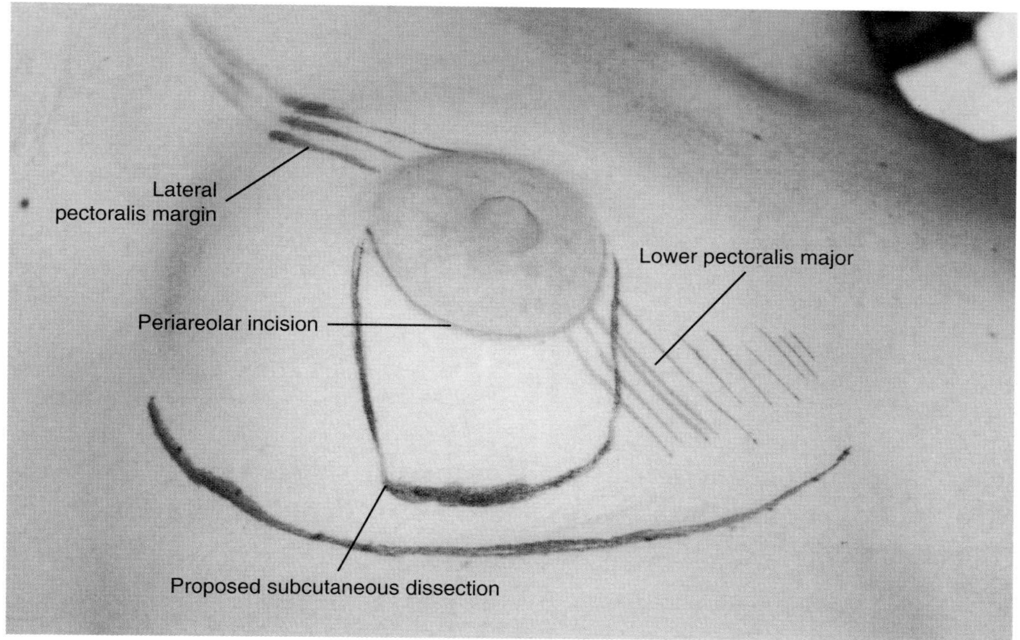

This patient has mammary hypoplasia with some involution. She has a relatively large areola of 5.5 cm diameter. ***The periareolar incision will be made at the junction of the areola with the skin along the lower margin of the areola. It is usually 3.5 to 4.0 cm long.*** When the nipple-areola has some asymmetry or needs to be repositioned, the incision can be placed elsewhere along the outer circumference of the areola and can include a crescent excision of some of the areola or the adjacent skin.

The markings also illustrate the lower lateral portion of the pectoralis major muscle and the limits of the submusculofascial dissection for the periareolar approach. A line is drawn around the lower half of the areola to mark the incision that will be made there. This approach gives adequate access for submusculofascial dissection. Although some breast tissue is invariably divided with this technique, the line of incision depicted below requires minimal parenchymal disturbance.

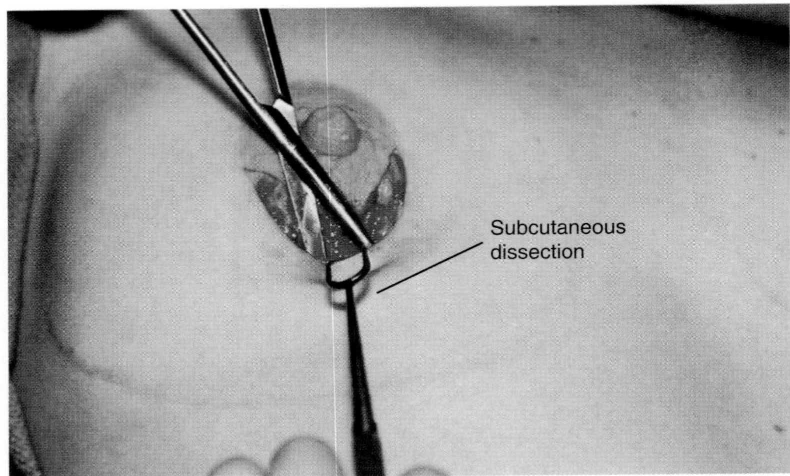

After the periareolar incision is made, superficial dissection at the level of the superficial layer of the superficial fascia is made down to the lower level of the breast.

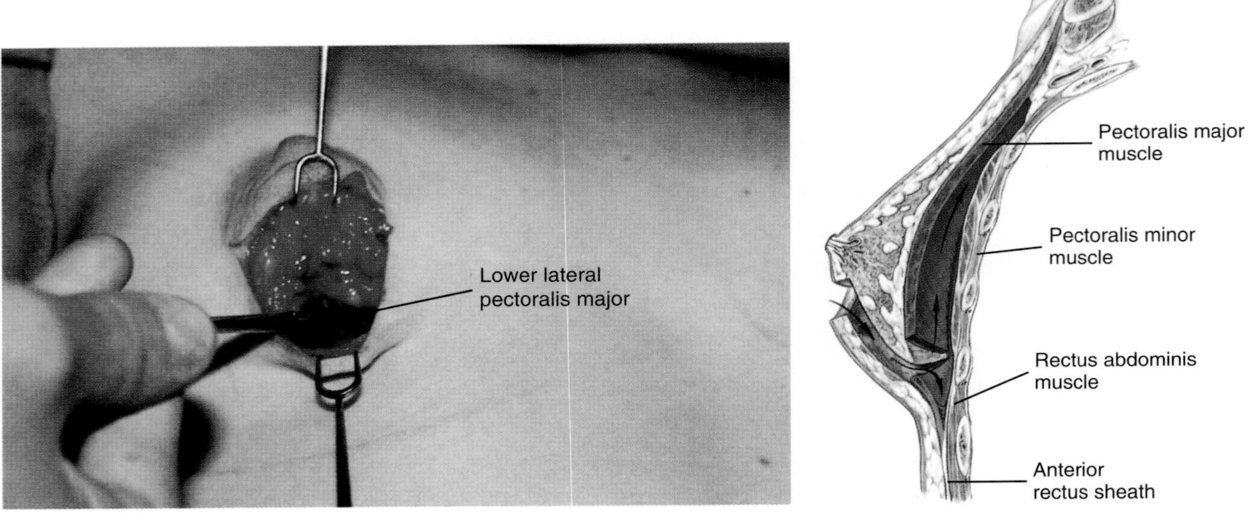

The width of the dissection must provide necessary access to make a deeper dissection. This means that it must admit two fingers. The incision is deepened around the lower pole of the breast and then upward on the deep fascia to the lower margin of the pectoralis major muscle. Lifting the breast upward "tents up" the pectoralis major muscle, and with blunt dissection the subpectoral space is entered and the pocket created. I also perform intraoperative expansion by lifting the breast and pectoralis major muscle away from the chest wall. The blunt dissection then sweeps laterally to develop the lateral pocket. When the intercostal neurovascular bundles are encountered, the dissection goes around them to preserve breast sensation.

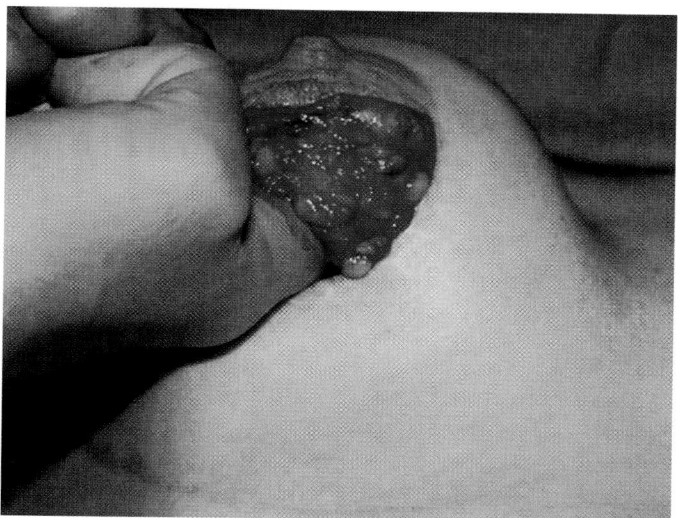

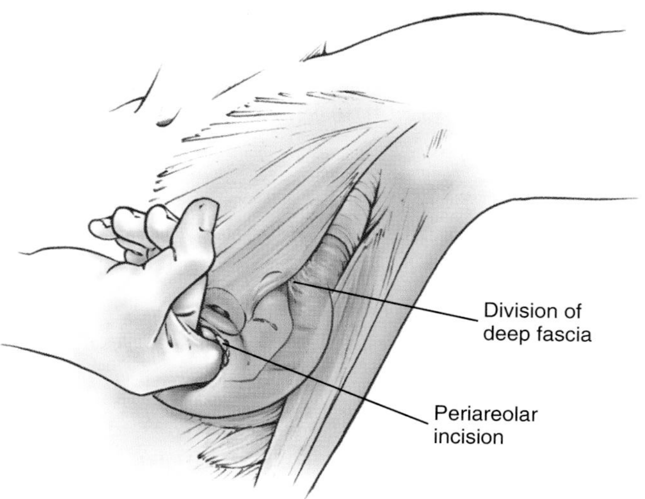

The dissection is then extended upward on the superficial layer of the deep fascia until the lower outer edge of the pectoralis major muscle is identified and its overlying deep fascia divided. The path of the dissection extends from the periareolar incision around the lower pole of the breast beneath the musculofascial level.

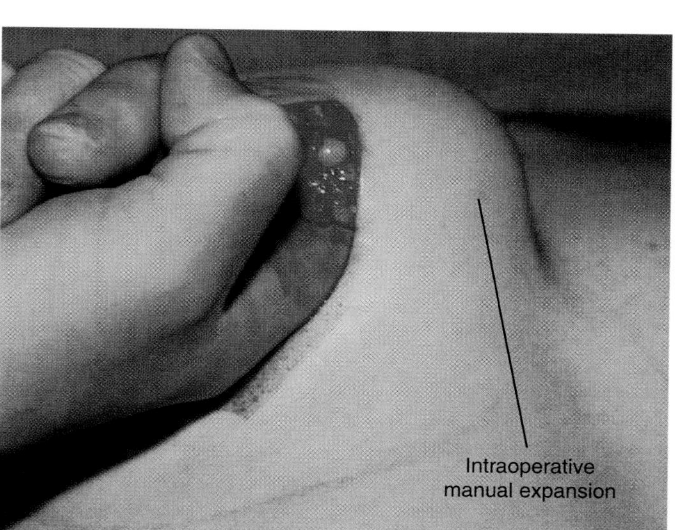

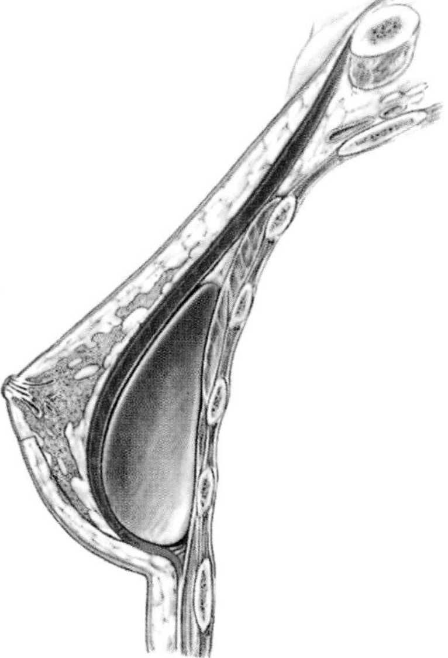

A pocket suitable for implant placement is created primarily by blunt dissection to the limits of the preoperative markings. This dissection is similar to that used for inframammary augmentation mammaplasty. It detaches the sternal origins of the pectoralis major muscle below the third intercostal space. The costal origins of the pectoralis major muscle are detached next.

When this is not possible, I use a lighted retractor and the electrocautery unit to divide these fibers; however, the endoscope enhances illumination and visualization. It is essential to perform an adequate lower dissection and to have the dissection properly defined for the proposed inframammary crease.

The pockets are checked for symmetry and hemostasis is ascertained. The lighted retractor is again helpful for visualizing specific areas that need to be released. The possibility of some bleeding from the breast parenchyma is more likely with the periareolar approach than it is with the inframammary approach. It is important to ensure that access to the pocket is sufficient for implant placement. Thus additional extension of the skin incision or additional breast dissection may be necessary. Implants are placed in the subpectoral position and checked for symmetry.

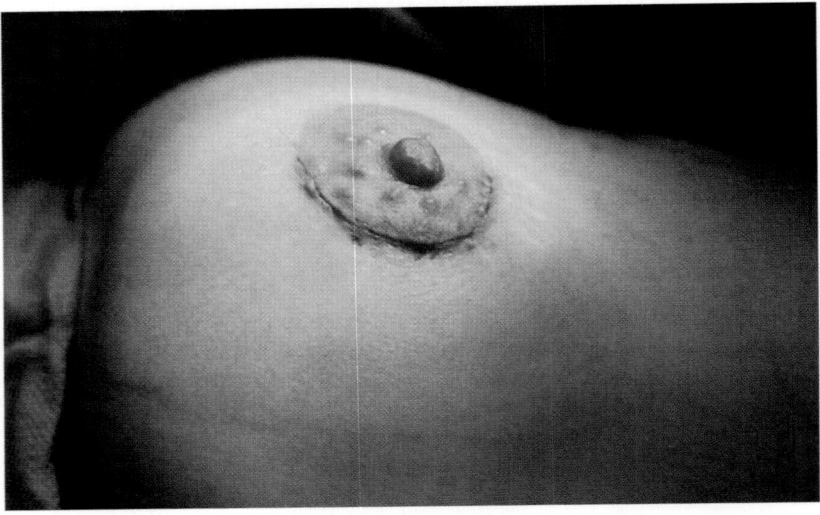

Before final closure the breasts are checked for symmetry with the patient in the upright position. ***Again, only by sitting the patient upright can the surgeon preview her appearance postoperatively and avoid asymmetries.*** The breast tissue is closed with running horizontal sutures, and the subcutaneous tissue and areolar skin layers are closed with intracuticular sutures.

Results

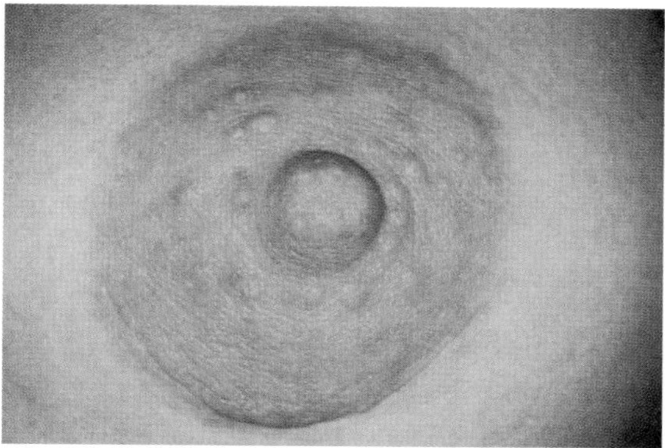

A lower periareolar scar is illustrated 1 year after augmentation mammaplasty. ***The scar placed at the junction of the areola and the breast skin has minimal visibility.*** If placed within the areola, this scar would appear light and depigmented. Incisions into the breast skin are avoided because these can become hypertrophic.

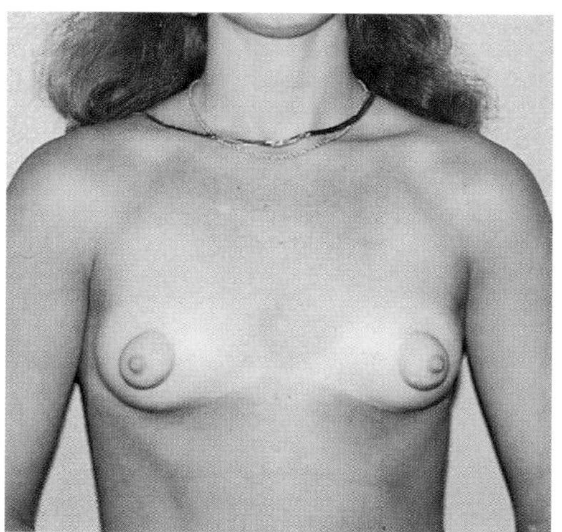

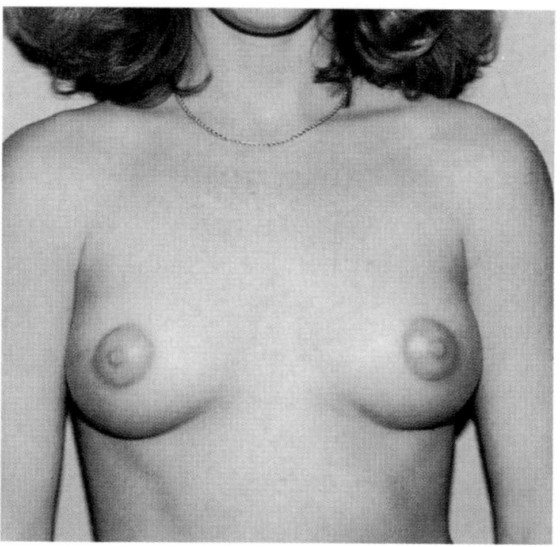

This 21-year-old patient has large areolae with some breast constriction and areolar prominence. A subpectoral periareolar breast augmentation was performed. Some tailoring of the lower breast parenchyma was necessary to reduce the areolar prominence. The inframammary crease was lowered about 2 cm by extending the subcutaneous dissection beyond the original inframammary crease. Intraoperative expansion permitted placement at the level of the new inframammary crease.

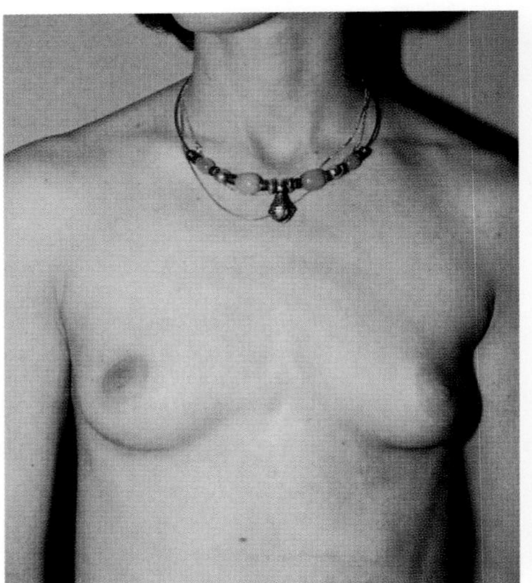

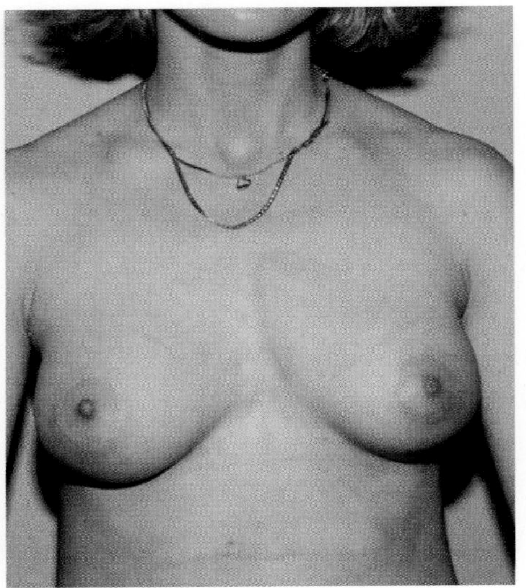

This 23-year old woman with mammary hypoplasia requested breast augmentation. Her breasts exhibited significant asymmetry, with the left breast positioned more laterally than the right. Her friend had a periareolar breast augmentation and she also wanted this approach used. A subpectoral periareolar breast augmentation was done with smooth-surface saline implants. The patient is shown 4 years following the procedure. She has mild capsular contracture on the left breast with some asymmetry.

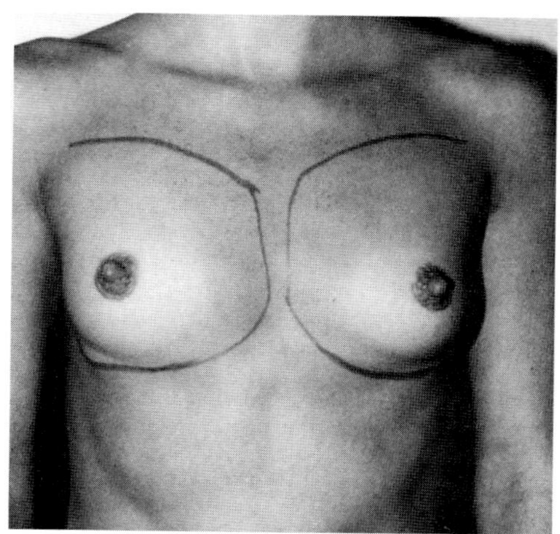
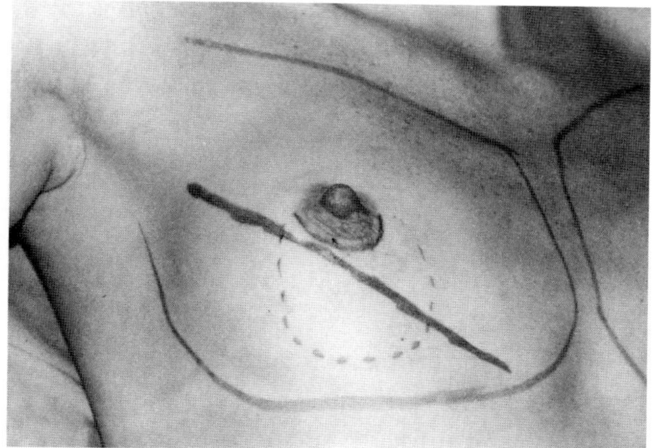

This nulliparous 22-year-old patient had size 32A breasts. She requested breast augmentation with periareolar incisions. The preoperative markings are shown. The markings, which were made while the patient was on the operating table, indicate the position of the periareolar incision, the amount of subcutaneous undermining, and the position of the lower margin of the pectoralis major muscle. The dissection proceeded from the top of the breast parenchyma to the inframammary crease and then around the inframammary crease and back up to the pectoralis major muscle. A 220 cc smooth-surface implant was positioned in the submusculofascial position.

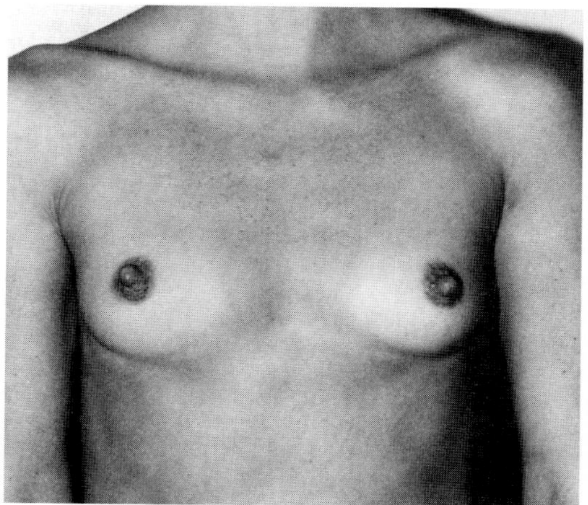
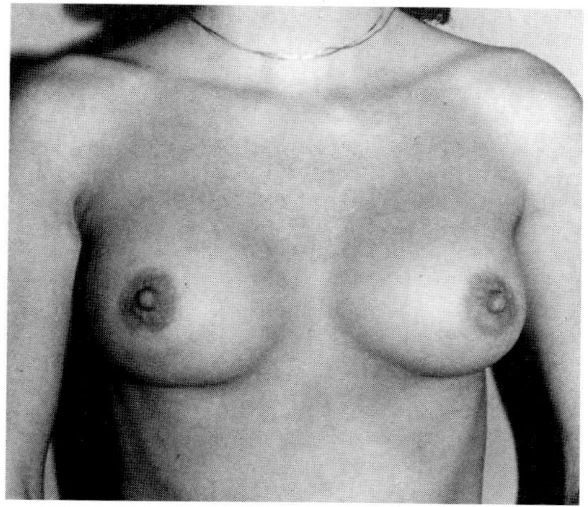

Two years following breast augmentation the scars have faded well; the preoperative asymmetry and nipple inclination, however, have been accentuated by the breast augmentation. There is some palpable breast firmness and some remaining asymmetry. Bilateral capsulotomies and placement of slightly larger implants could improve the result, but the patient is satisfied with her breast appearance and does not desire further revision.

SUBGLANDULAR PERIAREOLAR AUGMENTATION

Subglandular periareolar augmentation is usually selected for women who have mild breast ptosis and reasonably thick breast parenchyma. The breast is approached through the widened lower areolae, permitting the breast parenchyma to be draped over the implant and producing an elevated breast appearance. Rather than a total subglandular approach for implant positioning, I prefer upper subpectoral placement using a lower subglandular approach.

With this approach the superficial dissection is made toward the inframammary crease below the subdermal plexus. The breast parenchyma is retracted superiorly, and the retromammary pocket is dissected over the deep fascia. Next the implant is positioned in the submammary pocket, and the wound is closed in layers. In my experience, the rate of capsular contracture is higher when smooth-surface implants are placed in the subglandular position via a periareolar incision, possibly because of the increased potential for bacterial contamination when breast parenchyma is divided. Since I am also concerned about the performance, palpability, and rippling of textured-surface implants, I use this approach only if patients with thick skin cover request it.

Results

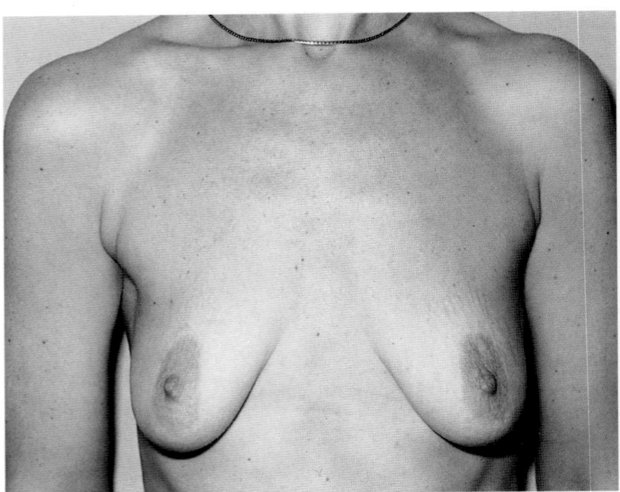

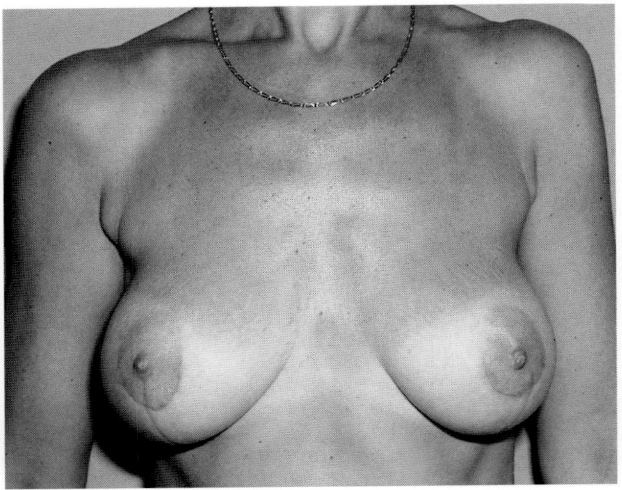

This 27-year-old woman had three previous pregnancies and breast-fed her children. She had low, mildly ptotic breasts and was most concerned about the postoperative involution and ptosis of her breasts. She inquired about breast mastopexy or breast augmentation and after initial discussions decided that breast implants were needed to meet her expectations for breast enhancement. Since her breasts were narrow, a mastopexy with a vertical excision was not indicated because it would only serve to further narrow her breasts. A periareolar approach was selected. The breasts were extensively undermined to create the subglandular pockets. Bilateral 220 cc smooth-surface implants were positioned and the breasts were redraped over them. The patient is pleased with her appearance. However, large implants would probably have given her more upper breast fill and a more satisfactory appearance. Patients with subglandular smooth-surface implants are encouraged to perform upward displacement exercises twice daily to keep the implants mobile throughout the extent of the large subglandular pockets.

Ancillary Procedures

A number of ancillary procedures can be executed at the time of breast augmentation to enhance the final result.

INTRAOPERATIVE EXPANSION

When the patient desires a volume increase greater than can be obtained at the initial procedure, I recommend several strategies to expand the pocket intraoperatively. The first option is manual intraoperative dissection, stretching, and expansion. After the breast implant pocket has been dissected in the usual manner and the lower and medial pectoral muscle fibers are divided, I place two fingers into the pocket and lift upward and outward in many areas of the pocket to stretch and expand the tissues. This maneuver usually results in a larger and less constricted pocket that will accommodate a larger breast implant. When an endoscopic procedure is used, the lower breast pocket is expanded with the large urethral or Agris-Dingman dissector elevated from the posterior aspect of the dissected pocket.

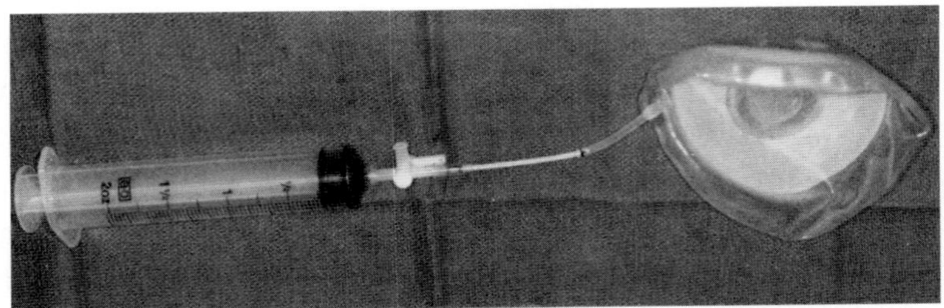

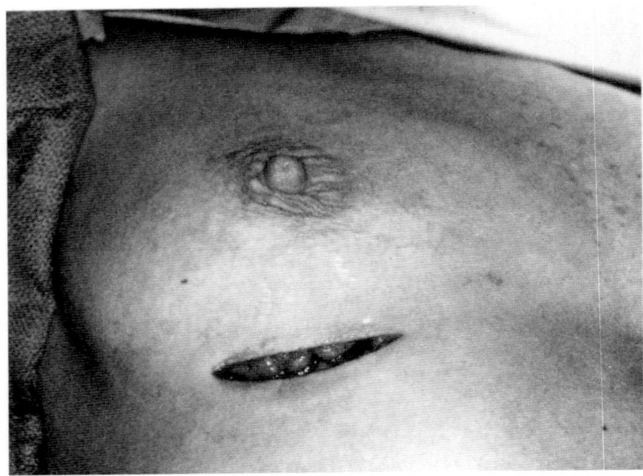

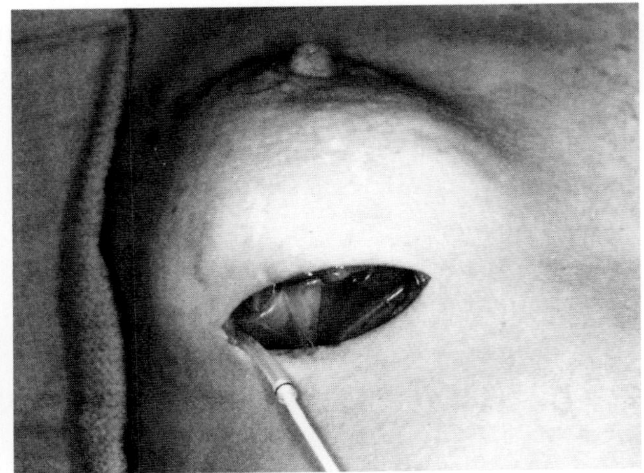

Alternatively, a tissue expander can be used. The larger device is placed in the implant pocket and inflated with air several times, gradually enlarging the pocket to accommodate a larger breast implant. Intraoperative expansion should not, however, be a substitute for creating the proper pocket initially with adequate dissection, release, and undermining.

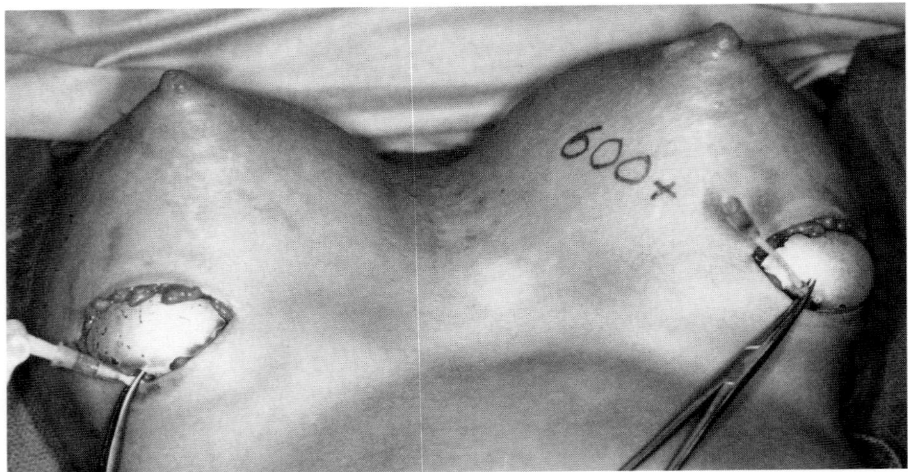

The volume injected into the tissue expander is checked; the amount that appears to be the appropriate volume to meet the patient's expectations for size is a helpful indicator in determining the appropriate size of the permanent breast implant.

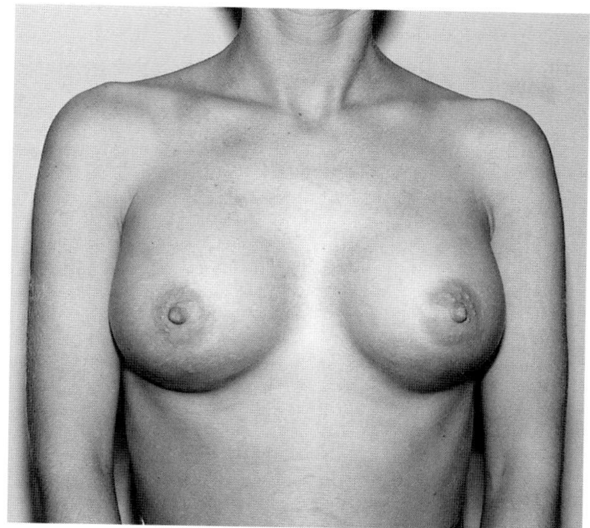

The patient is shown 6 months later; she was delighted with the significant enlargement of her breasts that was achieved with intraoperative expansion followed by placement of permanent implants. Although the expander is helpful, I have also found that the release of the pectoral muscle both inferiorly and medially combined with manual intraoperative expansion can stretch the breast and permit placement of satisfactorily large implants.

BREAST AUGMENTATION WITH LIPOSUCTION OF THE ABDOMEN OR ABDOMINOPLASTY

Some women request augmentation mammaplasty at the time of abdominal liposuction or an abdominoplasty. With the development of liposuction, fewer patients are having traditional abdominoplasty. The breast implant can be placed into the pocket from the abdominoplasty incision without leaving a breast scar. I have found that this strategy requires more upper abdominal dissection than I usually need for abdominoplasty. It is also more difficult to access the subpectoral region and to obtain symmetry. I usually advise these women to have breast augmentation through a more traditional incision if they already have a major abdominal incision. Transumbilical breast augmentation requires introduction of a smooth-surface implant through a tube in the umbilicus to the subglandular pocket. Although I have little experience with this technique, I believe more accurate subglandular dissection is possible through more established incisions, which can be reduced if the endoscope is used. However, I prefer the subpectoral implant position and transumbilical breast augmentation is not a satisfactory approach when this implant position is selected.

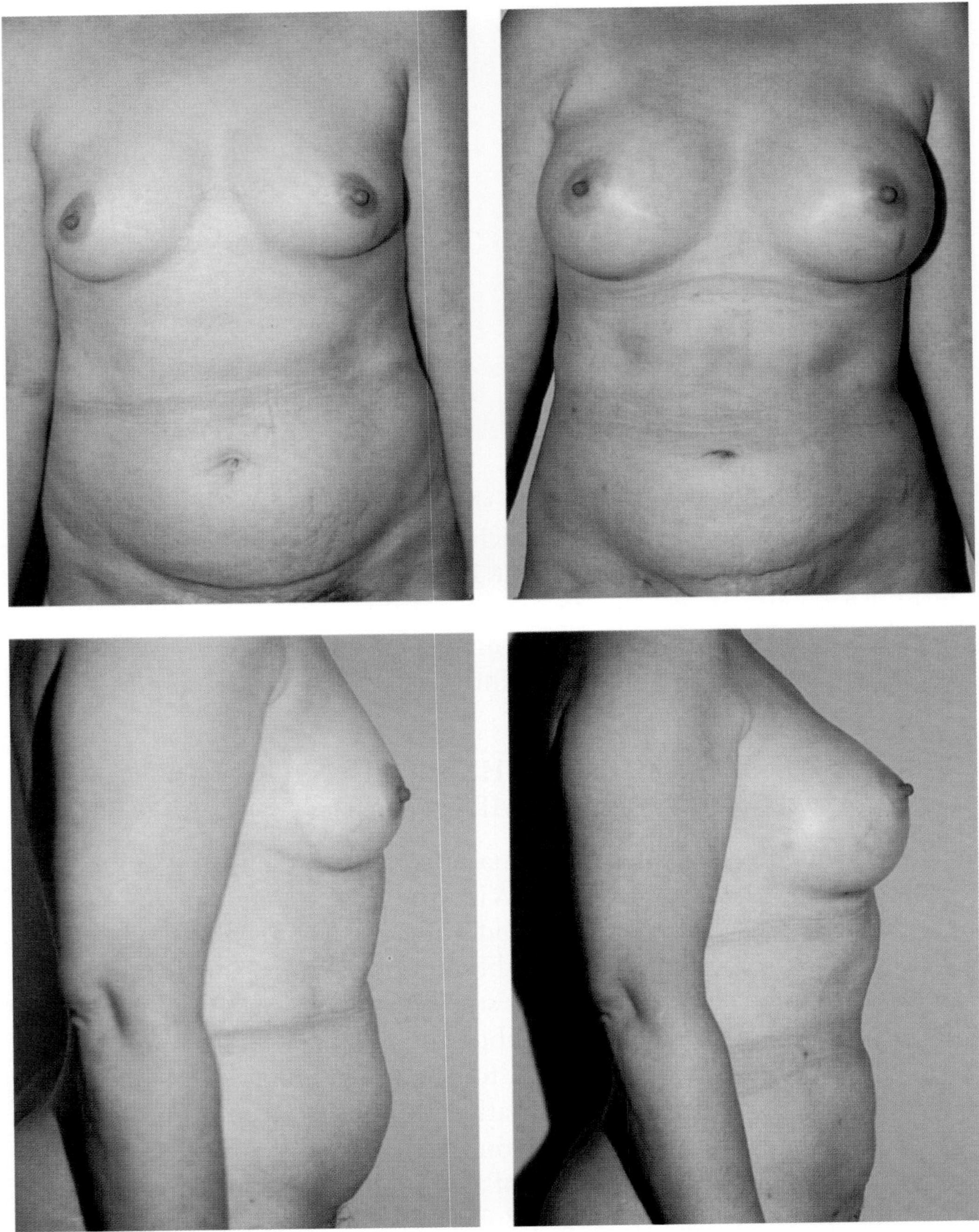

This patient is shown 3 months postoperatively. She underwent abdominoplasty at the time of endoscopic inframammary augmentation. The patient had requested larger breasts to match her wide chest dimensions. Postoperative morbidity was minimal and the patient is pleased with the projection and symmetry of her breasts.

BIOPSIES OF THE BREAST

Some women who request breast augmentation have breast masses. Since the incidence of breast cancer among young women is increasing, it is important for the aesthetic breast surgeon to have the best possible preoperative evaluation. ***All breast augmentation patients should undergo preoperative breast imaging if they are 30 years old and earlier if they are at high risk for developing breast cancer or if they have a dominant mass.*** An accurate diagnosis and consultation with a general surgeon are in order when there is a suspicious breast mass. When the mass seems to be a cyst and the woman has considerable cyclic changes, aspiration is diagnostic if the mass disappears completely when the cyst is drained. Fine-needle aspiration cytology is only helpful when positive for breast cancer; when there is a high probability of breast cancer, I prefer for the patient to be evaluated by a general surgeon. The aesthetic breast surgeon must always be vigilant not to do anything that can obscure, delay, or complicate the diagnosis or treatment of a breast cancer.

At other times some breast thickening will require a biopsy; if the mass is benign, the augmentation mammaplasty can be planned to coincide with the biopsy. With minimally invasive biopsies and modern imaging techniques, the diagnosis can usually be made without an open biopsy. I try to plan the biopsy incision to accommodate the implant placement when the mass is in the region of the axilla or periareolar region or near the inframammary fold. It is safest to perform the biopsy first and get a pathologist's evaluation of a frozen section of the specimen before entering additional deeper planes.

It is inappropriate, unnecessary, and ethically wrong to perform routine breast biopsies during augmentation mammaplasty.

FAT INJECTIONS: A CAUTIONARY NOTE

In my opinion fat should not be injected into the breasts. Although free fat usually reabsorbs, it can calcify and form nodules within the breast, potentially obscuring, confusing, or delaying the diagnosis of a breast cancer. Warnings have been issued against the use of free fat injections for management of small breasts by the American Society of Plastic and Reconstructive Surgeons.

Postoperative Considerations

The patient's incisions and breasts are checked periodically during the first hours after the operation for indications of a developing hematoma. Broad-spectrum antibiotics are given intravenously before the incision is made and an antistaphylococcal and antistreptococcal broad-spectrum antibiotic (usually cephalothin, 500 mg qid) is prescribed postoperatively to be continued for 2 days after the operation.

Ordinarily the patient is placed in a soft elastic brassiere after the operation. When the implants appear higher than desired, an elastic bandage such as an Ace bandage is placed circumferentially about the upper portions of the breast. This support is also used after axillary augmentation to prevent upward displacement of the breast implants. When the implants are low, a brassiere is worn at all times for implant elevation and obliteration of the lower extent of the pocket.

At the first postoperative visit after placement of smooth-surface implants I instruct the patient in a regimen in which she massages the implants gently throughout the extent of the pocket for several minutes three or four times a day. This movement enables the pocket to remain as large as possible, encourages a softer result, and reeducates the breasts to touch after the operation. Massage is especially helpful when there is hypesthesia and paresthesia, which can accompany the return of sensation and are often associated with actual "shooting sensations" throughout the area of nerve compromise. Massaging the breast decreases sensitivity, permitting the breasts to be touched more comfortably and with less anxiety by both the patient and significant others.

Steri-Strips are placed linearly in the direction of the incisions and are replaced periodically for about 2 months postoperatively. The pressure and support from the tape tends to reduce the incidence of thick, raised hypertrophic scars and also resists separation and widening of the supports and incisions. If there is a tendency to hypertrophic scars, I suggest that the patient use the tapes for several more months.

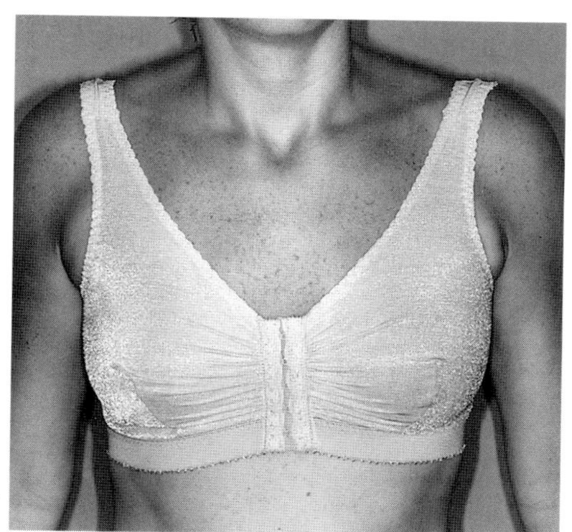

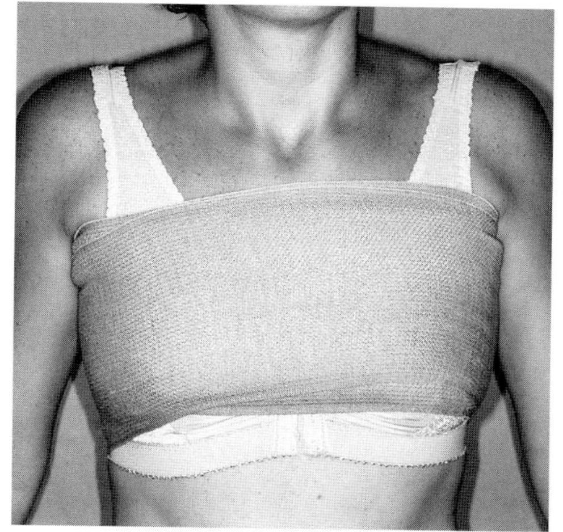

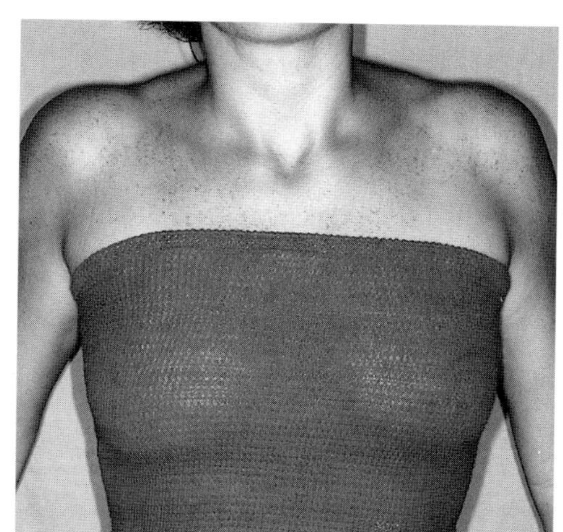

Capsular Contracture

Capsular contracture is the most common problem encountered after augmentation mammaplasty with breast implants. The spectrum of postoperative results ranges from breasts that look and feel normal to those that exhibit different degrees of unilateral or bilateral capsular contracture resulting in varying degrees of asymmetry, distortion, firmness, and discomfort.

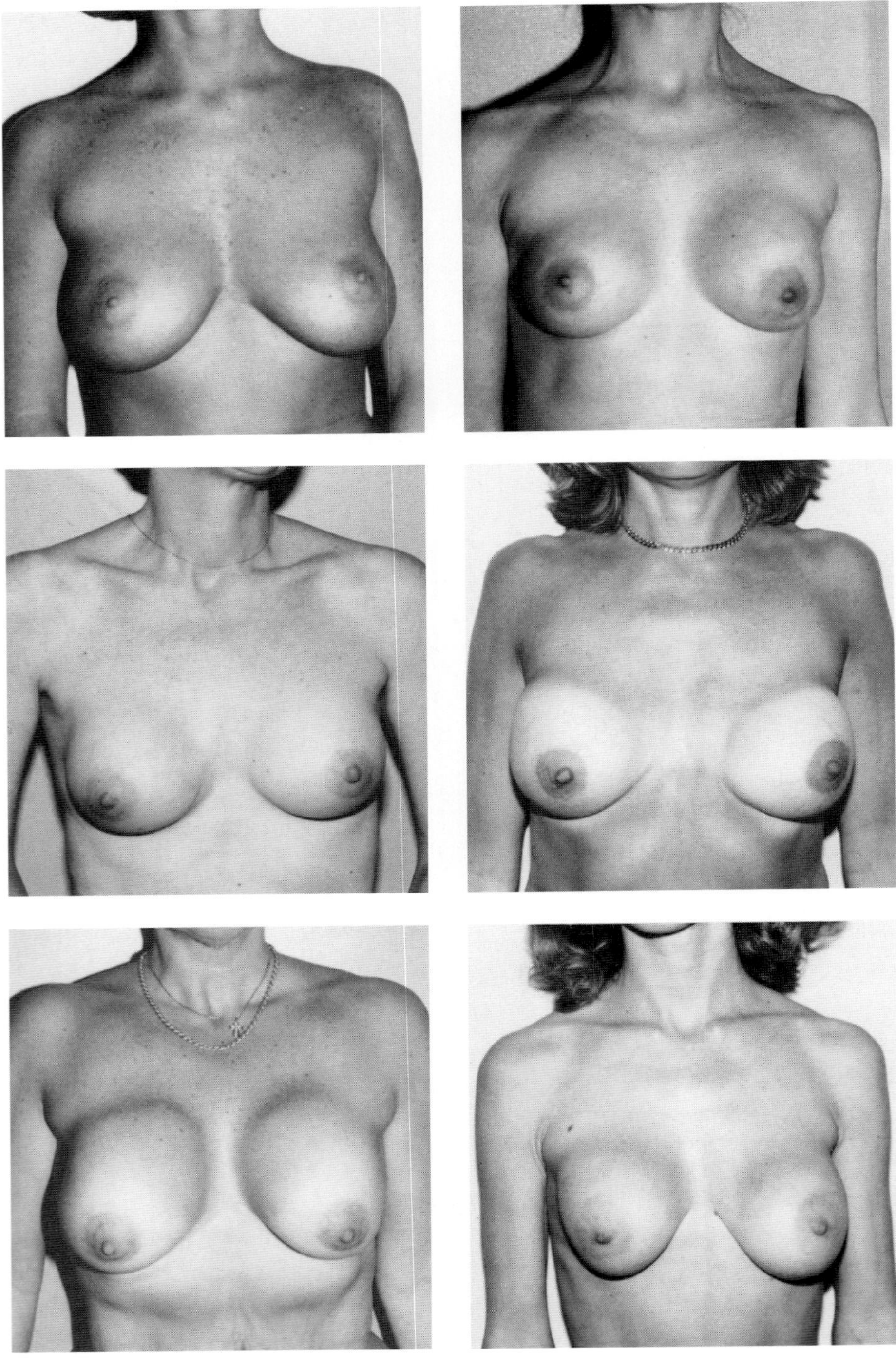

PREVENTION

A number of intraoperative and postoperative factors may be linked to capsular contracture and will be briefly discussed here. Unfortunately no well-controlled studies are available to scientifically document the specific cause or prevention of capsular contracture.

Type of Breast Implant (see Chapter 5)

Saline-inflatable breast implants have been reported to have a lower incidence of capsular contracture than traditional silicone gel–filled breast implants. There is less possibility of silicone bleed from the elastomer of a saline breast implant, double-lumen implant, and low-bleed implant.

Textured-surface saline breast implants are purported to reduce the potential for capsular contracture when placed in the subglandular position. Initial reports concerning textured-surface implants indicate a low incidence of capsular contracture when these implants are placed in the subglandular position in humans. Throughout the history of the use of silicone breast implants, early results have often been encouraging, but after some time the problems and incidence of capsular contracture were higher and more sobering.

Position of the Breast Implant

Most studies of smooth-surface breast implants indicate that they are more likely to remain soft and have a lower incidence of capsular contracture when placed in the subpectoral position. Continued softness of a smooth-surface implant in the subglandular position seems to be enhanced by maintaining a pocket through daily breast exercises. Textured-surface implants seem to have a lower contracture rate in the subglandular position provided that the patient has sufficient tissue cover to prevent problems of rippling and palpability. For breast imaging purposes and to ensure a lower incidence of capsular contracture, I generally prefer to place the breast implant in the subpectoral position.

Blunt Dissection

With blunt dissection there is less incidence of hematoma and less need to use the electrocautery, thereby resulting in less necrotic tissue. I also believe that the subpectoral position avoids lifting the breast parenchyma from the superficial layer of the deep fascia and opening lactiferous ducts that often contain bacteria. The subpectoral approach may also avoid devascularizing the deep surface of the breast parenchyma. These small areas of parenchyma can be the source of infection—a precursor of capsular contracture.

Avoidance of Infection

This topic is covered earlier in this chapter and also in Chapter 5.

Adequate Breast Implant Pocket

The breast implant should fit into the implant pocket without being tight and firm. Additional space is helpful for a smooth-surface implant to ensure mobility during massage and displacement exercises in the postoperative period, especially upward toward the clavicle. A pocket that is overly large, however, can permit an implant to drift outward beyond the normal confines of the breast. Since the textured-surface implants do not move as much, a "mega" pocket is not as necessary; however, an adequate pocket and intraoperative expansion can prevent early postoperative tightness.

TREATMENT

Capsular contracture is most commonly thought to be caused by infection. When a capsular contracture develops, a complete systemic evaluation is made to determine if there is a source of infection. I have had patients in whom capsular contracture developed coincidentally with paranasal sinus infection, respiratory infections, cystitis, or pharyngitis. These conditions should be diagnosed and treated before management of the capsular contracture, for it could develop again with a recurrence of the systemic infection. An appropriate course of antibiotics is prescribed in consultation with the appropriate colleague. After a capsular contracture becomes established, the prognosis for a permanently soft, normal-feeling breast is not good.

Closed Capsulotomy

Closed capsulotomy is used to reduce the breast firmness associated with capsular contracture, particularly when associated with a silicone breast implant in the subglandular position. External pressure with both hands grasping the breast can create a tear in the capsule, and the breast feels softer. After this maneuver the patient should perform daily forceful breast compression exercises to minimize the risk of capsular contracture and firmness recurring. Despite the use of massage, firmness will redevelop in most of these breasts, and another closed capsulotomy will be required.

My initial enthusiasm for the procedure has given way to a number of concerns. ***I now rarely perform closed capsulotomy. The likelihood of long-term success is small and the potential for problems is greater.*** I have noted a number of disturbing and serious problems that can be associated with this procedure. The breast capsule can tear eccentrically, thus creating an asymmetry. Sometimes only one closed capsulotomy is successful, and the breasts become asymmetric. A hematoma can develop following a closed capsulotomy, which can lead to additional firmness, pain, and distortion.

The silicone gel–filled breast implant elastomer shell can also be ruptured, causing extrusion and high-pressure injection of silicone gel into the breast or actually outside the confines of the breast. Rupture is more likely to occur with older thin-wall silicone breast implants. When an inflatable breast implant ruptures, the affected breast is soon deflated and flattened. A ruptured implant with silicone gel extrusion is serious, and if the silicone is not removed soon after the rupture, it can migrate regionally and throughout the body; it is then impossible to remove all remnants. The gel soon becomes the nidus of a siliconoma, a fibrous mass containing silicone that causes chronic inflammation. I have seen patients with silicone in the breast, upper abdomen, axilla, upper arm, and forearm and wrist after closed capsulotomy.

The aesthetic breast surgeon can also be injured performing closed capsulotomy. Injuries have often been reported to the metacarpophalangeal joints of the thumbs, a particularly painful and potentially disabling injury because it impedes the pinch mechanism.

A closed capsulotomy is not indicated for submusculofascial breast implants or for saline breast implants. Nor do I perform closed capsulotomy for capsular contracture after breast reconstructions.

When I see a patient in consultation with capsular contractures after breast augmentation by another surgeon, I do not perform a closed capsulotomy. If this procedure is ever done it should be performed by the aesthetic breast surgeon who did the initial procedure and who is prepared to exchange the implant or manage an implant rupture should a problem develop.

Open Capsulotomy

I occasionally do an open capsulotomy to improve a capsular contracture but more often to improve an asymmetry of implant position. It is most often successful when the capsular contracture is not intense, the capsule is mature, and there is an accompanying asymmetry, usually an elevation of the inframammary fold and a medially displaced breast implant. This condition is sometimes seen after axillary augmentation mammaplasty.

I generally use a smooth-surface saline implant because the skin cover is often thin and a textured-surface implant could ripple and be palpable. Of course these latter strategies require increasing degrees of operative intervention.

Capsulectomy

A capsulectomy is indicated when there is a firm, thick, or calcified capsule. The endoscope can be helpful in this situation by improving visualization of the calcified capsule. I prefer the optimal visualization provided by an inframammary incision when attempting this maneuver.

My strategy for capsular contracture and capsulectomy with a smooth-surface implant has long been subpectoral conversion if it was originally in a subglandular position or a capsulectomy to replace the smooth-surface silicone implant with a textured-surface implant. The restricted choice of breast implants makes this strategy less successful than formerly when polyurethane-covered breast implants were available. I have found that submuscular conversion is difficult and only partially successful when an established capsular contracture has compressed the pectoralis major muscle.

Most reports of calcified capsules have been associated with the older designs of smooth-surface silicone breast implants that had Dacron patches. These patches are densely adherent to the underlying pectoralis major muscle, and the capsulectomy involves some sharp and potentially bloody dissection.

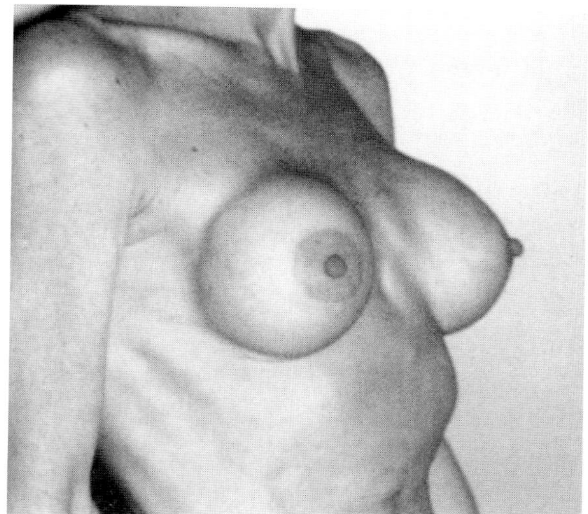

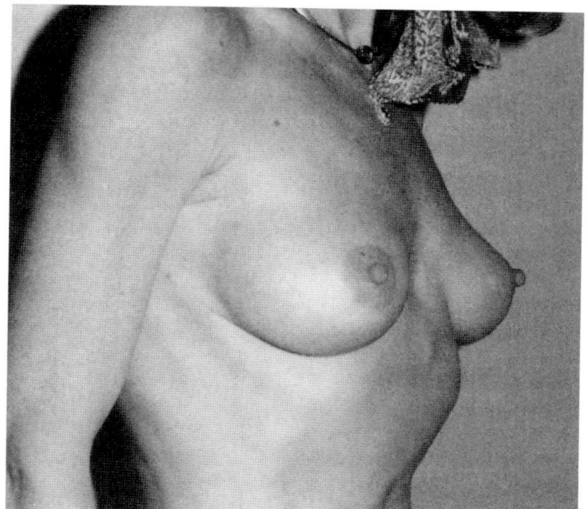

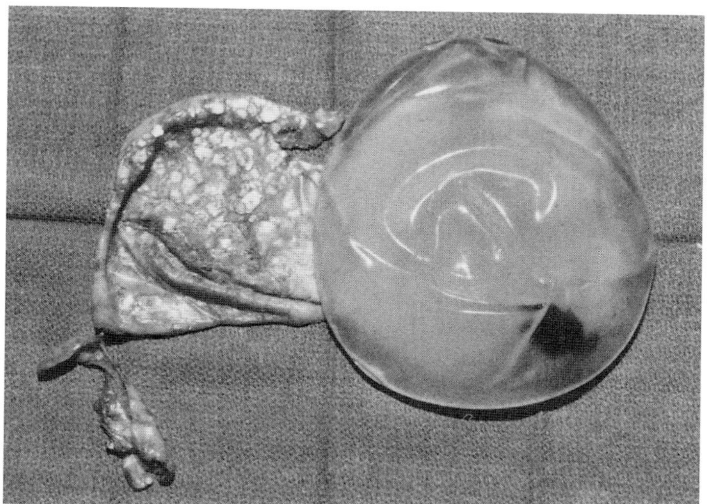

This patient had marked capsular contracture around Dacron-backed silicone implants. Preoperative mammography revealed calcifications around the implants. On palpation the capsules were found to be especially firm, indicating calcification. A total capsulectomy, including removal of the Dacron patches that involved the outer surface of the pectoralis major muscle, was done and smooth-surface breast implants used to replace the Dacron-backed implants. The patient was pleased with the overall improvement despite some postoperative firmness.

Subpectoral Conversion

Subpectoral conversion of the breast implant was one of the first successful strategies for producing softer breasts. It was useful when subglandular smooth-surface silicone breast implants were used primarily. With this approach the silicone breast implant is removed from the subglandular position and a selective capsulectomy performed, excising any capsule that deforms the breast. When calcification is present, the entire capsule is excised. When the entire capsule is left intact and a subpectoral conversion is done, a persistent seroma can develop in the retained capsule and create an asymmetry and resulting deformity.

An inframammary incision is used to approach the posterior surface of the breast implant and the lower margin of the pectoralis major muscle. The dissection goes bluntly around the lower pole of the breast and under the capsule to the muscle; the retractor then elevates the muscle and the breast implant. Blunt submusculofascial dissection creates a pocket in a deeper plane for the new implant.

The capsule is divided and the breast implants are removed. A partial lower capsulectomy removes some thickened scar on the lower portion of the breast.

Saline implants are then placed in the subpectoral position, and preplaced sutures are secured to protect the implant. Capsular contracture can thin the muscle and a tight capsule over it can also cause distortion. For this reason, this strategy is not used as frequently as when initially introduced.

The postoperative management is the same as for the initial procedure. Displacement exercises and avoidance of infection contribute to breast softness.

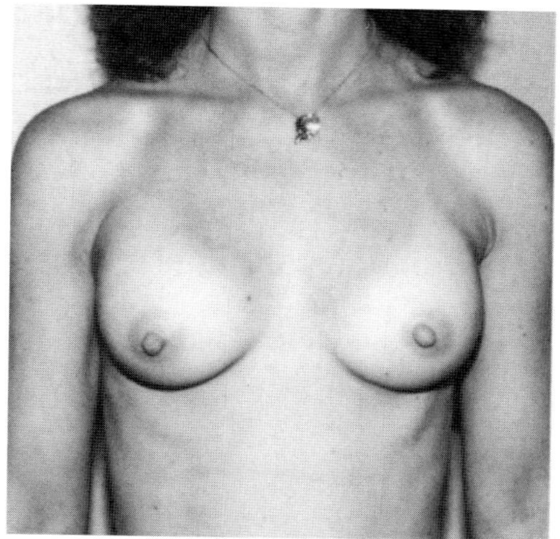
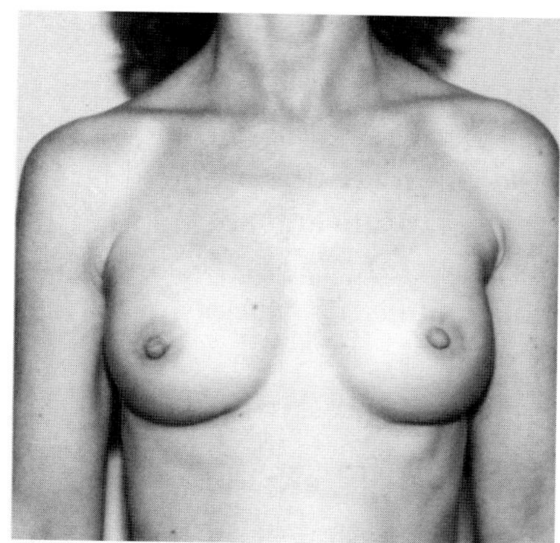

This patient had firm capsules 4 years after augmentation mammaplasty using periareolar incisions. The implants were converted to a submusculofascial position using the inframammary approach. The breasts have remained soft 4 years following this conversion. When established capsular contracture occurs after subglandular smooth-surface silicone implant placement, I now perform a limited capsulectomy and replace it with a saline implant. I have found subpectoral conversion to be of limited benefit because the pectoralis major muscle is often flattened and atrophic after years behind constricted implants. If a capsular contracture forms about a smooth-surface silicone implant in the submusculofascial position, the breast implant is removed, the deep pocket closed, and a smooth-surface saline implant placed in the subglandular position. If there is good implant cover, I use a textured-surface saline implant.

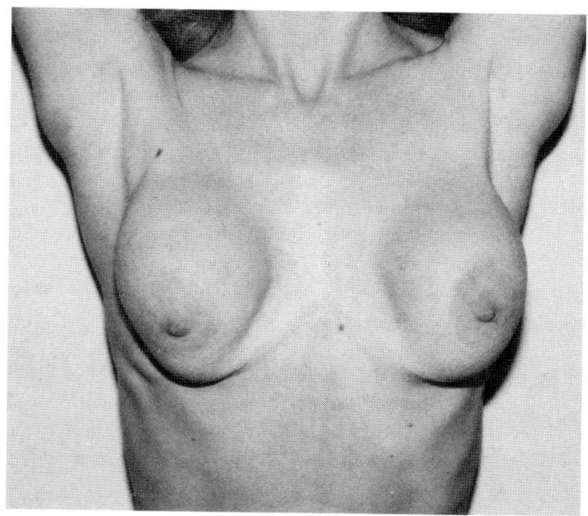
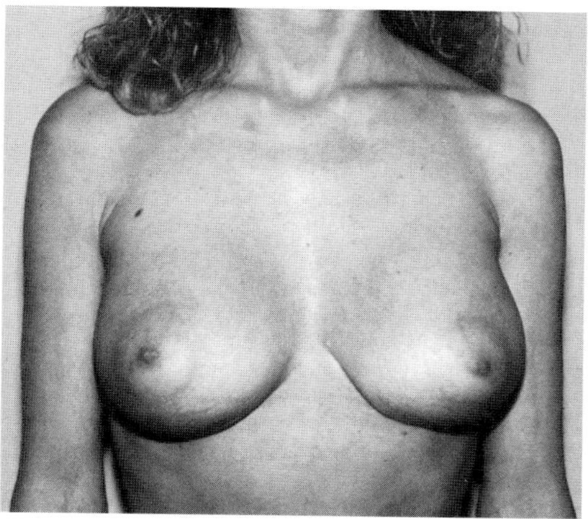

This patient had breast capsules 3 years after subglandular placement of a silicone gel implant. After capsulectomy, implants were placed beneath the pectoralis major muscle above and in the subglandular position below.

Capsulorrhaphy

At times, particularly with smooth-surface implants, the implant pocket can extend beyond the normal confines of the breast, creating an asymmetry. One solution for this problem is a capsulorrhaphy to locally excise or obliterate the capsule and suture the capsular edges to revise the contour of the implant pocket. Another solution calls for repositioning the implants, which are too mobile or will not hold their position.

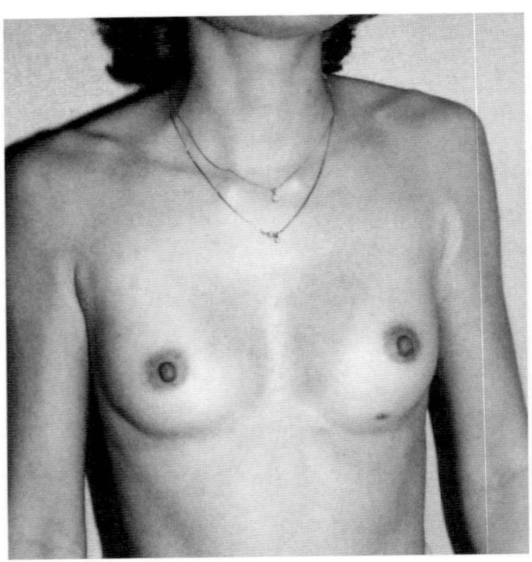

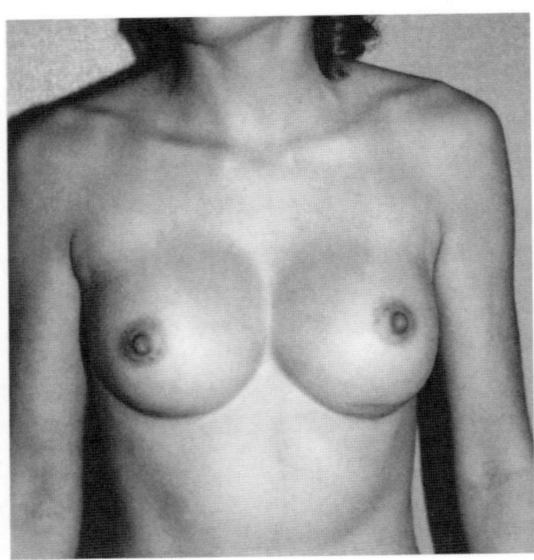

This 24-year-old patient had an inframammary crease dystopia following placement of submusculofascial breast implants via an inframammary approach. Three possible options are available for treating her problem:

1. A capsulotomy on the right breast to lower the right implant to the level of the left breast
2. A left capsulorrhaphy with elevation of the left inframammary crease
3. Replacement of the silicone gel implants with saline implants to help the breasts maintain their symmetric appearance

During capsulorrhaphy I resect the excess capsule and suture the edges with 2-0 polyglycolic acid sutures. I also instruct the patient to wear a brassiere at all times for the first month after this procedure to allow healing of the pocket without downward stress from the implant.

Implant Deflation or Rupture

When a saline implant deflates, there is usually a noticeable change in the appearance, size, shape, and feel of the involved breast. The breast volume diminishes as the saline solution is absorbed from the capsule. This usually occurs over a few days, and the implant should be replaced within a month to avoid the possibility of capsular contracture following the deflation.

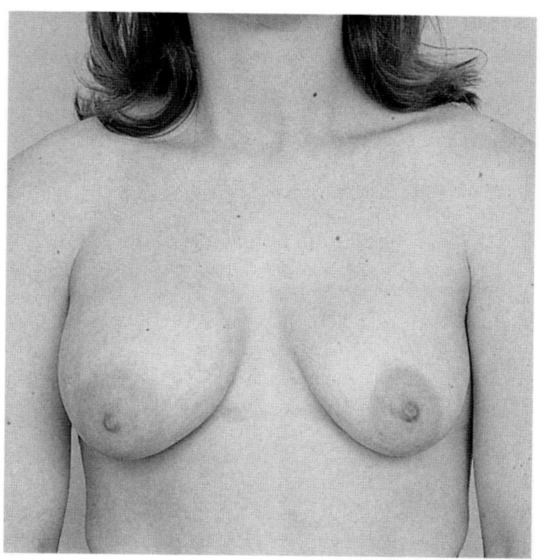

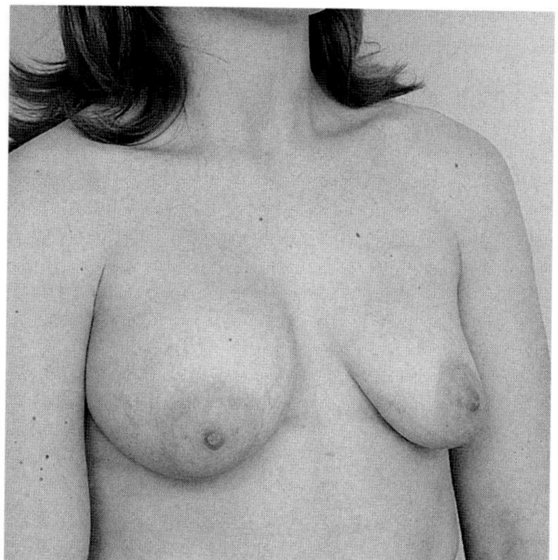

This 32-year-old woman had bilateral subpectoral inframammary breast augmentation with smooth-surface implants 5 years previously. Approximately 1 week before these photographs were taken her left implant developed a leak and she noticed that the breast was becoming progressively smaller until it approximated her preoperative size. Correction required bilateral implant replacement. The inframammary incisions were opened and the implants removed. Capsulotomies were then performed medially, laterally, and superiorly, and the implants were replaced with implants of a similar volume and shape. Postoperatively she did well and was satisfied with the correction. She has not experienced any subsequent problems.

When a silicone implant ruptures, the gel usually remains within the fibrous capsule and does not leak outside this capsule. If there is significant trauma at the time of rupture or there is a break in the capsule, the gel can migrate beyond the capsule into the breast as well as the surrounding tissues. The body's reaction to the silicone gel is usually inflammatory, with collagen deposited around the silicone producing a firm mass or distinct masses. These silicomas can occur in the breast, but more frequently they will gravitate to the axillary area or to the upper abdomen or the arm.

Magnetic resonance imaging is currently the best and most sensitive method for visualizing breast implants and determining implant integrity. With this approach the breasts are positioned inside a special breast coil and multiple views of the breast and implants are obtained. Drawbacks of this procedure include the need for specialized equipment, the length of the procedure, and expense.

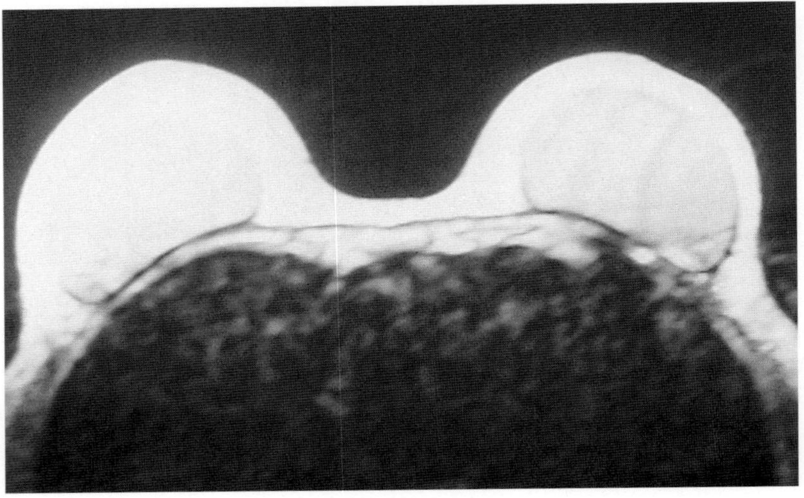

This MRI image shows capsular contracture of two silicone implants. These devices show no evidence of rupture.

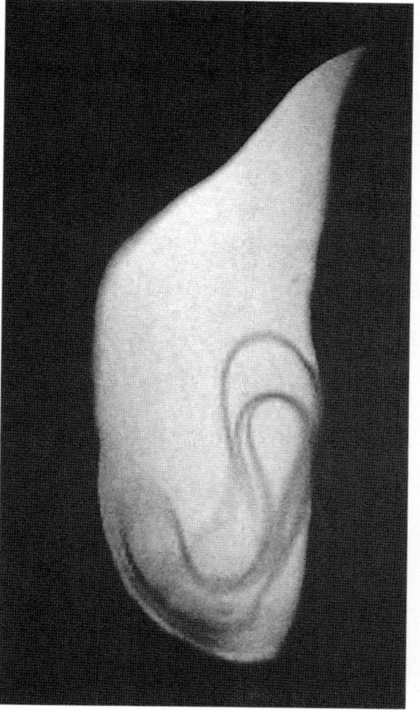

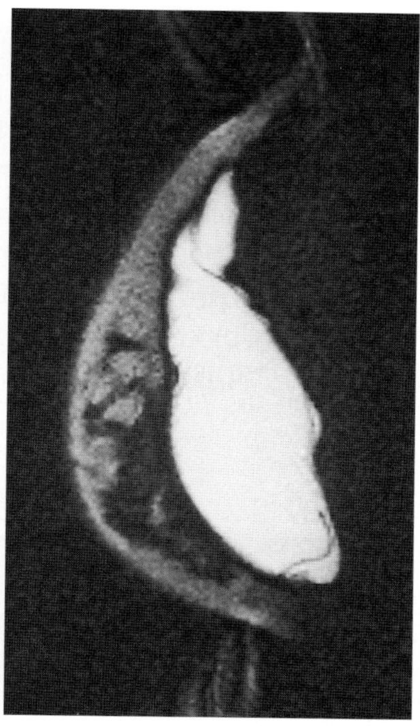

The MRI view on the left shows a ruptured silicone implant with some extrusion in its upper portion. Note the so-called linguini sign in the lower portion of this view in which the coiled implant elastomer resembles strands of pasta. The MRI view on the right demonstrates a ruptured silicone implant with gel extruded into the breast parenchyma. This is a very difficult situation to manage because the areas of fibrous tissue around each portion of the extruded silicone and the breasts are very nodular. Choices for management include explantation of the ruptured implant with removal of most of the extruded gel or subcutaneous mastectomy with reconstruction. This latter option is rarely recommended because even subcutaneous mastectomy may not successfully remove all of the extruded gel.

Other methods for assessing implant integrity include mammography, which can be used to detect a ruptured implant, particularly if silicone has leaked outside the capsule; ultrasonography, an adjunct to mammography; and computed tomography, which is usually not recommended for these diagnostic purposes because of the breast radiation involved and the increased accuracy and specificity of MRI.

Complications

HEMATOMA

The best treatment of a hematoma is prevention. ***Blunt dissection and direct visualization of any sharply dissected area with careful hemostasis are key to hematoma prevention.*** Another preventive measure is for the patient to avoid drugs that reduce platelet adhesiveness and prolong blood coagulation. Aspirin or other pain medications that affect platelet adhesiveness can prolong bleeding and promote hematoma formation and should be discontinued several weeks prior to the operation. A list of these drugs (see p. 10) is given to patients. This list should be updated frequently as new drugs become available.

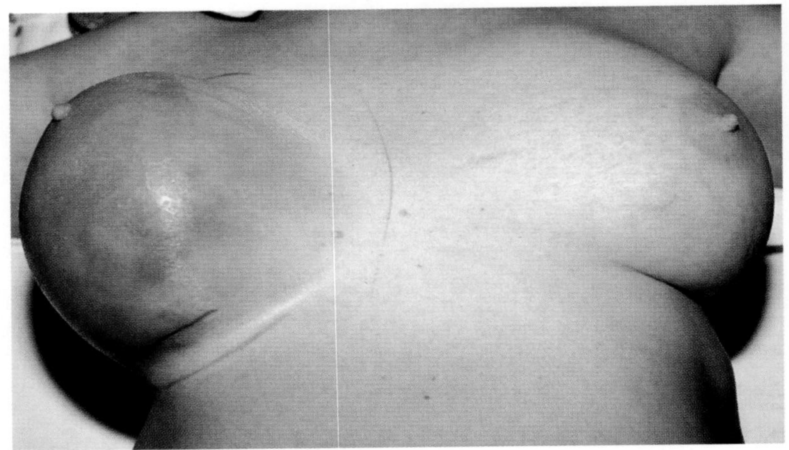

A hematoma in the immediate postoperative period should be treated by returning the patient to the operating room and evacuating the hematoma, controlling the bleeding, and replacing the breast implant. Unilateral breast pain and swelling are the primary indicators of a hematoma. An untreated hematoma is painful, can affect skin viability and wound healing, and may increase the probability of infection, capsular contracture, and asymmetry.

The patient may occasionally return for the first postoperative visit with a mild asymmetry related to a hematoma. It has been my usual practice to let these minor problems resolve naturally and not return the patient to the operating room to avoid the risk of infection. I also question whether the final result after reoperation will be an improvement.

A delayed hematoma can develop between 1 and 2 weeks after augmentation mammaplasty when the clots on the vessels lyse, resulting in considerable bleeding and a tight hematoma. If the hematoma is tight and expanding, it needs to be reexplored.

A late hematoma can develop weeks and even years later and is usually associated with some increased activity that causes a tear and subsequent bleeding of the breast capsule around the implant. These usually are seen some hours to days after the incident. When I see a patient with a tight painful breast shortly after a bleeding episode, I evacuate the hematoma in the operating room and allow a few days or weeks for the hematoma to resolve. I have noted, however, that a capsular contracture often develops and she will most likely eventually require a capsulotomy and implant exchange.

INFECTION

As with hematoma, avoiding an infection is the best strategy. Actually it is surprising that the rate of infection is no greater than it is considering the fact that the breast parenchyma is connected to the exterior of the body via the lactiferous ducts, and *Staphylococcus epidermidis* and other bacteria actually can be cultured from most breasts as well as from the implant pocket. I administer cephalothin intravenously before the incision is made and prescribe an oral cephalosporin antibiotic for 2 days postoperatively. I also irrigate the breast pocket with 5% povidone-iodine solution. It is important not to let an early infection go untreated or persist.

Treatment of infections caused by atypical mycobacteria with any type of breast implant requires complete capsulectomy, removal of the breast implant, and specific intravenous antifungal agents for several weeks. I consult with an infectious disease colleague when this type of infection is diagnosed. Prolonged drainage indicates a focus of foreign material or necrotic tissue that needs to be excised.

MONDOR'S DISEASE

Thrombosis of an upper abdominal wall vein, Mondor's disease is a self-limited condition that usually develops in 1% to 2% of cases, most often after inframammary augmentation mammaplasty. It poses no danger of systemic embolization of the thrombus. I reassure the patient that the condition will resolve; however, it will take a number of weeks.

This condition can also develop spontaneously and after reduction mammaplasty. It is characterized by a tender, inflamed cord extending from the inframammary fold at the area of the incision to the upper abdominal wall.

Long-Term Results

Initial proper implant placement influences the ability of the implants to remain soft over the long term without developing deforming capsular contracture. Breast appearance will be compromised by persistent capsular contracture. If this problem is long-standing, it can result in increased pressure within the breast, compression of the underlying ribs, thinning of the overlying breast parenchyma, and even exposure and extrusion of the breast implant. Not all contractures require correction. There are various degrees of firmness. Some women are pleased with the result of breast augmentation even at the expense of some firmness from capsular contracture and mild breast deformity. Although capsular contracture is the main deterrent to satisfactory long-term postoperative results, changes in weight, the effects of pregnancy, lactation, and involution, and the development of breast hypertrophy or ptosis can also affect the long-term appearance.

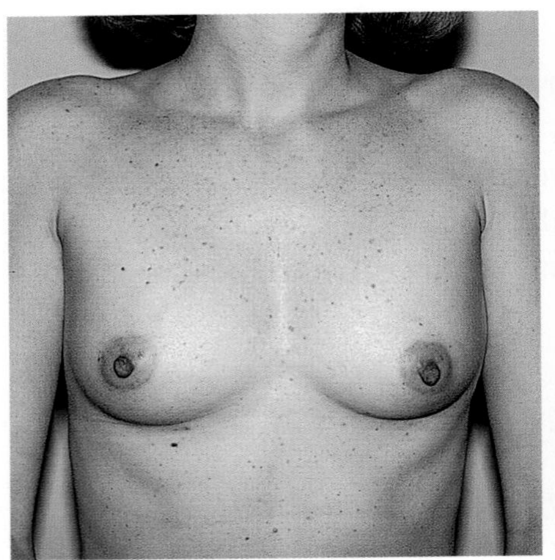

Preoperative

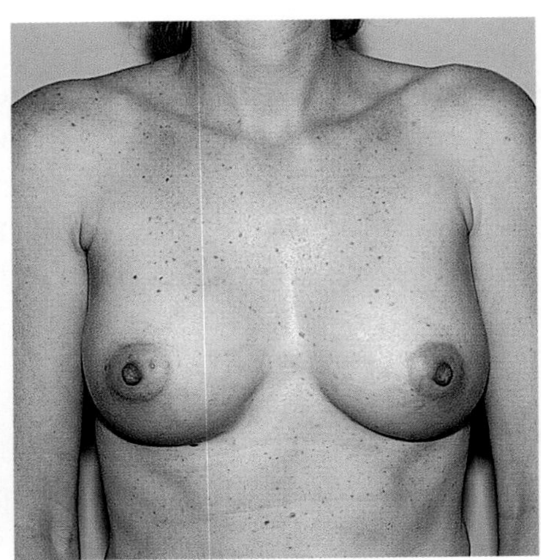

1 year

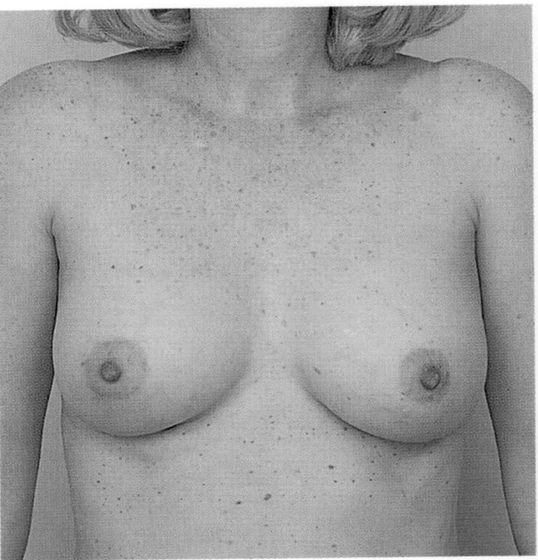

11 years

This young woman had hypoplasia with minimal breast development. She had breast augmentation with 280 cc smooth-surface double-lumen implants when she was 24 years old. She is shown 1 year and 11 years following breast augmentation through an inframammary approach. Although she had some implant firmness, she does not find it disturbing and remains pleased with the result, which has had a positive impact on her body image and her feelings about herself.

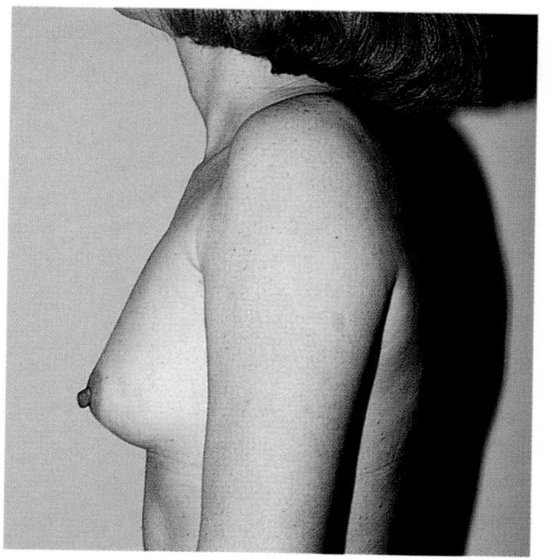
Preoperative

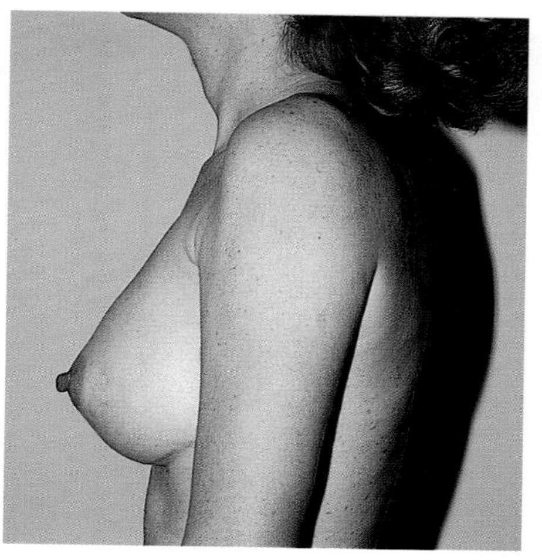
1 year

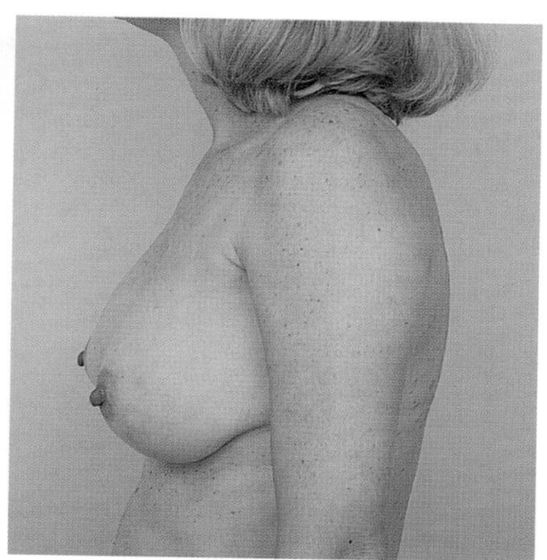
11 years

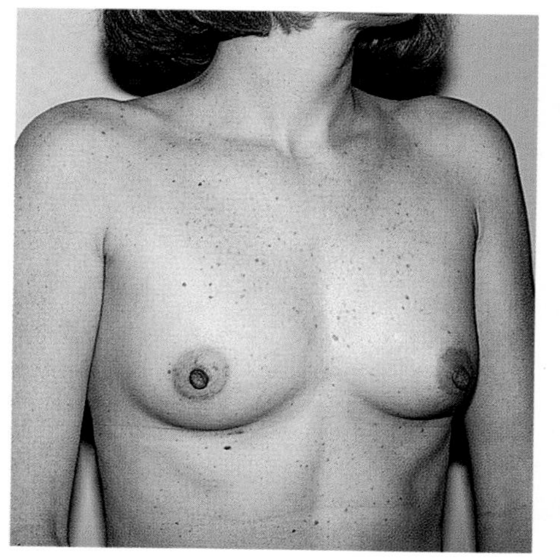
Preoperative

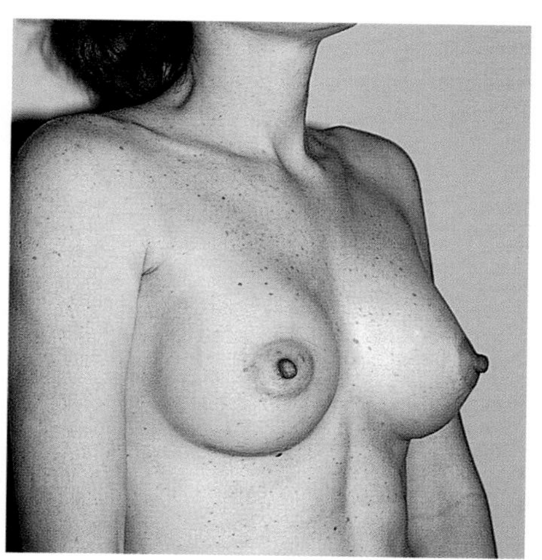
1 year

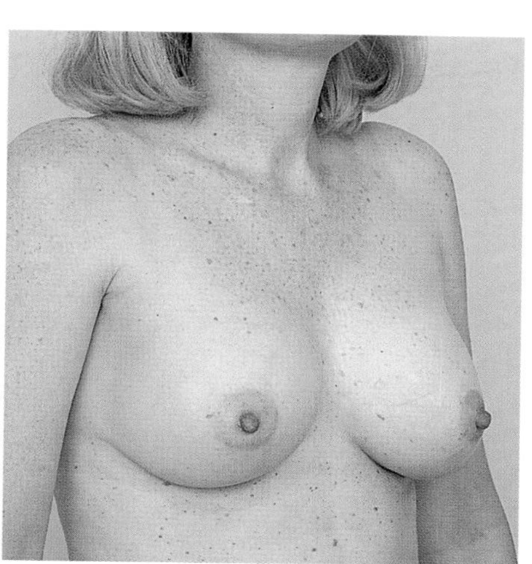
11 years

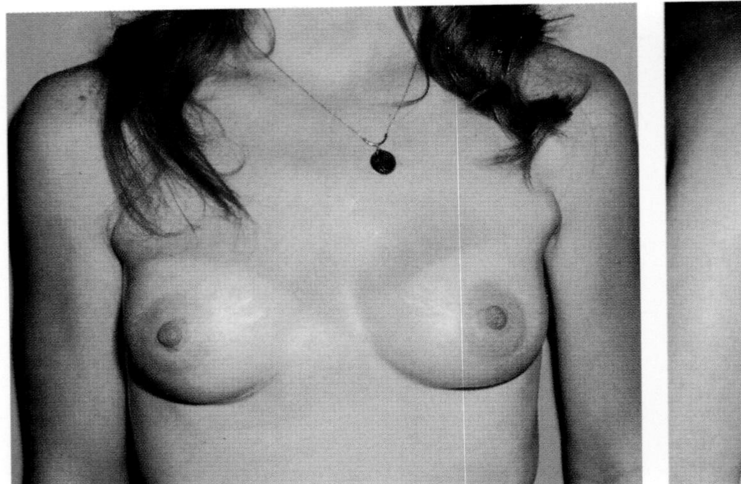
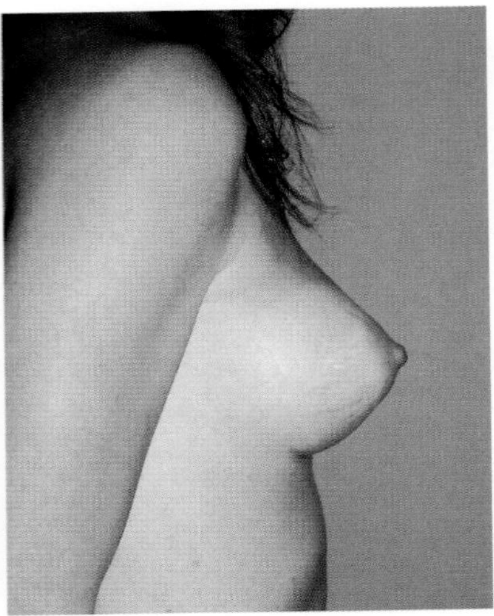

This patient is photographed 6 months following breast augmentation via the inframammary approach with placement of 210 cc smooth-surface implants in the subglandular position.

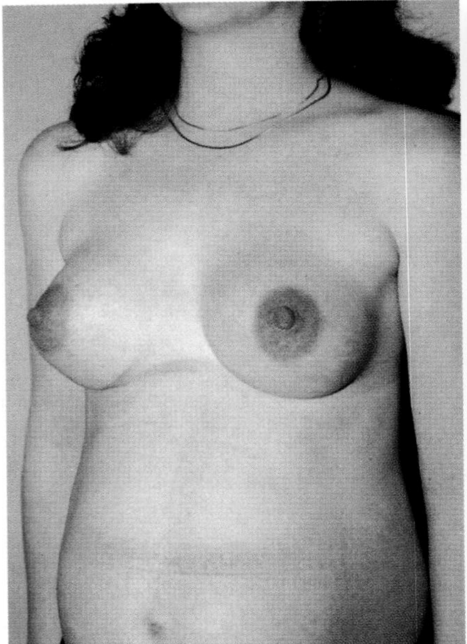
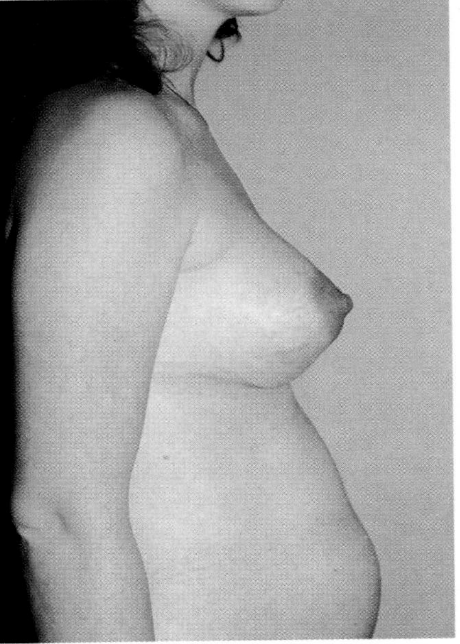

She is shown 2 years later in her eighth month of pregnancy. Note the breast enlargement and pigmentation of the nipple-areola.

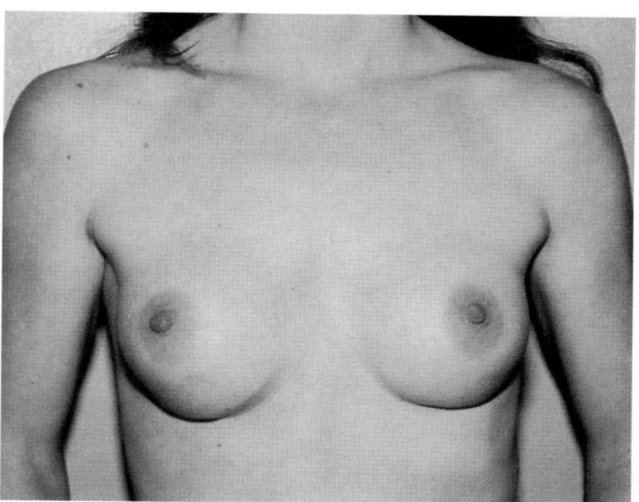
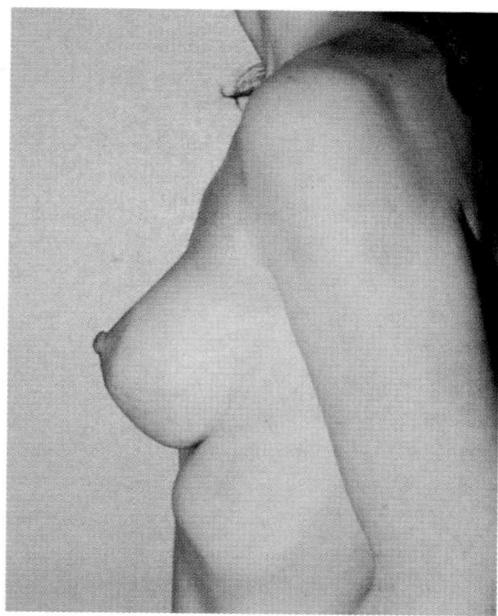

The patient is shown 5 years following the breast augmentation. She has mild breast firmness on the right; otherwise she is pleased with her appearance and the results of breast augmentation.

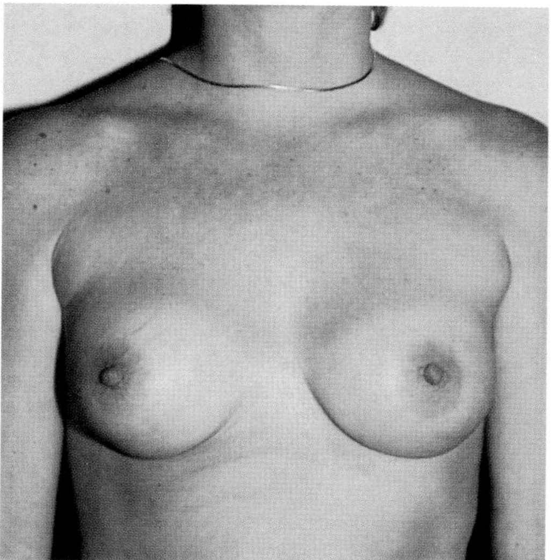
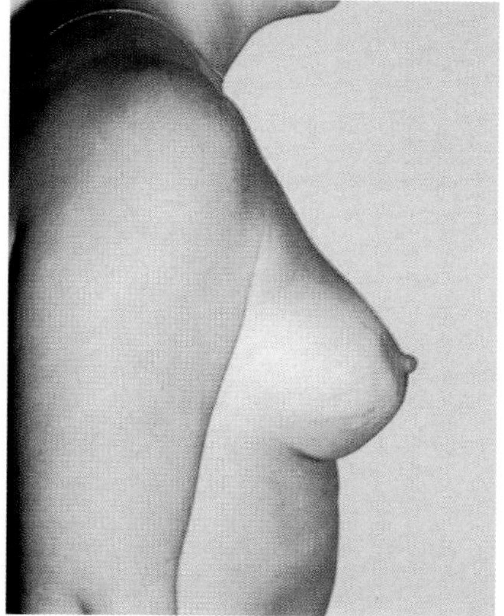

The patient is shown 12 years following breast augmentation. She has gained about 20 pounds. There is some breast enlargement and mild breast firmness. There are no breast masses, and the patient continues to be satisfied with her breast augmentation.

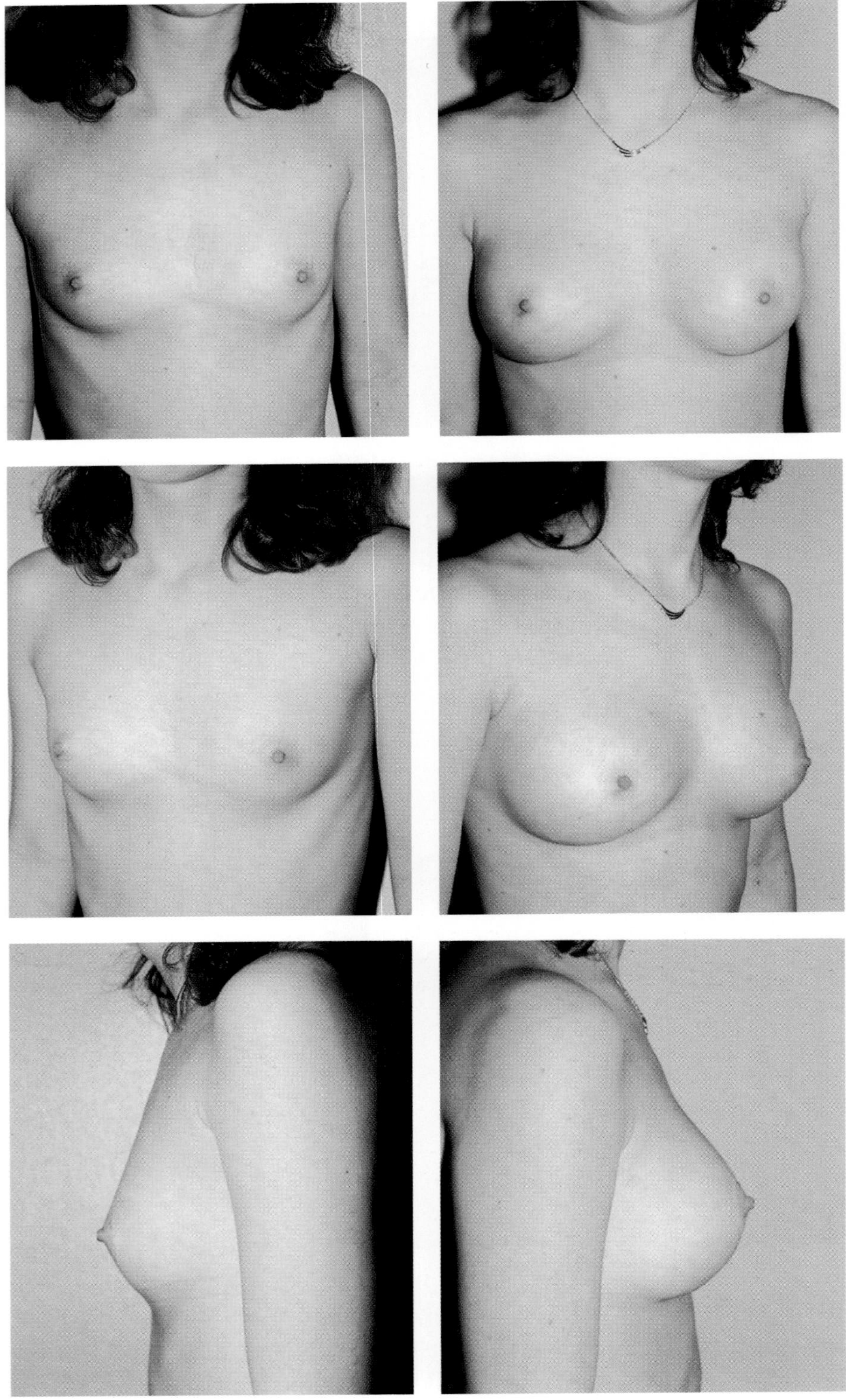

This patient was seen initially at age 18 years with breast hypoplasia. She requested breast augmentation without breast scars. She is shown 5 years after submusculofascial axillary breast augmentation. The breast implants have remained soft.

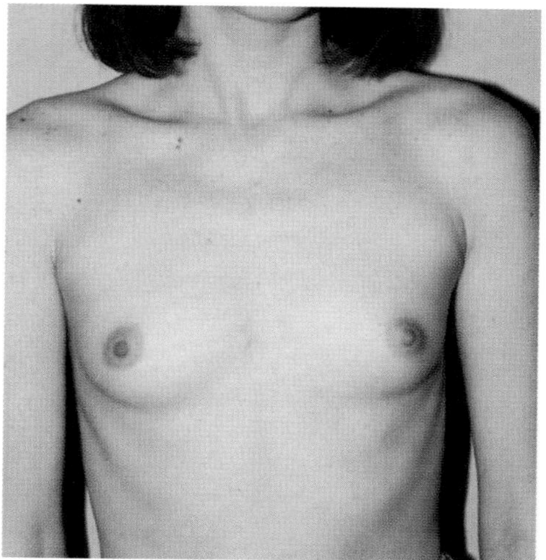

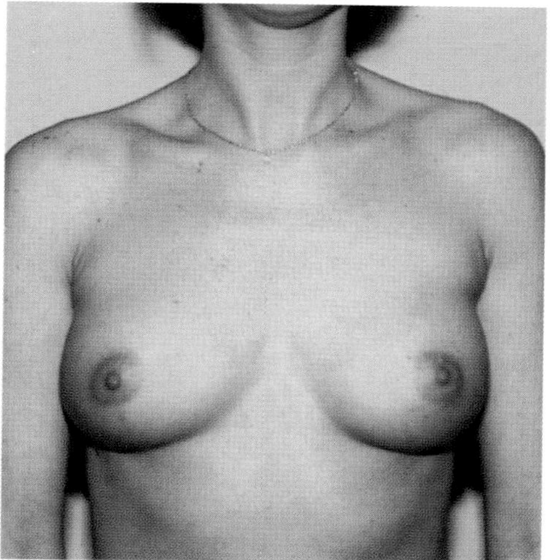

This patient was first seen when she was 21 years old. She had breast hypoplasia and requested breast augmentation without visible scars. She had a submusculofascial axillary breast augmentation with 240 cc smooth-surface implants. She had no postoperative problems and her breasts have remained soft during the 4-year postoperative period. She has continued to perform the displacement exercises daily.

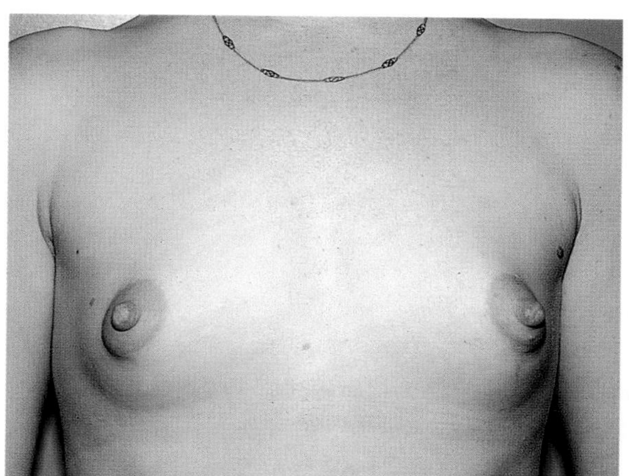

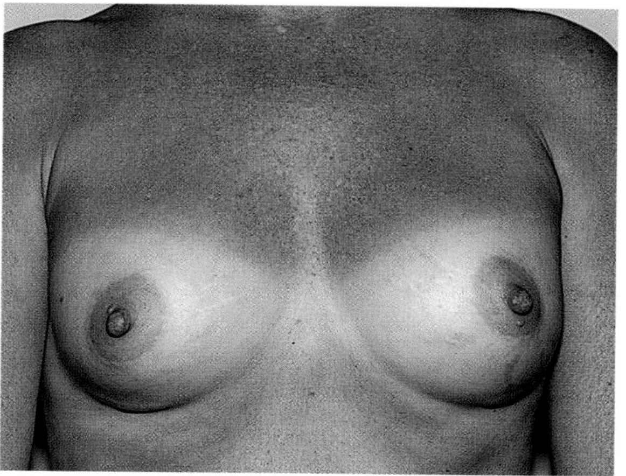

This 31-year-old woman requested breast augmentation. She had two children and had breast-fed them as infants. She noted that her breasts were now smaller than before her initial pregnancy. Her breasts were augmented via an inframammary approach with placement of smooth-surface implants in the subpectoral position. She is shown 13 years following this operation. The implants have maintained a satisfactory position with no significant capsular contracture. The patient is pleased with the overall appearance and feel of her breasts.

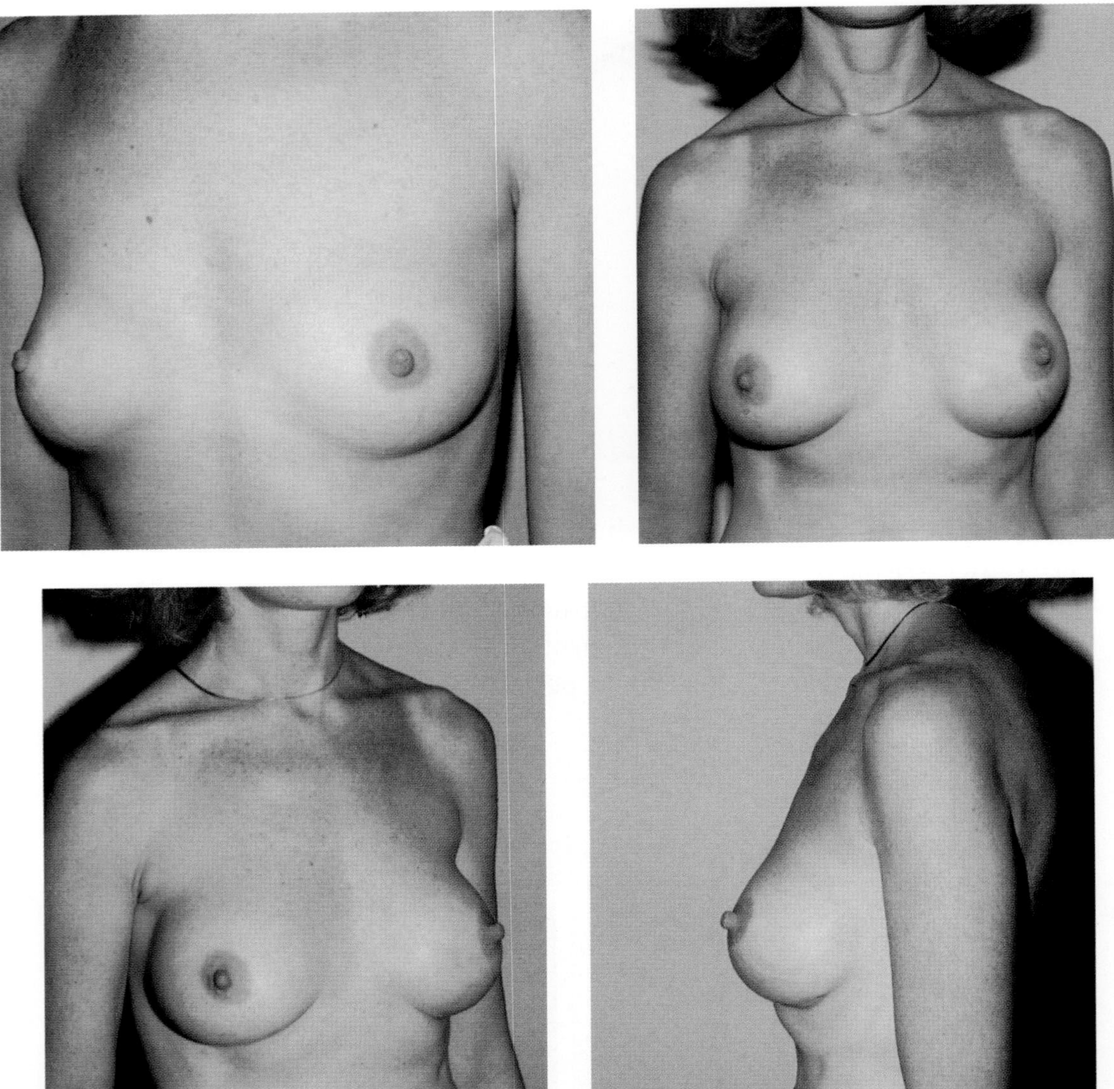

This patient was seen originally with mammary hypoplasia at 24 years of age. She had subglandular inframammary breast augmentation with 220 cc smooth-surface implants. She is shown 11 years later after the birth of two children, both of whom she nursed without difficulty. She has some breast firmness but continues to be satisfied with the improvement from her breast augmentation. Mammography reveals no breast abnormalities.

REFERENCES

Addington DB, Mallin RE. Closed capsulotomy causing fractures of the scar capsule and the silicone bag of a breast implant. Plast Reconstr Surg 62:300, 1978.

Baker JL Jr, Bartels RJ, Douglas WM. Closed compression technique for rupturing a contracted capsule around a breast implant. Plast Reconstr Surg 58:137, 1976.

Baker JL, Kolin L, Bartlett E. Psychosexual dynamics of patients undergoing mammary augmentation. Plast Reconstr Surg 53:652, 1974.

Beale S, Lisper HO, Palm B. A psychological study of patients seeking augmentation mammoplasty. Br J Psychiatry 136:133, 1980.

Beale S, Hambert G, Lisper HO, Ohlsën L, Palm B. Augmentation mammaplasty: The surgical and psychological effects of the operation and prediction of the result. Ann Plast Surg 13:279, 1984.

Becker H, Springer R. Prevention of capsular contracture. Plast Reconstr Surg 103:1766, 1999.

Biggs TM. Augmentation mammaplasty: A comparative analysis. Plast Reconstr Surg 103:1761, 1999.

Biggs TM, Cukier J, Worthing LF. Augmentation mammaplasty: A review of 18 years. Plast Reconstr Surg 69:445, 1982.

Bostwick J III, Eaves FF III, Nahai F. Endoscopic Plastic Surgery. St. Louis: Quality Medical Publishing, 1995.

Brinton LA, Malone KE, Coates RJ, Schoenberg JB, Swanson CA, Daling JR, Stanford JL. Breast enlargement and reduction: Results from a breast cancer case-control study. Plast Reconstr Surg 97:269, 1996.

Brody GS. Breast implant, size selection and patient satisfaction. Plast Reconstr Surg 68:611, 1981.

Burkhardt BR, Schnur PL, Tofield JJ, Dempsey PD. Objective clinical assessment of fibrous capsular contracture. Plast Reconstr Surg 69:794, 1982.

Cohen IK, Scheflan M, Monteiro IC. Transaxillary subpectoral breast augmentation. Presented at the Fiftieth Annual Meeting of the American Society of Plastic and Reconstructive Surgeons. New York: October 1981.

Courtiss EH, Goldwyn RM, Anastasi GW. The fate of breast implants with infections around them. Plast Reconstr Surg 63:812, 1979.

Cronin TD, Gerow F. Augmentation mammaplasty—A new "natural feel" prosthesis. In Transactions of the Third International Congress of Plastic Surgeons. Amsterdam: Excerpta Medica, 1964.

Deapen DM, Pike MC, Casagrande JT, Brody GS. The relationship between breast cancer and augmentation mammaplasty: An epidemiologic study. Plast Reconstr Surg 77:368, 1986.

Dempsey WC, Latham WD. Subpectoral implants in augmentation mammaplasty. Plast Reconstr Surg 42:515, 1968.

Eaves FF III, Bostwick J III, Nahai F, Murray DR, Stylo TM, Carlson GW. Endoscopic techniques in aesthetic breast surgery: Augmentation, mastectomy, biopsy, capsulotomy, capsulorrhaphy, reduction, mastopexy, and reconstructive techniques. Clin Plast Surg 22:683, 1995.

Ellenberg AH, Braun H. A 3½-year experience with double-lumen implants in breast surgery. Plast Reconstr Surg 65:307, 1980.

Gifford S. Emotional attitudes towards cosmetic breast surgery: Loss and restitution of the "ideal self." In Goldwyn RM, ed. Plastic and Reconstructive Surgery of the Breast. Boston: Little, Brown, 1976.

Goin JM. High-pressure injection of silicone gel into an axilla—A complication of closed compression capsulotomy of the breast: Case report. Plast Reconstr Surg 62:891, 1978.

Gorczyca DP, Brenner RJ. The Augmented Breast: Radiologic and Clinical Perspectives. New York: Thieme, 1997.

Gruber RP, Friedman GD. Periareolar subpectoral augmentation mammaplasty. Plast Reconstr Surg 67:453, 1981.

Gruber RP, Jones HW. Review of closed capsulotomy complications. Ann Plast Surg 6:271, 1981.

Handel N, Jensen JA, Black Q, Waisman JR, Silverstein MJ. The fate of breast implants: A critical analysis of complications and outcomes. Plast Reconstr Surg 96:1521, 1995.

Hartley JH Jr. Specific applications of the double lumen prosthesis. Clin Plast Surg 3:247, 1976.

Hoehler H. Breast augmentation: The axillary approach. Br J Plast Surg 26:373, 1973.

Hörl HW, Feller AM, Steinau HU, Biemer E. Autologous injection of fatty tissue following liposuction—Not a method for breast augmentation. Handchir Mikrochir Plast Chir 21(2):59, 1989.

Howard BJ. The role of endoscopy and implant texture in transaxillary submuscular breast augmentation. Ann Plast Surg 42:245, 1999.

Johnson M, Lloyd HED. Bilateral breast cancer 10 years after an augmentation mammaplasty: Case report. Plast Reconstr Surg 53:88, 1974.

Laughlin RA, Raynor AC, Habal MB. Complications of closed capsulotomies after augmentation mammaplasty. Plast Reconstr Surg 60:362, 1977.

Liebman AJ. Imaging of complications of augmentation mammaplasty. Plast Reconstr Surg 93: 1134, 1994.

Little G, Baker JL Jr. Results of closed compression capsulotomy for treatment of contracted breast implant capsules. Plast Reconstr Surg 65:30, 1980.

Malata CM, Feldberg L, Coleman DJ, Foo IT, Sharpe DJ. Textured or smooth implants for breast augmentation? Three-year follow-up of a prospective randomized controlled trial. Br J Plast Surg 50:99, 1997.

McCain LA, Jones G. Endoscopic techniques in aesthetic plastic surgery. Plast Surg Nurs 15:145, 1995.

McGrath MH, Burkhardt BR. The safety and efficacy of breast implants for augmentation mammaplasty. Plast Reconstr Surg 74:550, 1984.

Nelson GD. Update. Complications from the treatment of fibrous capsular contracture of the breast. Plast Reconstr Surg 68:969, 1981.

Netscher DT, Sharma S, Thornby J, Peltier M, Lyos A, Fater M, Mosharrafa A. Aesthetic outcome of breast implant removal in 85 consecutive patients. Plast Reconstr Surg 100:206, 1997.

Oneal RM, Argenta LC. Late side effects related to inflatable breast prostheses containing soluble steroids. Plast Reconstr Surg 69:641, 1982.

Papillon J. Pros and cons of subpectoral implantation. Clin Plast Surg 3:321, 1976.

Perrin ER. The use of soluble steroids within inflatable breast prostheses. Plast Reconstr Surg 57: 163, 1976.

Peterson HD, Burt GB. The role of steroids in prevention of circumferential capsular scarring in augmentation mammaplasty. Plast Reconstr Surg 54:28, 1974.

Pickrell KL, Puckett CL, Given KS. Subpectoral augmentation mammaplasty. Plast Reconstr Surg 60:325, 1977.

Price CI, Eaves FF III, Nahai F, Jones G, Bostwick J III. Endoscopic transaxillary subpectoral breast augmentation. Plast Reconstr Surg 94:612, 1994.

Redfern AB, Ryan JJ, Su CT. Calcification of the fibrous capsule about mammary implants. Plast Reconstr Surg 59:249, 1977.

Regnault P. Partially submuscular breast augmentation. Plast Reconstr Surg 59:72, 1977.

Rheingold LM, Yoo RP, Courtiss EH. Experience with 326 inflatable breast implants. Plast Reconstr Surg 93:118, 1994.

Robles JM, Zimman OA, Lee JC. A larger subpectoral pocket for breast implants. Plast Reconstr Surg 61:78, 1978.

Rohrich RJ, Kenkel JM, Adams WP. Preventing capsular contracture in breast augmentation: In search of the Holy Grail. Plast Reconstr Surg 103:1759, 1999.

Sarwer DB, Barlett SP, Bucky LP, LaRossa D, Low DW, Pertschuk MJ, Wadden TA, Whitaker LA. Big is not always better: Body image dissatisfaction in breast reduction and breast augmentation patients. Plast Reconstr Surg 101:1956, 1998.

Shah Z, Lehman A Jr, Tan J. Does infection play a role in breast capsular contracture? Plast Reconstr Surg 68:34, 1981.

Shipley RH, O'Donnell JM, Bader KF. Psychological effects of cosmetic augmentation mammaplasty. Aesthetic Plast Surg 2:429, 1978.

Shipley RH, O'Donnell JM, Bader KF. Personality characteristics of women seeking breast augmentation. Comparison to small-busted and average-busted controls. Plast Reconstr Surg 60: 369, 1977.

Spear SL, Baker JL Jr. Classification of capsular contracture after prosthetic breast reconstruction. Plast Reconstr Surg 96:1119, 1995.

Thomas WO III, Harper LL, Wong SW, Michalski JP, Harris CN, Moore JT, Rodning CB. Explantation of silicone breast implants. Am Surg 63:421, 1997.

Truppman ES, Ellenby JD. A 13-year evaluation of subpectoral augmentation mammaplasty. In Owsley JQ Jr, Peterson RA, eds. Symposium on Aesthetic Surgery of the Breast, vol 18. St. Louis: CV Mosby, 1978.

Widdice L. The effects of breast reduction and breast augmentation surgery on lactation: An annotated bibliography. J Hum Lact 9:161, 1993.

Williams C, Aston S, Rees TD. The effect of hematoma on the thickness of pseudosheaths around silicone implants. Plast Reconstr Surg 56:194, 1975.

Woods JE. Unusual complications of submuscular placement of implants in breast surgery. Plast Reconstr Surg 73:972, 1984.

Worton EW, Seifert LN, Sherwood R. Late leakage of inflatable silicone breast prostheses. Plast Reconstr Surg 65:302, 1980.

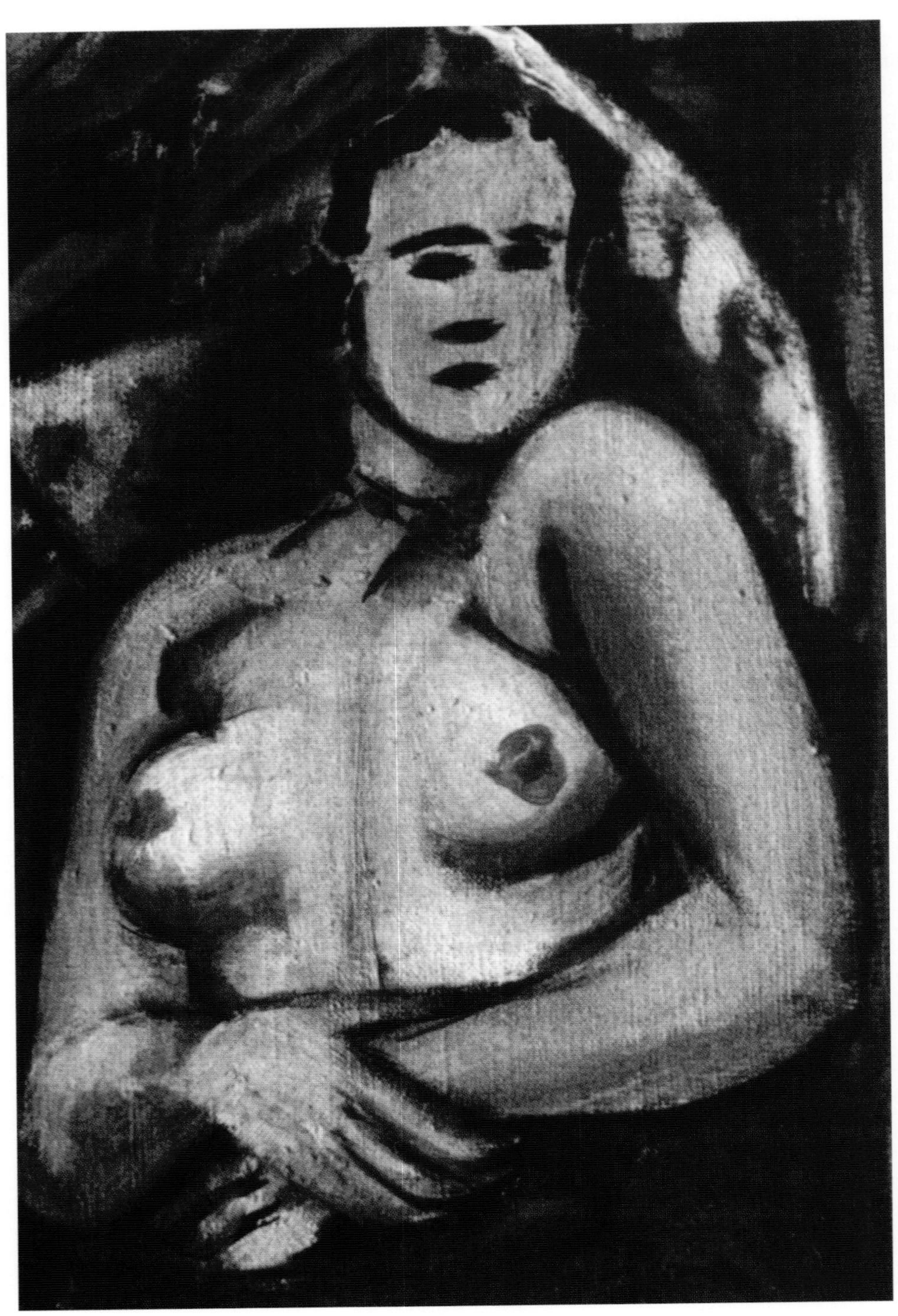

7 Reduction Mammaplasty

Key Topics

Areas and Amount of Skin and Breast Reduction

Vertical Mammaplasty With Liposuction

Superior Pedicle Technique

Superior Medial Pedicle Technique

Inferior Central Pedicle Technique

Free Nipple Graft

Reduction-Augmentation for Upper Breast Fullness

Liposuction for Lateral, Axillary, and Presternal Fullness

Liposuction for Abdominal Contouring

Special Problems

Problems and Complications

Long-Term Results

Observations

For many women, breast reduction offers a resolution of the functional and aesthetic problems associated with large breasts. That is why this operation is associated with high patient acceptance and satisfaction. Individuals who request this operation usually have given careful consideration to their decision for surgery and their desire for smaller breasts is self-motivated. These women readily incorporate their new, smaller breasts into their body image and rapidly adjust to their changed appearance.

When treating breast hyperplasia patients, I find the major challenge, and one shared by my colleagues, is determining the patient's desired breast appearance, specifically just how small she wants her breasts to be. The tendency in reduction is to underestimate the amount of tissue resection required, resulting in failure to remove enough breast parenchyma. A woman's breasts will look much smaller when she is supine on the operating table than when she is upright after surgery. Careful preoperative markings with the patient upright and discussing the proposed changes and her expectations for breast size will help ensure a more accurate reduction. It is frustrating to the reduction patient to have to return for more surgery because her breasts are still too large and her symptoms have not been alleviated.

Patient Assessment and Selection

Patients requesting reduction present with a variety of different problems—from the young girl with virginal hypertrophy and embarrassingly disproportionate breasts to the elderly woman with large, uncomfortable, sagging breasts with associated breast pain and irritation, back and shoulder pain, and even numbness of her hands. ***Understanding their motivations and their expectations is crucially important in deciding which patients are good candidates for this operation.***

PATIENT PROFILES

Teenagers

Giant virginal hypertrophy is a condition in which young girls (generally at puberty) develop massive breasts out of proportion to their normal body and chest size; patients are usually 11 to 15 years old. This condition can have a devastating impact on a young girl's body image and self-confidence during the early teen years, which are difficult times fraught with insecurity and self-consciousness, even in the absence of such an anomaly.

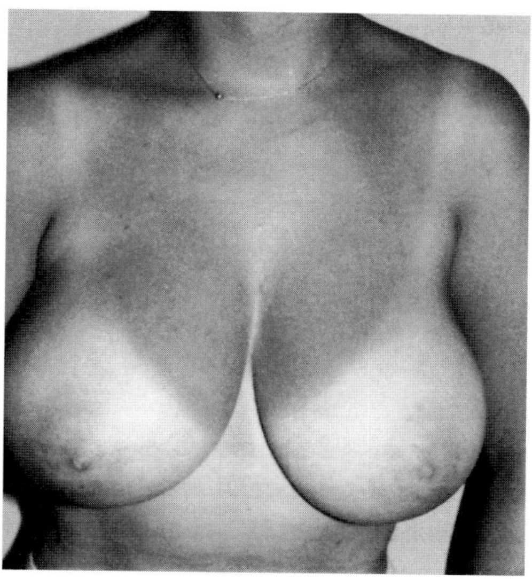

In such cases I believe that breast reduction is indicated despite the risk of additional breast growth postoperatively, which may necessitate a secondary correction. The large breasts are already a major problem; any further growth will compound the problem and will also be more difficult to manage later.

Most patients and their mothers would rather accept the risk of additional surgery in the future than to live with the hypertrophy a few more years. When they come to the plastic surgeon's office, they are ready for a breast reduction. These operations are usually done on an outpatient basis or require an overnight hospital stay; a second procedure, if necessary, can be done through the same incisions on an outpatient basis. I prefer to deal with the young teenager's potential for breast regrowth when and if it occurs rather than consider hormonal therapy to prevent it. In my opinion the risk of a second operation is less odious than the unknown risk of administering large doses of hormones to a young woman. Furthermore, in some of the cases I have seen the administration of hormones does not completely halt or suppress breast growth, and these young patients can still experience enough regrowth to require a secondary reduction.

Some girls experience sudden and substantial breast growth during their mid- to late teens. This is not the massive growth and malproportion that exists with giant virginal hypertrophy, but it is troubling nevertheless. At a time when they are struggling with their emerging female identity and the transition to young womanhood, their large breasts propel them physically far beyond their psychological development and their capability to cope with their body image. This is a major psychological and emotional problem for them. Their large breasts are a source of embarrassment and a focus of jokes and comments by other teenagers who stare and make unkind remarks. They may also experience back, shoulder, and breast pain. These young girls are not prepared for this type of attention; they want to be considered normal, to fit into the crowd. Typically, they have problems finding properly fitting clothing. Athletic activities are hampered by their large breasts. Swimsuits that provide sufficient cover and do not accentuate their breasts are difficult if not impossible to find.

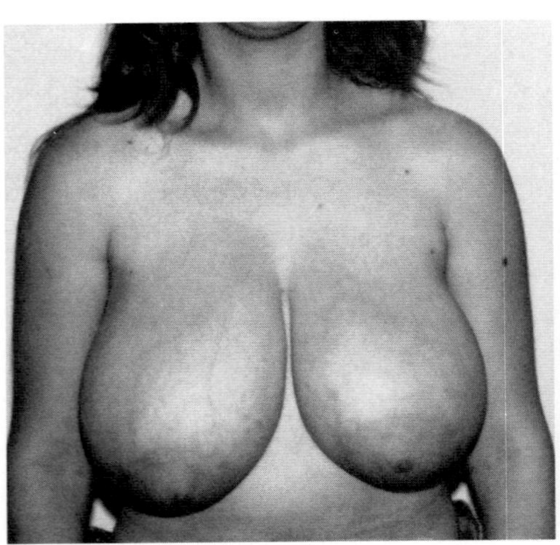

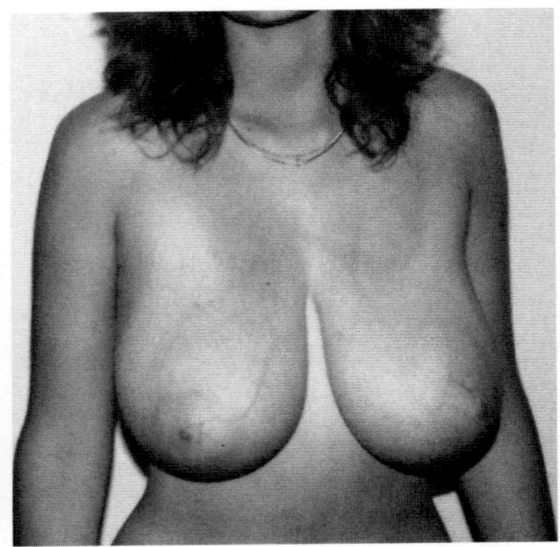

These 16-year-old fraternal twins demonstrate some of the variations seen with breast hypertrophy in the adolescent. Teenage breast reduction patients want their breasts to be "normal" in size. For them that usually translates into a "B" or "C" cup brassiere. They want breasts in proportion to their bodies that do not attract undue attention. Frequently they are somewhat overweight, and sometimes this excess weight is retained as a conscious means of minimizing the visibility of their disproportionately large breasts. ***Overreduction should be avoided in these patients; many of them will lose weight following surgery and their breasts can then become quite small.*** The teenage patient is a good candidate for breast reduction surgery; she quickly incorporates her smaller breasts into her body image and is very appreciative of her new breast profile and more normal appearance.

Women After Childbearing

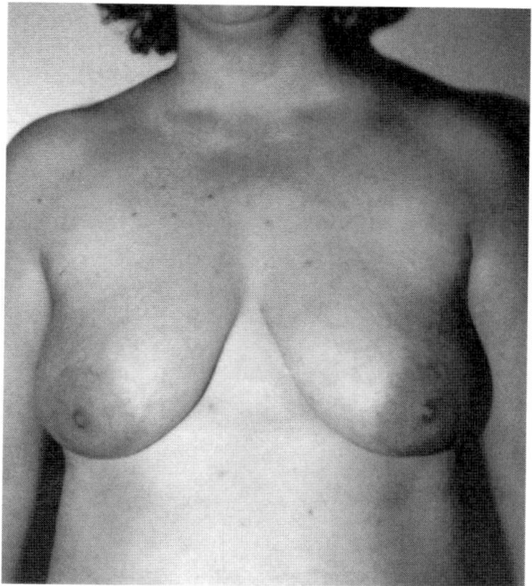

Women who request breast reduction after their childbearing years often exhibit more than the normal degree of ptosis and upper breast flattening; they also may have gained a few additional pounds during their reproductive years and their drooping breasts only accentuate this problem. The additional breast volume can cause the breasts to descend and rest on the upper abdomen.

Frequently these women had large breasts before pregnancy but with some upper breast fullness and minor ptosis. Since they were not interested in breast reduction before their pregnancies, they often are not as distressed with their large breasts as younger patients are. They seek reduction to relieve chronic symptoms related to large breasts. Some of these women do not want a large volume removed, and a major reduction would result in breasts disproportionate to their body habitus, particularly if they are somewhat overweight.

Estimating the proper size reduction for these women is somewhat more difficult than for the younger group of women. Some who request reduction may in fact simply desire less fullness below and more upper breast fullness. A reduction without upper breast resection may be considered for these women. Sufficient volume reduction can be achieved with breast liposuction in some women requesting only a small reduction. Others truly desire to be smaller. Ptosis can be present to such a degree that practically all of the breast parenchyma is below the inframammary fold. This is an area where the plastic surgeon must rely on his knowledge of body and breast proportions to judge what the woman really wants to accomplish by surgery: What is the "look" and size that she is requesting? The chest wall, lateral breast region, and even abdominal wall must be carefully evaluated before developing a surgical plan.

Women After Menopause

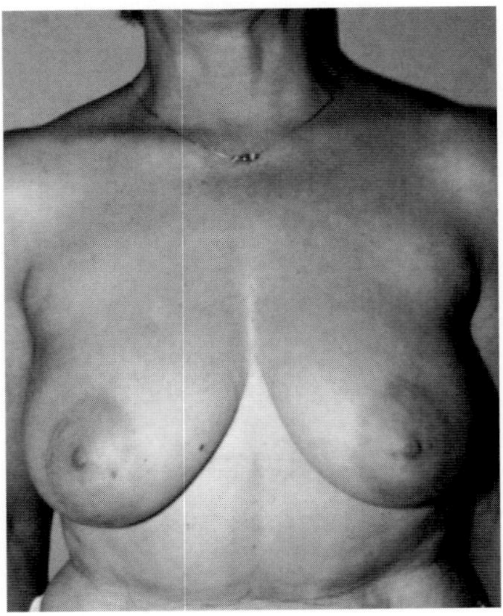

Women who request breast reduction after menopause usually exhibit significant symptoms related to excessive breast weight. Deep brassiere strap grooves can cause pressure on the brachial plexus and produce upper extremity numbness and motor symptoms. Often a rash and irritation beneath the breast develops because of skin-to-skin contact. These women have had large breasts for many years and admit to being "tired" of the weight and physical limitations they impose. They do not consider their breasts as "sexy" or alluring; they are usually realistic in their expectations and request enough tissue removal to ease their discomfort. Frequently they request that their breasts be made small enough so that they do not need the support of a brassiere.

Women With Sexual Identification Problems

Some women reject their breasts as symbols of femininity. They recognize this to varying degrees. Some admit to a masculine orientation and will tell the surgeon that they no longer want breasts. Others will not openly reveal their desire for a more masculine appearance, but instead will be intensely disappointed with a result that the surgeon and the surgical team judge to be an appropriate proportional breast reduction. They truly do not want more than a minimal masculine breast projection. They are not transsexuals but are women who do not want to have a full-figured feminine appearance. It is important to identify these patients before the operation. When they say they want to be "flat," they usually mean it. I devote considerable time to determining if they desire such a radical reduction. These women can have major underlying sexual identification problems that indicate the need for psychiatric evaluation during the preoperative decision-making process. Some are not satisfied with anything short of total mastectomies. These patients should be very carefully evaluated before they are selected for surgery. A strong possibility exists that their problems will not be resolved by surgery.

Concerns of Patient and Surgeon

BREAST SIZE

The major concern of most breast hyperplasia patients is whether their breasts can be made small enough. This is a legitimate concern. The most frequent complaint of women after this operation is that their breasts are "still too big." To meet this expectation for size and avoid reoperation, careful preoperative evaluation and planning and good communication with the patient are essential. It may be helpful to have her view photographs of other breast reduction patients who have had varying degrees of breast reduction and see which appearance most appeals to her. The surgeon also wants to avoid the distress caused when the patient feels she is too small, particularly when correction may require a breast implant and all of the associated considerations.

When the patient is overweight, it is best for her to lose weight before the breast reduction to ensure that her breasts will be the size she has requested. Preferably the woman's weight should not exceed 30 pounds over her ideal weight. Sometimes weight loss can reduce breast size sufficiently to obviate the need for a breast reduction. In addition, anesthesia-related as well as pulmonary and venous complications are higher in obese patients. The patient's overall appearance will also be improved if she loses weight. If she plans to lose weight after breast reduction, she is told that she will likely lose breast volume, but to an unpredictable degree, and that breast ptosis can develop. Often, however, the breasts become slightly elevated when they are less heavy. The estimated loss of breast volume following weight loss is influenced by the parenchyma-fat ratio in the breast. For example, a young patient who is somewhat overweight with a high percentage of breast fat would be expected to have smaller breasts if she loses weight, whereas a woman whose breasts are composed primarily of fibrous stroma and glandular tissue will not experience a comparable change in breast size after weight loss.

SCARS

Traditionally, breast reduction techniques required relatively long, significant scars around the nipple-areola, down the breast, and in the inframammary crease. Today, with the availability of short scar techniques such as vertical mammaplasty, surgeons are able to reduce or eliminate the scarring in many patients. Frequently the scar in the inframammary fold can be eliminated altogether. Although I use the periareolar purse-string approach for mastopexy and mastopexy-augmentation, I do not think it is a good choice when a significant breast reduction and nipple reduction and elevation are needed. ***When consulting with patients who request reduction mammaplasty, it is important that the location and length of possible scars be shown and described to them.*** I sometimes mark the future scars with a washable marker. Evidence of previous scar hypertrophy should be elicited and discussed with the patient who has healed with unattractive scars in the past; significant scar hypertrophy can be a reason to forego the breast reduction, or if the patient still wants to pursue this course, the surgeon should try to perform the breast reduction with shorter inframammary fold scars or use the vertical mammaplasty technique. ***Periareolar and vertical scars generally heal with less hypertrophy and widening than inframammary fold scars, especially the medial and lateral aspects of these scars.***

The size and location of scars seem to be particular concerns of the smaller breasted woman requesting minor changes in her breasts. The short scar techniques are ideal for some of these patients since it is more difficult to conceal the scars in women with small breasts.

SYMMETRY

Most breasts are asymmetric, as is the chest wall on which they are located. As a consequence, residual asymmetry is to be expected after surgery, and the patient should be so advised of her preoperative asymmetry as well as anticipated postoperative asymmetry. Many times women who request reduction mammaplasty are unaware of preexisting breast asymmetries, even though there may be a 200 gm discrepancy or more. Using photographs that I have taken or by viewing her mirror image, I show the patient that her breasts do not match and explain that while my goal will be to reduce the amount of asymmetry I cannot guarantee that symmetry will be achieved. In fact, the only guarantee that I can offer is that "she will not be perfectly symmetric," and if that is her goal, she will surely be disappointed and should reconsider her decision to have breast reduction.

When one breast is larger than the other, I try to make this breast equal to the other breast or slightly larger. It is difficult for many women to go from a larger left breast to a larger right breast. The degree of asymmetry can affect the technique selected to provide the best postoperative symmetry. (See Chapter 6 for additional discussion of this frequent area of patient concern.)

LACTATION POTENTIAL

Lactation potential seems less of a concern for the teenage breast reduction patient than it is for her mother or for the plastic surgeon. Many teenage breast reduction patients tell me they are not interested in breast-feeding. Despite their protestations, I believe it is important to preserve lactation potential. These young women can change their minds later when they mature and face the possibility of breast-feeding. ***The potential for lactation function is maximized when a major portion of the parenchyma and breast ductal system is preserved beneath the nipple.*** This is why I prefer breast reduction techniques that preserve some central breast parenchyma and ductal system and resect more breast tissue peripherally and tangentially from the breast parenchyma.

SENSATION

It is surprising how many reduction patients report minimal sensation in their breasts preoperatively. Although there are many parameters of sensation (touch, cold, heat, and vibratory), basically I take into consideration generalized touch and two-point discrimination and erogenous sensation. When the areola is distended by marked breast hypertrophy, it is left with even less sensation. The nipple usually is relatively insensitive in comparison to the areola. Sensation must be discussed with each patient before an operation is planned to determine her perception of current breast sensitivity and the importance she attaches to it. I tell my patients that general "feeling" to touch will probably be diminished right after surgery but will gradually increase in the next few weeks to months. Full sensation does not return in a small percentage of patients (usually those with large reductions) and they report a continued numbness.

Preservation of the erogenous quality of nipple-areola sensation is difficult to measure as well as predict because significant psychological and emotional factors influence the patient's perception. If, during the preoperative discussion, the patient stresses that this quality of sensation is essential to her happiness and satisfaction, I hesitate to perform the reduction. Sensation can be lost postoperatively either because of division of the nerves or because of the patient's psychological reaction to the operation—some patients do not want to touch their breasts or have them touched after breast operations. Partners, too, can be disturbed by the breast scars.

BREAST SHAPE

Breast shape is a definite focus for reduction patients; most women have specific desires for breast contour. Some women want flat chests and will only be happy with a significant volume reduction with minimal projection. Others want upper breast fullness and lower breast resection without ptosis, a difficult goal to achieve without shifting lower breast parenchyma to the upper breast region or using an implant to create the upper fullness. These desires should be thoroughly examined before an operation is planned. ***A woman's expectations for breast form will influence the planning of the operation because breast shape depends on preservation of the parenchyma in the desired areas with resection in the hypertrophic areas.***

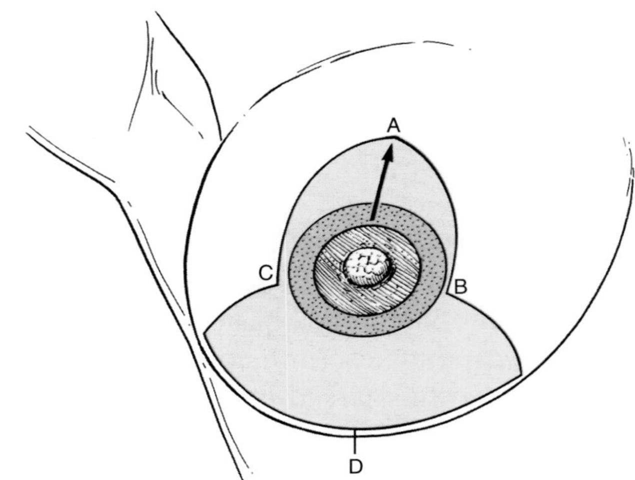

Superior pedicle technique

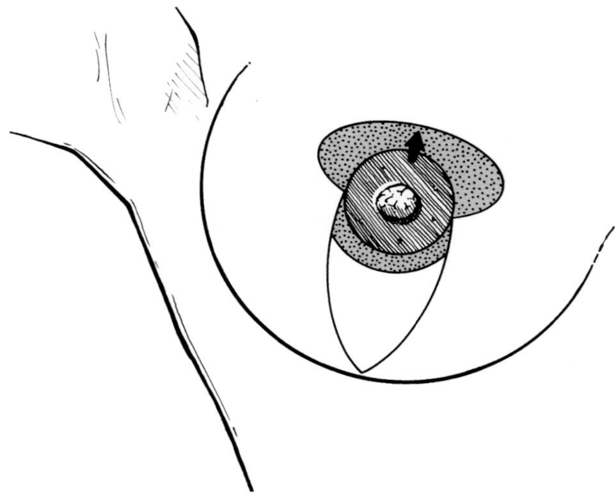

Vertical mammaplasty technique

Different techniques produce different breast shapes. ***The central pedicle technique provides central and lower projection while preserving lower breast tissue. The superior pedicle technique preserves upper and central tissue and can produce wider, boxier breasts with less lower parenchyma to droop later. The vertical approach resects lower central tissue and narrows the breast shape.*** Liposuction can further reduce the lateral chest wall and breast parenchyma and produce a nicely contoured breast shape.

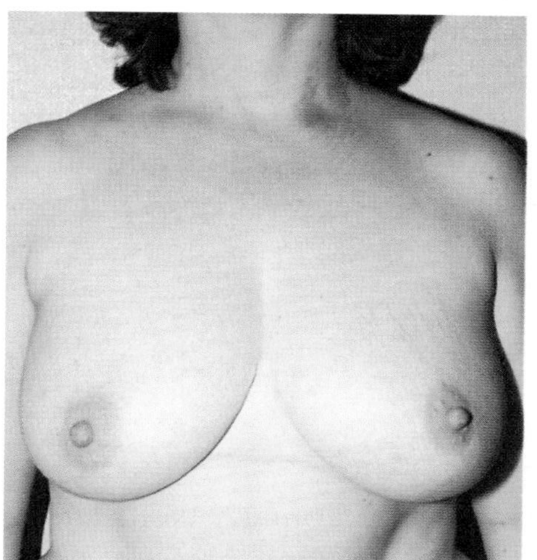
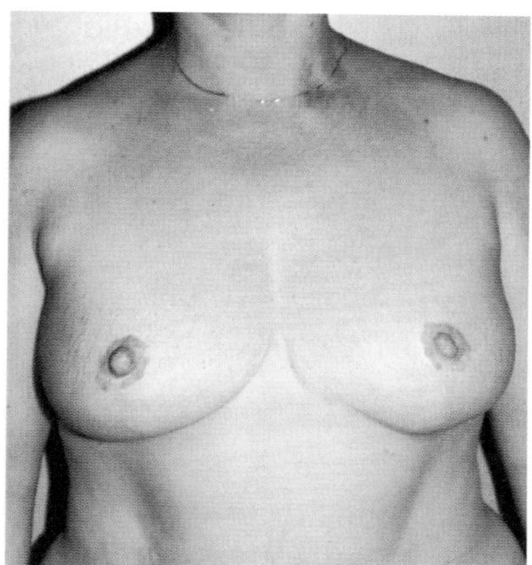

Breast shape after superior pedicle technique

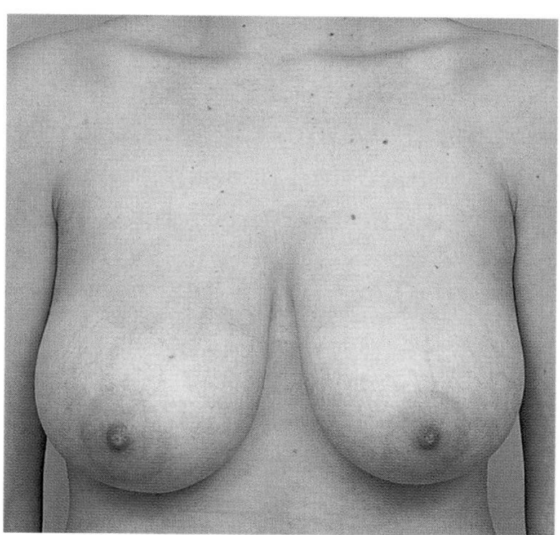
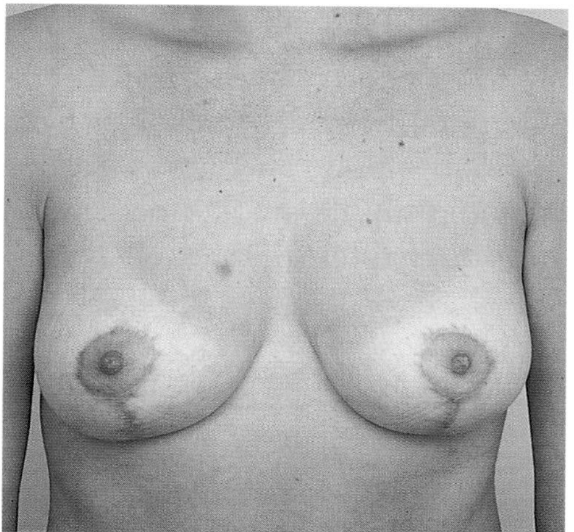

Breast shape after vertical mammaplasty technique

ONCOLOGIC CONSIDERATIONS

Many women worry about the effect of the operation on the ability to detect a breast lump or cancer on mammograms. These worries are particularly intense if a woman is past menopause or other factors place her in a high-risk group (see Chapters 10 and 18 for risk factors). Patient and physician awareness with careful preoperative, intraoperative, and postoperative monitoring is the best method for avoiding a delayed or missed diagnosis of breast cancer. This includes preoperative screening, physical examination, and mammography. I suggest mammography before breast reduction for women 30 years or older. A follow-up mammogram is then obtained 6 to 12 months postoperatively to determine and establish the postoperative baseline. Changes are usually noted on postoperative images; these can include scarring, pedicle folds, calcifications related to the operation, and fat necrosis related to liposuction. If liposuction has been used, breasts will also appear more dense.

Planning

Surgical planning focuses on skin removal, excision of fatty tissue and excess breast parenchyma, areas and volume of breast resection, areas of lateral and abdominal fullness, scar length and placement, preservation of breast function and nipple-areola sensation, and nipple-areolar size and position. A successful result and avoidance of major complications depend on the preservation of the blood supply supporting these structures. The most carefully contrived surgical plan can fail because of tissue necrosis. Most reduction techniques today depend on the upward mobilization of the nipple-areola on its underlying central breast parenchyma and secondarily on its subdermal blood supply. Therefore knowledge of the blood and nerve supply of the breast and nipple-areola is essential to ensure a safe and predictable operation (see Chapter 2).

SKIN REMOVAL

Skin excisions are necessary primarily to adjust the skin envelope to the reduced breast volume and to reposition the nipple-areola to gain access for the parenchymal excision; secondarily breast skin removal provides breast support. Excess skin is removed to conform to a smaller or more uplifted breast contour. ***Removal and tightening of breast skin should not be relied on to control and shape the breast; the actual volume removed and its location as well as the contouring and shaping of the breast parenchyma are most critical for achieving this goal.*** In fact, skin and scar contraction over the reduced breast parenchyma is necessary for the final result when using short incision techniques. If the breast skin is tightened to shape the breast during breast reduction, it often results in separation of the incisions or widening of the scars and the "T" vertically and spreading of the scars in the postoperative period.

Skin for the breast reduction is usually removed through a combination of vertical and horizontal skin excisions. I have found three basic approaches to skin removal to be most effective for different degrees of reduction: vertical, horizontal, and periareolar. I increasingly rely on the vertical approach.

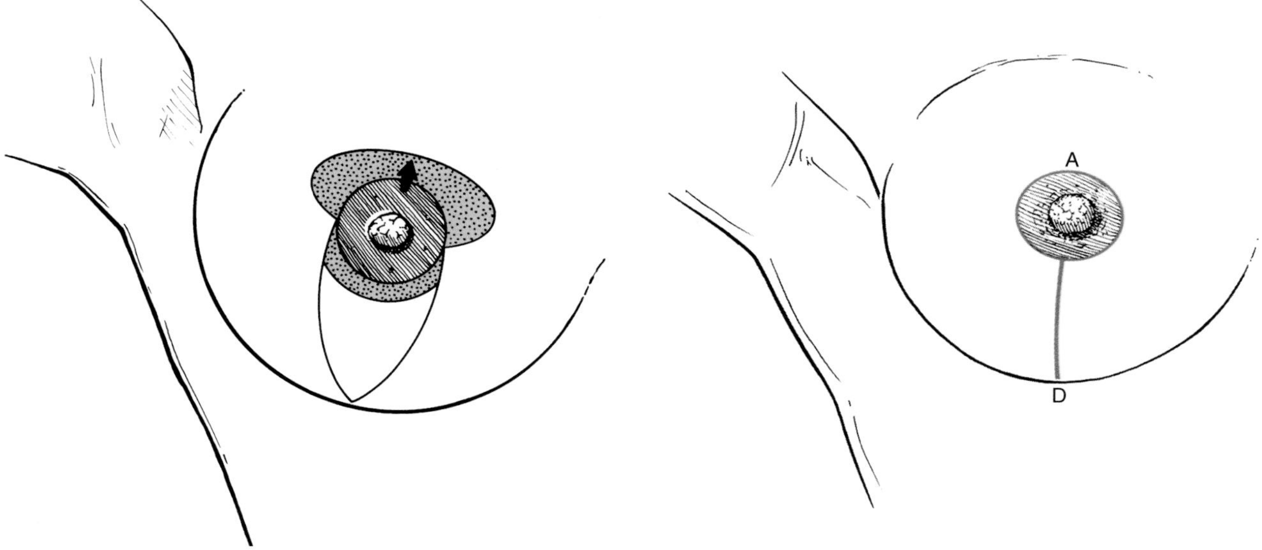

The vertical approach permits removal of the lower region of breast parenchyma and the lower breast, and when combined with liposuction, it permits significant breast reduction. A periareolar and vertical skin excision will elevate the nipple-areola and the breast to correct ptosis. The excess breast parenchyma is excised through the vertical excisions as well as both central, inferior, inferomedial, and lateral excisions. The horizontal incision is made 1 to 3 cm above the initial inframammary fold. Lower breast skin is converted to upper chest skin.

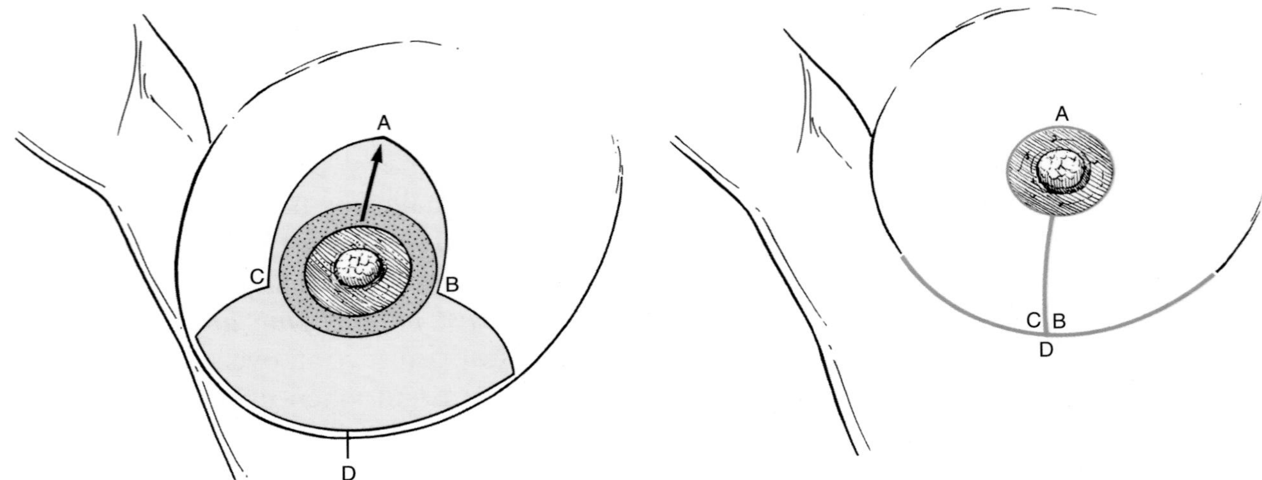

For larger breast reductions the traditional wide vertical and horizontal ellipse provides versatility in removing excess skin and contouring the breast. The skin is excised in three planes, but primarily in a vertical and horizontal orientation as well as above the areola. These skin excision techniques permit the surgical correction of a wide variety of breast deformities. By tightening the lower pole of the breast they contribute to the creation of a conical breast shape while minimizing ptosis. An inverted T closure completes these excisions. With this approach the surgeon can control the distance from the clavicle to the nipple-areola and from the nipple to the inframammary crease; the width of the breast can also be controlled from the nipple-areola downward to the inframammary fold.

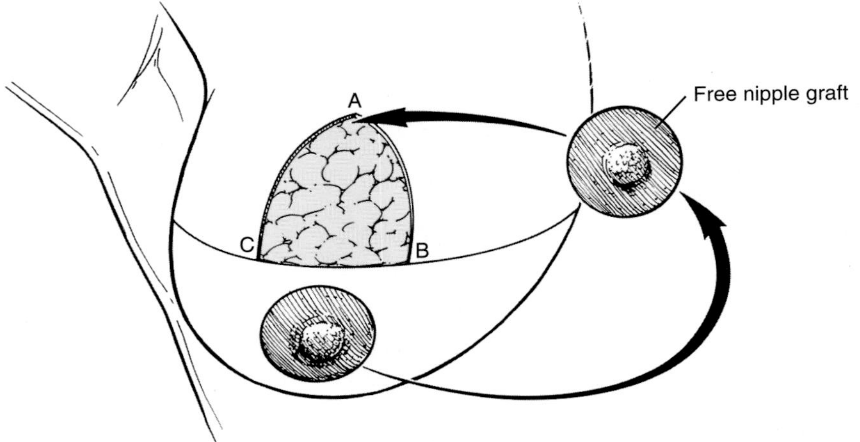

Similar inverted T excisions are used with the free nipple graft technique. The parenchyma is usually excised from the lower as well as the central or lateral breast regions to correct breast ptosis and narrow the breast.

AREAS OF BREAST RESECTION

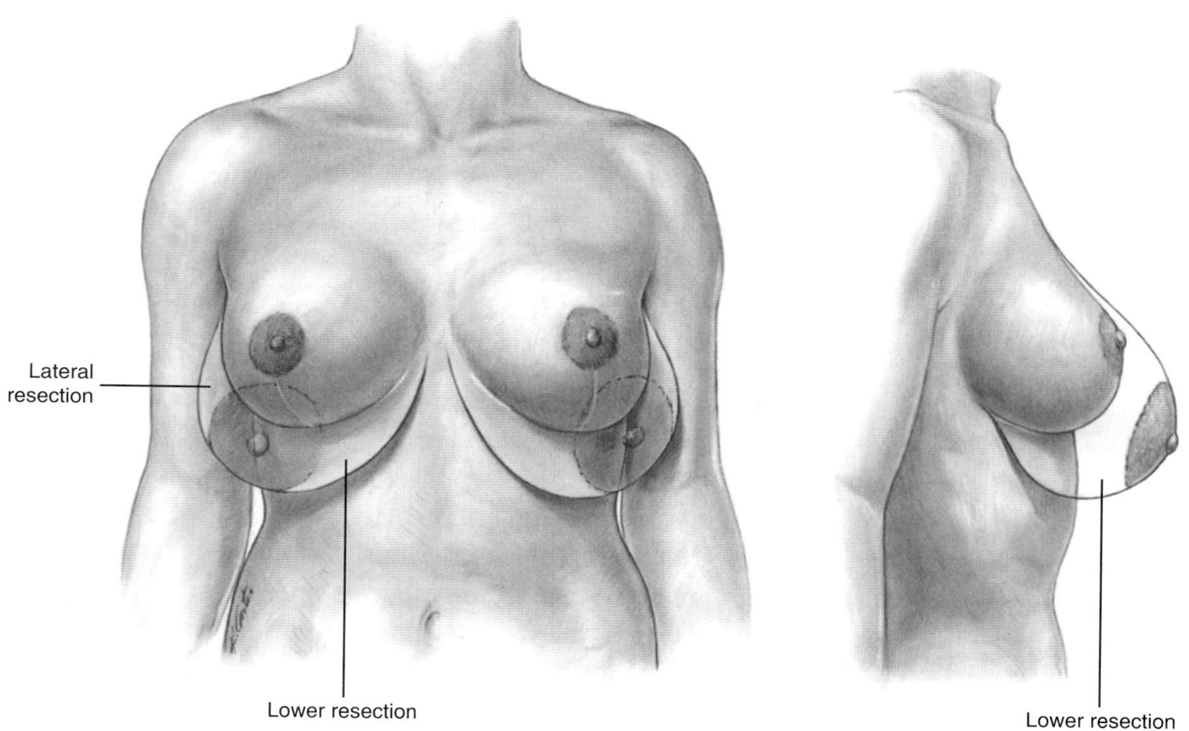

Removal of breast parenchymal volume in areas of excess improves early breast form and also increases the likelihood of a long-lasting correction that does not rely on taut skin. Because most breast reduction patients have acceptable or even deficient upper breast tissue (this tissue has often fallen and the upper breast fullness characteristic of the youthful breast has been lost), I avoid removing breast parenchyma from the upper, medial, and central breast areas. Liposuction at the time of the reduction can be used to further contour those areas where there is considerable hypertrophy, thereby permitting shorter incisions and promoting postoperative wound contraction and tightening.

AMOUNT OF BREAST REDUCTION

The patient's current breast volume and the proposed percentage of reduction and intended volume after reduction should be estimated. Determination of size is made in concert with the patient to most accurately ensure that the volume of her reduced breasts will meet her expectations. It is helpful to understand how brassieres are sized because that is the way most women conceptualize, discuss, and explain their desired breast size.

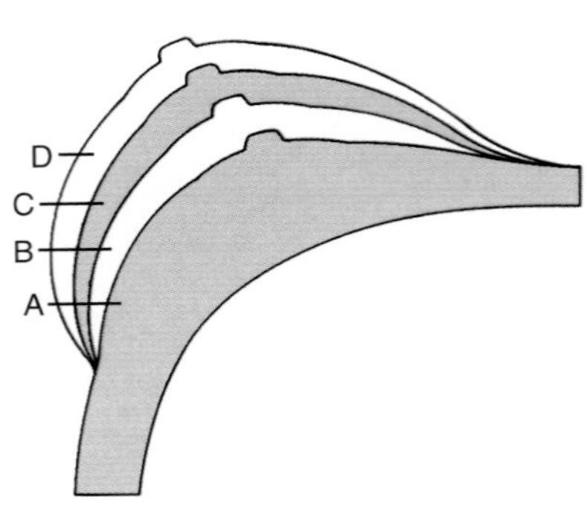

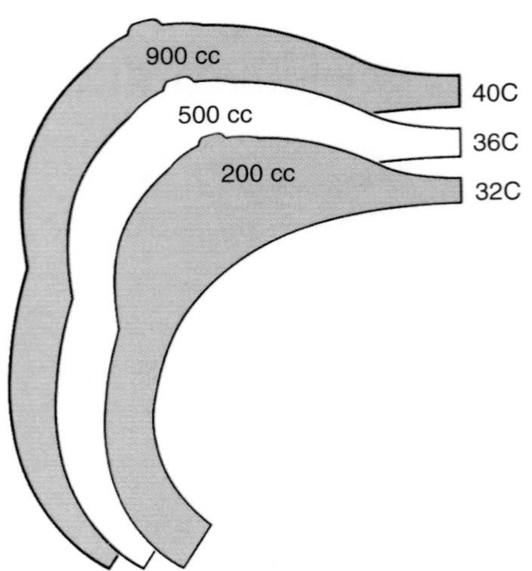

Although there is no sizing standard for brassieres, most manufacturers seem to follow the general rule that as the chest circumference increases, the brassiere cup must allow for progressively greater volume for each lettered brassiere size. Therefore a woman with a 40-inch chest circumference and size D breasts would require a relatively larger reduction to become a size 40B than if her chest circumference were 34 inches and her breasts were size D. These are only approximations. I never promise or guarantee a postoperative brassiere size because of the variations among manufacturers, individual variations and preferences, and various brassiere fittings.

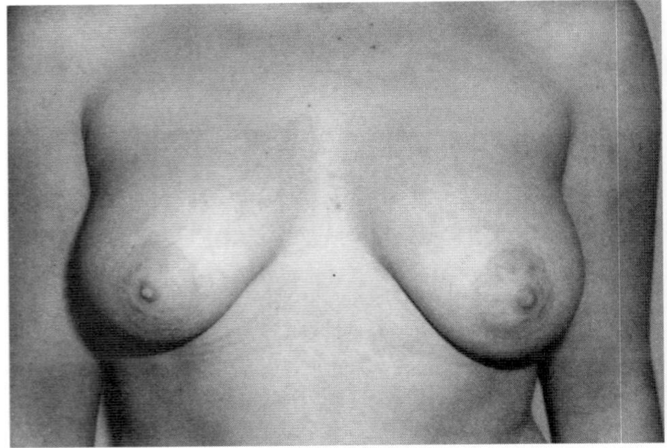

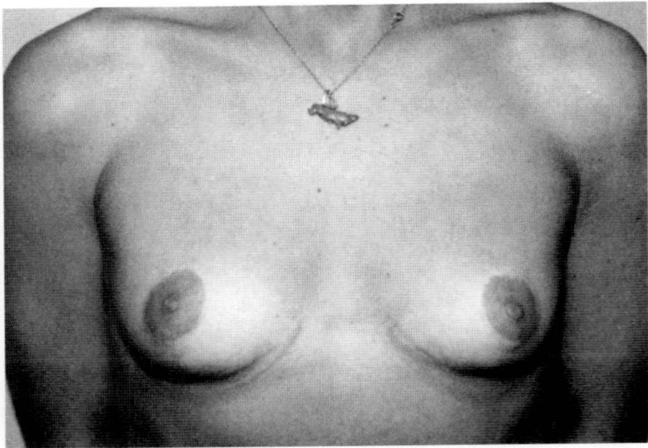

This 19-year-old patient is 5 feet 6 inches tall and weighs 120 pounds. Her chest circumference is 34 inches and she wears a 34D brassiere. Reduction of 300 gm in each breast made her a size 34B postoperatively.

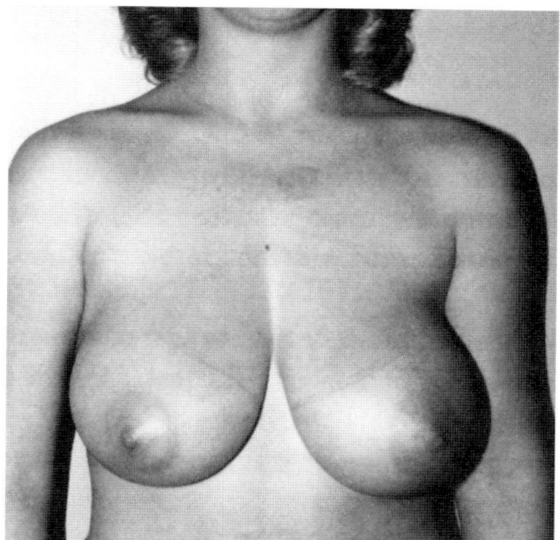

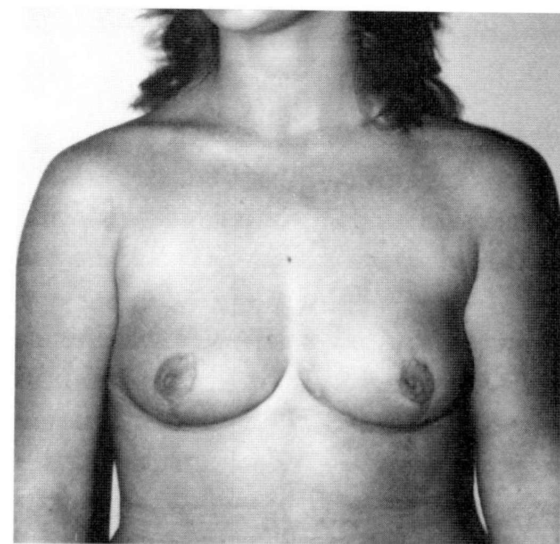

This 20-year-old woman wanted to wear a smaller size than the 40D brassiere she now required. A reduction of 800 gm in each breast gave her size 40B breasts.

Frequently third-party providers request a preoperative estimate of the volume to be resected; a minimum weight of 500 gm per breast or greater is required for inclusion under the provider contract. In an effort to reduce reimbursements for these operations they classify smaller reductions as mastopexies, which are not reimbursed because they are considered "cosmetic" procedures. This size limitation is unfortunate and clinically questionable because smaller women may derive significant relief from removal of volumes of breast parenchyma less than 500 gm per side. ***The plastic surgeon should make a practice of documenting the volume of breast reductions and of mastectomies as well as estimates of the breast implant volumes. These estimates, along with experience, will help in determining the expected volume of the breast reduction.***

Judging volume discrepancy is helpful in planning resections for asymmetric breasts. It is not the amount of tissue that is removed but rather the amount to be preserved that is key to producing a balanced result. Regardless of the volume resected, the most important concern for the patient is that the proper amount of parenchyma is preserved in the proper location so that her breasts are aesthetically contoured to her satisfaction. If one side is larger preoperatively, I try to let it remain the larger side postoperatively. It is more difficult for the woman's body image to transfer sides of an asymmetry. When there is a breast asymmetry, I usually mark the anticipated additional resection in grams on the larger breast. This marking is a reminder that more should be removed from this side; it also affords me the opportunity to check my estimates of breast volume.

INCISION LENGTH AND PLACEMENT

I use a spectrum of incisions to resect breast parenchyma and to remove and recontour the skin cover after the resection. For smaller breast reductions (up to 500 to 1000 gm per breast) requiring minimal nipple elevation with closure of the nipple defect and vertical excess skin resection, I use a vertical scar technique that results in scars extending as much as 7 to 8 cm below the areola and occasionally 1 or 2 cm beneath the inframammary fold. (These scars will contract and shorten postoperatively with skin and wound contraction.) This approach is particularly appropriate for younger women who have better skin elasticity and whose scars tend to heal with more hypertrophy.

As the skin excess increases, there is more breast ptosis and breast hypertrophy. When the volume of reduction is greater than 500 to 1000 gm per breast or smaller in older women with poor skin elasticity, a horizontal limb is added to the vertical limb, shortening the vertical distance and removing excess skin laterally. The horizontal incision also gives additional access for resection of the lower pole. Traditionally, this horizontal scar was marked in the inframammary crease with the patient standing. ***A shorter scar can be created, however, if the incision is marked with the patient supine, which causes the inframammary fold to rise slightly, permitting the medial and lateral extents of the excision and scar to be better contoured to fit the new, smaller breast shape.*** It is important, however, to resect medial and lateral parenchyma beneath the scars to avoid bulges in these regions postoperatively.

In selected patients with good skin elasticity who require a small reduction, the short horizontal incision is moved upward another 1 to 2 cm, further shortening the scars. ***Incisions should be placed so that the resulting scars are out of the patient's vision on frontal or lateral view when she is standing.***

LATERAL AND ABDOMINAL FULLNESS

When the entire lateral chest and breast have become full and ptotic as a unit, sometimes extending around to the back, especially in cases of mild to moderate obesity, lateral breast fullness must be addressed. I generally use liposuction for these areas because this lateral breast tissue often cannot be fully resected. This approach results in shorter incisions and a better postoperative contour by reducing the breasts laterally, providing some lateral breast definition, and giving the appearance of narrower breasts. If only the central breast is to be reduced and the lateral breast preserved, this considerable lateral fullness persists and looks disproportionately wide and large compared to the smaller, reshaped breasts.

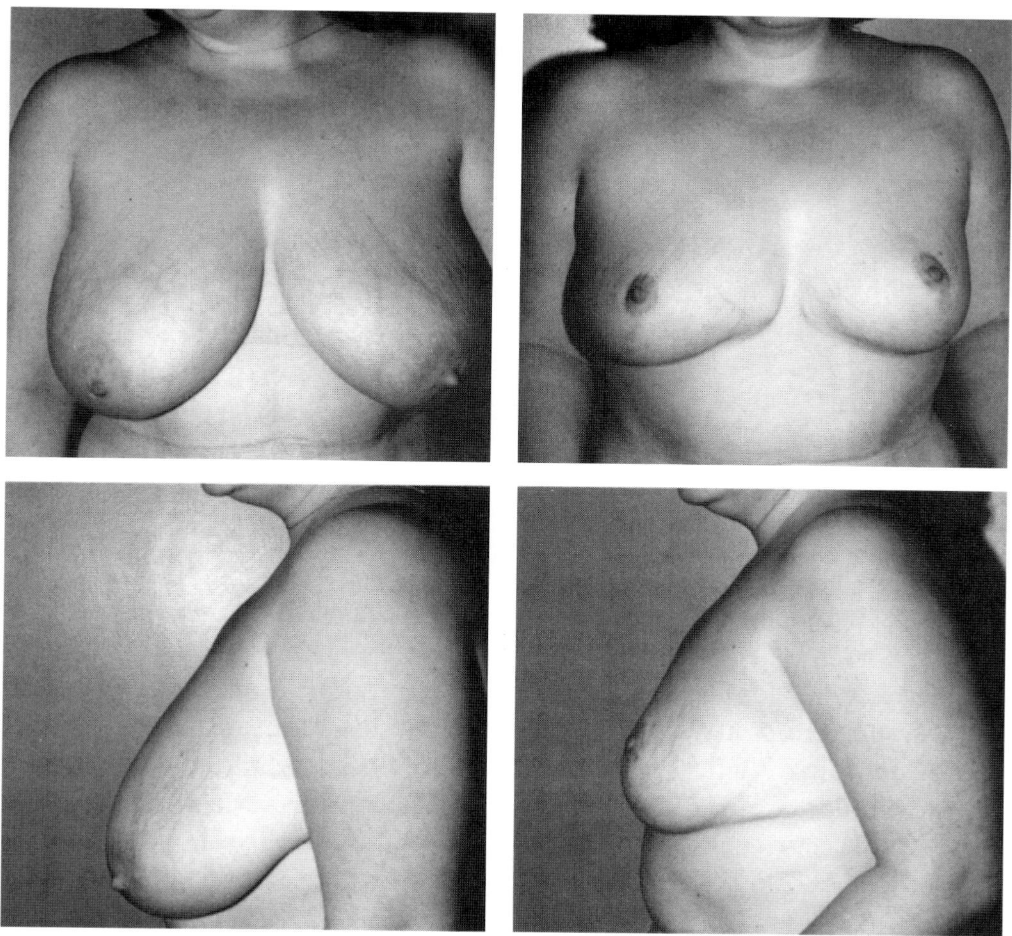

This 35-year-old woman had excess lateral chest wall and breast fullness. The reduction mammaplasty incisions were extended laterally to enable additional lateral resection and a smooth contour of the lateral chest-breast junction. Liposuction was also used to reduce and contour this lateral tissue.

Since proportion involves the entire torso, the abdominal contour should also be considered before reduction and discussed with the patient to avoid postoperative distress. She should understand that if her abdomen is protuberant, reducing and lifting the breasts off a full upper abdomen can reveal or seem to accentuate this condition. That is another reason for suggesting preoperative weight loss for the heavy patient. Alternatively, abdominoplasty or liposuction of the abdomen is planned in conjunction with a breast reduction or at a secondary operation.

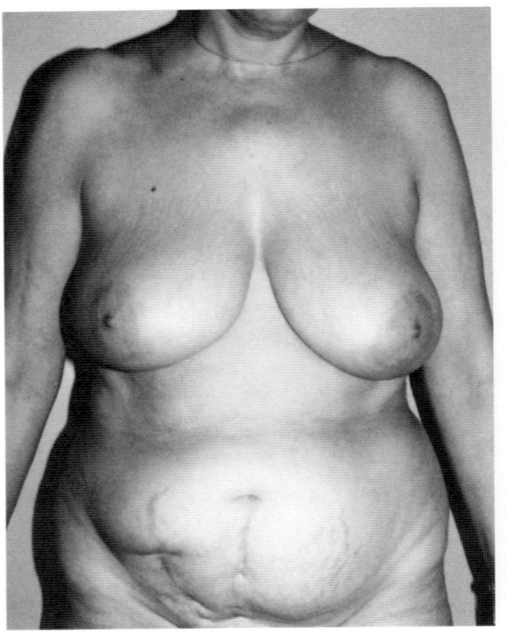 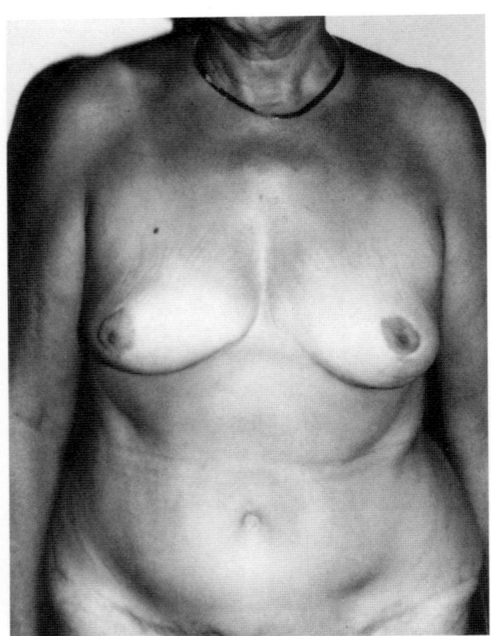

This 45-year-old woman requested breast reduction; however, her abdominal scars and deformity were so marked that she requested an abdominoplasty be combined with the breast reduction. She is delighted with the overall improvement, and the abdominoplasty is an important component of the result.

PRESERVATION OF BREAST AND NIPPLE SENSATION

Most breast reduction techniques depend on the cutaneous blood supply entering from the breast periphery and breast base via the intercostal perforators and external mammary artery. Sensory nerves accompany most of these segmental vessels within the breast. The fourth anterior lateral and medial intercostal nerves are important for nipple-areolar innervation; with careful dissection, these nerves and vessels can be identified extending through the breast to the areolar region. Additionally, there is significant overlap from the adjacent third and fifth anterolateral segments and from similar levels of anteromedial intercostal segmental nerves.

Techniques that preserve the breast on its deep, posterior, or medial attachments usually have a predictably satisfactory nipple-areolar innervation. Although sensation may be decreased in the postoperative period, it often returns a few weeks or months later.

The innervation of the skin of the upper and central chest comes from the cervical plexus and supraclavicular nerves. When a free nipple graft technique is used, the graft is placed on this deepithelialized skin. Within a few weeks of the operation most patients report a return of sensation with reinnervation of the nipple through the skin graft dermal bed.

SIZE AND POSITION OF NIPPLE-AREOLA

Breast reduction permits alterations of the areolar diameter and level, adjustment of nipple-areolar inclination, reduction of a protruding nipple, and correction of nipple inversion. Most patients with breast hypertrophy also have expanded, enlarged areolae. Although there will be a natural decrease in areolar diameter when the underlying breast volume is reduced, after appropriate discussion with the patient, I often suggest additional reduction of the areolar diameter at the time of breast reduction to make it proportional to the new breast size. The woman's preference for areolar diameter is considered in planning; usually a diameter of 4.0 to 4.5 cm is considered attractive for the smaller reduced breast and 4.5 to 5.5 cm for larger breasts.

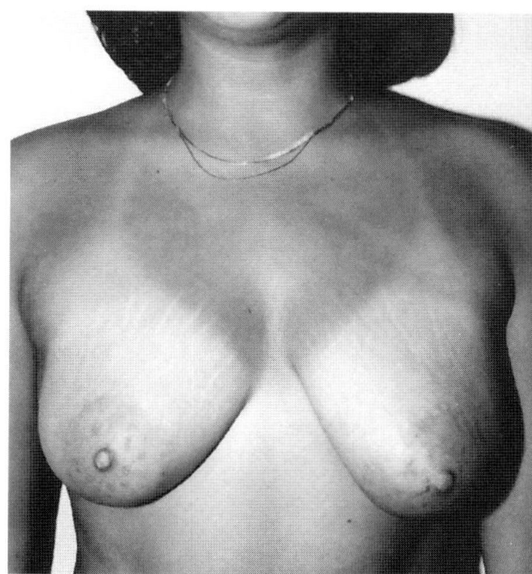

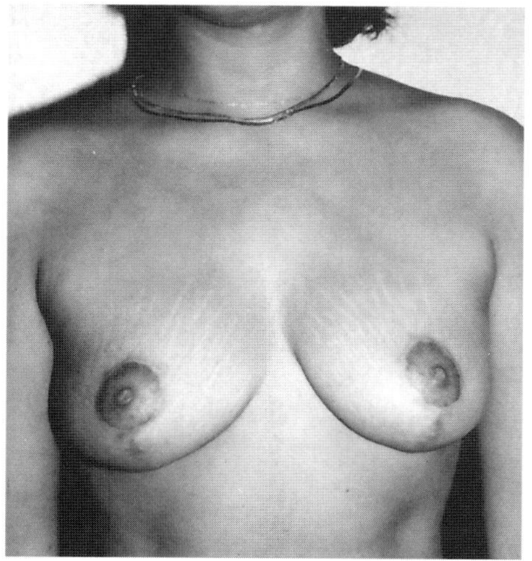

Reduction of areolar size should be proportional to the new breast volume. The scar around the areola should be a fine line, just as thin as that for a periareolar augmentation. To ensure a fine line the nipple-areola should move to the new site easily, without skin tension or underlying parenchymal tightness or restriction that could cause nipple inversion. ***Tension on the skin closure is also avoided; this is accomplished by cutting the areolar diameter larger than its planned final diameter.*** The more the areola is expanded over a tight breast, the more it will usually contract. I prefer to cut the recipient area for the areola about 2 to 5 mm smaller in diameter so that the skin edges are lightly approximated and the closure is without tension. To minimize the lower skin removal, periareolar short scar techniques reliant on removal of excess central breast skin are avoided. These techniques often result in a tight central periareolar closure, central breast flatness, and an unattractive wide scar as a focal point on the newly reduced breast. The distance from the nipple to the inframammary crease also varies as the breasts enlarge. The length varies from 7 cm for 32B breasts to 10 cm for 42C breasts.

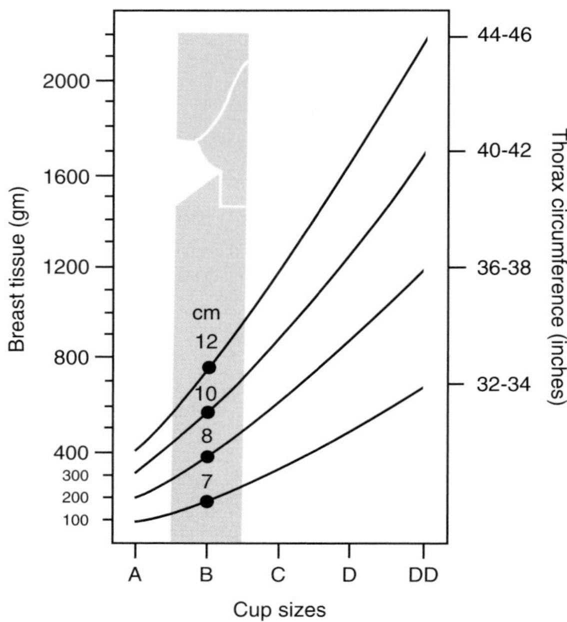

Relationship of nipple to inframammary fold distance with increasing breast volume

The distance from the nipple to the inframammary crease must be progressively longer as breast volume increases. For example, an 800 gm breast, size 42B, would have a greater distance from nipple to inframammary crease than a size 36B with a 7 cm distance. These distances apply to the inverted T techniques. The reduced breasts tend to "settle" down and increase in length postoperatively, especially when the inferior pedicle technique is used. This length can be a few centimeters longer with the vertical scar technique because the lower parenchyma has been resected and the scar tends to contract and shorten in the postoperative period.

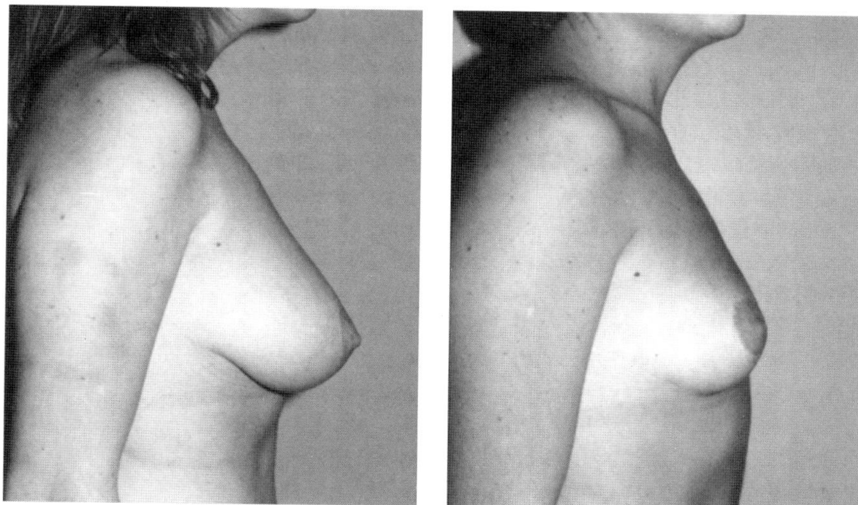

This patient's postoperative brassiere size is 34B; the distance from her inframammary crease to nipple is 7 cm.

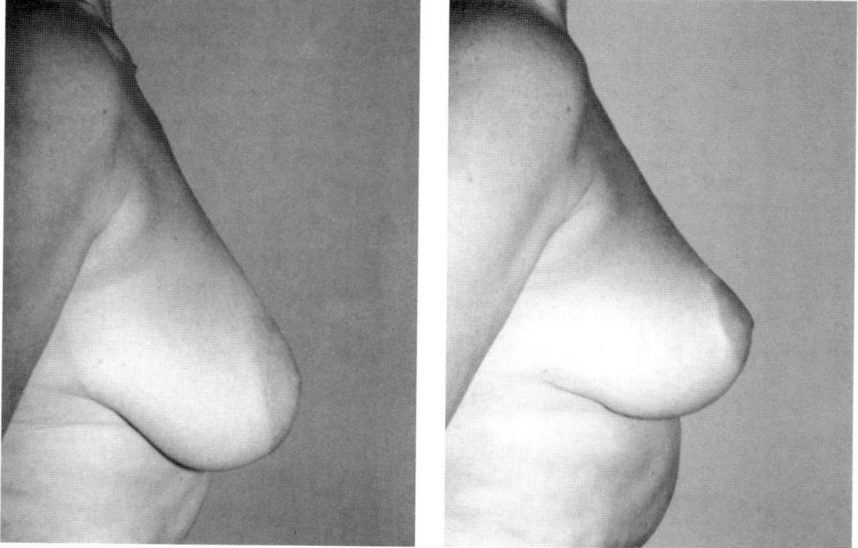

This patient's postoperative brassiere size is 38C; the distance from her nipple to inframammary crease is 9 cm.

REDUCTION MAMMAPLASTY WORKSHEET

PATIENT DATA
Name: ______
Age: ______ Height: ______ Weight: ______
Married: ______ Single: ______
Nulliparous: ______ Pregnancies: ______
Children: ______ Nursing: ______

ONCOLOGIC INFORMATION
Family history of breast CA: ______
Prev. breast cancer: ______
Prev. breast surg.: ______
Mastodynia: ______
Fibrocystic chg.: ______
Breast disease: ______
Mammogram: ______
Masses: R ______ L ______
Biopsies: R ______ L ______

MEDICAL INFORMATION
Systemic disease: ______
Diabetes: ______
Bleeding problems: ______
Allergies: ______
Medications: ______
Smoking (pk-yr): ______
Alcohol/wk: ______
Other: ______

______

PHYSICAL EXAMINATION
Chest wall:
Pectus defor.: ______ Scoliosis: ______
Asymmetries: R ______ L ______
Constriction: R ______ L ______
Tubular: R ______ L ______
Striae: R ______ L ______
Breast scars: ______
Neurologic exam:
Normal: ______ Problem: ______

INFORMED CONSENT
Verbal explan.: ______ Signed form: ______
Bleed sheet: ______ Preop. mamm.: ______
FDA info.: ______ Mfg. info.: ______

EXPECTATIONS ______

______

SPECIFIC DESIRES
To achieve: ______

______

To avoid: ______

______

SYMPTOMS ______

______

MEASUREMENTS AND PLAN

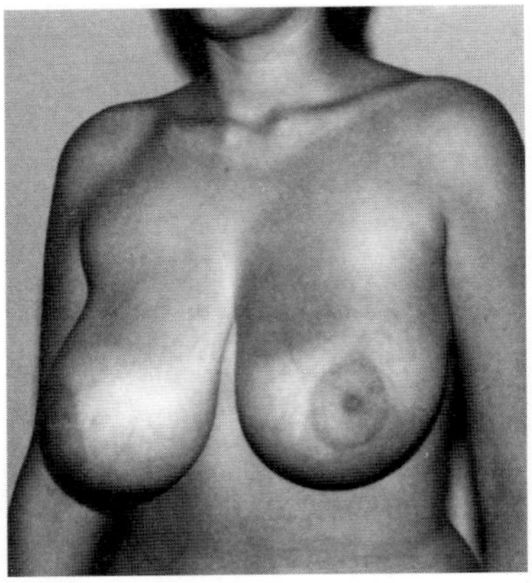

Chest circum.: ______
Bra size: ______
Breast width:
R ______ cm L ______ cm
N → infr. cr.:
R ______ cm L ______ cm
SN → N:
R ______ cm L ______ cm
Vol.: R ______
L ______

PLANNED REDUCTION
Resection: R ______ L ______
Areolar diameter: R ______ L ______
Lateral folds: ______
Abdominal excess: ______

TECHNIQUE
Vertical pedicle: ______
Superior pedicle: ______
Inferior pedicle: ______
Free nipple graft: ______

______

Liposuction: SAL: ______ UAL: ______

IMPRESSIONS AND NOTES ______

______

PLAN ______

______

______

SURGICAL OPTIONS FOR BREAST REDUCTION

VERTICAL MAMMAPLASTY

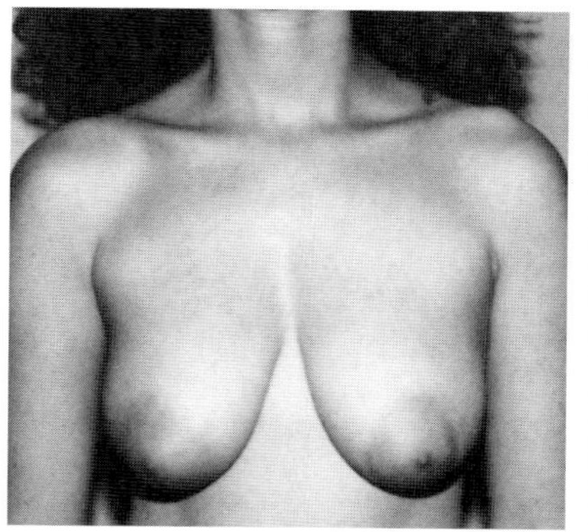

Age: Young (premenopausal)
Skin quality: Elastic
Breast size: <800 gm
Nipple elevation: <5 cm

SUPERIOR PEDICLE

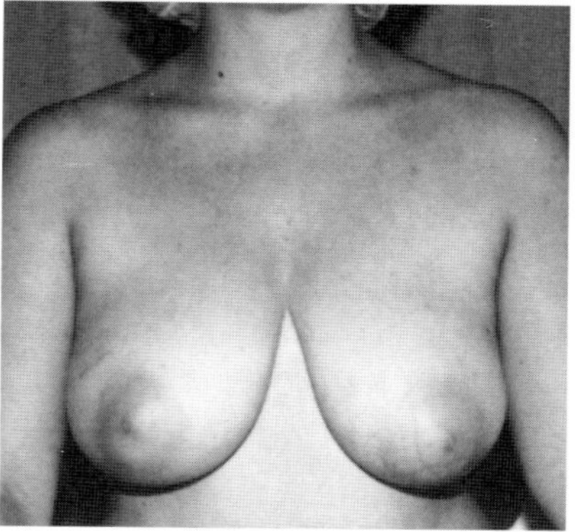

Age: Any
Skin quality: Elastic
Breast size: <800 gm
Nipple elevation: <7 cm

SUPERIOR MEDIAL PEDICLE

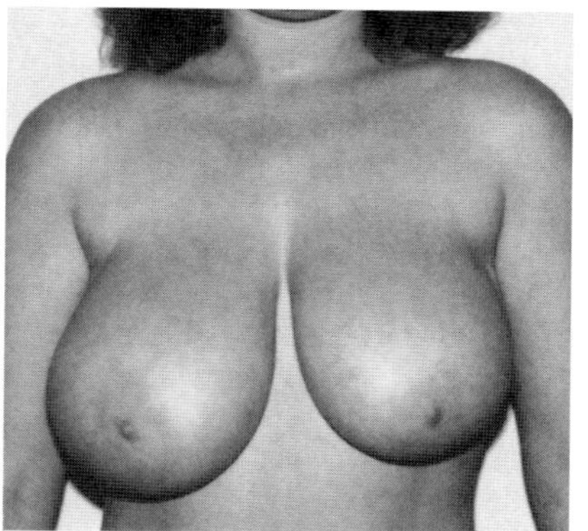

Age: Any
Skin quality: Any
Breast size: <2000 gm
Nipple elevation: >5 cm

INFERIOR CENTRAL PEDICLE

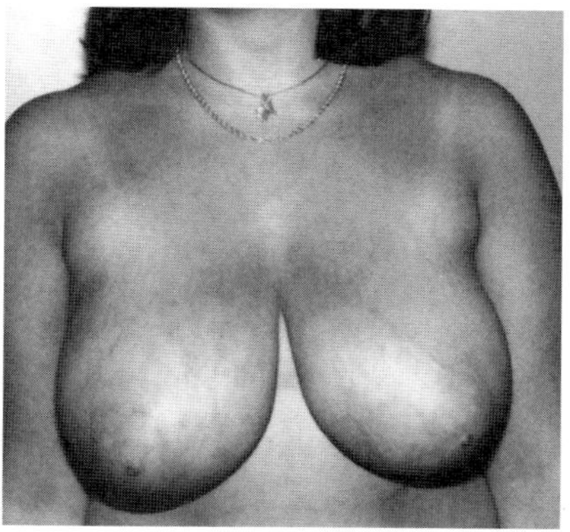

Age: Any
Skin quality: Any
Breast size: Any
Nipple elevation: Any

FREE NIPPLE GRAFT

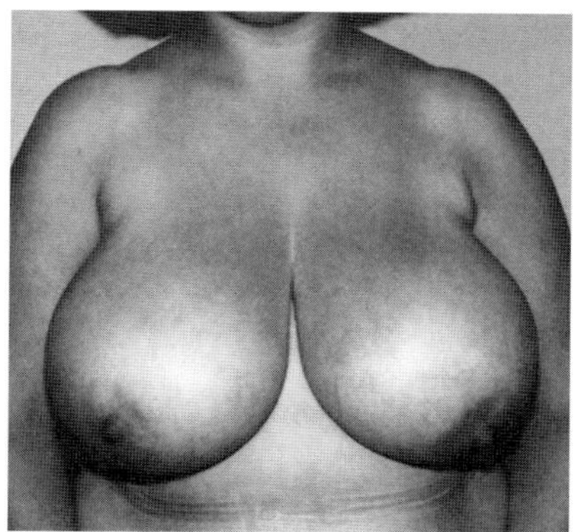

Age: Postmenopausal
Skin quality: Any
Breast size: >800 gm
Nipple elevation: >7 cm

Surgical Approach: Matching the Technique to the Problem

Because the specifications for breast reduction will vary with each patient, depending on age, skin quality, breast size, nipple position, and desire for change, the surgeon needs to be skilled in a number of different techniques that can be applied or modified for each individual.

Most breast reduction techniques in which the vertical or inverted T closure is used elevate the nipple-areola toward the clavicle. The nipple-areola must move to the new position upward and medial and remain attached to the underlying central breast parenchyma. A more medial inclination of the elevated nipple-areola on a smaller breast should be considered in preoperative planning. Preoperative mobility of the nipple-areola and underlying breast parenchyma also influences selection of the technique.

Options for breast reduction
- Vertical mammaplasty with liposuction
- Superior pedicle
- Superior medial pedicle
- Inferior central pedicle
- Free nipple graft

Patients whose breasts are soft with elastic, mobile skin and underlying breast parenchyma require minimal external and parenchymal incisions to elevate their nipple-areolae. These patients are candidates for vertical techniques or transposition of the nipple-areola on a superior central breast parenchymal pedicle (superior pedicle technique). These techniques are also useful for the full, wide breast that does not need much upward mobility of the nipple.

In patients with tighter, dense parenchyma there will be greater resistance to upward nipple-areolar movement. More mobility of the nipple-areola will usually require additional breast parenchymal releases. In addition to vertical mammaplasty techniques, the superior and superior medial parenchymal pedicle transfer (superior and superior medial pedicle techniques) are suitable for these patients.

The mobility of the nipple-areola on the inferior central parenchymal pedicle (inferior pedicle technique) is appropriate for women with larger, wider, pendulous breasts requiring larger breast reductions (500 to 2000 gm) with higher density requiring transposition from a greater distance. These women should have good microcirculation. This technique is also useful for reducing the breasts of women with smaller, firmer breasts whose nipple-areola would be elevated with difficulty. The greater versatility and ease of nipple-areolar positioning and preservation of function and sensation make this technique a possible option for all types of breast reductions. However, experience has shown that the inferior central pedicle technique does not always provide the long-term correction anticipated because the preserved lower breast parenchyma can "bottom out" and descend below the inframammary fold.

For patients with good skin elasticity and thickness (usually younger patients) or those requiring smaller reductions with good upward mobility of the nipple-areolae on the parenchyma, the vertical mammaplasty technique is used. Liposuction is a useful adjunct for reducing additional volume throughout the breast as well as the periphery of the breast. If the parenchyma is reduced appropriately and the skin is elastic, this short scar technique produces the desired result and leaves well-concealed scars. It can enhance shape while correcting ptosis, providing some upper fill and narrowing a wide breast. A young woman who has a relatively small reduction will not be pleased with the aesthetic result if she is left with long hypertrophic scars.

When the patient's breasts are large and ptotic with the likelihood of deceased or compromised parenchymal blood flow and increased risk of fat necrosis (older patients, those with fatty postmenopausal breasts, and patients who smoke cigarettes), the inferior and lateral resection combined with the free nipple-areola graft technique (free graft technique) can be a good, safe choice that is frequently selected. To achieve more reduction, additional parenchyma can be removed with liposuction. These patients often have striated breast skin that is thin and inelastic and lacks sufficient resiliency to contract and tighten optimally after the short scar technique. For these individuals the traditional longer inverted T reduction incisions are preferred to produce the best early shape and to contour the breast skin. Fortunately scars in older women tend to heal as fine lines if closed without unnecessary tension.

Lactation potential is lost when the free graft technique is used. Many women with very large breasts, however, report little preoperative sensation and minimize its importance in relation to the benefits gained from smaller, more comfortable breasts. They frequently report sensation in the grafted nipple-areola. The graft is probably reinnervated from the underlying de-epithelialized skin. Safety is ensured if the skin is not elevated from the underlying gland, which contains large vessels in the subdermal plexus. The ability to shape a smaller breast is also less restricted when pedicles for the nipple-areola are not developed.

VERTICAL MAMMAPLASTY WITH LIPOSUCTION

Lejour has been a major force in popularizing the vertical mammaplasty technique. After learning of the technique from Lassus, she demonstrated that the vertical reduction technique could be combined with liposuction to remove breast fat in all of the hypertrophic areas to produce an aesthetically contoured breast. ***This vertical technique narrows the breasts, removes fat and lowers ptotic tissue through inframammary and central lower breast resections, and avoids the undesirable medial and lateral incisions by using a vertical accordion closure.*** The width of the breast is reduced horizontally, shortened vertically, and reduced significantly by using this technique. This approach also decreases the base circumference of the breast as well as the lateral width and elevates the inframammary crease. A significant volume of breast parenchyma can be removed through excision of the lower breast parenchyma, and the inframammary fold elevation decreases the amount of skin traditionally resected, resulting in shorter vertical scars. Elevation of the inframammary fold converts lower breast skin to chest wall skin and makes the breasts appear elevated and more youthful in appearance.

Liposuction is performed prior to resection to tailor fatty areas. The percentage of fat within the breast is variable, and it is difficult to predict preoperatively how much can be removed. As with all breast surgery, preoperative examination, including oncologic evaluation and breast imaging, is necessary for all patients 30 years or older. After liposuction the breasts are bruised for 3 to 4 weeks and remain tender, swollen, and firm for several more months. The breasts will appear more dense on mammograms and calcifications can form. I tend to reserve liposuction for younger women. Many women note that there is more pain and discomfort in the areas of liposuction than in the areas of actual surgical breast reduction.

This technique is appropriate for small as well as for larger breasts. It can be successfully used in young women with full, nonptotic breasts with excellent skin elasticity who are to have a reduction of up to 1500 gm in each breast. ***Younger women with good skin elasticity and full breasts particularly benefit from liposuction as part of this procedure.***

This technique is somewhat more technically and artistically demanding and the beginner should start with mastopexies and smaller resections. The inframammary fold skin may require subsequent revision. Lejour reports that 10% of her patients undergo secondary revision of the lower scar.

OPERATIVE OVERVIEW

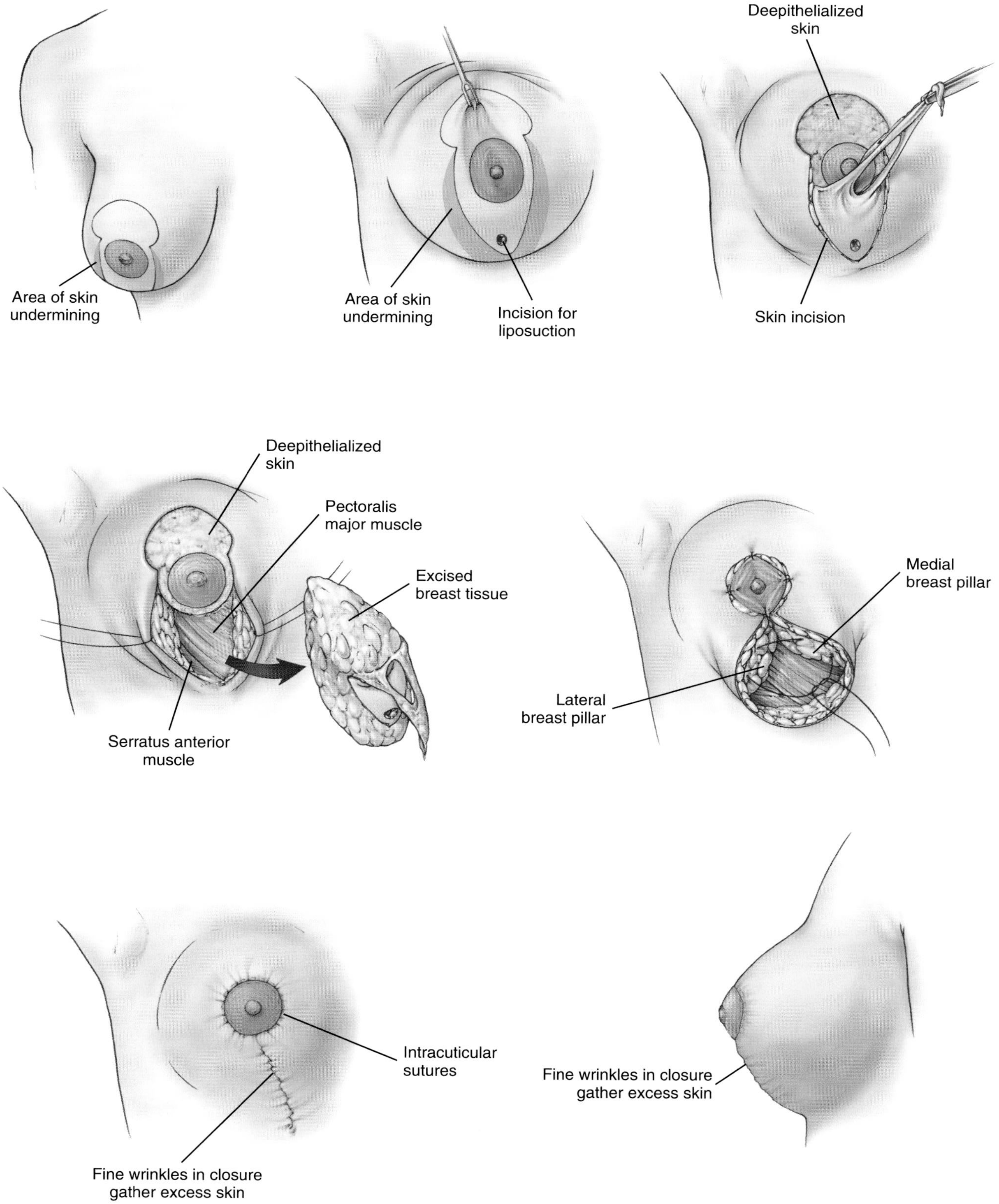

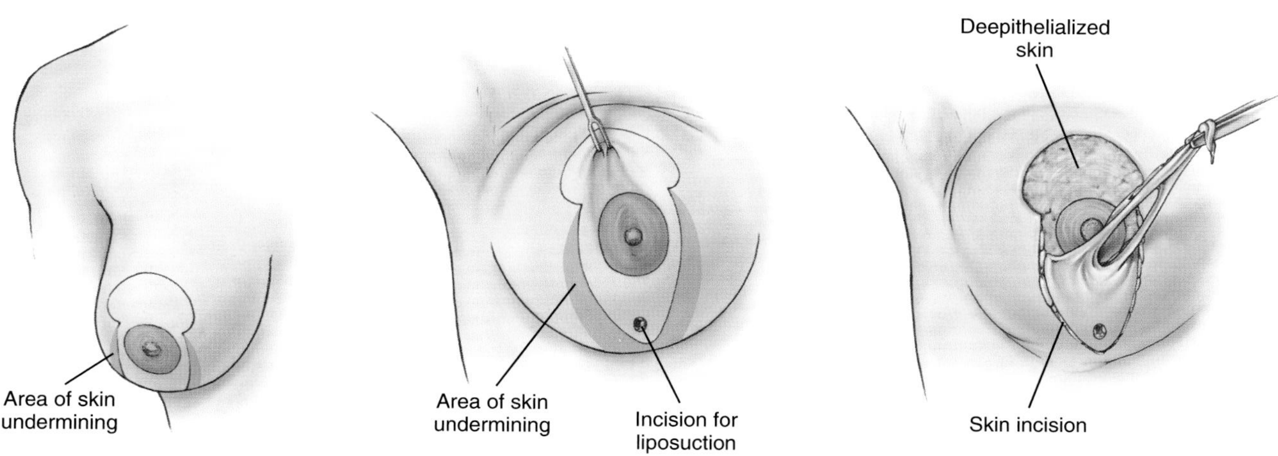

Markings and Technique

The markings for vertical breast reduction are made with the patient in an upright position. This can either be done preoperatively with the patient sitting up or with the anesthetized patient on the operating table and elevated to a sitting position.

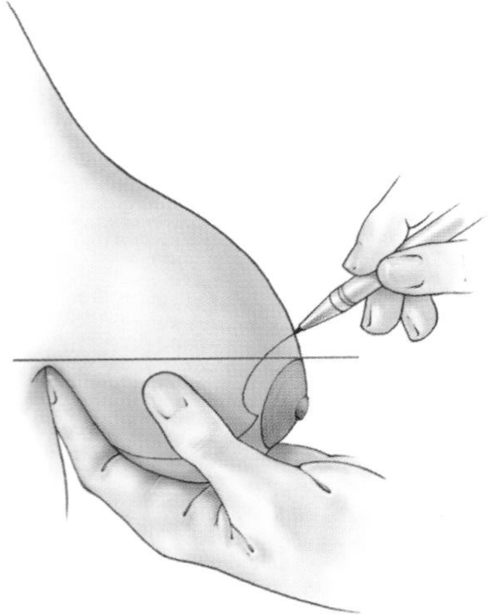

The top of the future areola is marked; it should be located about 2 cm above the inframammary fold. The diameter of the final nipple is determined; this is usually around 40 to 45 mm. A point is chosen on the breast line about 2 to 3 cm above the inframammary fold.

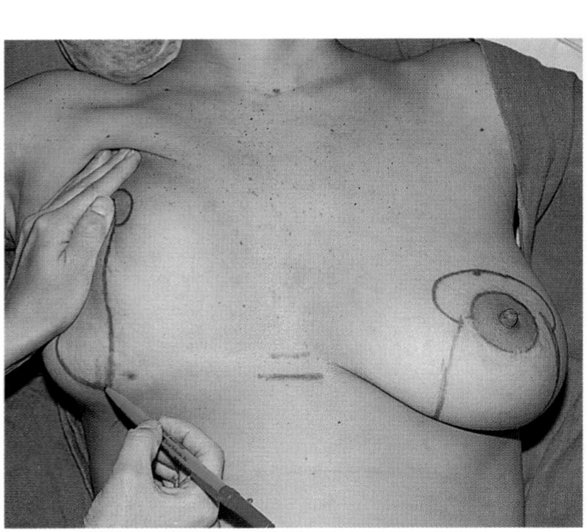

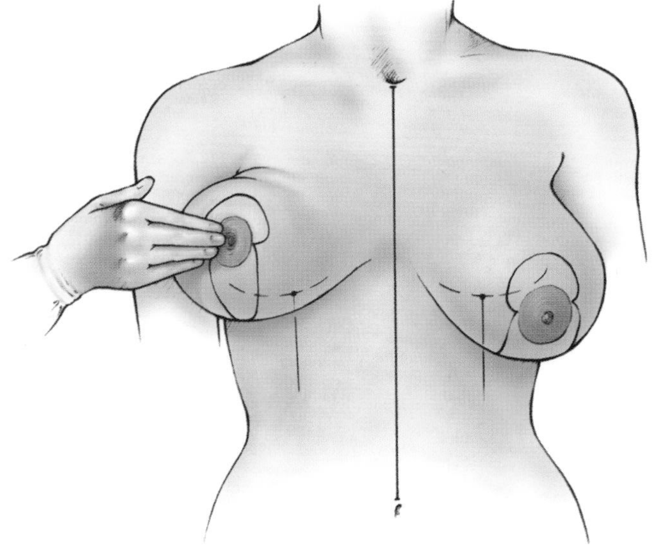

The vertical limbs of the breast incision are marked next. Starting about 40 mm inferior to the proposed top of the areola, with the breast displaced medially with the hand (more inferiorly than superiorly), the vertical line is drawn from the upper point to the inferior point just above the inframammary fold. This completes the medial line.

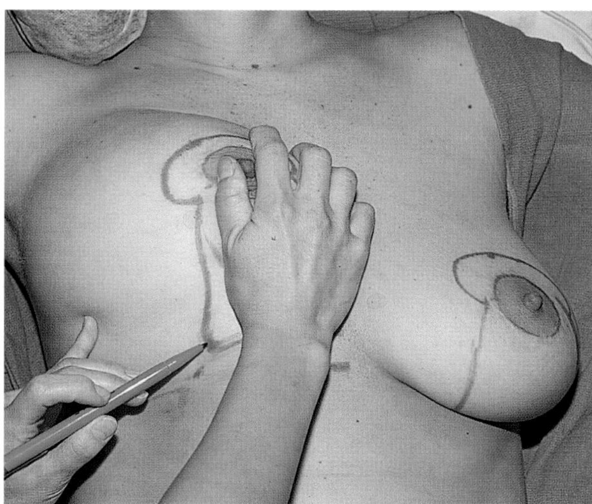

The lateral line is then drawn as the lower marking. The lateral line is a vertical line drawn from 40 mm below the level of the new areola to the point where the breast is displaced medially (more inferiorly than in the upper portion of the breast). ***The amount of force placed on the displaced tissue will be reflected in the corresponding tightness of the closure.*** The displacement should not be so firm if more skin is required for the closure. The position of the upper areola is marked, and an ellipse the width of the areola is drawn upward to connect the medial and lateral lines.

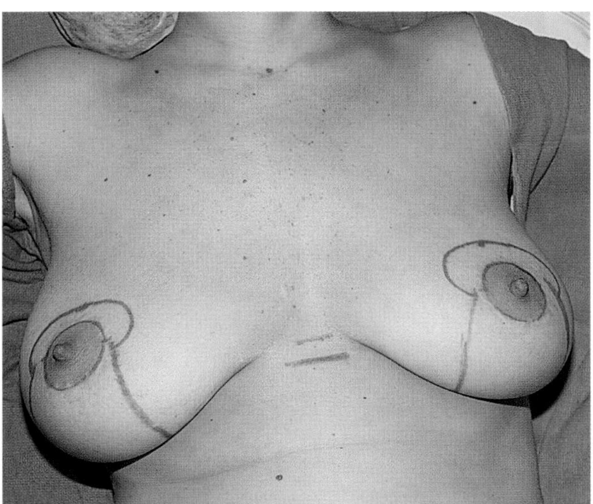

The patient is prepped and draped on the operating table. Her arms are abducted and secured to arm boards so that she can be elevated to an upright position during the operation.

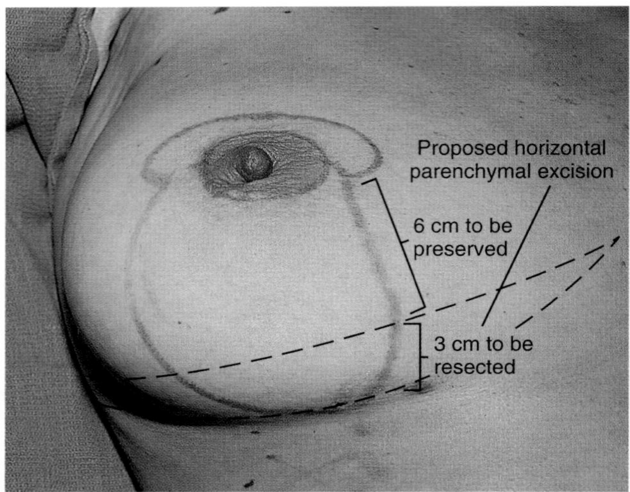

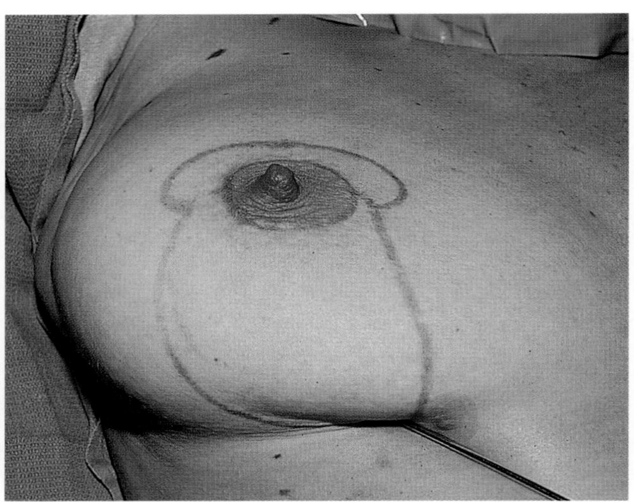

The vertical extent of the breast parenchyma of the reduced breast to be preserved is then determined. This is usually 5 to 6 cm below the future areolar site. This point is marked and an ellipse is drawn below this point toward the inframammary fold to delineate the amount of transverse parenchymal resection.

Wetting solution is infiltrated lateral to the breast to facilitate liposuction of this area. Some additional wetting solution is also infiltrated in the breast parenchyma, particularly along the areas to be resected, to reduce bleeding intraoperatively. A solution containing 1000 ml Ringer's lactate, 1 ml of 1:1000 epinephrine, and 25 ml of 1% lidocaine is used. The solution is introduced through a blunt 2 mm cannula and injected with a Byron pump.

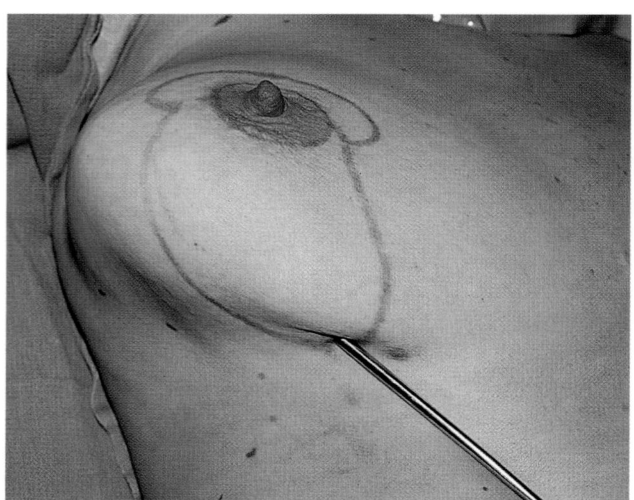

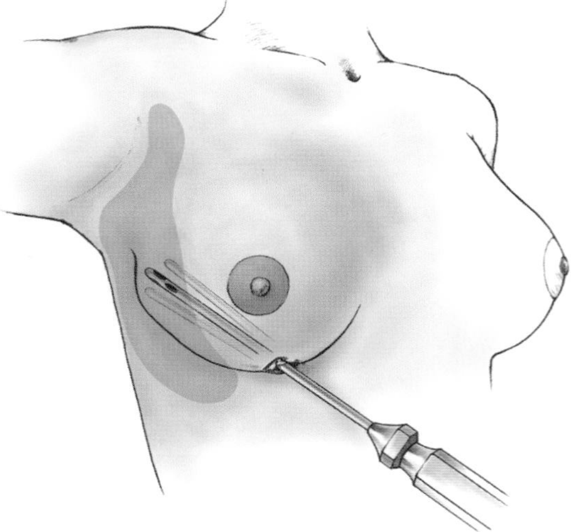

Liposuction is used to remove any excess fatty tissue laterally. This helps define the lateral breast line and narrows the breast. It is also used when the breast parenchyma is quite fatty and additional parenchymal resection is necessary.

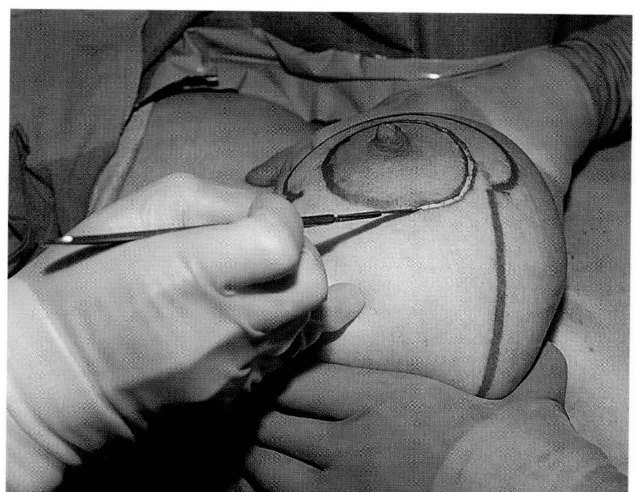

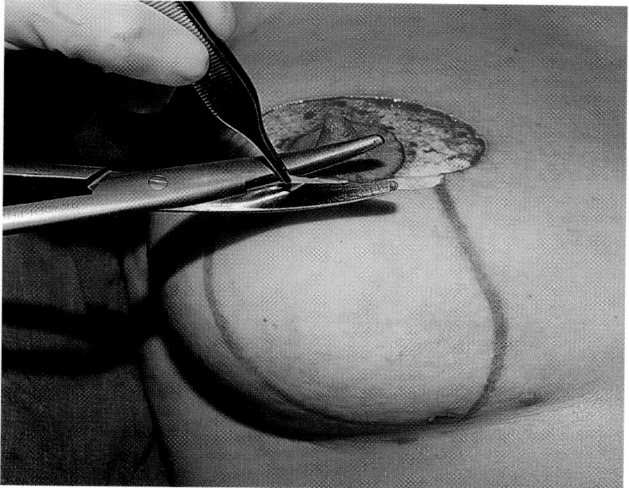

The operative procedure is started by making an incision into the deep dermis of the periareolar area. The subdermal plexus is spared to preserve the subdermal blood supply to the areola. The outer skin and deep dermis of this breast region are then deepithelialized with curved scissors. Care is taken not to go beneath the dermis to avoid injury to the subdermal plexus, which could reduce the nipple-areola blood supply.

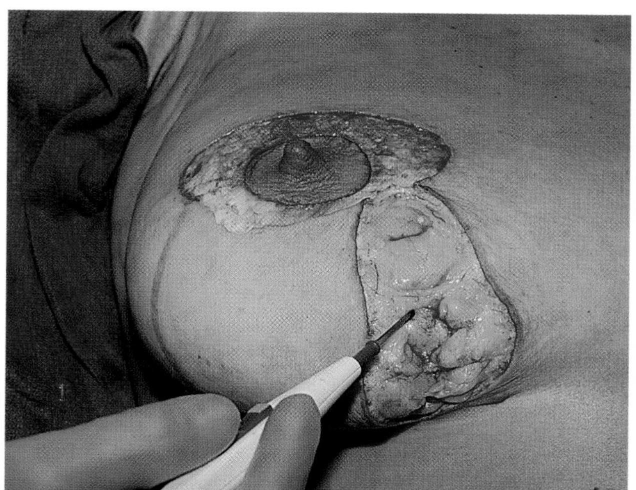

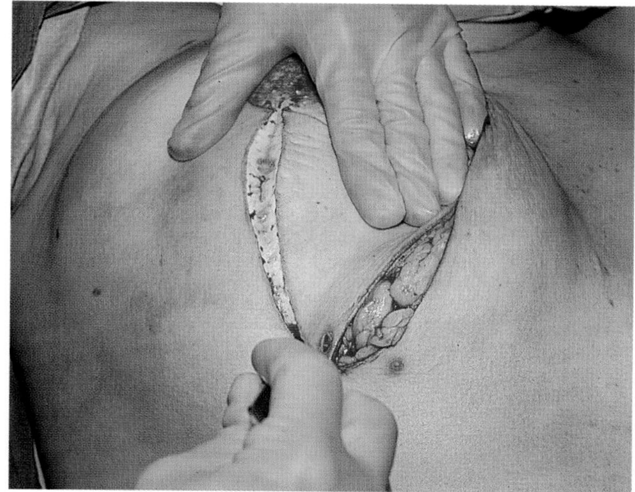

With the breast displaced laterally the medial breast parenchyma is incised vertically from the lower areola marking downward to the point of the V. Similarly, with the breast displaced medially a second vertical incision is made in the lateral breast parenchyma. Both of these incisions extend down to the fascia over the pectoralis major muscle and the serratus anterior muscle. These incisions define the resection of the lower breast parenchyma.

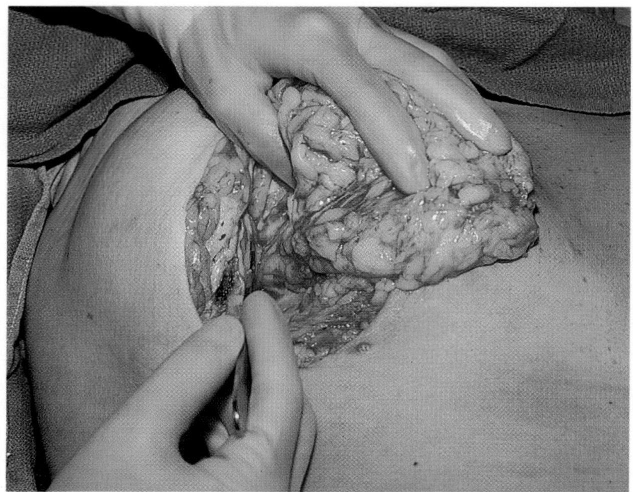

After the V is incised and reflected, additional subcutaneous tissue is resected beneath the lower point in the inframammary fold region and the tissue is then lifted off the fascia up to beneath the areola.

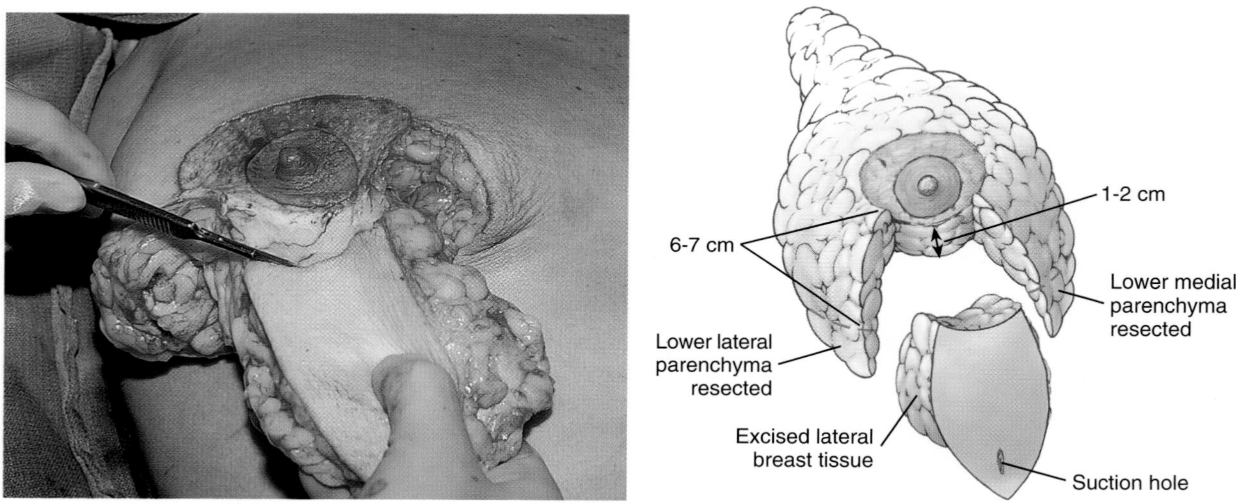

Starting just below the areola, a vertical incision is made to excise the lower breast parenchyma, leaving approximately 1 to 2 cm of breast parenchyma under the areola to preserve central breast projection and areola blood supply.

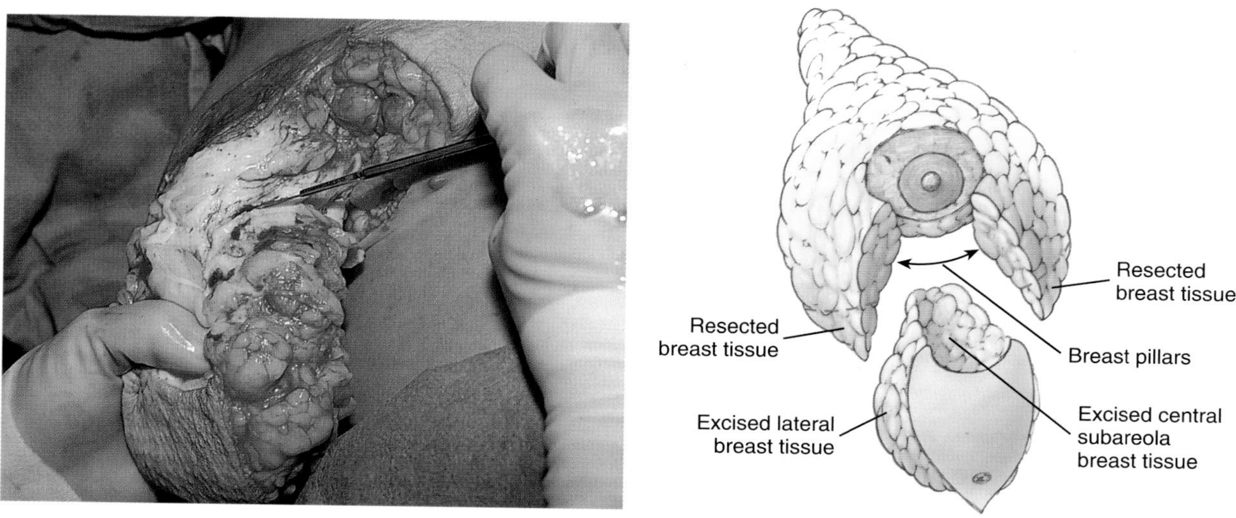

To remove additional breast volume the resection is taken deep to the areola toward the upper breast area and laterally in the breast parenchyma.

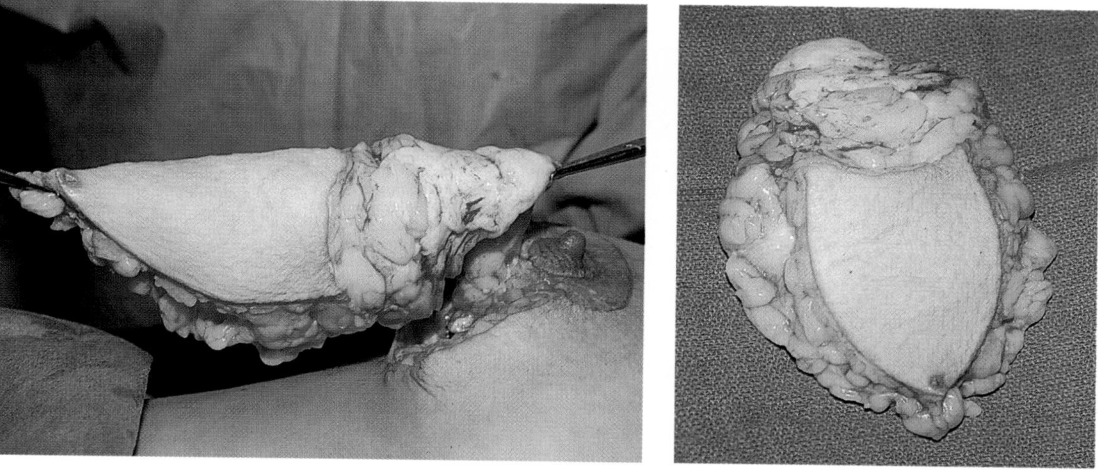

The amount of tissue removed from the lower V and from the subareolar area is demonstrated. These resections reduce breast projection, width, and volume. The vertical resection is shown. Closing the pillars will narrow the breast after removal of the ptotic breast tissue. This tightens the lower breast and reduces the ptosis.

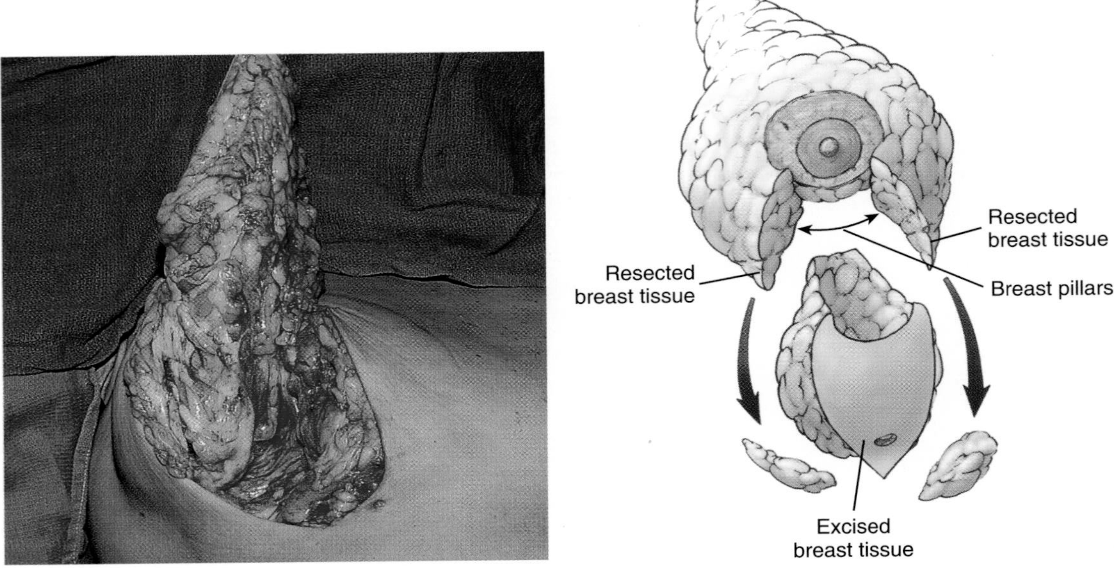

By lifting the breast off the lower deep fascia, the surgeon can assess the medial and lateral pillars of the breast. If additional breast tissue requires resection, deep lateral tissue is usually removed to reduce lateral breast volume and fullness.

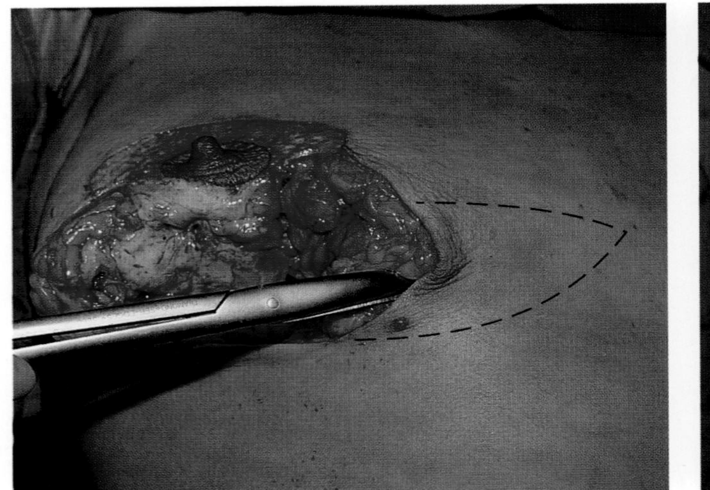

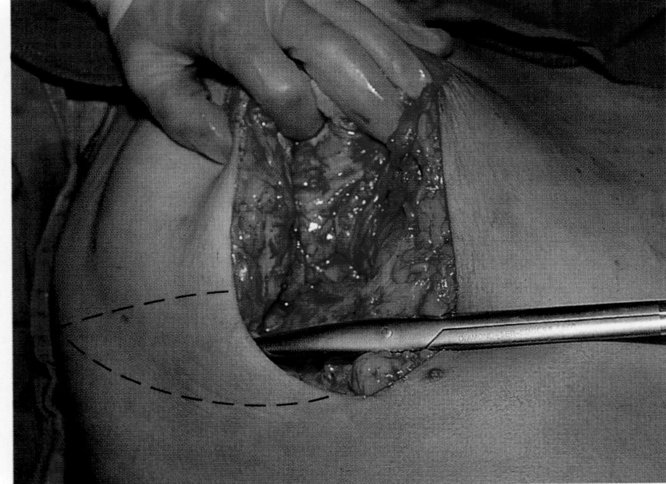

The lower breast skin just above the inframammary fold is undermined in preparation for removal of the medial and lower lateral breast parenchyma. The lower 3 to 4 cm of breast skin is undermined both medially and laterally.

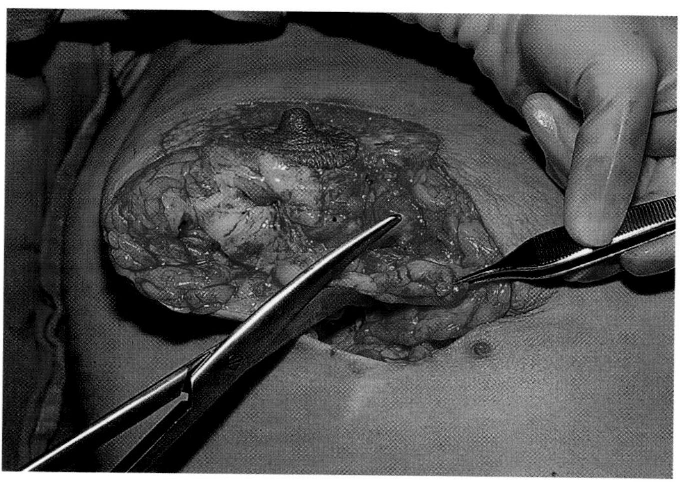

The lower breast parenchyma is resected to leave 5 to 7 cm vertical breast pillars medially and laterally. This provides the proper proportions for the lower reduced breast.

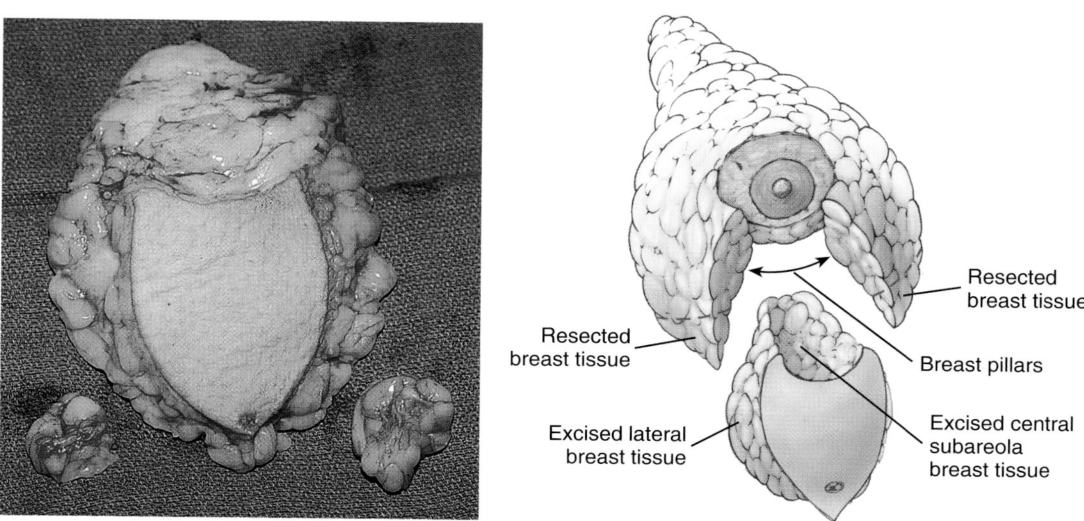

The medial, lateral, and central resections are shown. Most of the resection is done centrally in the lower breast, which is the breast parenchyma that is responsible for most ptosis.

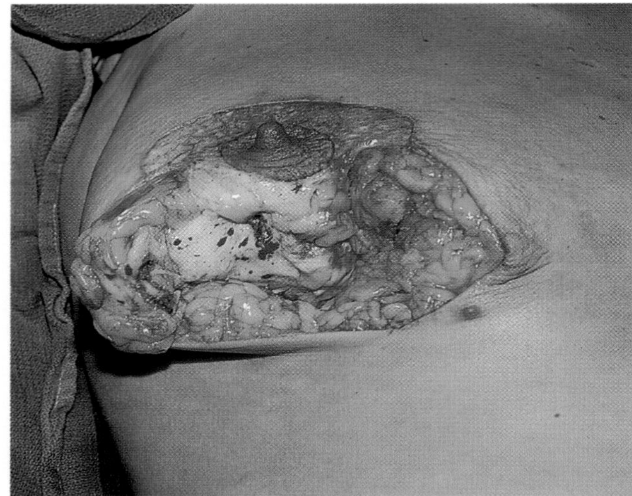

After the lower resection the breast is somewhat shortened vertically and the 6 cm long vertical pillars of the breast are left intact.

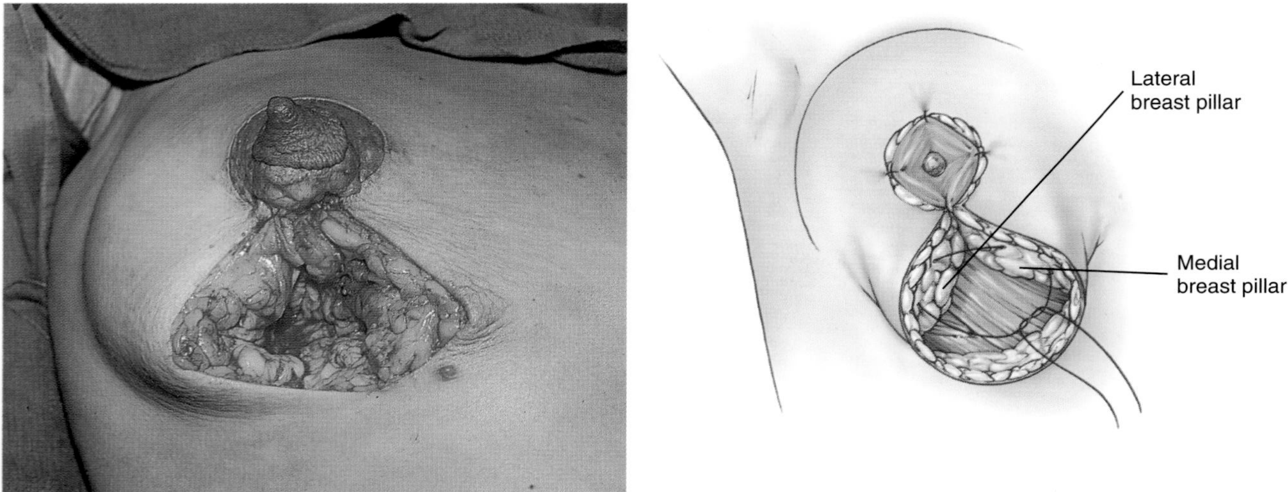

The pillars of the breast are then approximated, starting first at the lower portion of the areola. The nipple-areola is moved to its new position, and large absorbable 2-0 sutures are used to approximate the pillars firmly from the point of the areola down to the lower point of the incision.

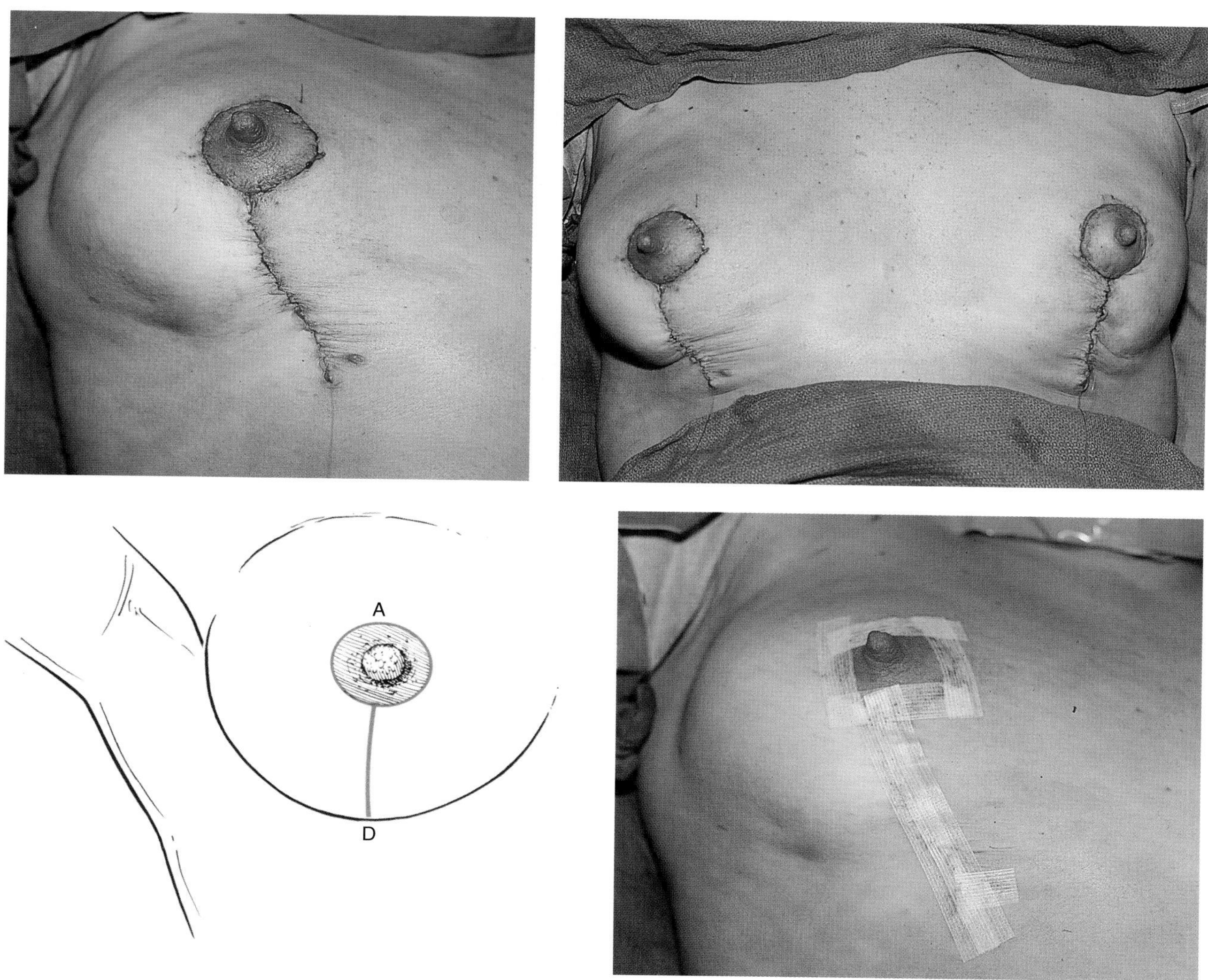

The wound and the incision around the areola are closed with intracuticular 3-0 to 4-0 absorbable sutures. The vertical limb is closed first with 3-0 absorbable sutures and then with intracuticular 3-0 clear PDS placed with small passes to minimize skin rippling. This suture can be cinched tight to reduce the vertical limb to an appropriate and attractive length. Steri-Strips are applied to the lower breast region.

Results

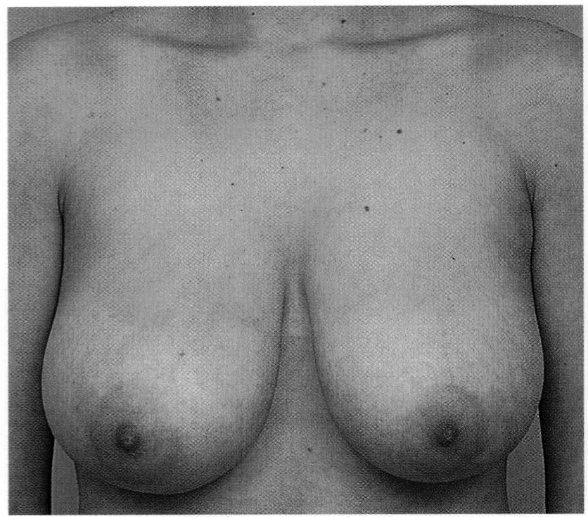
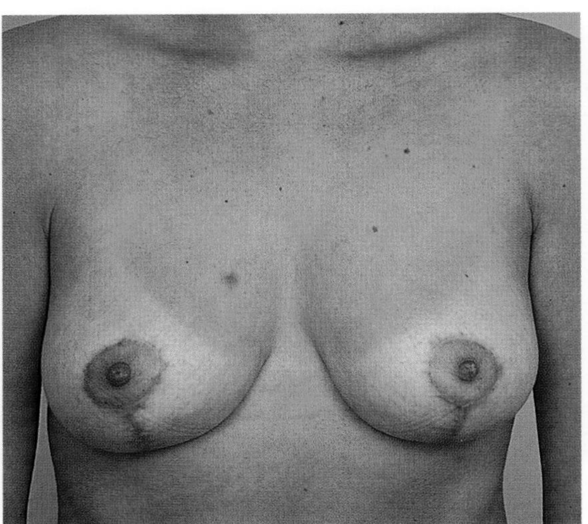

This 26-year-old woman's heavy breasts produced back and shoulder pain as well as breast pain. The skin under her breasts was irritated and moist. She complained that her breasts were just too full and too low and disliked how the fullness extended under her arms and over the sides of her bra. She requested breast reduction with minimal scars. She had tried weight loss and exercise but was unable to reduce the size of her breasts and ameliorate her symptoms. Her general health was good, and no dominant breast masses were found on mammography or on physical examination. A vertical reduction technique with liposuction was selected. Liposuction was first performed in the axillary and lateral breast regions as well as within the breast parenchyma. Next the breast was resected inferiorly along the inframammary fold and centrally. A total of 700 gm was removed on each side. The patient is shown 3 months after surgery. Early postoperative healing is satisfactory. The symptoms of back and shoulder pain have been alleviated and she has been able to resume normal activities. The breasts have been reduced, elevated, narrowed, and rounded, thus giving a more attractive, youthful appearance.

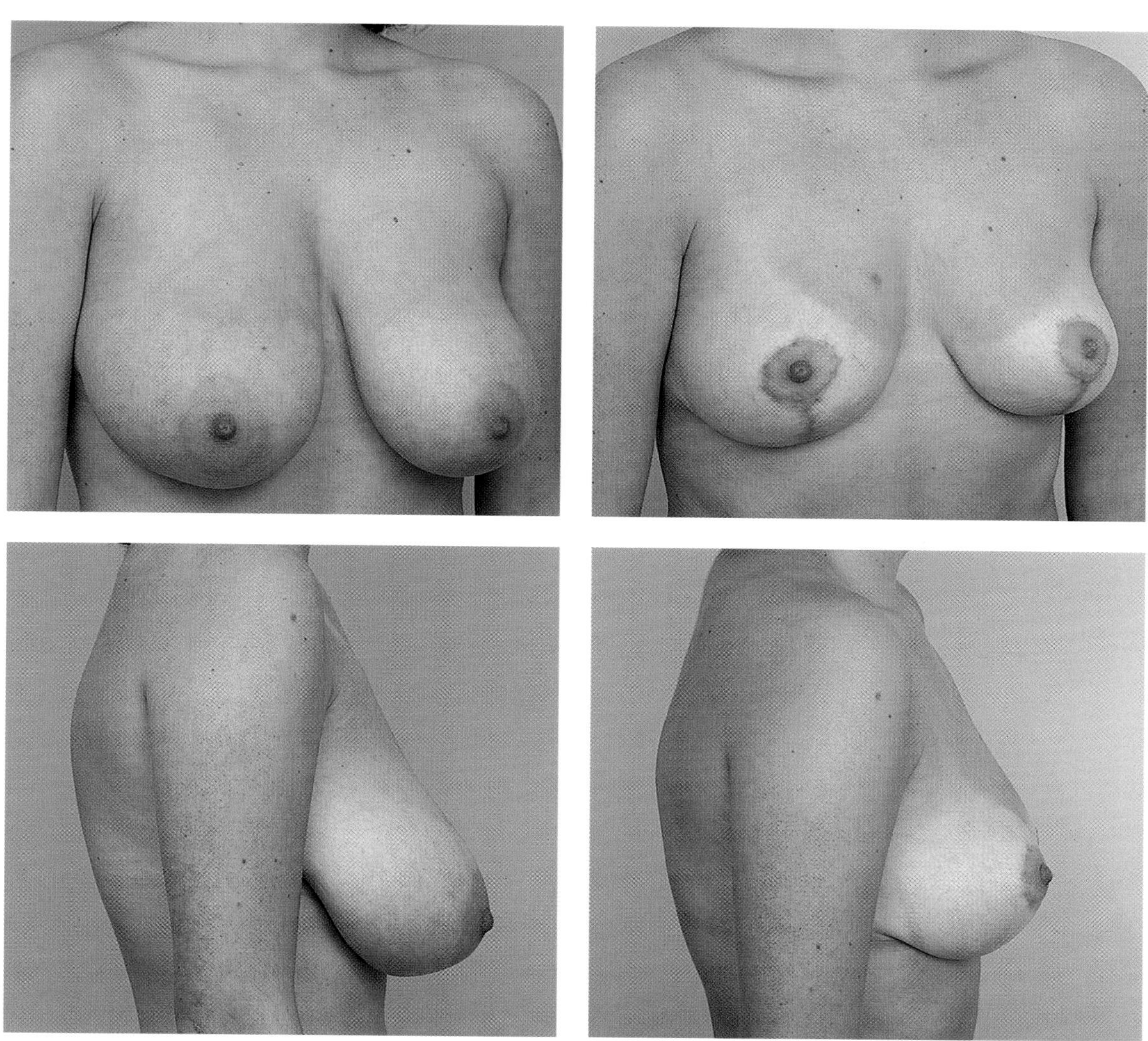

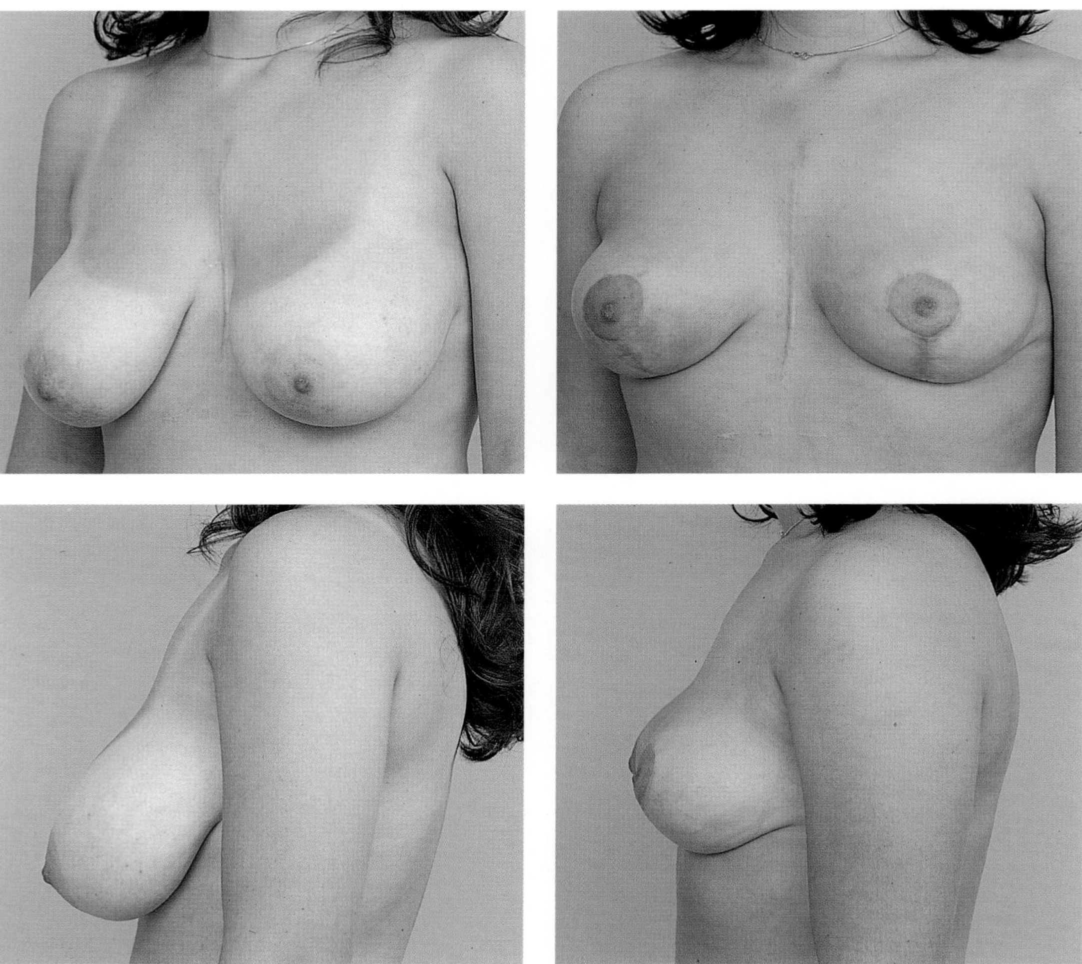

This 23-year-old woman was concerned about the fullness and heaviness of her breasts. She also felt that her breasts were too wide, too ptotic, and too full laterally. She had back pain, shoulder pain, and irritation beneath her breasts. Despite losing 10 pounds, her breasts were still heavy and uncomfortable. She requested breast reduction. A vertical mammaplasty approach was selected. Liposuction was used to reduce the breast laterally as well as centrally and additional breast parenchyma was resected centrally and inferiorly. A total of 600 gm per side was removed. She is shown 3 months after surgery; her breasts are more elevated and the lateral fullness has been eliminated. Her symptoms have been alleviated.

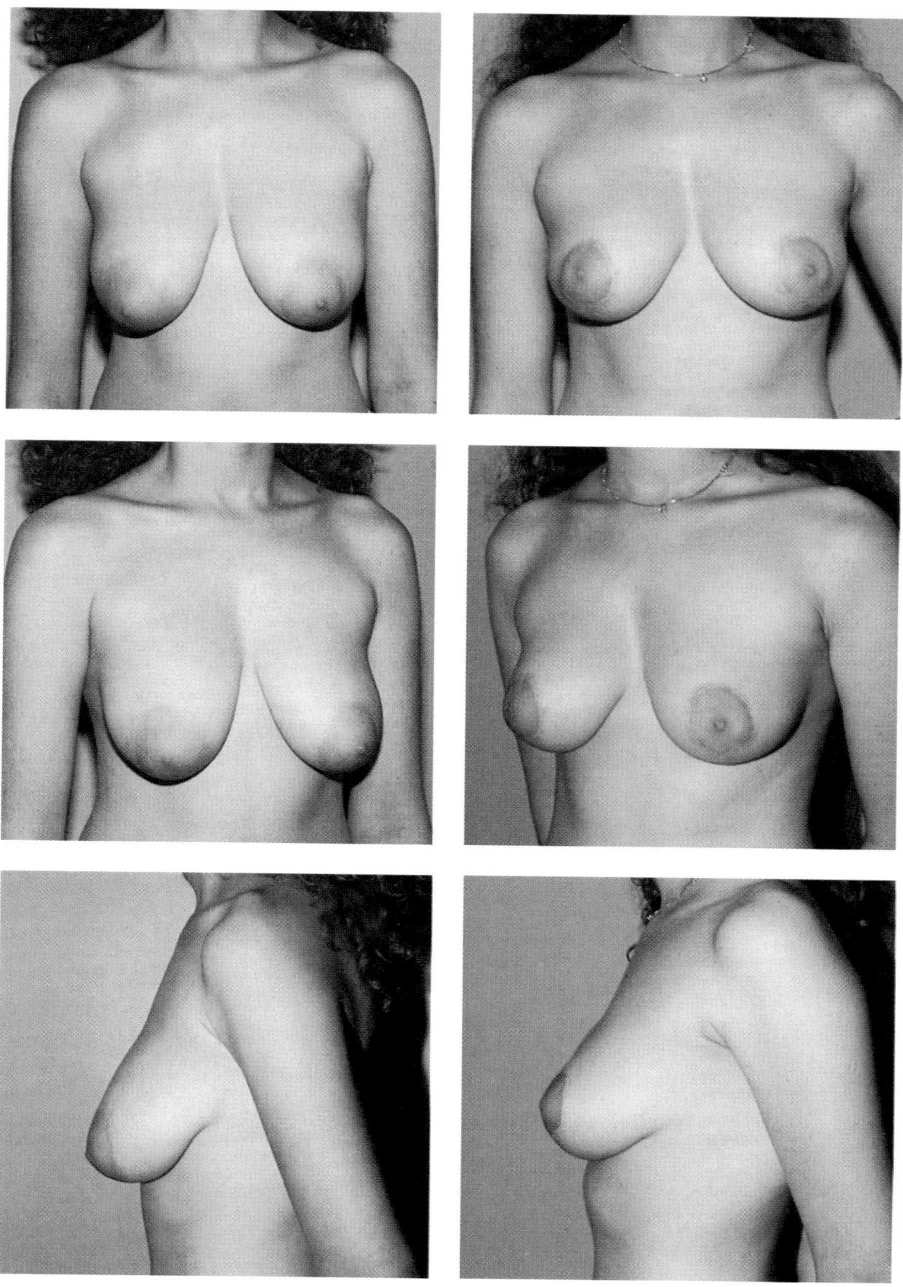

Fourteen months after a vertical mammaplasty this woman is satisfied with the amount of reduction and new contour of her breasts. Her brassiere size has gone from 36D to 36C. She is particularly pleased with the inconspicuous short scars. The areolae have stretched somewhat more than they would have with other techniques because of the central skin excised. The amount of breast elevation is somewhat less than that achieved with other techniques in which more skin is resected; however, this patient feels that the short scar technique was her best option. The vertical incision has shortened about 2 cm during the postoperative period, and the erythema should continue to fade.

WOMEN WITH LARGER BREASTS

The vertical approach can be extended to larger breasts, particularly if there is satisfactory skin elasticity. The combination of liposuction and resection serves to further reduce and narrow the breasts by removing the lateral breast fullness. Additional liposuction within the breast parenchyma will further reduce the breasts. This approach is usually appropriate for younger women with full breasts without significant ptosis and with good skin elasticity.

Markings and Technique

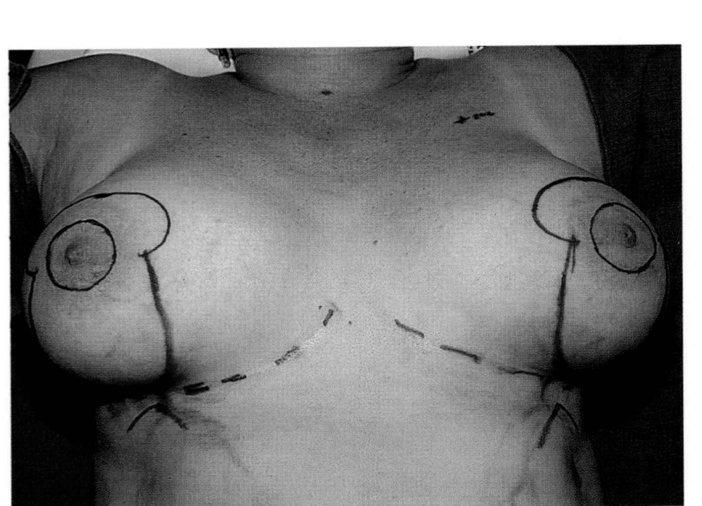

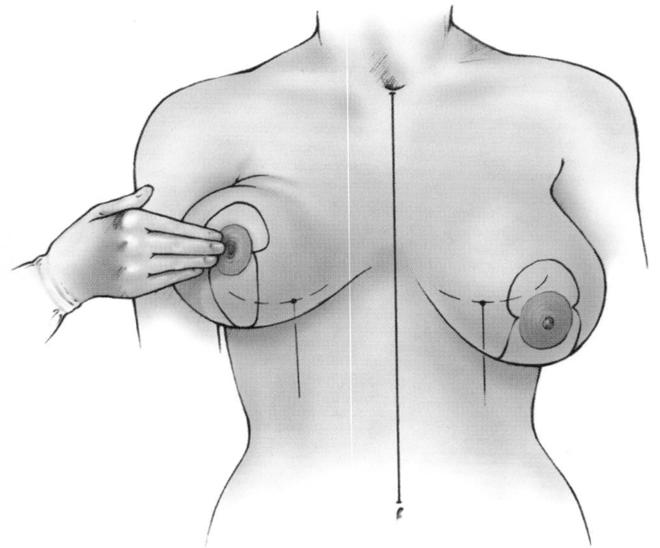

This 32-year-old woman with size 38DD breasts requested breast reduction with minimal scarring. She had significant back and shoulder pain and described her breasts as quite uncomfortable. She disliked the lateral breast fullness as well as the significant breast ptosis. To meet her request for minimal incisions a vertical reduction was planned. She is shown after the initial preoperative markings have been drawn.

Surgical plan

- General breast reduction combined with liposuction
- Reduction of lateral breast region with liposuction to reposition nipple-areola to appropriate level
- Resection of breast parenchyma inferiorly and centrally
- Resection of breast parenchyma along inframammary fold
- Closure of vertical pillars to narrow breast
- Closure of skin leaving periareolar and vertical scars

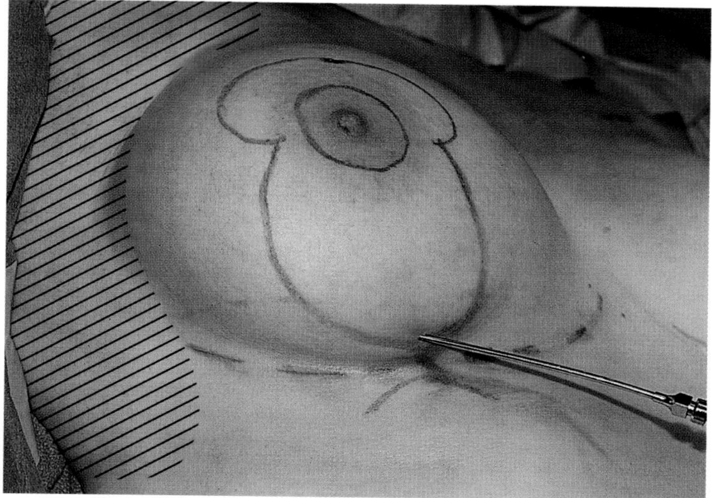

Approximately 500 ml of wetting solution is infiltrated laterally and inter-parenchymally, particularly in the area of breast parenchyma resection.

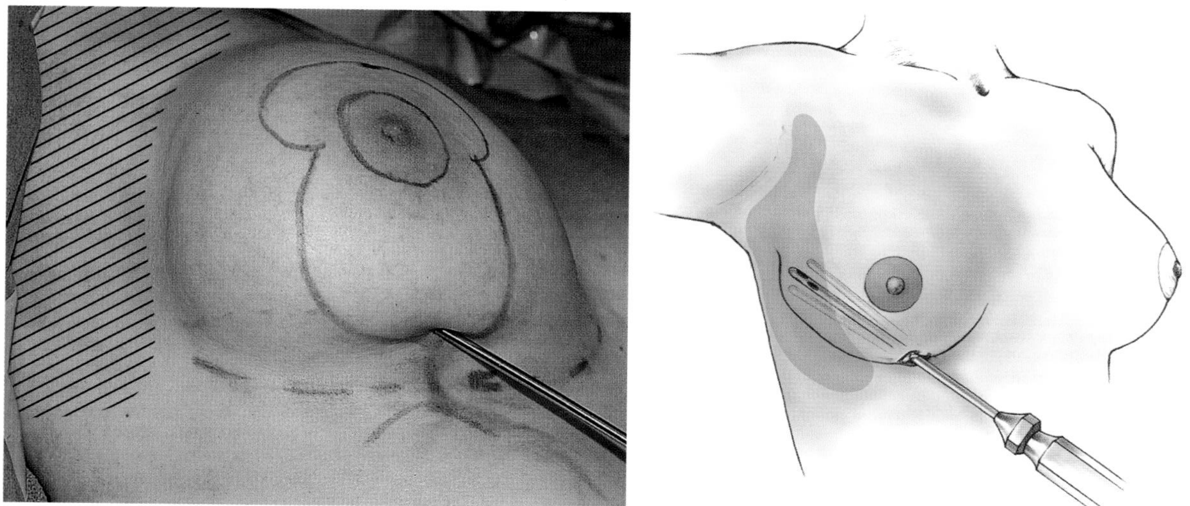

Liposuction is then performed on the lateral breast tissue and within the breast parenchyma to reduce the fatty tissue.

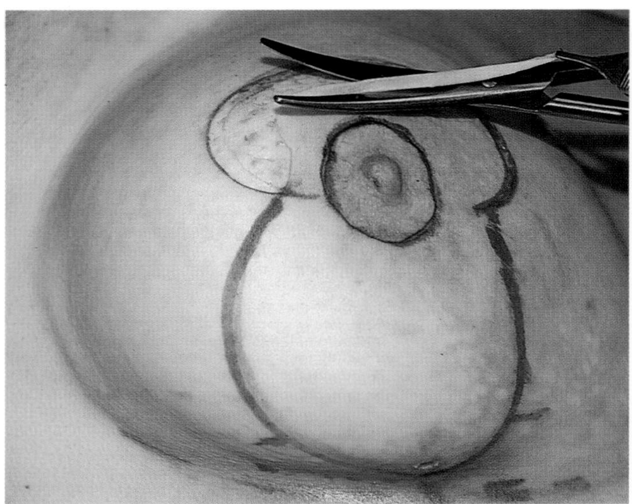
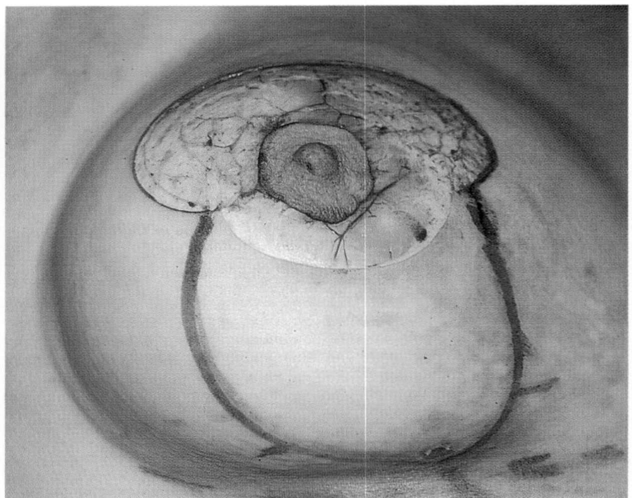

An incision is made around the areola. The upper breast skin is deepithelialized as well as a strip of skin approximately 1 cm below the areola. ***Care is taken to avoid injury to the subdermal plexus. This plexus as well as the blood supply coming from the deeper parenchyma provides an additional margin of safety.***

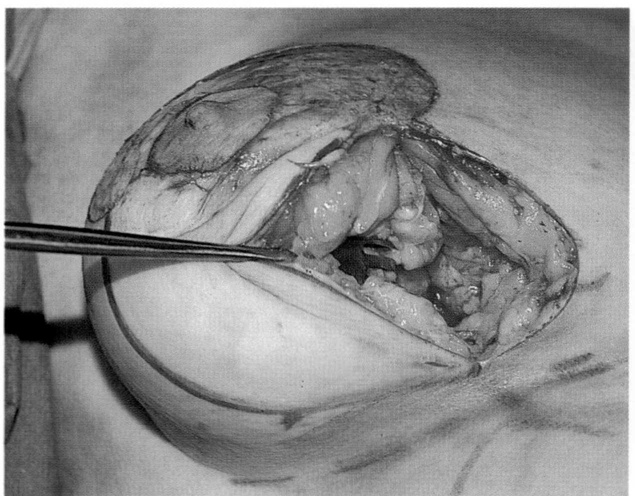
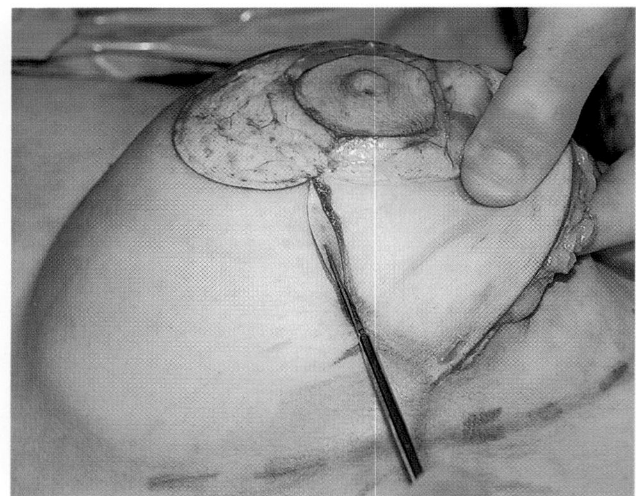

The vertical incision is made in the breast from the lower areolar marking to the lower point of the resection. This incision goes down to the external outer fascia over the pectoralis muscle layer. This incision is also made vertically to create the lateral breast pillar. It extends down to the lower point of the resection.

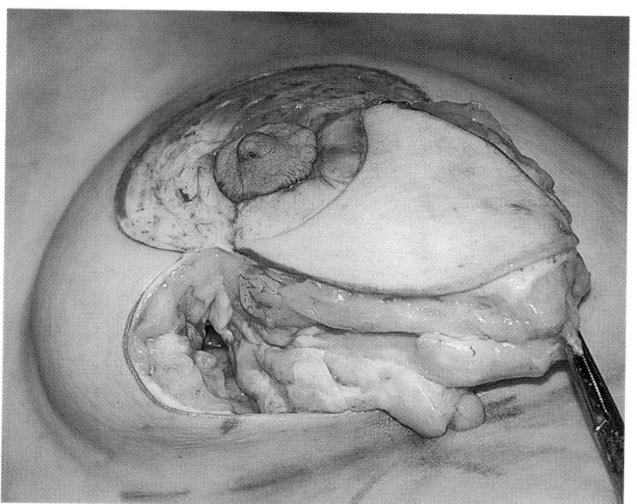

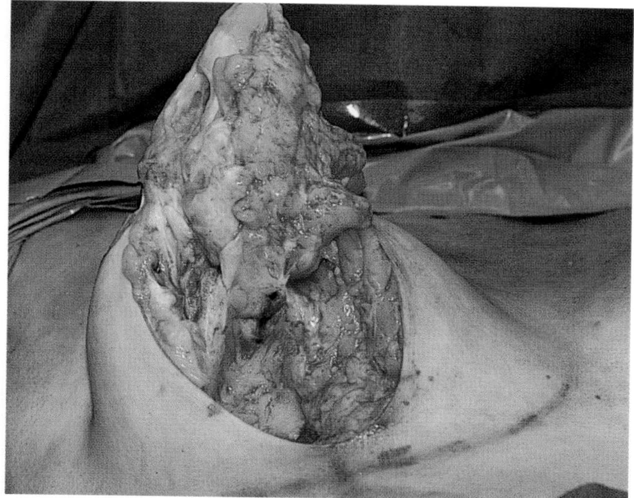

The tissue for the proposed resection is then freed up as a lower triangular segment and is lifted off the deep fascia in preparation for removal. Care is taken to remove all the tissue in the lower triangle to prevent fullness at the future inframammary fold. The triangular portion of the lower breast is then elevated in preparation for the resection.

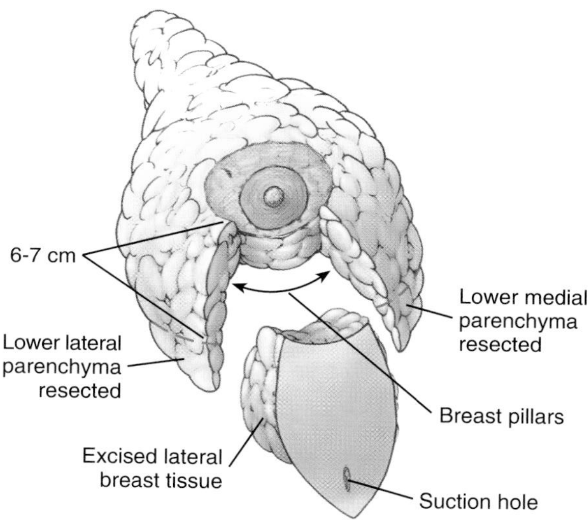

The resection removes the lower triangle. The resection line inferior to the areola is along an arc about 1 cm below the areola. Additional resection can be done from the depths of the breast centrally and laterally.

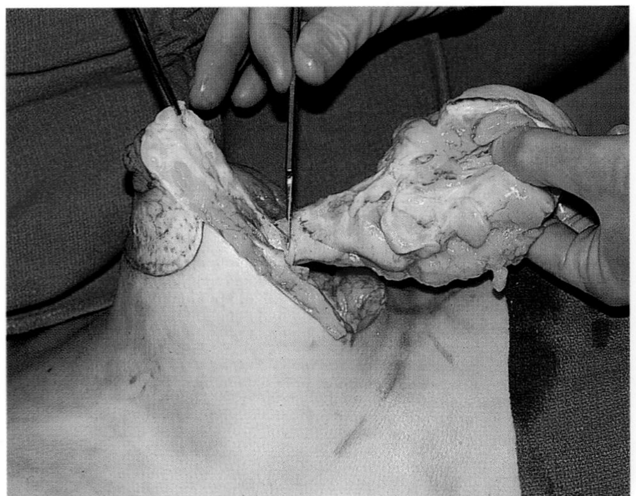

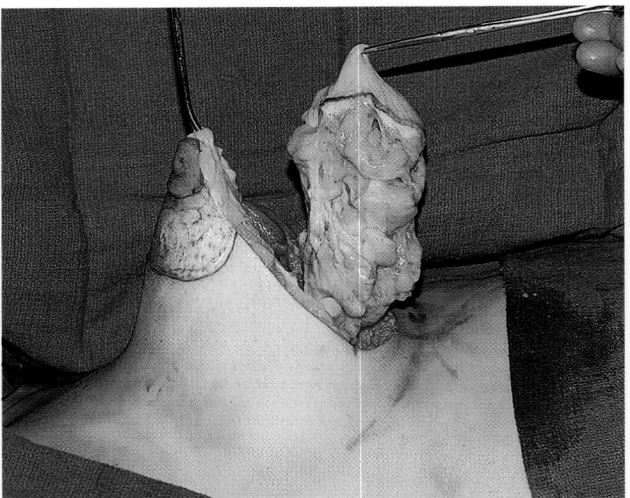

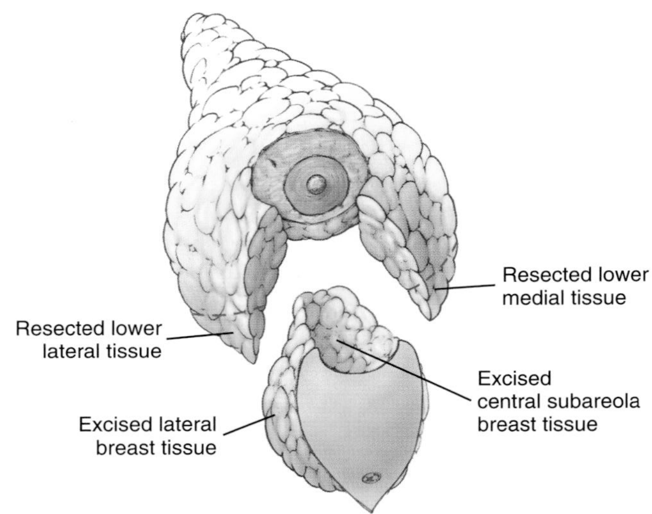

This triangular segment is resected vertically and additional tissue is removed from the subareolar area, leaving at least 2 cm of tissue beneath the areola to provide additional parenchymal blood flow to the areola.

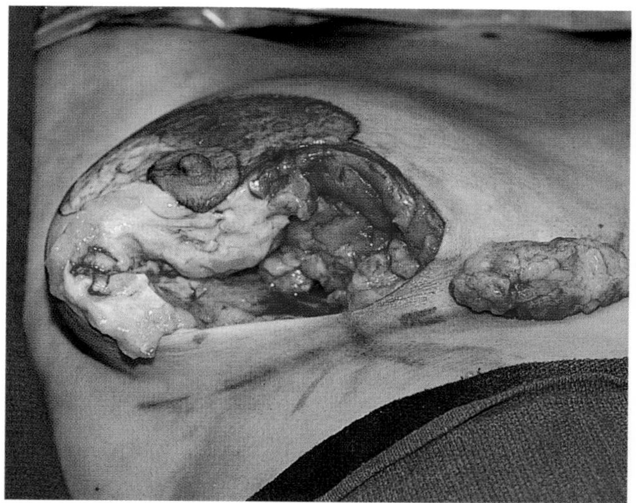

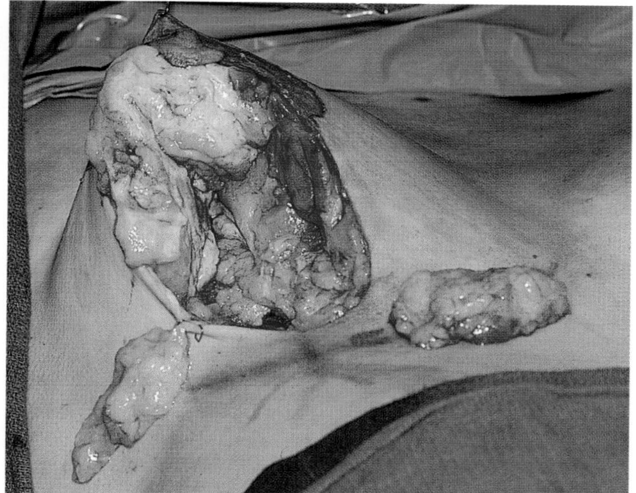

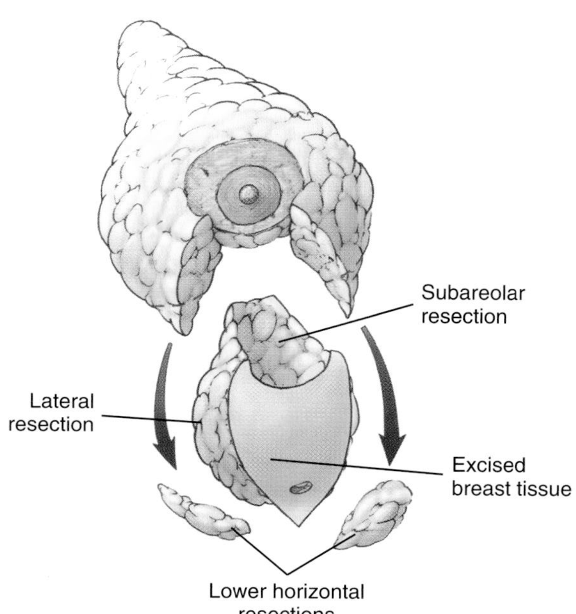

The lower breast skin is lifted off the lower breast parenchyma and medial and lateral strips of parenchyma are resected to preserve at least 6 cm limbs of vertical breast pillars.

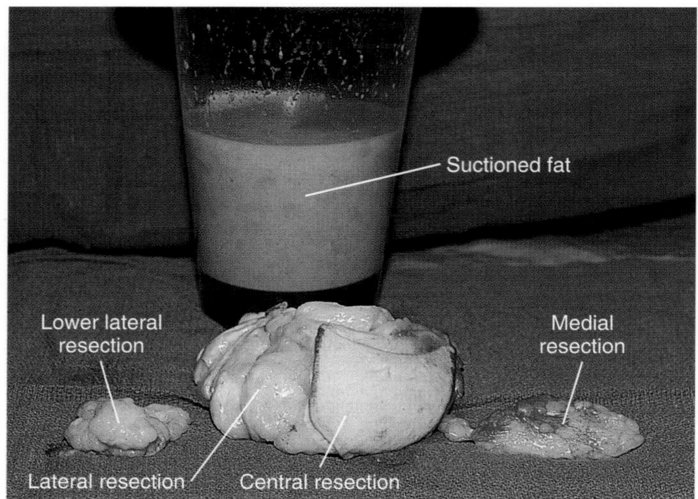

The tissue resected from the central, medial, and lateral breast is shown. The fat suctioned from each breast is recorded. As illustrated, approximately 500 cc of fatty material is suctioned from the right breast in addition to the resected tissue, making the total amount of tissue removed 1100 gm.

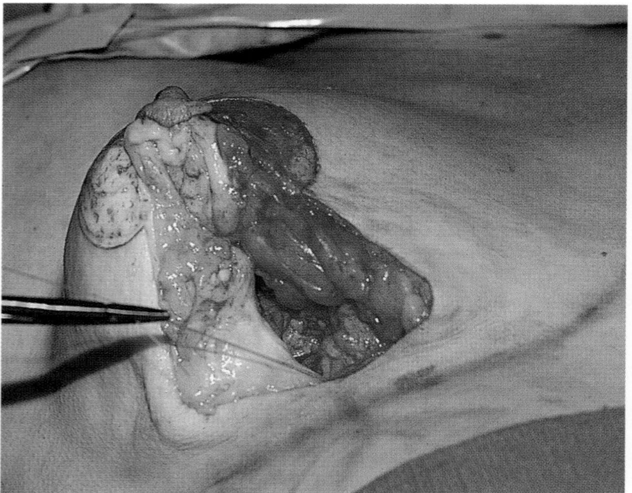

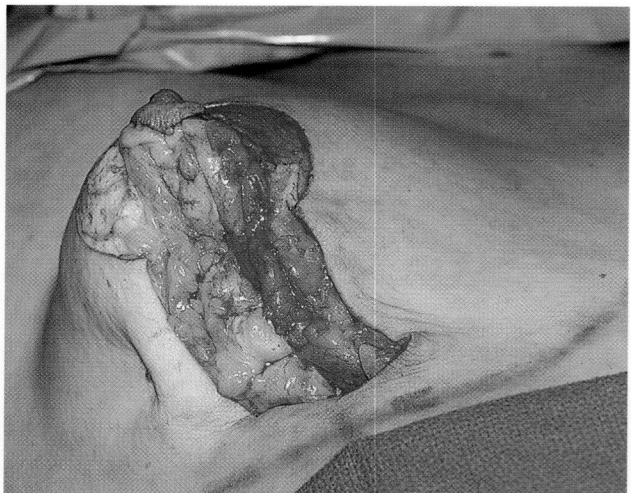

The areola is moved to its new position, and the pillars of the breast are approximated with two layers of absorbable sutures.

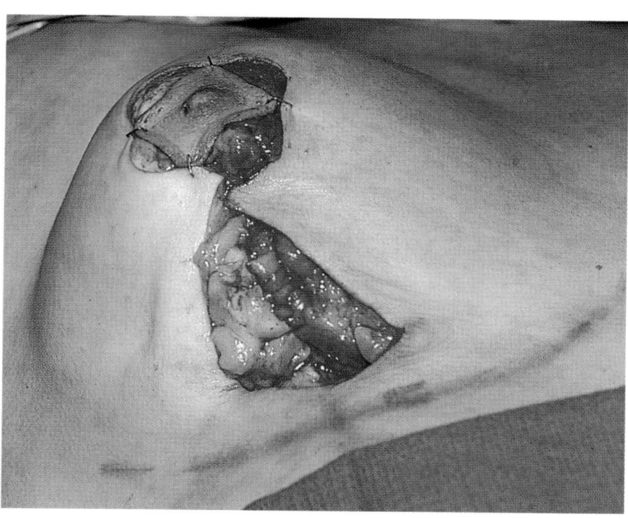

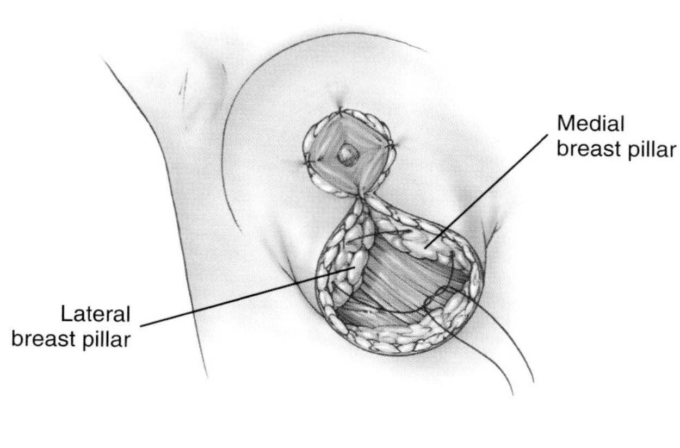

The outer subcutaneous tissue is approximated prior to vertical limb closure.

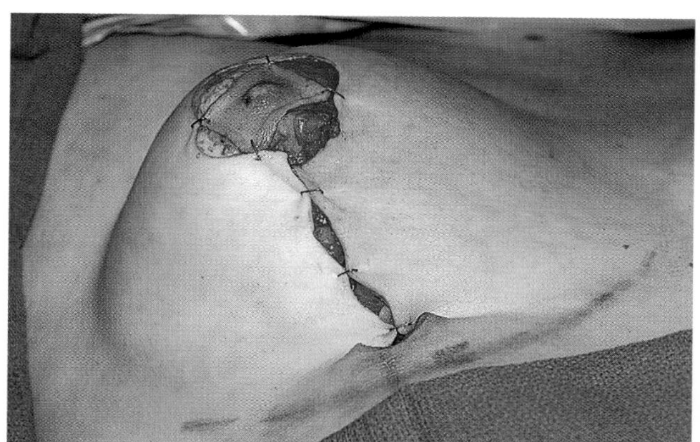

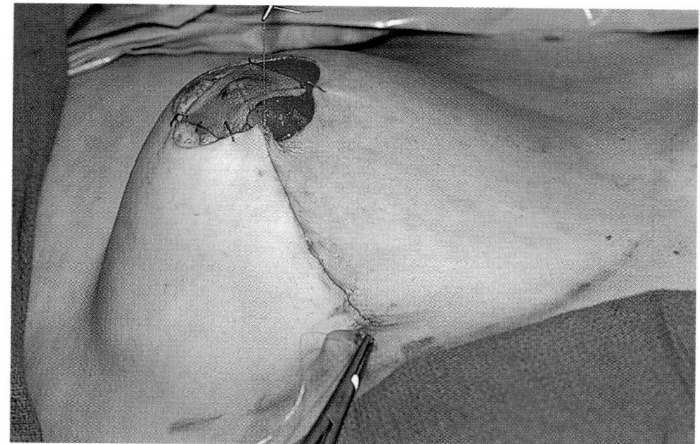

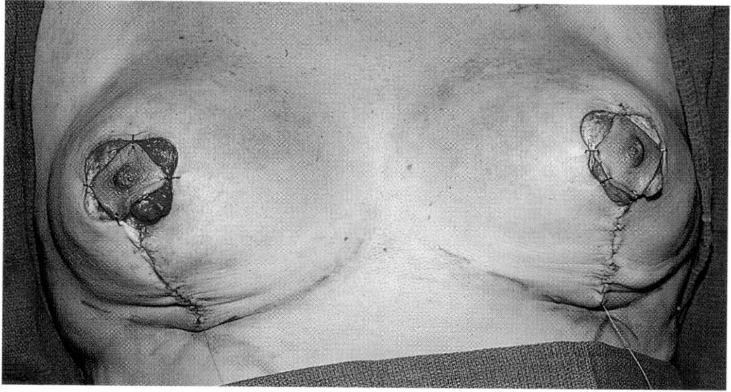

The initial vertical closure proceeds from the lower areola to the inframammary fold using deep dermal 3-0 absorbable sutures and then 3-0 clear PDS, pulled in an accordion-like manner to shorten the vertical limb. Excess skin is gathered in the lower portion of the scar rather than the upper portion.

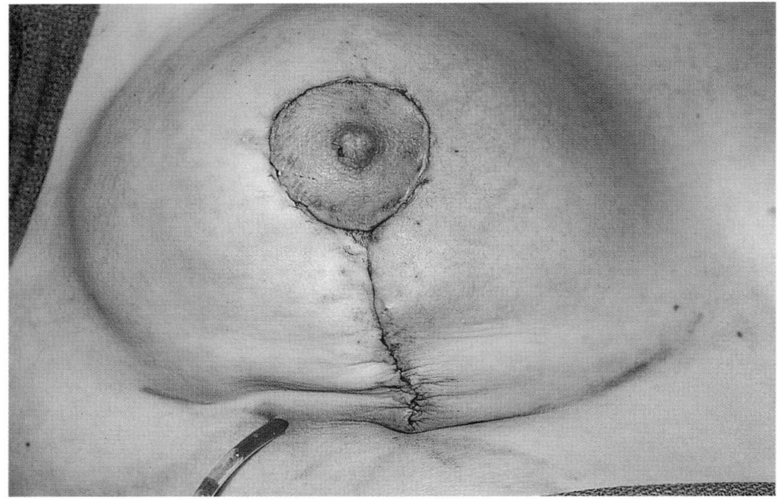

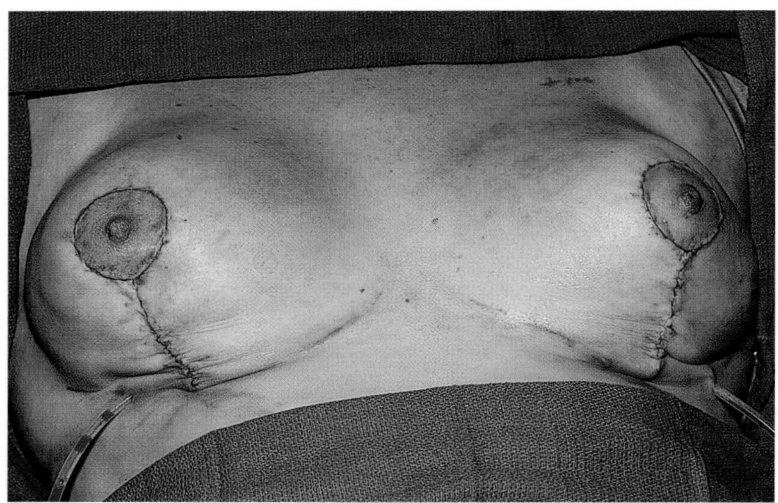

Drains are placed through a small lateral approach or through the lower incision. The scar has been shortened to approximately 7 cm. Because the excess breast tissue has been resected, there is little evidence of ptosis immediately postoperatively.

Results

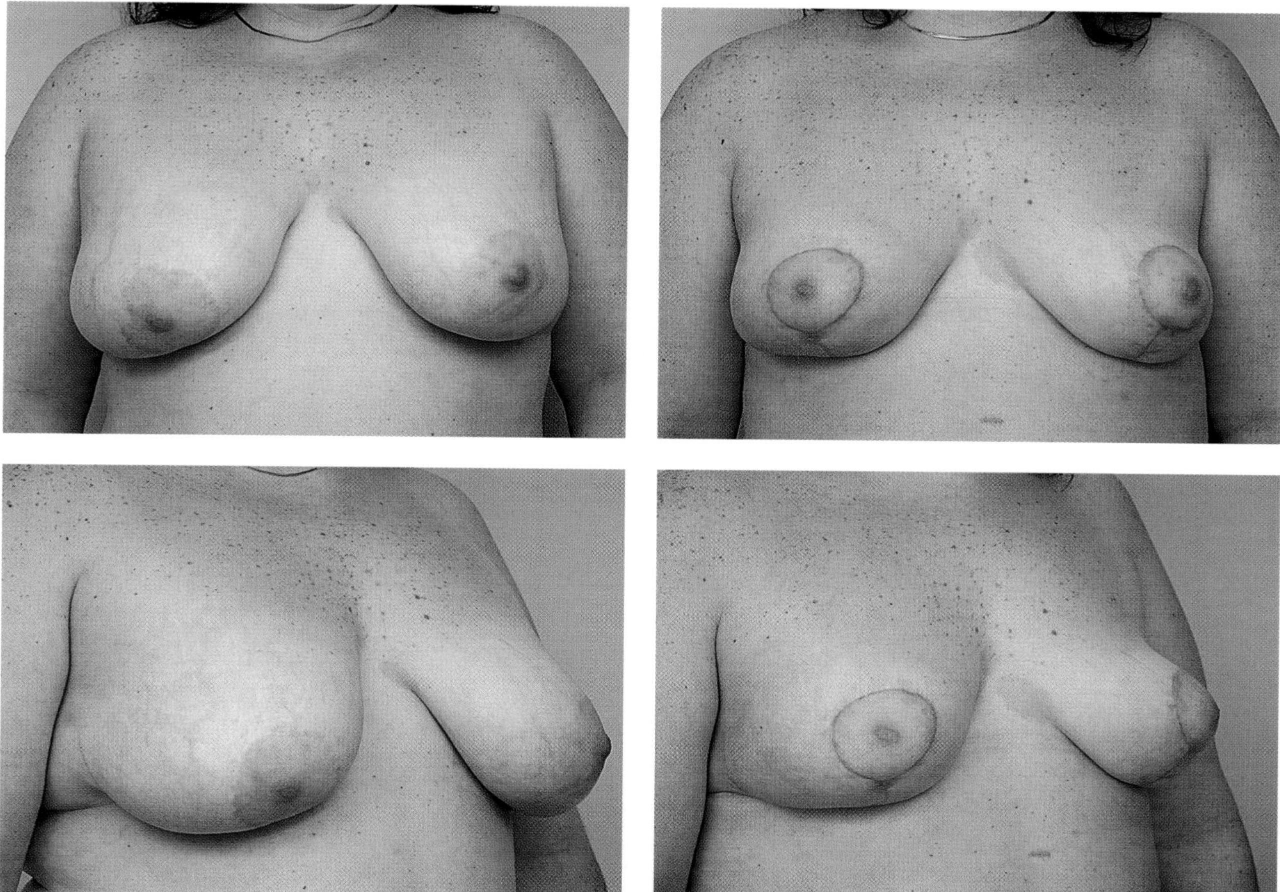

This 35-year-old woman had heavy, uncomfortable breasts and she complained of shoulder grooving from her brassiere straps. She requested a breast reduction technique that would reduce and narrow her breasts, particularly in the lateral aspect. Liposuction was used to reduce the lateral portion of her breasts in the axillary region. Approximately 400 ml of fatty tissue was resected in this area and another 150 gm of breast parenchyma removed during liposuction and lower breast resection. She is shown 4 months after surgery. She is pleased with the appearance of her breasts and particularly likes the improvement in breast ptosis and breast fullness.

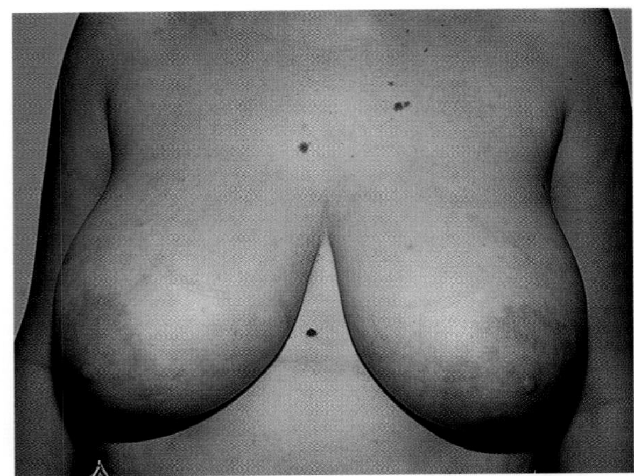

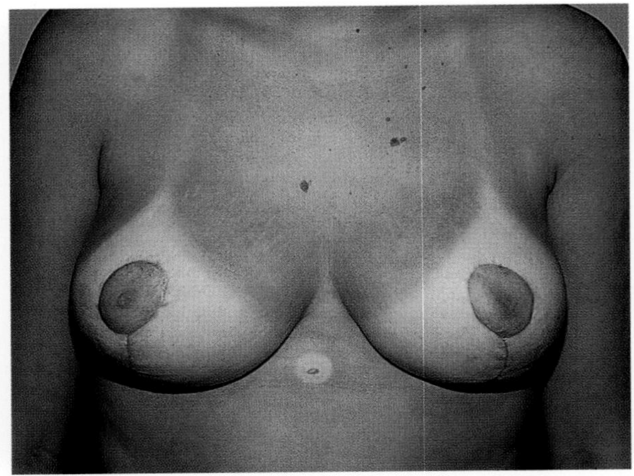

This 27-year-old woman had heavy breasts. She had been unsuccessful in efforts to lose weight and reduce her breast size. She complained of significant symptoms from back and shoulder pain as well as pain in her breasts. She requested breast reduction with short scars. Her general health was good and she had no masses in her breast and no family history of breast cancer. The vertical approach was used. Liposuction laterally as well as in the subaxillary region removed approximately 400 cc of fatty tissue. An additional 400 gm of tissue was removed during breast resection. Postoperatively she is very pleased with the narrowing of her breasts as well as the reduced tissue under her arms and in the subaxillary region. She has satisfactory areolar sensation and feels that her new 36C breasts are appropriate to her size.

SUPERIOR PEDICLE TECHNIQUE

The superior pedicle technique provides acceptable breast reduction for patients with mild hypertrophy requiring reductions of 500 to 2000 gm or less and minimal to moderate (no more than 7 to 10 cm) upward repositioning of the nipple-areola. When this procedure is used, ideally the breast tissue is soft and pliable and the nipple should be readily and easily elevated to its new position. Mobility is tested preoperatively to determine how difficult it is to position the nipple-areola upward. ***With the superior pedicle technique, breast parenchyma is removed primarily from the inferior and lateral aspect of the breast.*** The majority of the excess breast tissue is removed by horizontal resection and a deep upper lateral resection to narrow the breast and remove ptotic breast parenchyma prior to closure of the inverted T incision. The nipple-areola is moved on the superior central breast parenchyma. The periareolar vascular plexus is also preserved to enhance and supplement the blood supply to the nipple-areola from the underlying breast parenchyma; however, the dermis can be divided along the limits of the upper V to facilitate mobility. The nipple-areola is moved to its new, elevated position after the breast is reduced in width and volume and contoured to an improved natural, lifted, narrowed conical shape.

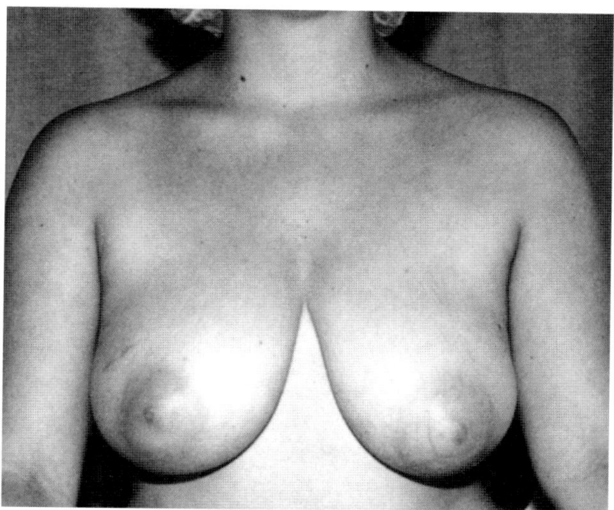

This 19-year-old patient had mild breast hypertrophy with some asymmetry. The preoperative nipple-areolar position is within the upper V. Her breasts are soft and mobile and the nipple-areola moves upward easily. The superior pedicle technique is selected to reduce the heaviness inferiorly and laterally.

Surgical plan

- Preoperative markings to define new nipple position as well as width of central breast and horizontal ellipse of skin to be excised
- Liposuction of lateral breast region to remove any extra fullness
- Resection of inferior breast region
- Resection of lateral breast parenchyma, reassembling of breast with clips, and transfer of nipple-areola superiorly to its new position
- Closure leaving inverted T scar and periareolar scar

Markings and Technique

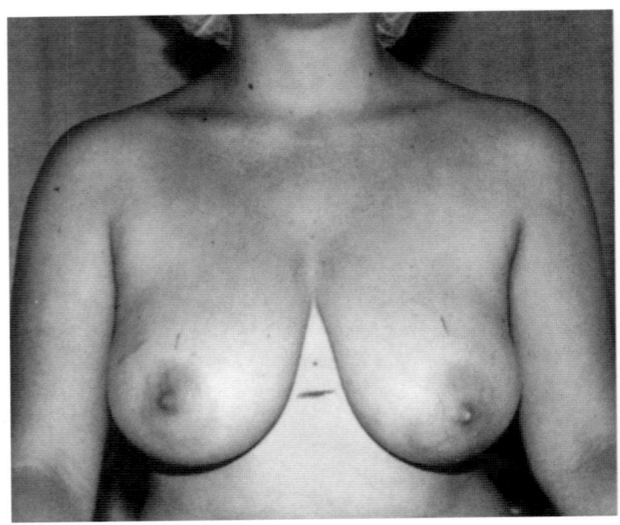

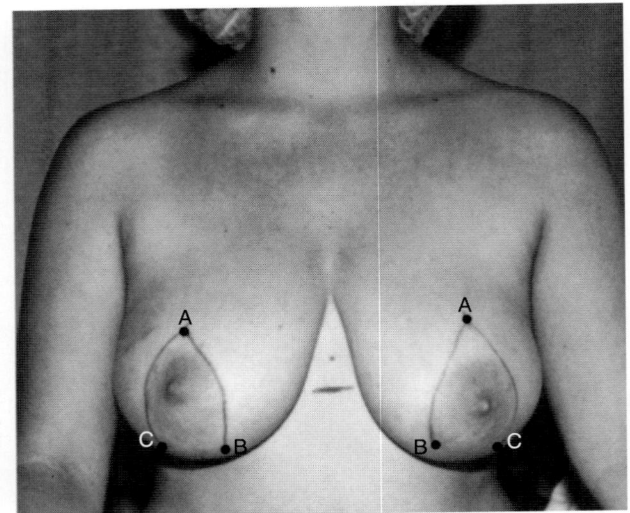

The new location for the upper margin of the areola is determined. The midbreast line (midclavicle to nipple) and inframammary crease are marked with the patient upright. The new nipple position will be located on a point on this midbreast line, approximately 19 to 21 cm from the sternal notch with the weight off the breast. When there is a medial or lateral inclination of the nipple away from this line, the true line is from the midclavicular point to the anterior superior iliac spine. ***The nipple's relationship to the inframammary crease is more important as a reference point for nipple placement than are the measurements taken down from the clavicle. It is better to measure up than to measure down! The breast weight should be lightly supported when the anterior projection of the inframammary crease onto the midbreast line is marked or the areola may be too high postoperatively.*** Usually the location for the top of the areola is 1 to 2 cm above the inframammary crease when final breast volume is 300 to 500 gm. For a larger volume the point will be closer to the level of the inframammary crease because the breast skin and areola site tend to move upward when the weight of the lower breast parenchyma is removed. Fixed distances should not be used for all breast reductions. Consideration should be given to the proportions and size of the patient's body and breasts.

Next, the upper V angle is identified by pushing a small portion of the breast upward approximately 7 cm below the proposed nipple position or 9 cm below the upper margin of the areola. The lateral and medial skin is brought together in a 9 cm arc below the future nipple site and then downward until it meets easily near the inframammary crease. The arc length can be 10 to 11 cm when the breasts are larger. Then points B and C are marked. The distance from the proposed areolar apex to the T is indicated by the 9 cm measurement. When points B and C are approximated, the patient can see the changes in breast size and contour.

Markings for the midbreast line begin at its intersection with the inframammary crease at point D. The lowest points of the V (B and C) are brought toward point D, and the inframammary line is marked. I position these points for conservative skin excision to avoid making the skin closure too tight. ***It is important to remember that lower skin tightness does not shape the breast and it can predispose to separation of the skin, especially at the T point. Breast shape and contour are influenced by resection of breast parenchyma.*** More skin can always be removed at the final stages of the operation if necessary.

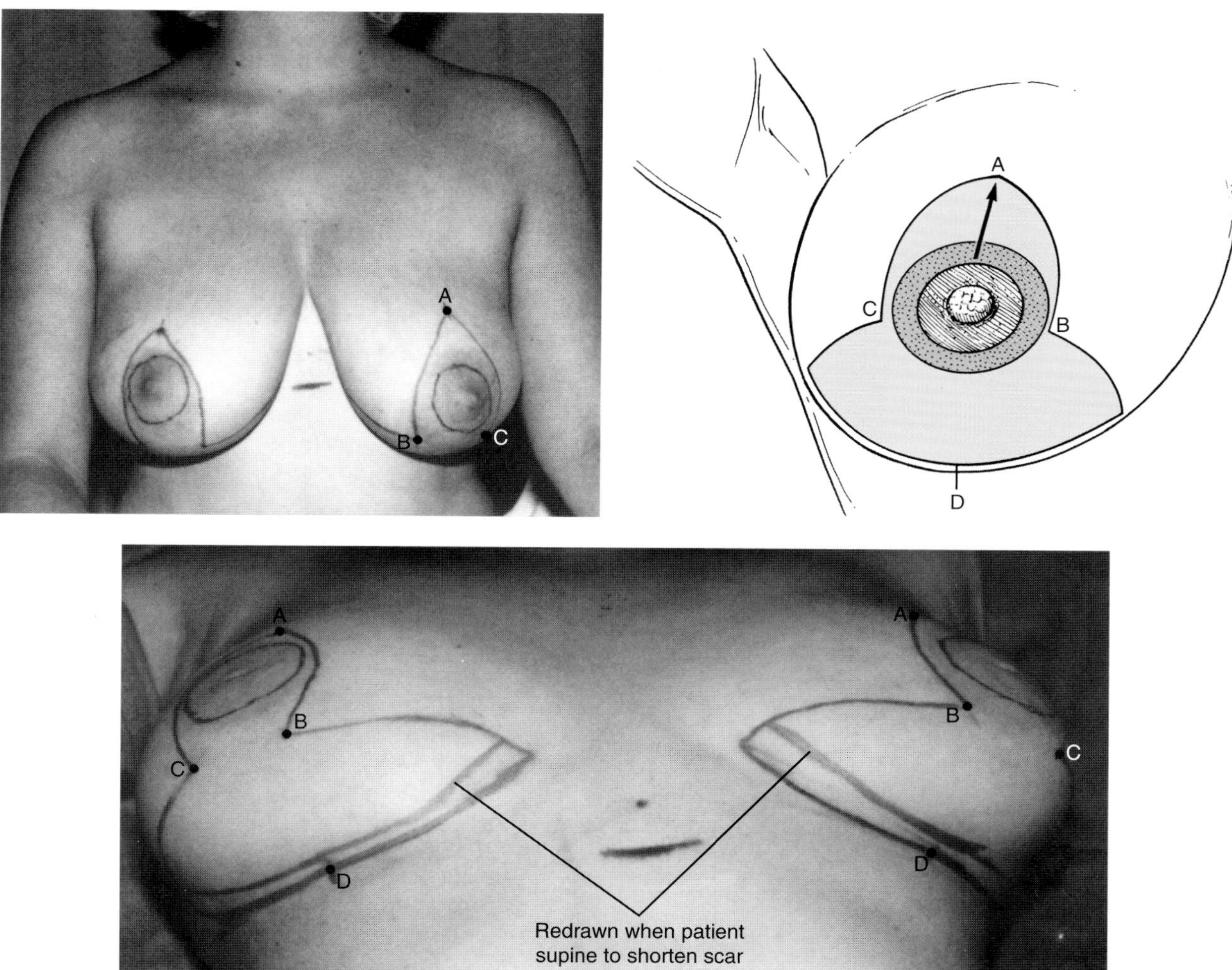

The lines are then connected to the inframammary crease lines medially and laterally. Curved or lateral and medial S lines to help shape the breast should be avoided because they create unnecessary tension during final closure and can cause wide scars. A 42 to 46 mm diameter circle is drawn within the areola. This should be marked with the areola at rest and not distended. The areolar diameter should be a proportional size. The inframammary crease lines are re-marked when the patient is supine. This shortens them and places them along the new inframammary fold.

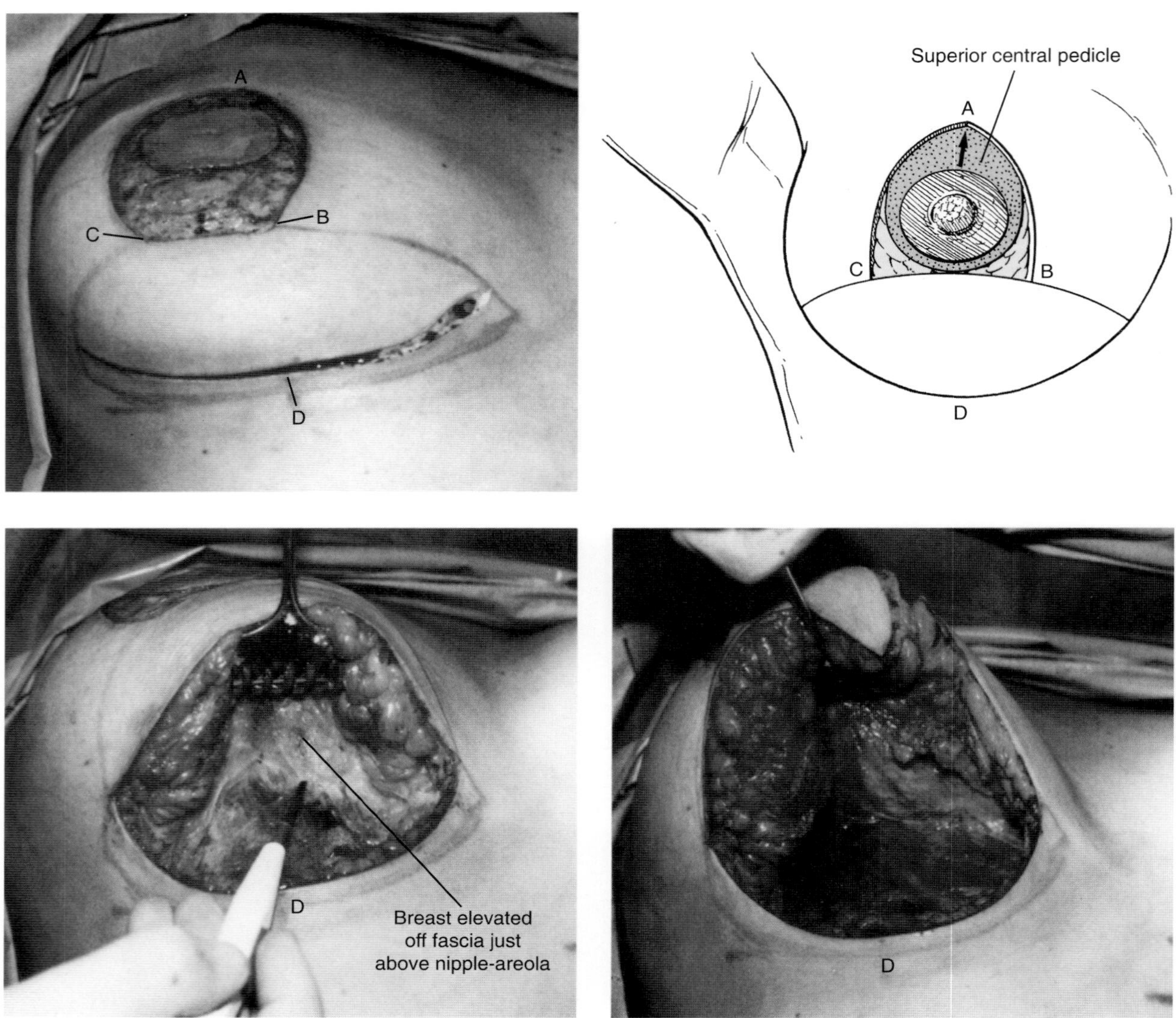

The initial incision is made around the areola line with a knife. Large scissors are used to deepithelialize the upper V. The nipple-areolar attachment to underlying central breast tissue, lactiferous ducts, and nerves is preserved for functional and circulatory reasons.

The inframammary incision is made down to the deep fascia and then around the lower breast to elevate it from the superficial layer of the deep fascia up to the nipple-areolar level. When perforators supplying a portion of the central breast parenchyma are encountered, they are controlled.

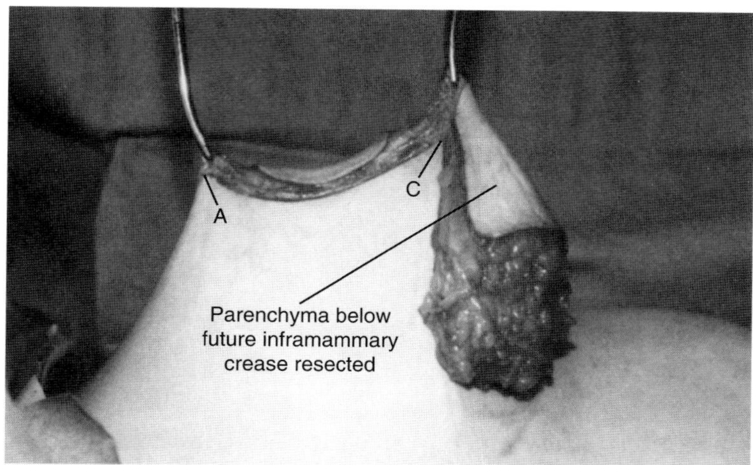

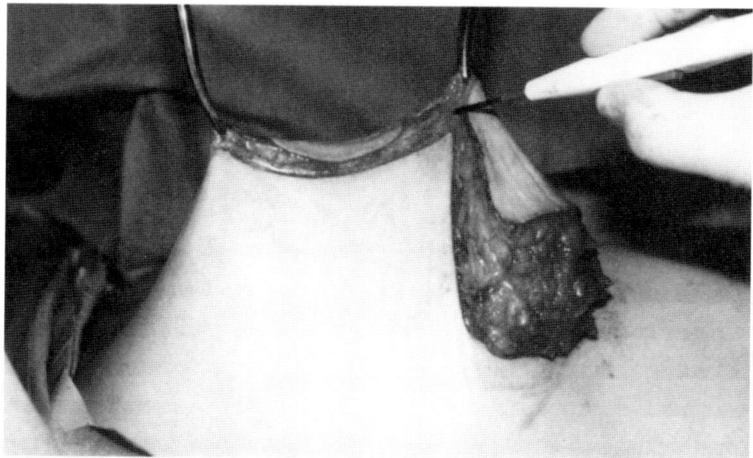

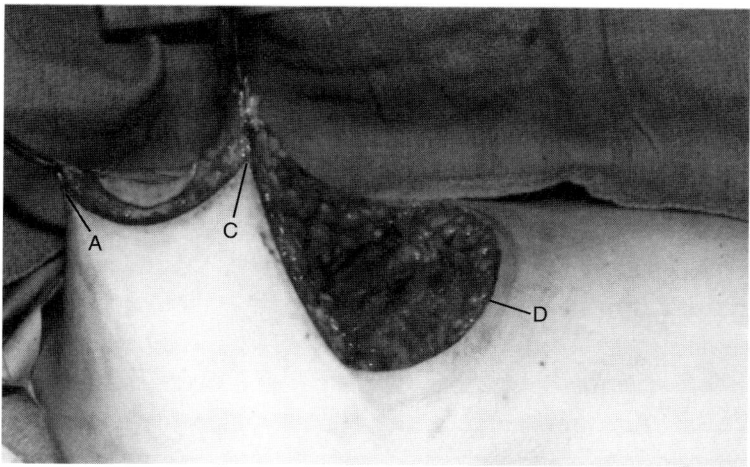

The breast is lifted perpendicularly to the chest wall. The lower portion of the breast, which projects below the final inframammary crease, is resected to remove the lower ptotic breast parenchyma below the inframammary fold when the woman is standing. Preservation of an adequate breast volume is ensured by elevating the breast at the top of the V and at the center of the lower resection line.

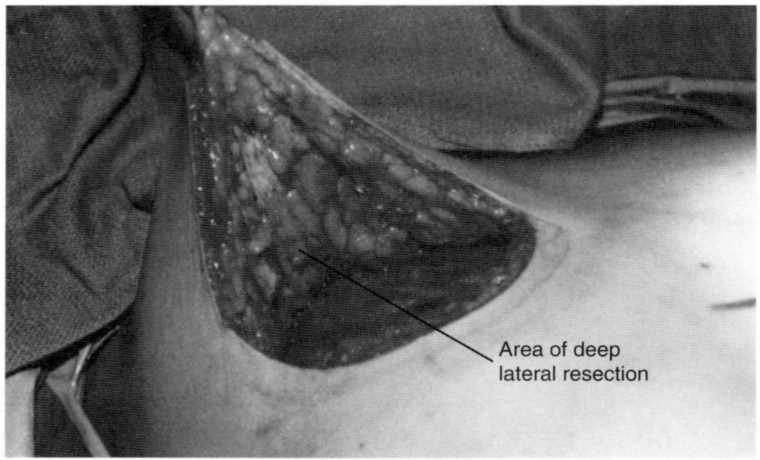

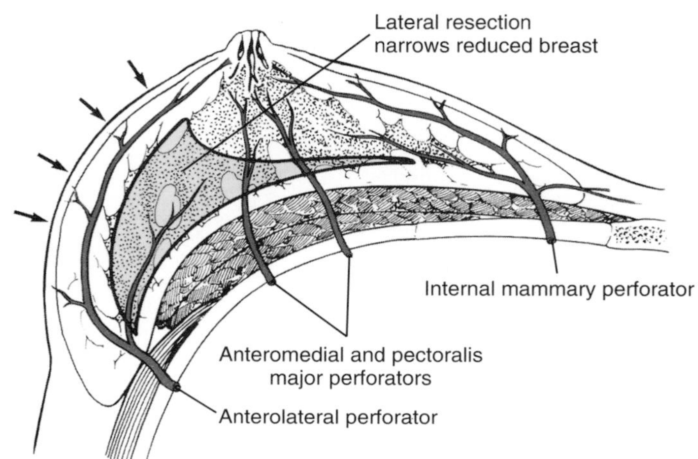

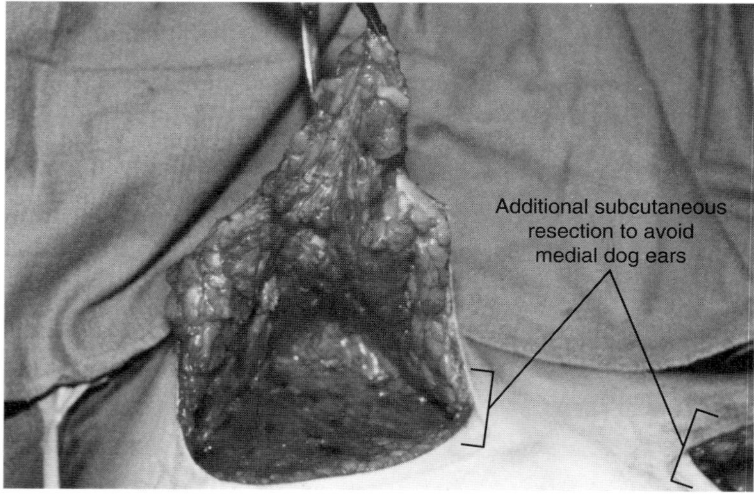

The upper breast width and projection are then addressed. ***The breast is narrowed and reduced to its eventual size and shape by resecting a wedge of lateral breast parenchyma and if necessary a tangential disk of deep central tissue.*** This reduces the breast further as well as reducing central breast projection.

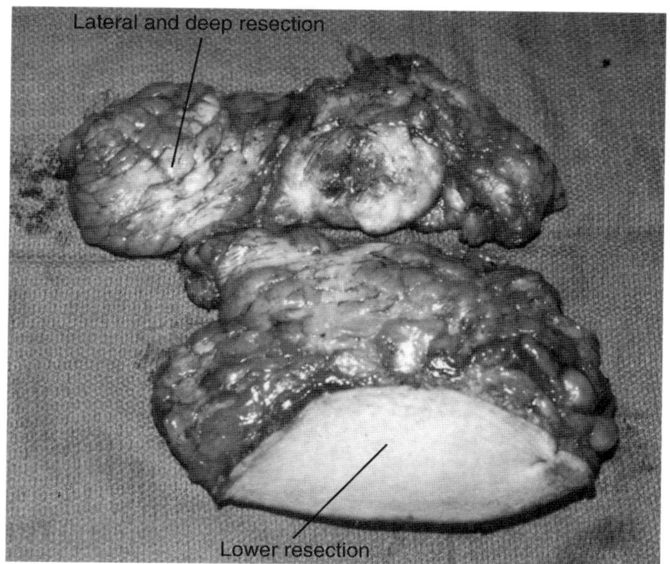

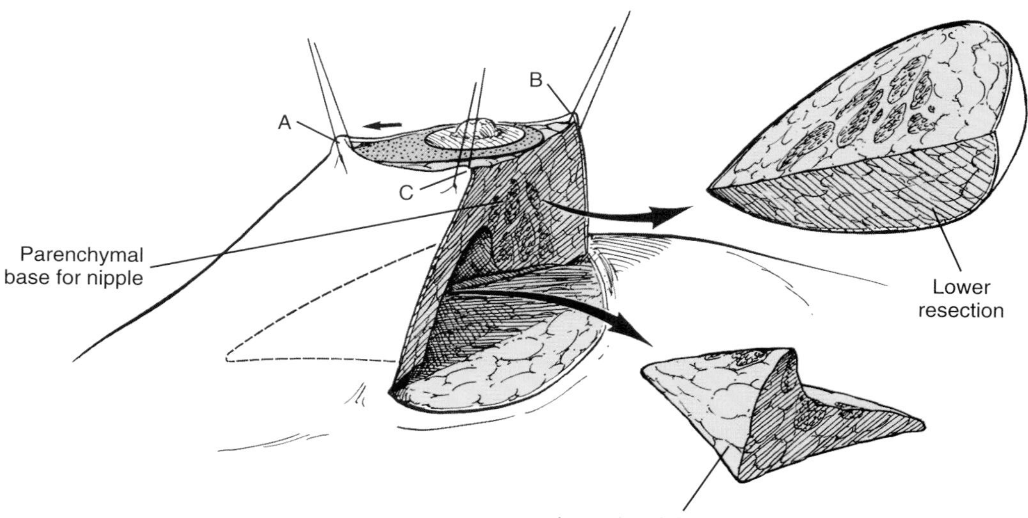

The resected specimen from the lower breast and deeper lateral area are shown, and the appearance of the reduced breasts before final closure is demonstrated. The tissue has now been resected from the inferior and lateral portions of the breast. The resected breast parenchyma extended below the inframammary crease and also contributed to increased breast width and fullness. This procedure removes the lower and lateral breast tissue and most of the lower outer quadrant, which is responsible for breast heaviness and hypertrophy. Once this lower breast parenchyma is resected, this problem does not usually recur. The well-vascularized upper breast, which nourishes the nipple-areola, is preserved to produce cleavage and central volume.

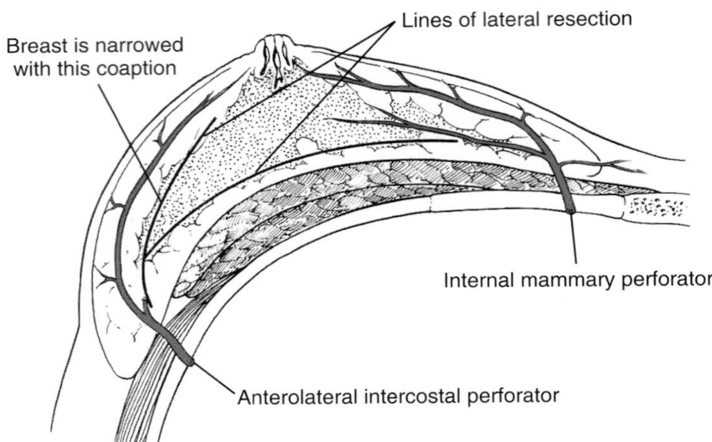

Despite the division of some lower central musculocutaneous perforators (which are preserved using the central pedicle technique) during the deep lateral resection, the vascularity of the remaining breast is good. Perforators are preserved medially, laterally, and superiorly and in the upper central region, especially the larger blood vessels, the second intercostal perforators from the internal mammary artery and the external mammary artery from the axilla.

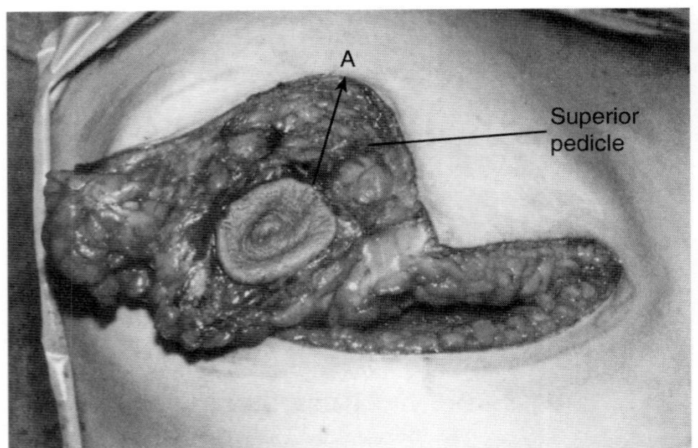

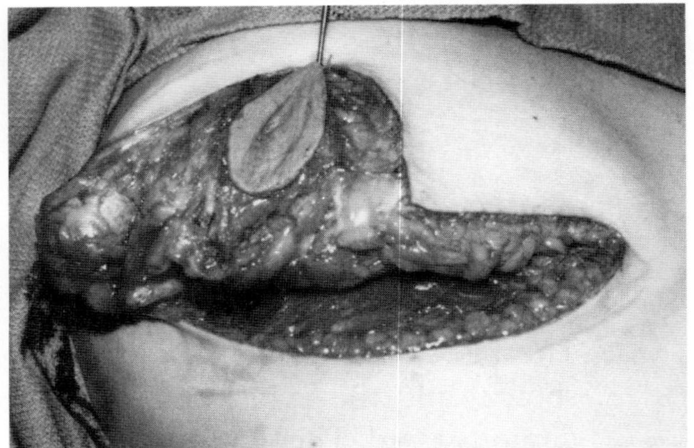

The nipple-areola should be easily moved to its new position. This can be facilitated by releasing and undermining the skin superiorly and dividing the dermis medially and laterally in the V. The nipple should be easily repositioned and rest there without undue tension. Some of the lower dermal attachments of the nipple-areola can be released to allow it to move upward more easily.

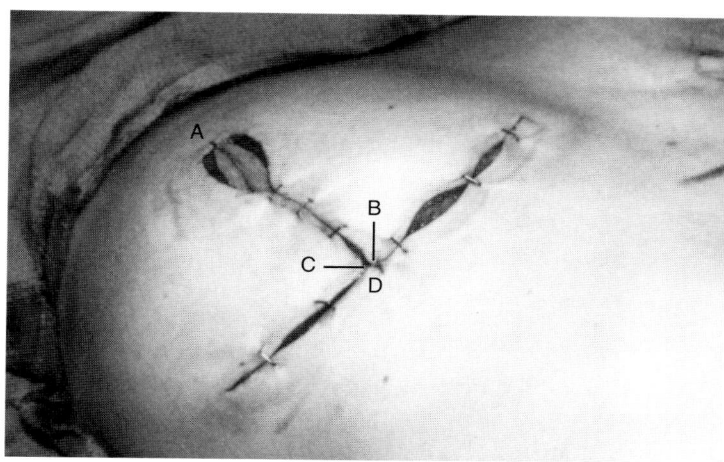

The areola apex is then secured to point A, and the breasts are checked for symmetry with the patient sitting up on the operating room table. The surgeon should be sure that each breast has the same volume before they are reassembled with clips. It is usually obvious when there is more tissue or fullness in one or the other. The resected volumes should be checked against the preoperative asymmetry as well as the size and appearance of each specific breast quadrant. I try to be sure that the breasts are symmetric before I close and suture them. ***Rather than completing one breast and closing, I feel it is easier to obtain symmetry by adjusting both breasts at the same time with wide exposure.***

Temporary clips are used to close the inframammary incision from the periphery to point D, and the breasts are rechecked for symmetry. If excess skin persists, it is removed centrally from point A to point D along A to B and A to C, taking care to avoid tight skin closure. No dog ears or excess underlying breast parenchyma should remain at the medial and lateral limits of the inframammary incision. The medial and lateral resections are checked to determine if sufficient underlying soft tissue has been removed, thus avoiding problems with lateral fullness, contour irregularities, and dog ears.

The proposed areolar position is prepared by marking a circle with a diameter 2 to 3 mm smaller than the preserved nipple-areola. The skin is excised full thickness. The larger areola is fit into this smaller circle, thereby avoiding tension on the areolar suture line. Closure of these incisions proceeds along the vertical line (A to D) up to 5 cm above point D. The placement of the nipple-areola is determined with the patient upright on the operating table. The nipple-areola should be pointing approximately 5 degrees downward with its lower margin about 4.5 to 5.5 cm above the inframammary crease for a breast reduction of 300 to 500 gm. A longer crease-areola distance is needed for larger breast reductions. The position for the nipple is marked, and a 38 to 42 mm circle is drawn around it. The lower portion of this circle is 5 cm above point D.

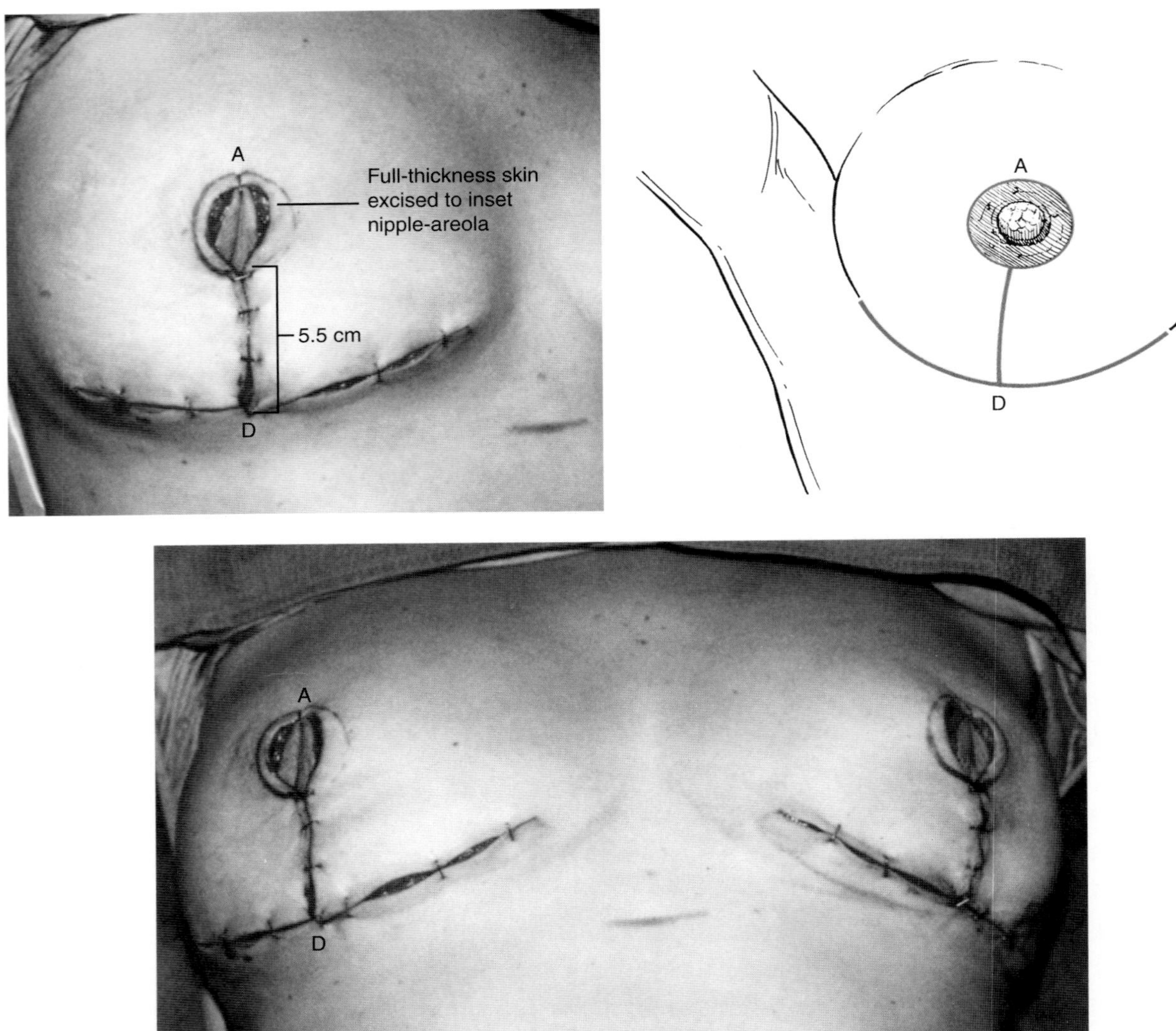

Intracuticular sutures are used to close the nipple-areola; deeper sutures should include the underlying layer of superficial fascia and dermis. Effective hemostasis is essential, but drains are usually unnecessary. A light dressing is required postoperatively, and the patient wears a brassiere the next day.

Results

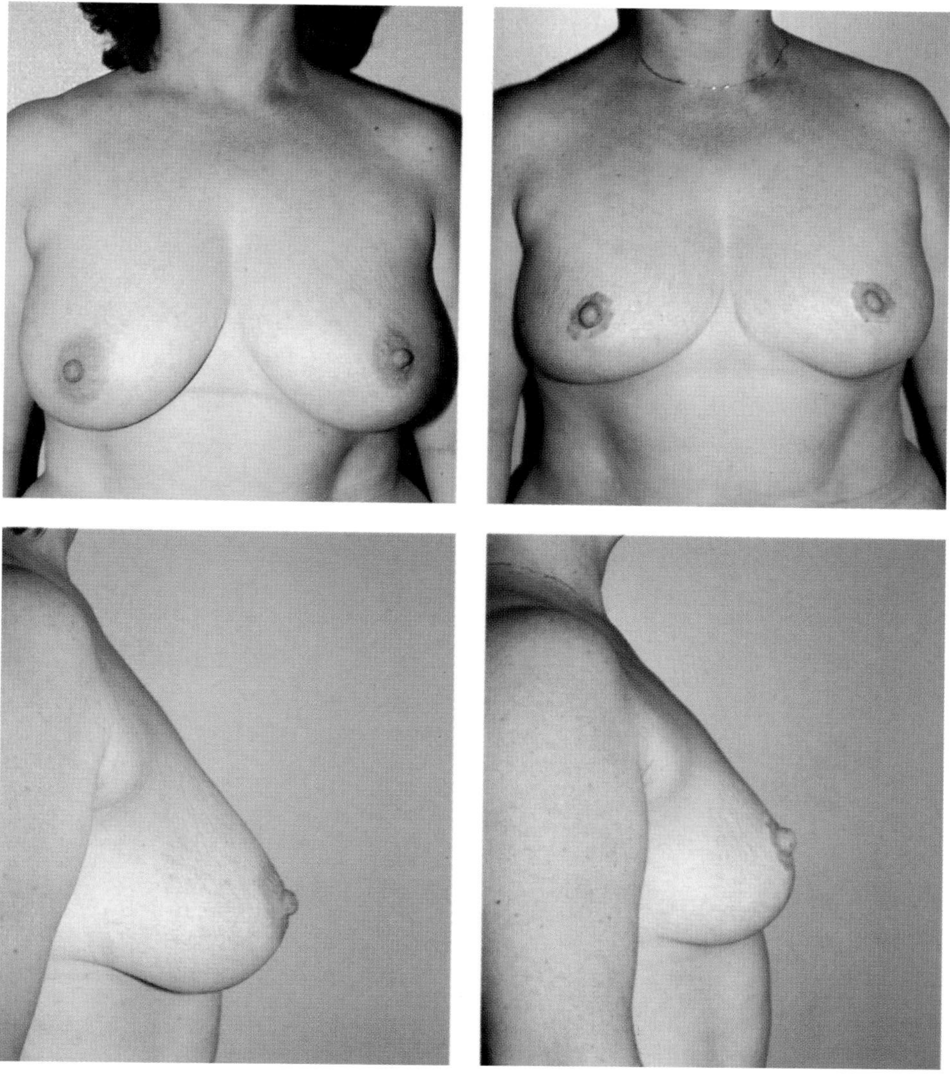

This 38-year-old woman complained of heaviness and discomfort caused by the weight of her breasts. The superior pedicle technique was used to remove 400 gm from each breast. This satisfied patient is shown 3 years following breast reduction. Note that the scars have faded and fall within the inframammary fold. Since the patient is mildly overweight, the reduction was consistent with her body proportions. She did not request abdominal liposuction, but this procedure could have enhanced her torso configuration. Additional lateral resection may have produced more breast narrowing.

SUPERIOR MEDIAL PEDICLE TECHNIQUE

The superior medial pedicle technique is selected when nipple-areolar elevation is restricted and the superior pedicle technique is not suitable because of firm, dense breast parenchyma or the nipple-areola needs to be moved a greater distance upward than the superior pedicle technique permits. This is a reliable technique because it incorporates the intercostal perforator blood supply with some of the primary blood flow to the breast from the upper medial perforators. I do not, however, use it for women who are likely to have impaired microcirculation, such as 60+ pack-year cigarette smokers, women who are markedly obese, or those with collagen vascular disease. ***The superior medial pedicle technique removes the lower ptotic breast tissue as well as some lateral and upper lateral breast tissue to narrow the breast.*** The preserved upper breast tissue is much less prone to ptosis postoperatively.

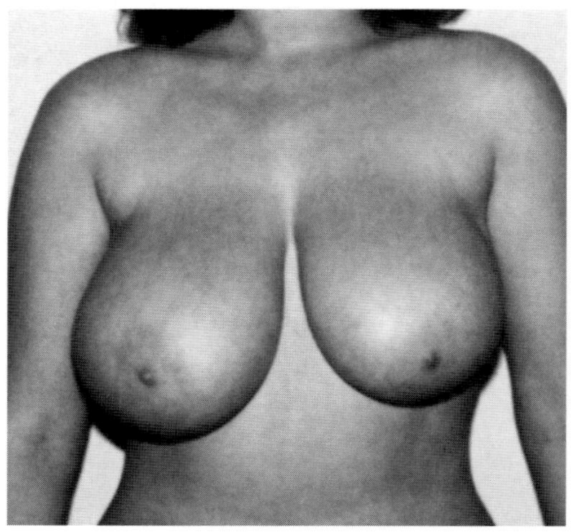

This 19-year-old woman has hypertrophic, asymmetric breasts. The breast parenchyma is somewhat firm, and the nipple-areola does not move easily to the new nipple position. A superior medial pedicle technique was selected because the nipple-areola required only modest elevation and the asymmetry could best be corrected by resecting skin from the upper mammary fold and vertically.

Surgical plan

- Preoperative markings to define new nipple position as well as width of central breast and horizontal ellipse of skin to be excised
- Liposuction of lateral breast region to remove any extra fullness
- Resection of inferior breast region
- Resection of lateral breast parenchyma, reassembling of breast with clips, and transfer of nipple-areola superomedially to its new position
- Closure leaving inverted T scar and periareolar scar

Markings and Technique

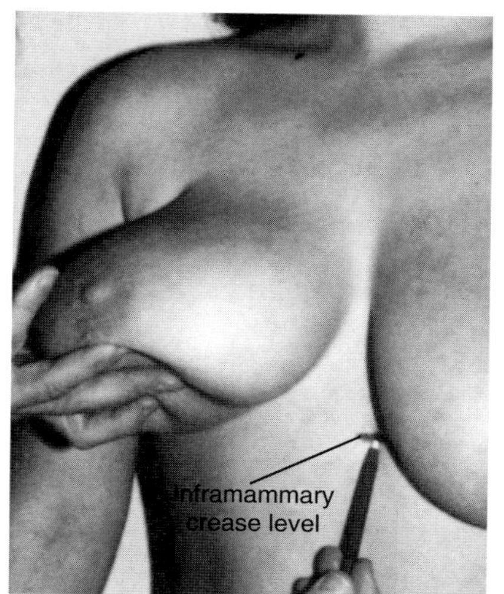

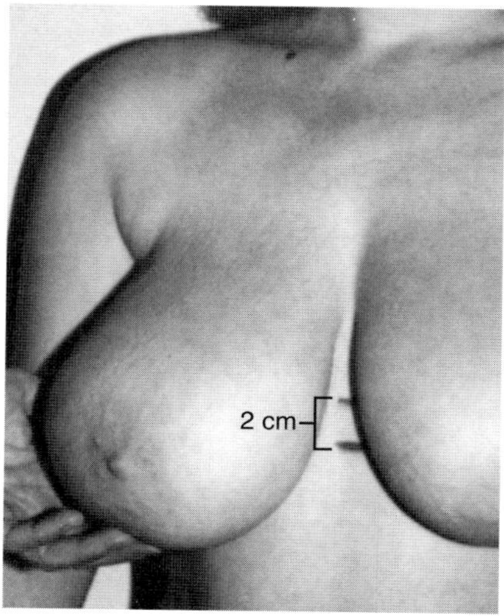

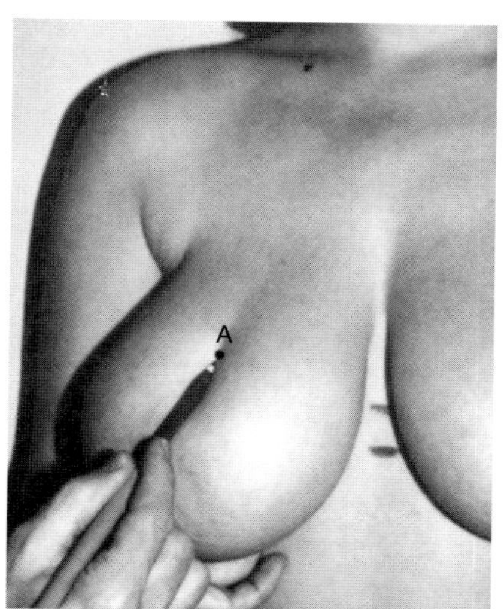

Markings are the same as for the superior pedicle technique. They are drawn preoperatively with the patient upright. The point for the placement of the upper portion of the areola is determined. The projection of the inframammary crease at the midline is marked, and a second line 2 cm above this line is also marked. With the breast lifted somewhat, this point can be identified by the projection of a finger through the breast on the midbreast line.

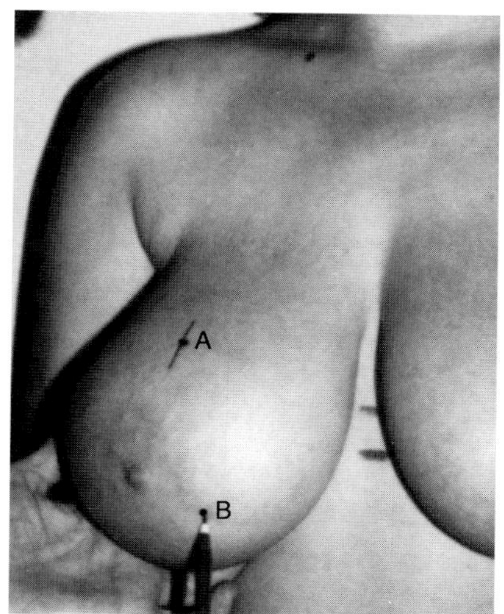

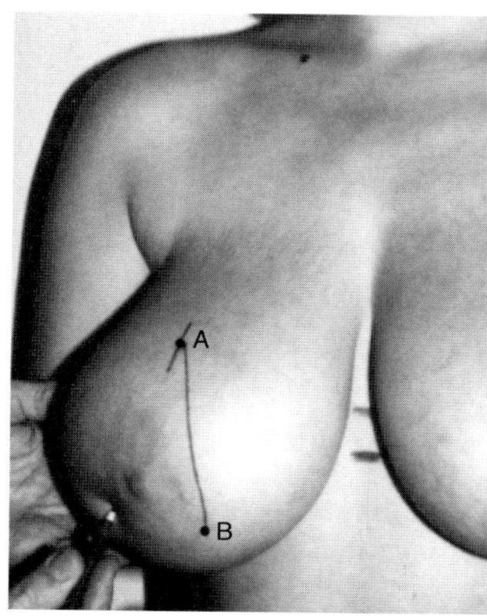

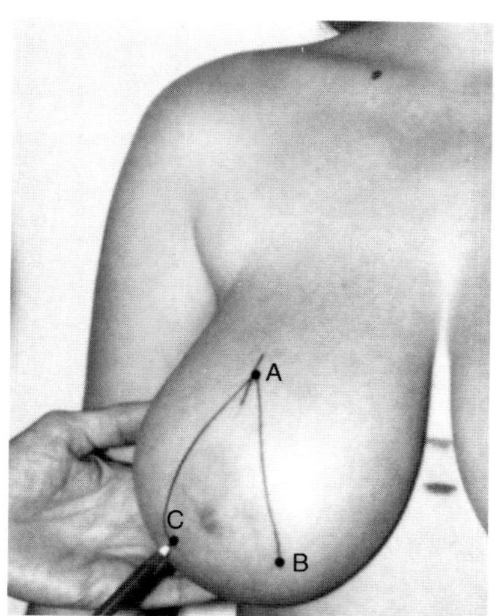

The upper V is marked. A safer strategy is to limit the angle of the V to the width of the areola. More skin can be removed later during closure if necessary and there is less chance of excess tightness at the T point. The distance from the top of the new areola to point D is 10 cm.

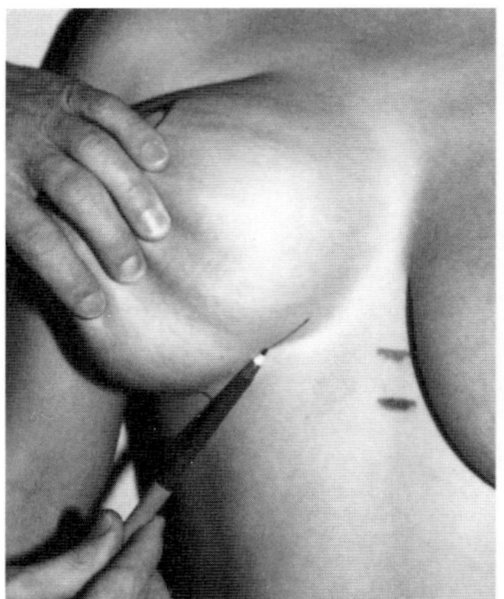

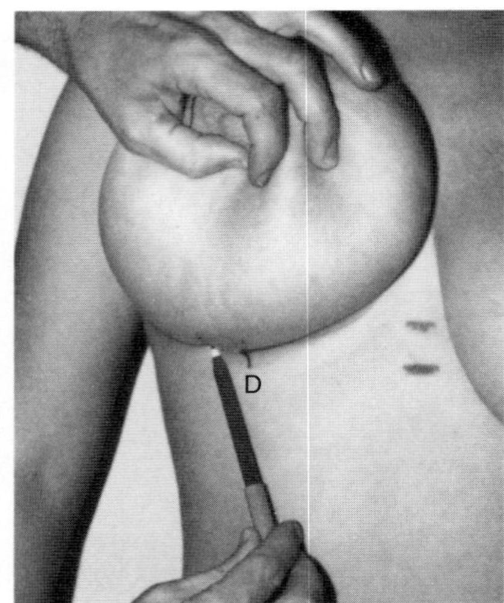

With the weight off the breast the limits of the inframammary crease are marked medially and laterally. I try to keep these incisions as short as possible to control the width of the final result.

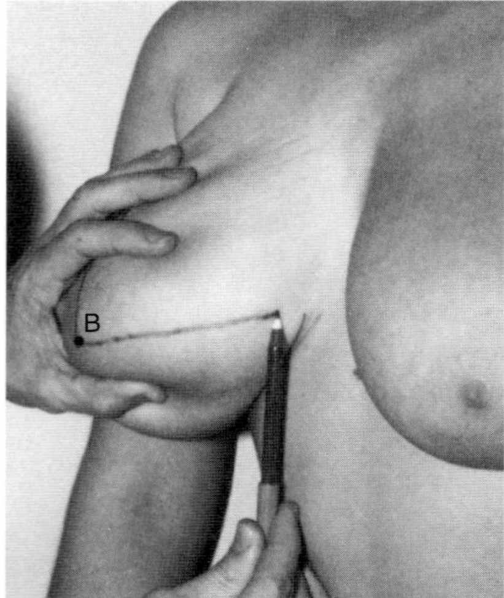

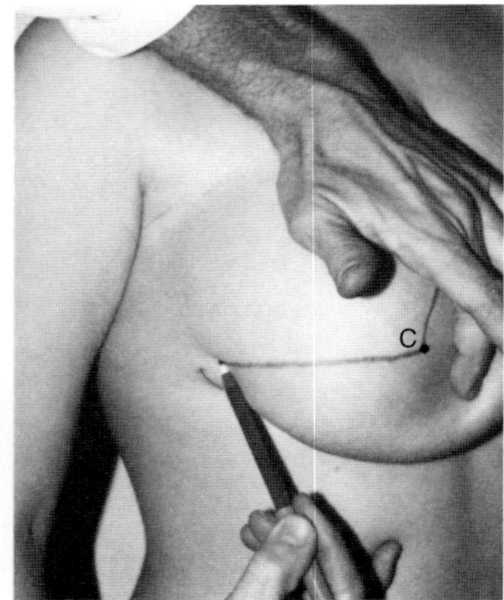

The medial and lateral lines are marked by displacing the breasts centrally and connecting the inferior points of the V to the medial and lateral junctures of the inframammary crease. This should not be too tight. ***It is better to leave some lower skin and tailor it postoperatively.***

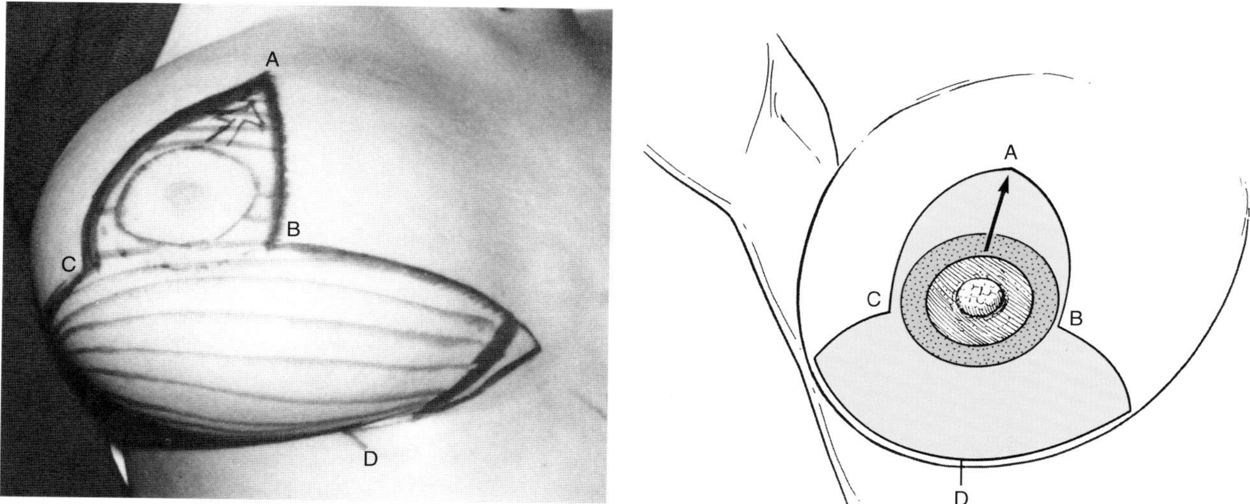

With the patient supine the inframammary fold is re-marked to minimize the length of the scars and to ensure that they fall in the new inframammary fold. I infiltrate up to 500 ml of wetting solution laterally in the region in which liposuction will be performed as well as in the lower breast to minimize bleeding. The breasts tend to fall laterally and this permits the medial incision to be redrawn to shorten the horizontal scar. Liposuction of the lateral breast region is performed first.

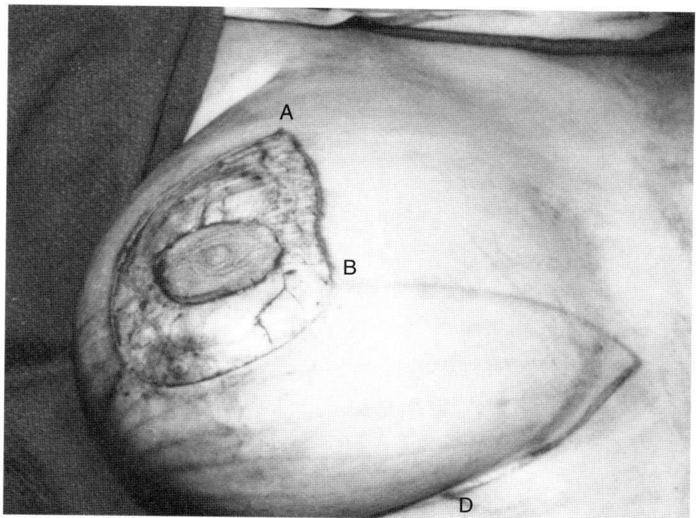

Incisions are made in the upper V and around the areolar markings. The upper V and the subdermal plexus surrounding the nipple are deepithelialized. The subdermal plexus must be preserved to enhance areola blood supply. In some women the superficial veins can be visualized and some of these preserved to ensure excellent venous drainage.

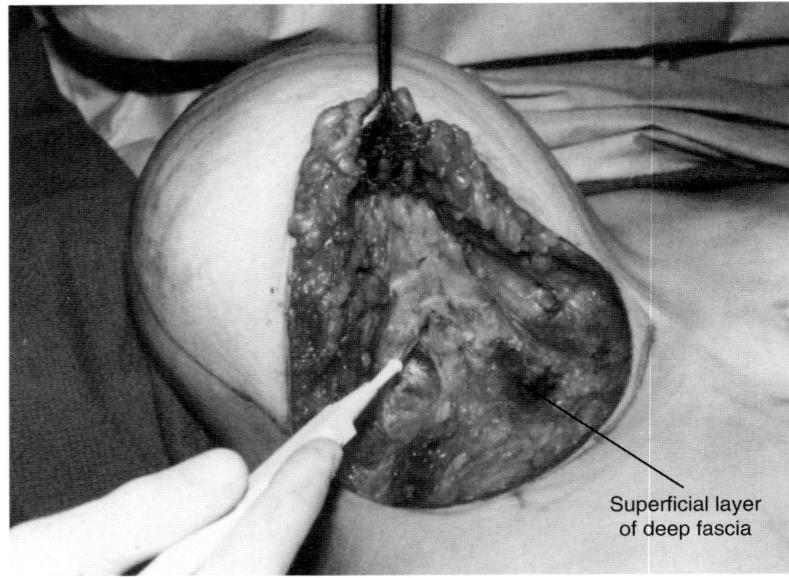

The operation begins with the patient in the supine position to provide better visualization. The inframammary crease incision is made, and the breast is lifted off the deep surface of the superficial fascia over the lower pectoralis major, serratus anterior, rectus abdominis, and external oblique muscles and up to the level where the areola will be repositioned.

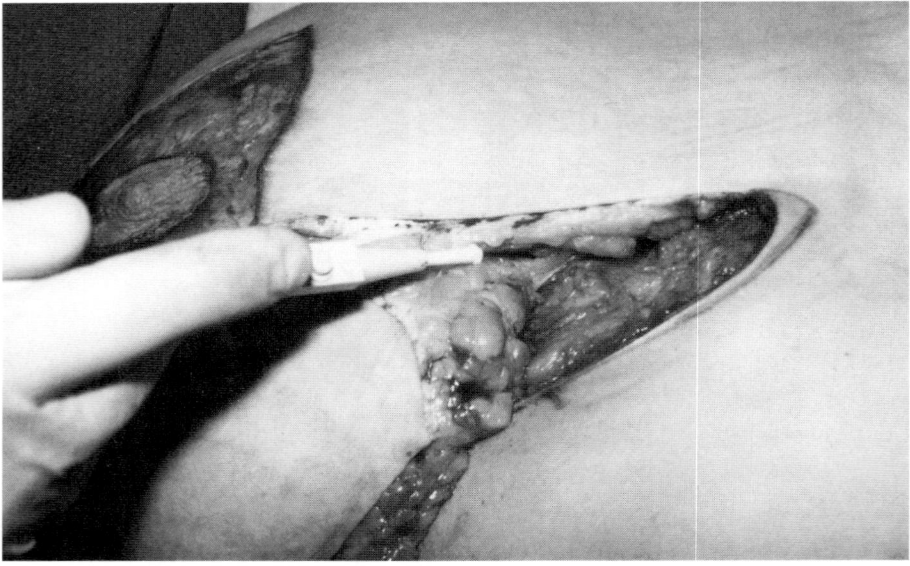

The medial portion is resected by beveling the breast parenchymal resection 45 degrees superiorly with the breast flat on the chest wall. Preservation of medial breast tissue obviates flattening in this area postoperatively.

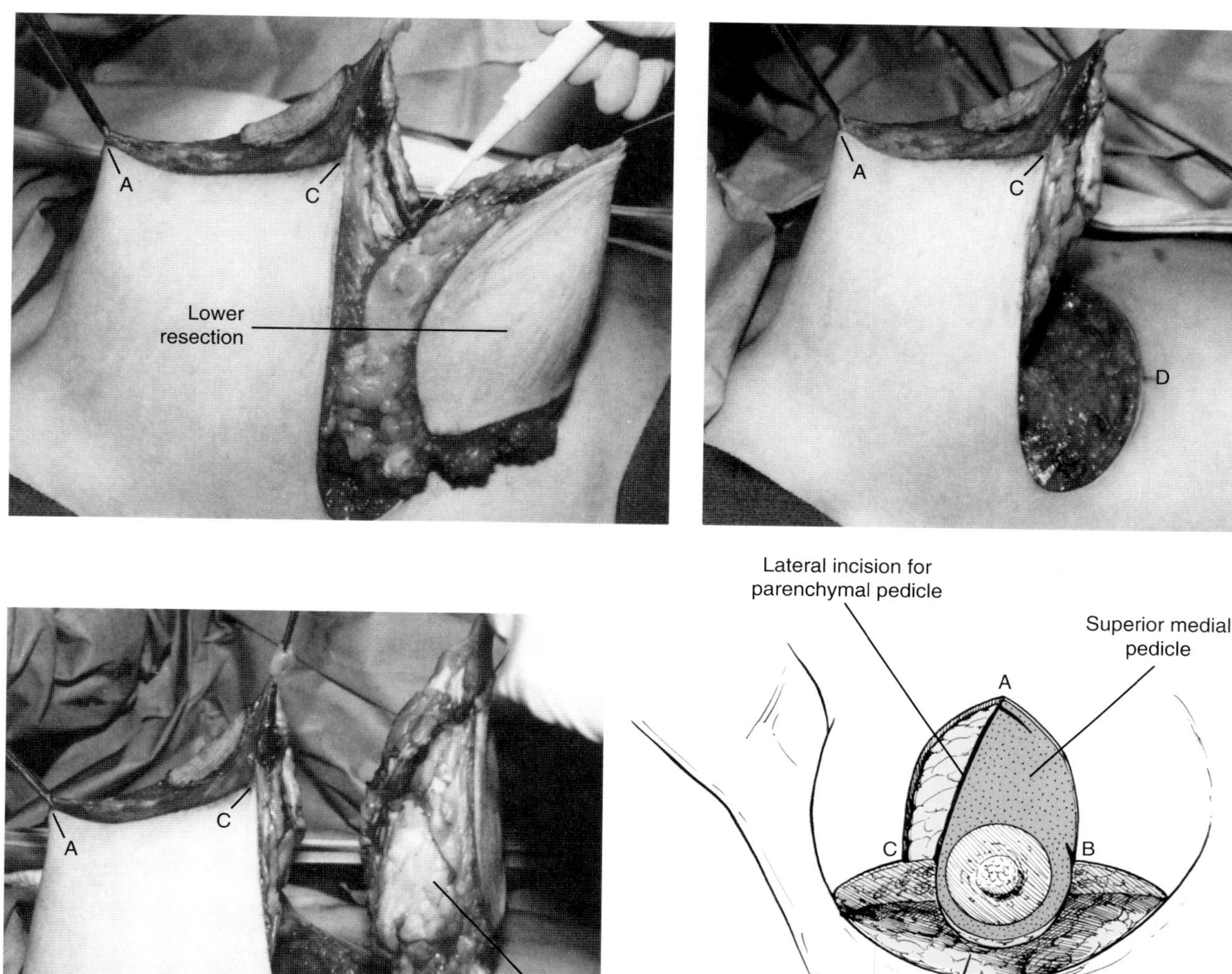

With the breasts elevated off the chest wall at points A and between B and C, the lower breast tissue is resected transversely below the future inframammary crease. This approach removes the heavy, ptotic breast parenchyma that can contribute to recurrence of hypertrophy and sagging. The upper parenchyma required to shape the future reduced breast is preserved. ***The tissue that hangs below the crease while the patient is standing is removed to minimize the possibility that ptosis will recur.***

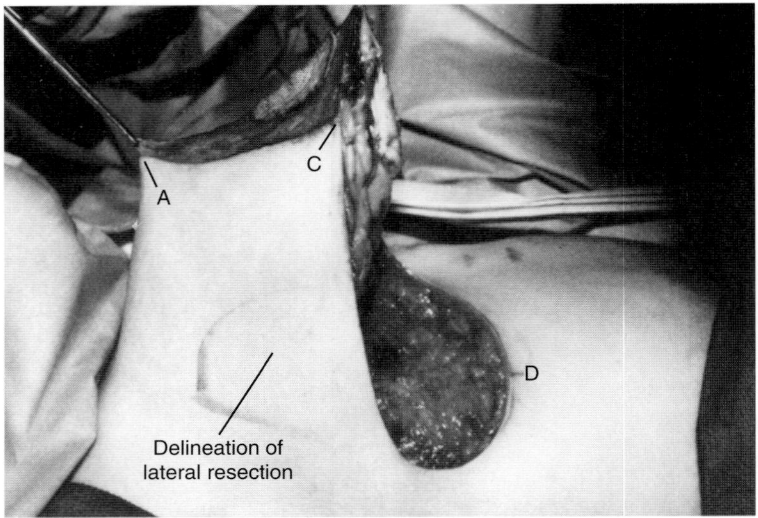

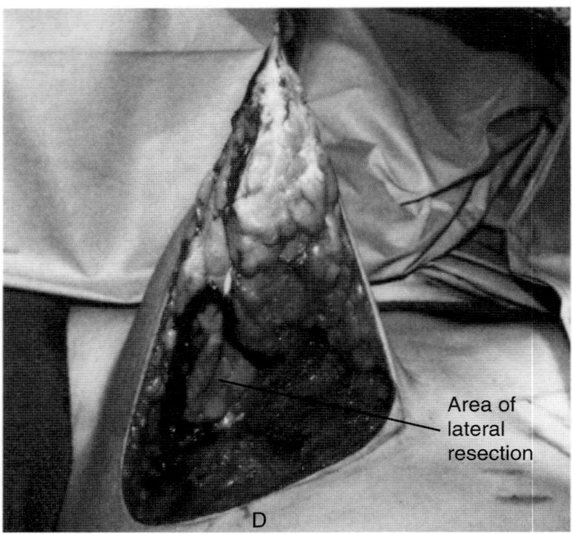

The area for the lateral resection is marked. ***This lateral parenchymal resection will narrow the breast and reduce the superior lateral fullness when the breast skin is closed.*** This resection allows further reduction in the region of breast fullness and hypertrophy while preserving the functional components of the breast.

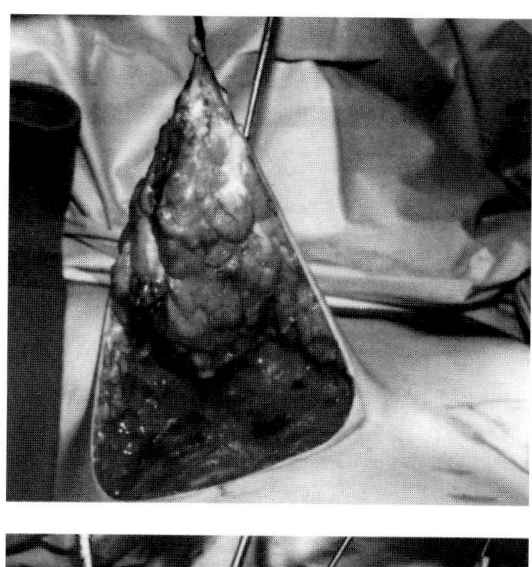

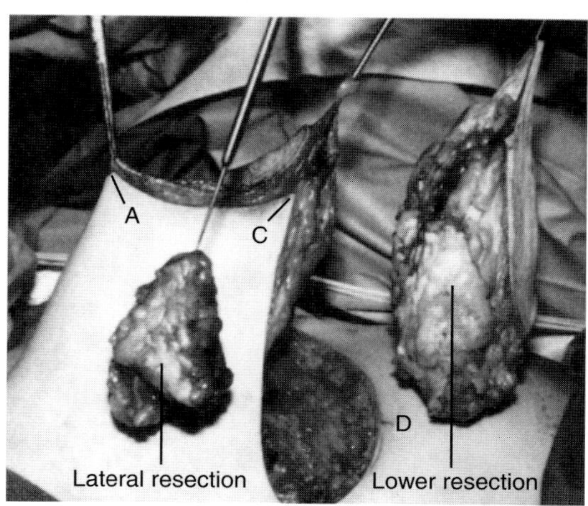

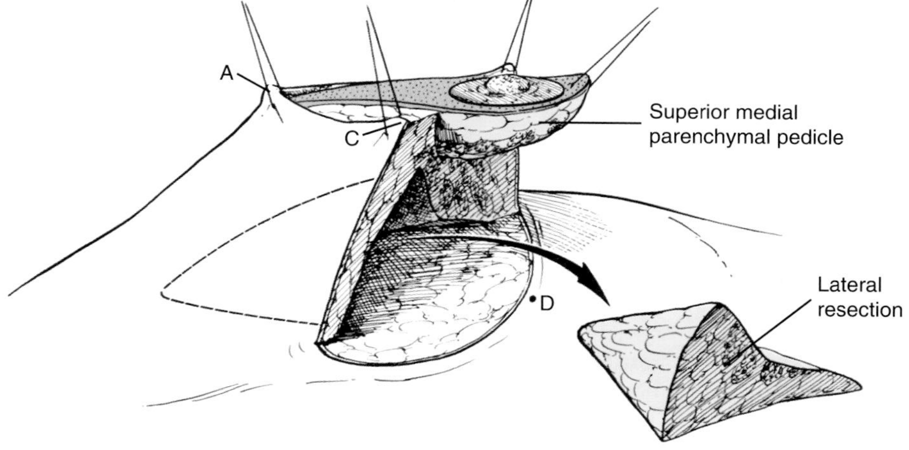

The breast has now been resected both inferiorly to reduce future ptosis and laterally to reduce breast width.

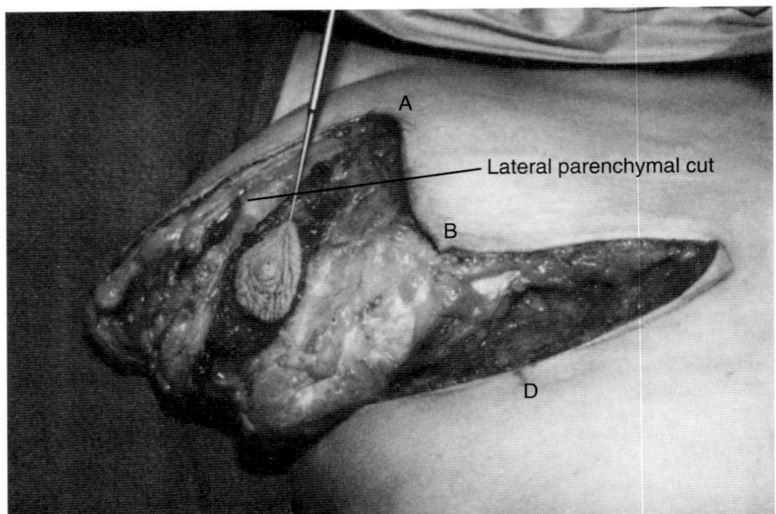

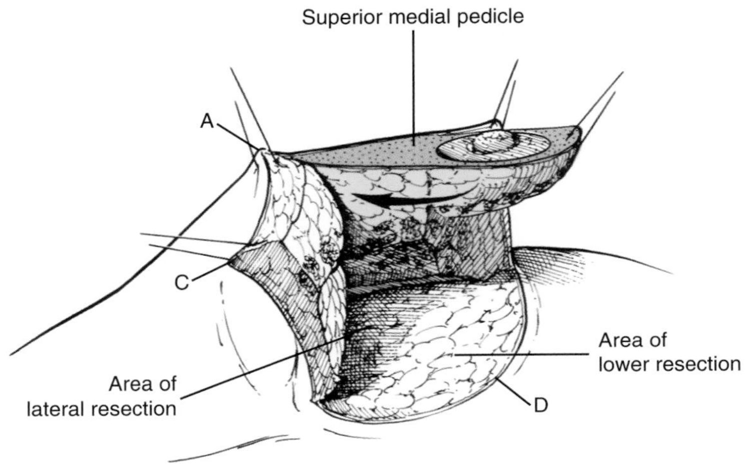

Before moving the nipple-areola upward to its new position, the mobility of the tissue is again checked. If the tissue is mobile and the nipple-areola can be moved upward, then the superior pedicle technique is used rather than the superior medial pedicle technique. Otherwise a full-thickness cut is made through the breast parenchyma laterally within the V from the future inframammary crease area, line B to C, up to the nipple-areola site at point A. A small backcut of about 1 to 2 cm along the medial border is also made. The upper breast skin in the area of the future nipple-areola site is undermined. A cut of about 1 cm is made on the medial portion of the V upward from the inframammary crease area at point B. This creates a medially based portion of breast parenchyma supporting the nipple-areola at its lower pole. The nipple-areola and the superior medial pedicle are then rotated upward until the nipple-areola is at the proposed site at point A. To enhance pedicle transposition some of the medial dermis but not the subdermal vessels can also be incised.

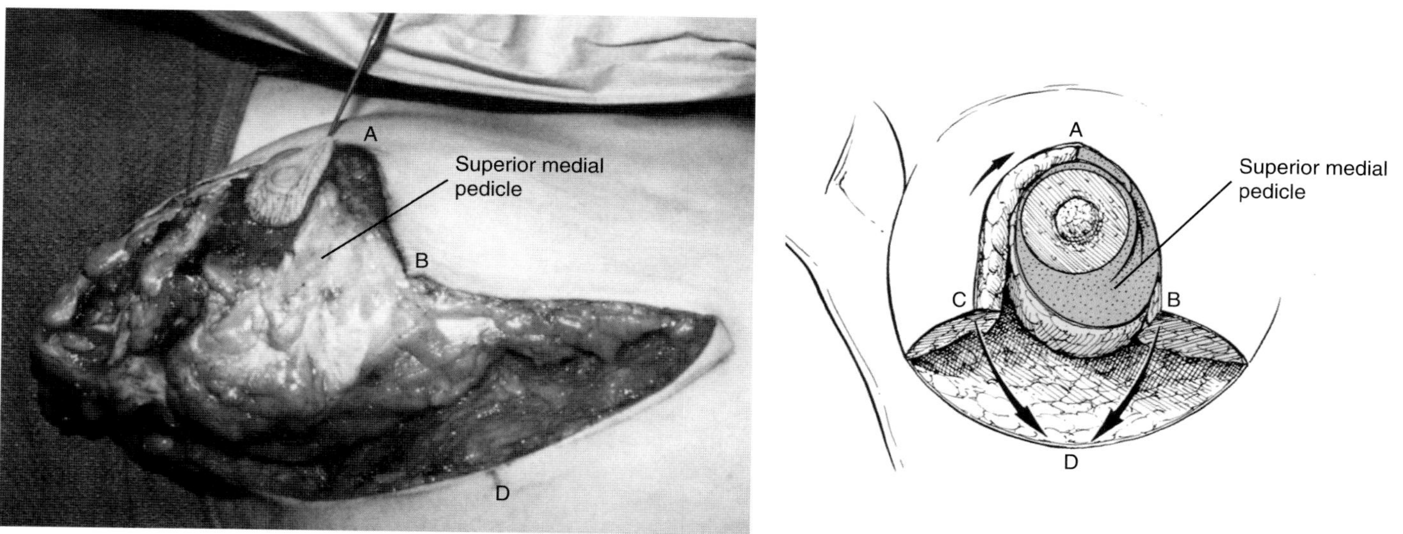

Rotation is actually easier when the pedicle is longer, and the breast is larger because the length of the arc of the pedicle increases. The lateral to medial inframammary fold closure fills the deficit left by upward pedicle transposition. The nipple-areola is inset as described earlier.

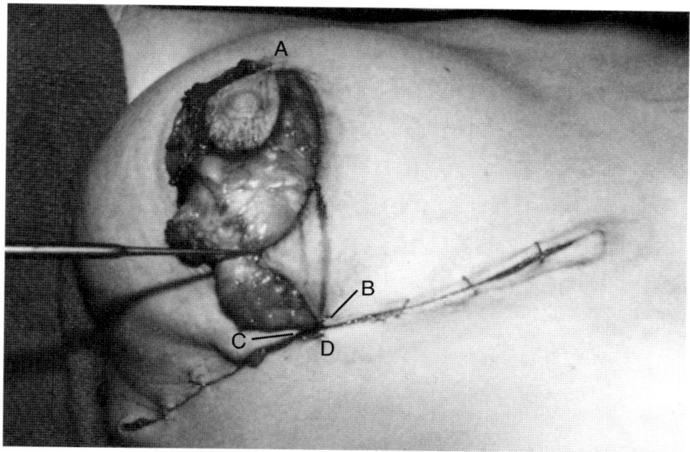

With the nipple rotated to its new position and secured, the incision is closed from lateral to medial toward the center T. Excess skin is resected medially for a gentle skin closure without tension to minimize the potential for separation of the T incision postoperatively.

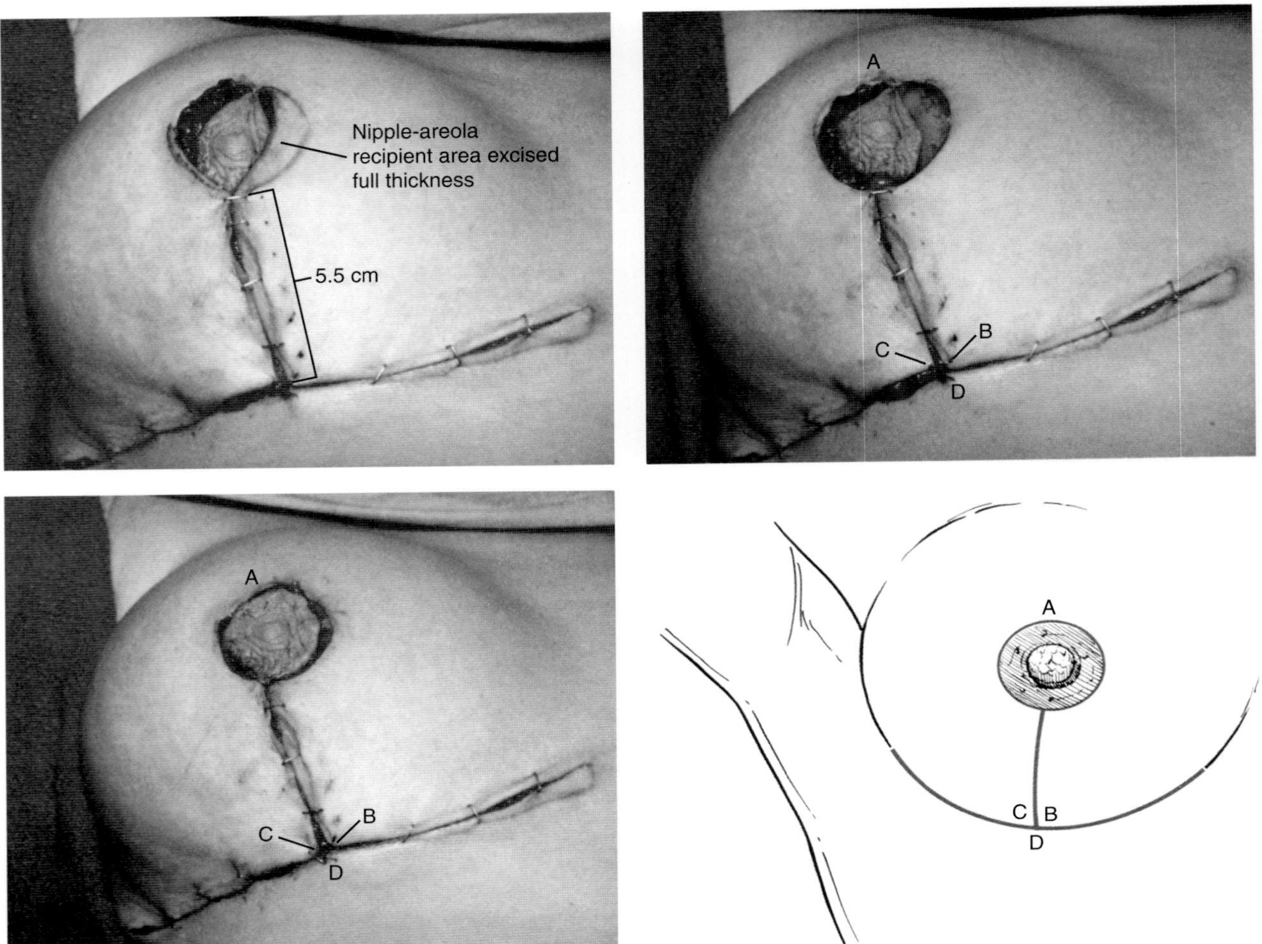

The diameter of the nipple-areolar recipient site is marked a few millimeters smaller than the incised diameter of the nipple-areola, usually 38 to 44 mm. It is also positioned to restore its medial inclination. Closure is effected with intracuticular sutures and the surgical clips removed.

Results

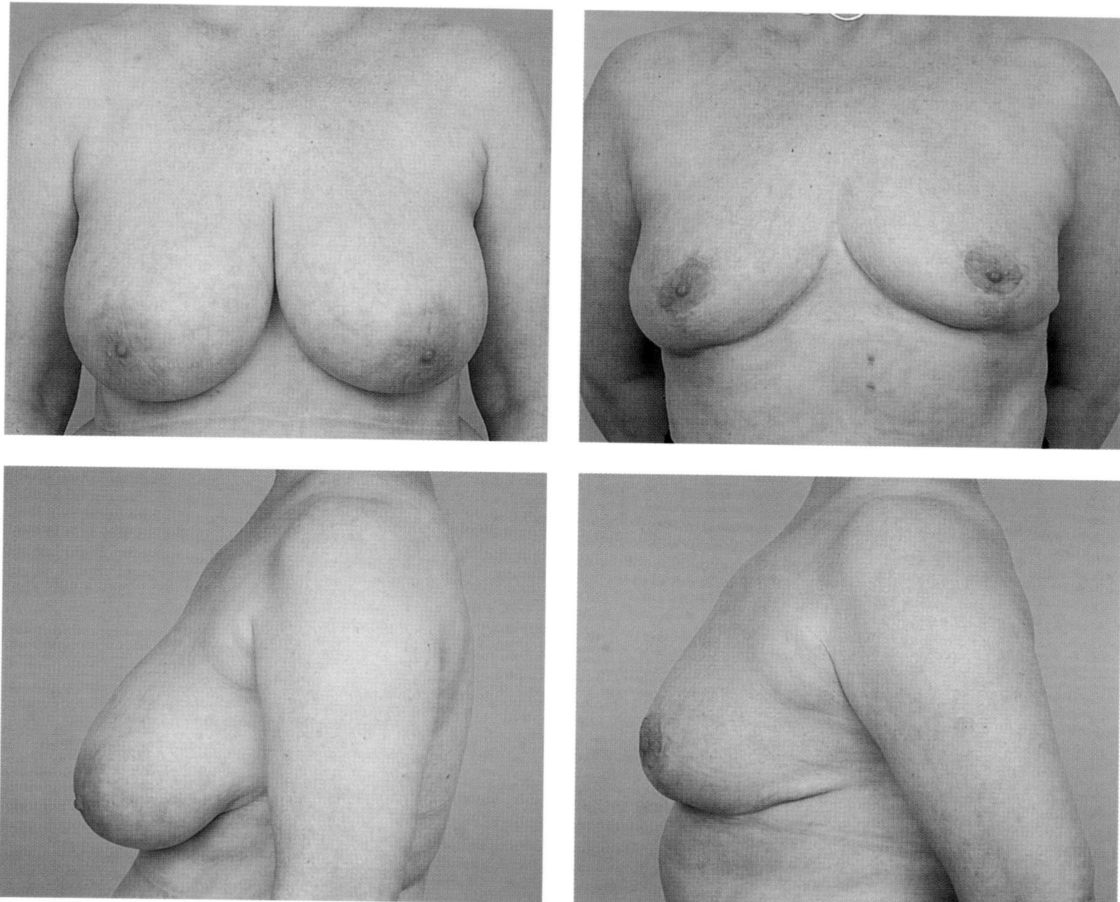

This 62-year-old woman was in good health, but her heavy breasts were a growing cause of concern. She had pain and shoulder grooving as well as a rash beneath her breasts. She requested breast reduction as well as removal of the lateral breast fullness. A superior medial pedicle technique was chosen. She was not a smoker and had evidence of good microcirculation. Wetting solution was infiltrated in the lower portion of her breasts as well as the lateral breast areas. Approximately 400 cc of fatty tissue was suctioned from each lateral breast region. Approximately 800 gm of tissue was resected from the inferior and lateral breast areas to remove ptotic breast tissue and narrow the breasts. She is shown 1 year postoperatively. Her breasts are now size 38B.

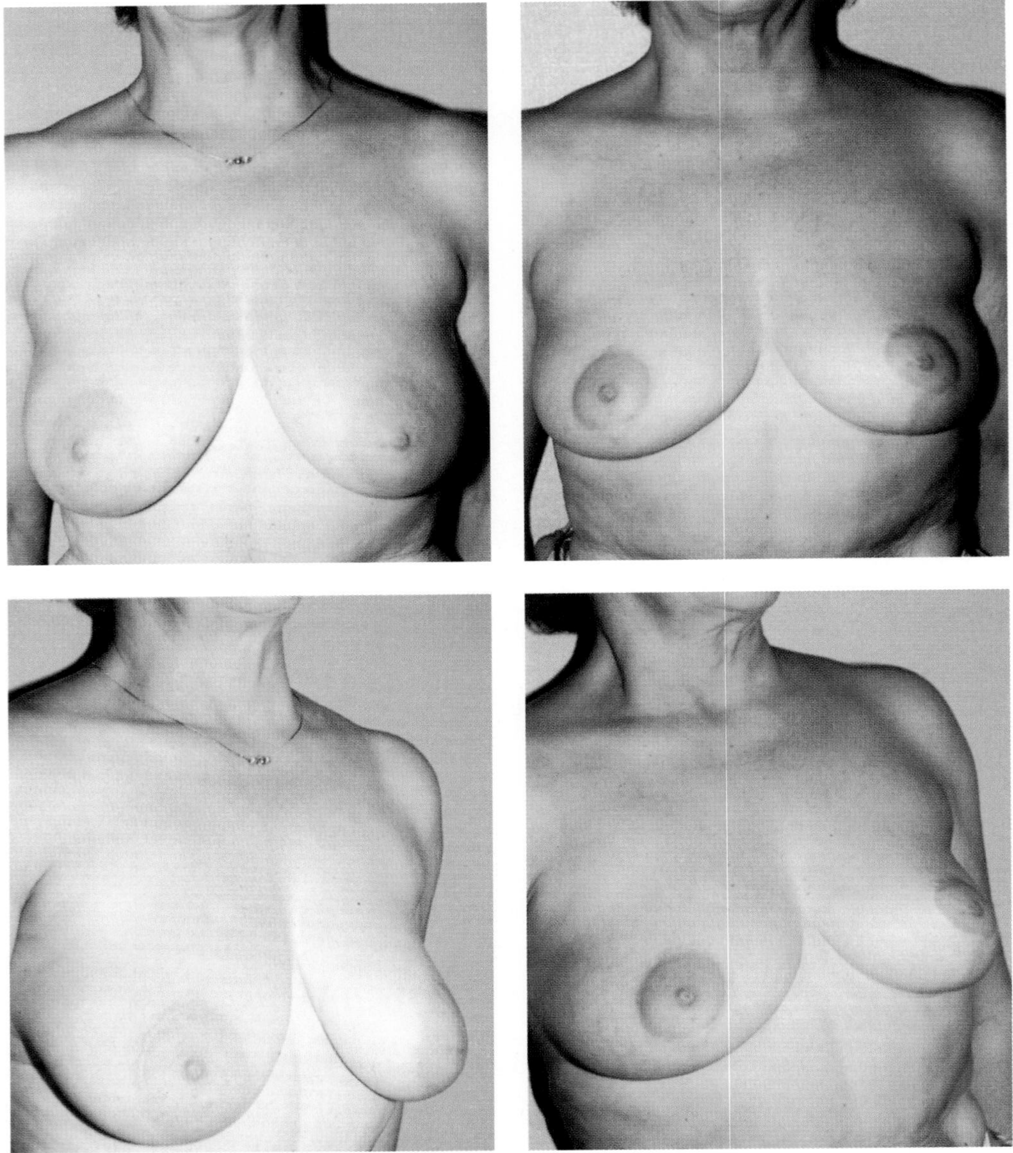

This 52-year old woman requested breast reduction. She had a small scar on her right breast from a biopsy several years earlier. This scar had healed with a thin line, indicating that she probably would have minor scarring after breast reduction. A superior medial breast reduction was planned. Her breasts were resected inferiorly as well as laterally. A total of 400 gm was removed from each breast. She is shown 2 years after breast reduction. Since the blood supply to the nipple comes from the underlying breast parenchyma, the biopsy scar posed no threat to periareolar vascularity or sensitivity. Although at the time I used the superior medial approach for this patient, today I would opt for the vertical mammaplasty technique to achieve a similar result without the horizontal incision.

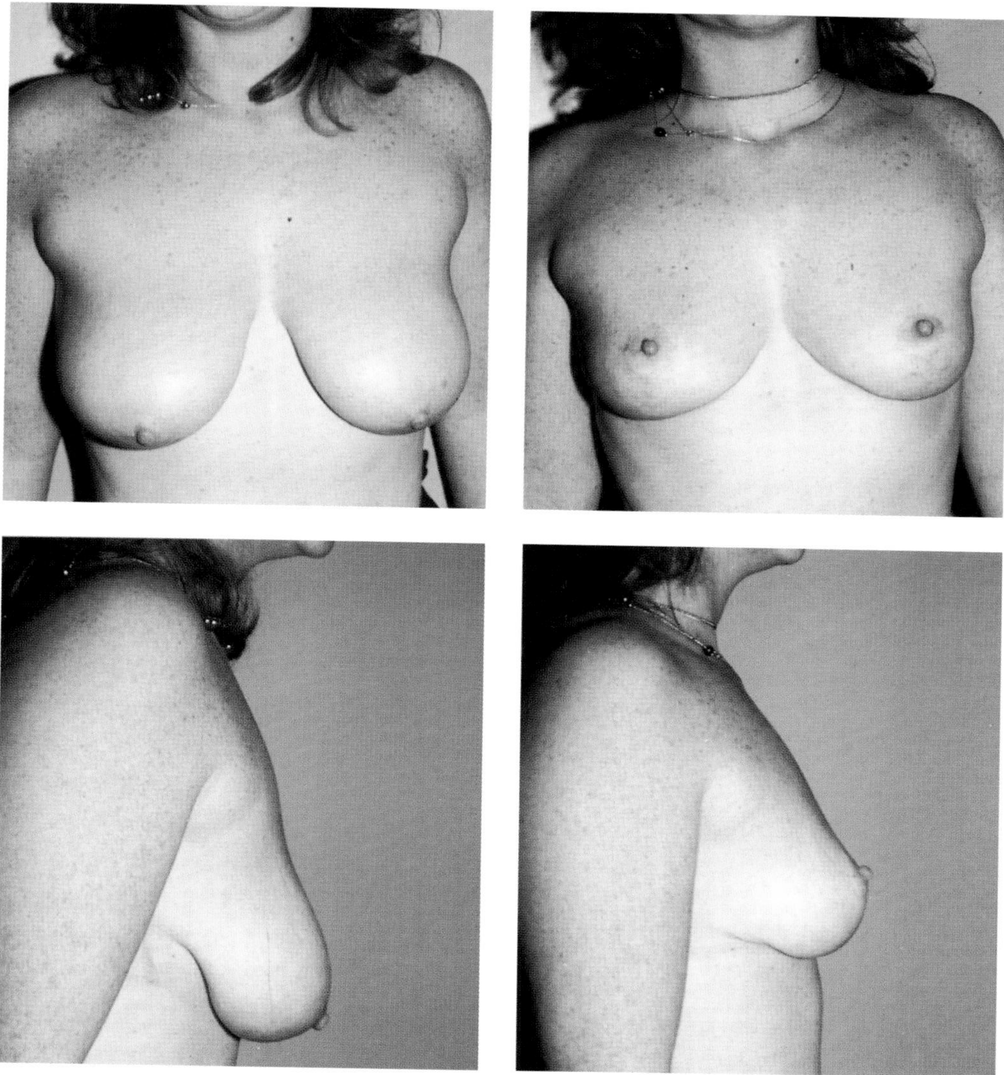

The superior medial breast reduction technique was selected for this 22-year-old woman because her nipple-areola did not move easily to the proposed new position when tested preoperatively. The patient is shown 2 years following breast reduction in which 400 gm was removed from each breast. Her scars have faded and she is delighted with her smaller, narrower breasts that have retained nipple-areola sensation. Resection of the breast inferiorly and laterally and retention of upper breast tissue have prevented recurrence of ptosis. Today, however, I would use liposuction to contour these areas and a vertical reduction technique.

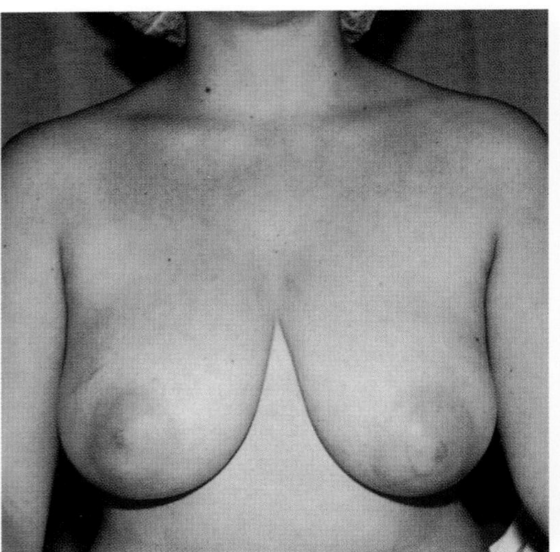

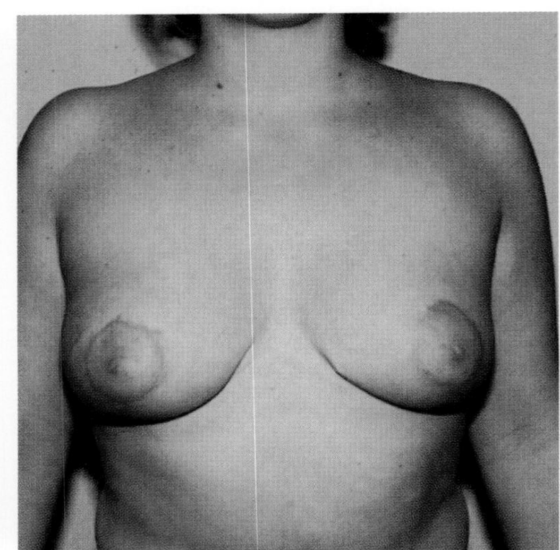

This 25-year-old woman requested reduction of her heavy breasts. She had a scar in the upper right quadrant of her right breast from a previous biopsy of the upper right quadrant of her breast when she was only 17 years of age. She requested breast reduction to reduce the heaviness of her breasts and to alleviate some of the symptoms related to her large breasts. A superior medial breast reduction with inverted T incisions was done. The areolae were left at 4.5 cm in diameter. Liposuction of the lateral area was unnecessary, and 350 gm was resected from each breast. The patient's symptoms of breast heaviness and back pain were alleviated. She is shown 6 months postoperatively. She now wears a 36C brassiere instead of the 36DD she wore previously. Her breasts have been reduced, narrowed, and lifted. The incisions were placed well within the inframammary fold and have healed without scar hypertrophy. There is no evidence at this time that atrophy will occur or that ptosis will recur. This procedure was done before I adopted the vertical approach. Now I probably would use vertical mammaplasty with liposuction for this woman.

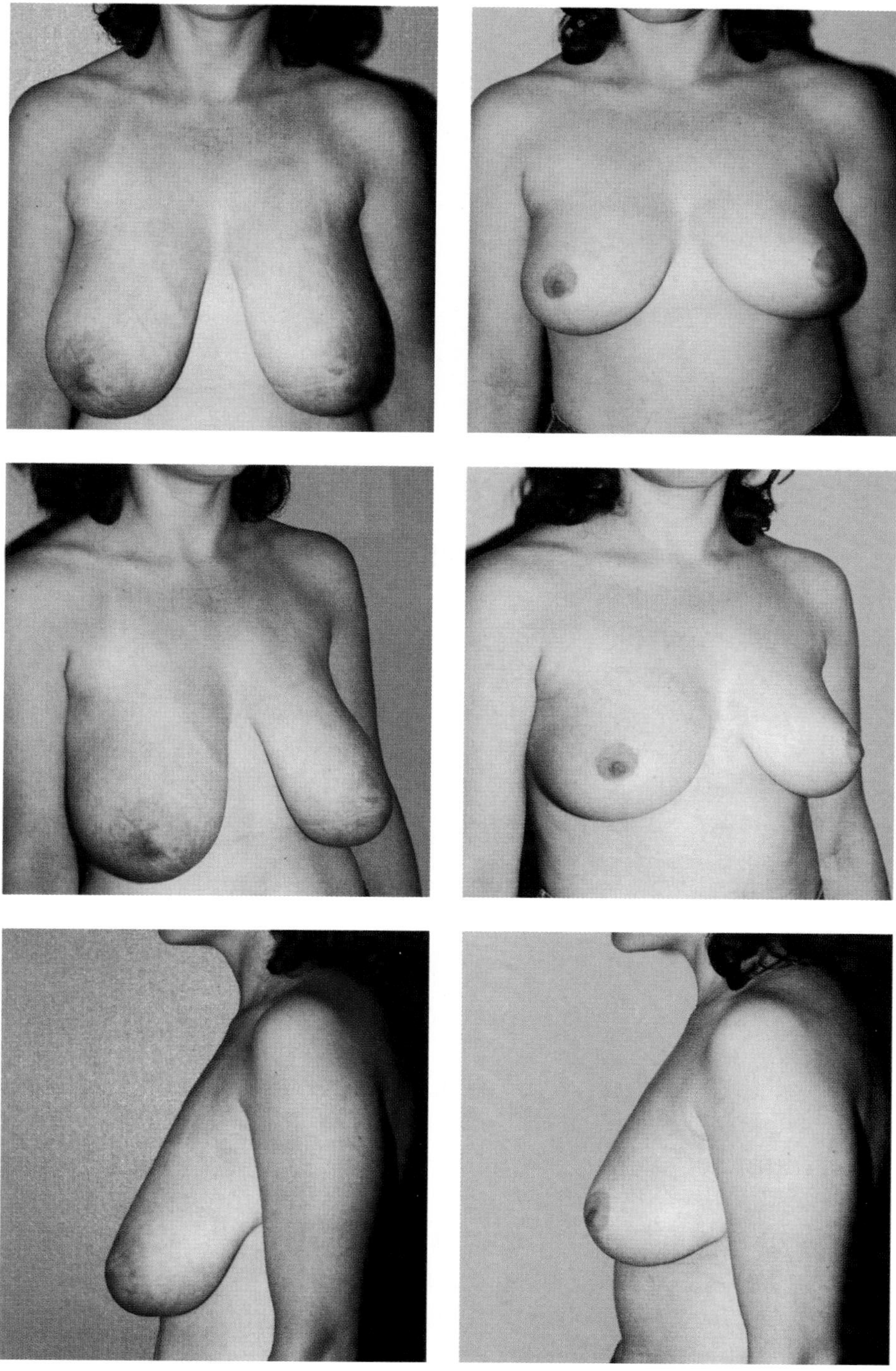

This 19-year-old patient had very full, heavy breasts with dense parenchyma. She is shown 1 year following the procedure. Her brassiere size is now 38C rather than 38DD. She is pleased with the appearance and size of her breasts, and the incisions are healing and fading appropriately. Incision scars are contained within the inframammary crease. Nipple-areola sensation has been preserved.

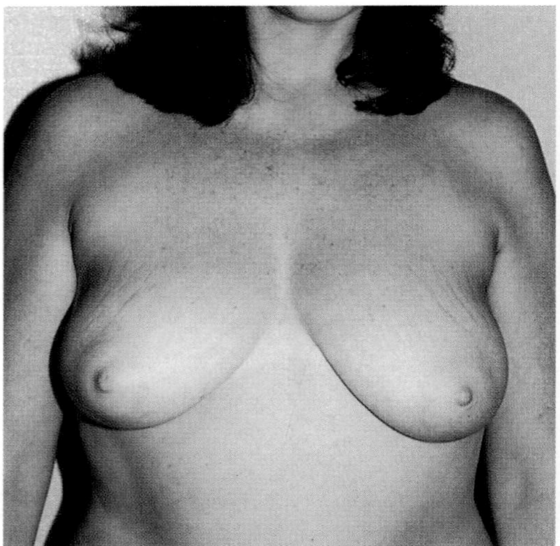

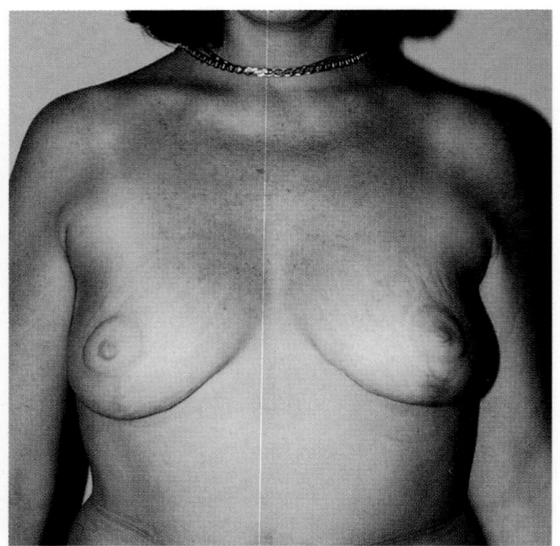

This 28-year-old woman had size 40D breasts and requested a breast reduction to relieve symptoms of breast heaviness and correct breast ptosis. She is shown 1 year following reduction with the superior medial pedicle. She now wears a size 40C brassiere. There is still some scar erythema; however, the breasts are symmetric and the incisions are contained beneath the inframammary folds. I operated on this patient before I began using liposuction for lateral axillary fullness or the vertical mammaplasty technique, which would have enhanced her result.

INFERIOR CENTRAL PEDICLE TECHNIQUE

The inferior pedicle technique preserves an inferior central breast mound to maintain the blood supply to the nipple-areola. ***This is a popular, versatile, and safe technique that relies primarily on the chest wall blood supply and allows breast shaping in all quadrants.*** The breast parenchyma is nourished by lower perforating intercostal arteries and by medial and lateral and direct intercostal arteries. As an option, an inferior dermal pedicle may also be preserved on the lower portion of the central pedicle to enhance the nipple-areola blood supply from the periareolar plexus.

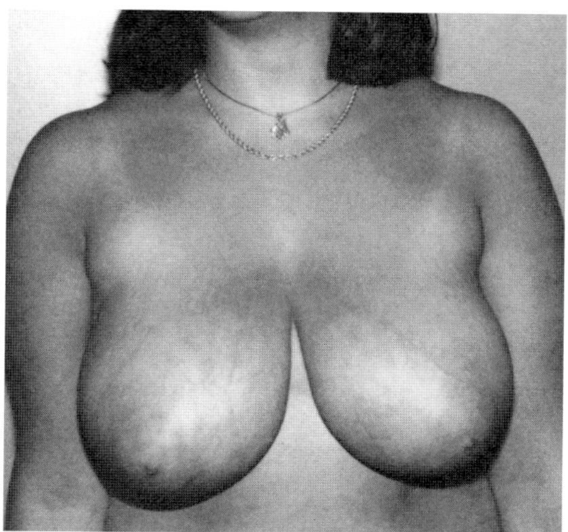

Although the technique as first described used an inferior dermal pedicle, the primary blood supply is derived from the vascularity of the central mound of breast parenchyma. The superior tissues (those above the future inframammary crease line) are elevated as thick (at least 1.5 to 2.0 cm) flaps, and breast tissue is removed tangentially, medially, laterally, superiorly, and inferiorly from the superficial surfaces of the central breast mound tissue. More tissue is removed from the primary area of breast hypertrophy, the lateral and inferior portions of the central mound. The breast parenchyma attached to the resected skin in the lower portions of the breast constitutes a sizable portion of the tissue resection. Conservatism is the wisest course of action. ***Overresection of breast parenchyma from the upper and medial breast area can create flattening and deformity in an area where most women prefer some fullness.*** It is also an area that is visible in certain clothing and sportswear. To obtain the final contour the thinned breast flaps are draped over the central breast mound and topped by the nipple-areola.

The inferior pedicle technique preserves the breast's sensation and lactation potential and permits more versatility in moving the nipple-areola than is possible with the superior pedicle techniques. It can narrow wide breasts somewhat and provides considerable flexibility for controlling breast size, shape, and volume. Resections in several areas of the breast make this procedure more complex and obtaining symmetry more challenging than those described previously. ***Care is taken to preserve equal volumes of skin and breast tissue to ensure that the result is symmetric.***

Surgical plan

- Projected amount of reduction and future shape of breasts
- Preoperative markings to denote future site of nipple-areola as well as inframammary incisions
- Liposuction of lateral breast region if excess fullness present
- Preservation of nipple-areola with 38 to 42 mm diameter and epithelialization of upper V
- Resection of breast parenchyma and skin from lower and upper breast regions
- Preservation of thick skin in breast parenchyma flaps; reflection of flaps to identify central pedicle
- Resection of central pedicle from inferior and lateral portions primarily to obtain new breast base shape
- Closure of skin and repositioning and closure of nipple-areola
- Closure of inverted T incision

Markings and Technique

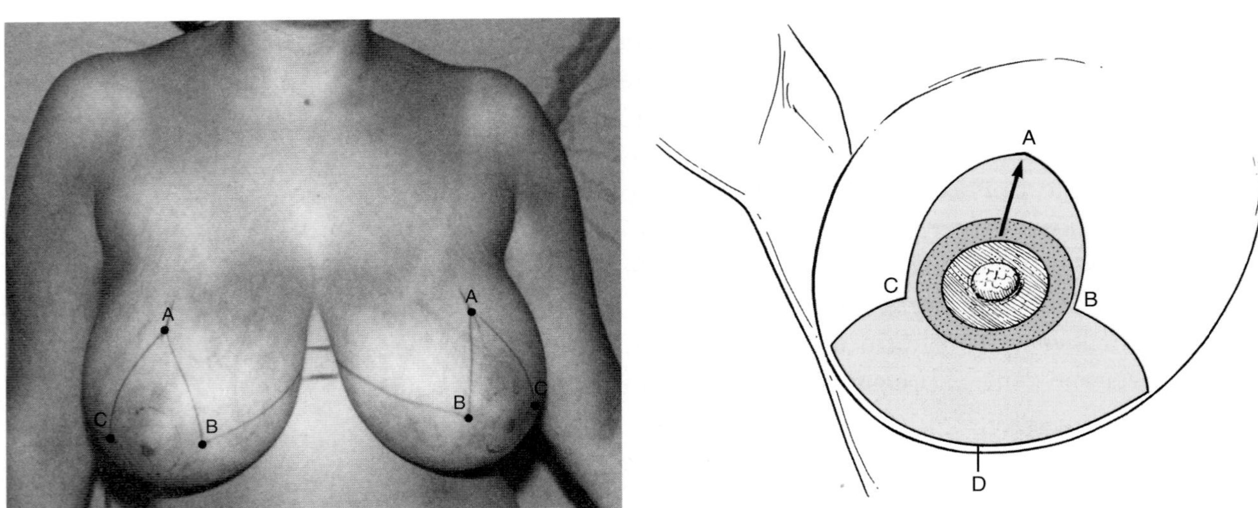

Markings for the inferior pedicle technique are similar to those described for the superior pedicle technique. The new nipple-areolar position is marked on the central breast line; marking the width of the V too wide is avoided to ensure breast closure of points B and C to D at the inframammary fold.

To accommodate the central pedicle the central V (B and C points) should diverge only enough to encompass the areola. Additional central breast skin along A to C and A and B within this V is removed at the conclusion of the procedure to avoid a tight T closure.

During the initial steps of the operation, including the markings for the inferior pedicle and the actual breast resection, the patient is in the supine position with the breast positioned vertically and anatomically over the chest wall. In this position there is no ptosis, and the perforators from the underlying musculofascial layer will enter directly into the breast. The nipple-areola is positioned centrally over the breast at the fourth intercostal space.

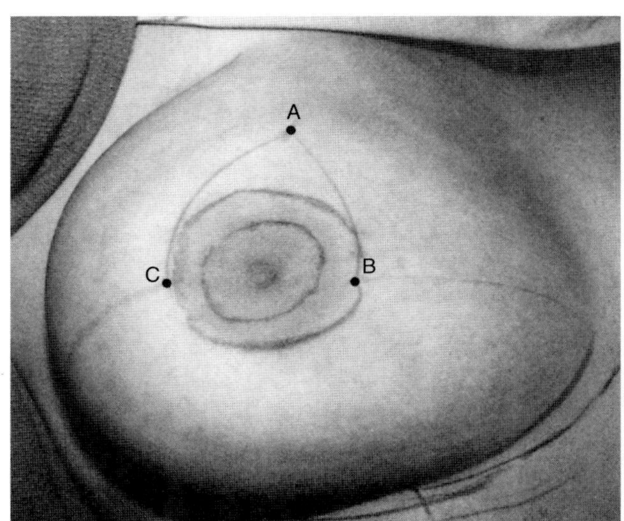

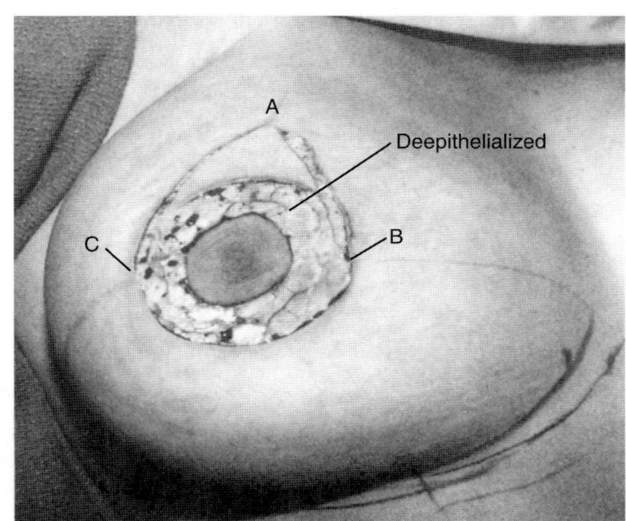

The nipple-areolar diameter is marked at about 45 mm with the areola relaxed. With the nipple-areola positioned centrally above the breasts and chest during the resection, an incision is made around the areola, and the circumareolar area is developed by deepithelialization using the scissors or knife. The main source of blood supply to the nipple-areola will be the underlying breast parenchyma and perforating underlying vessels; however, some additional blood supply is provided by the subdermal plexus.

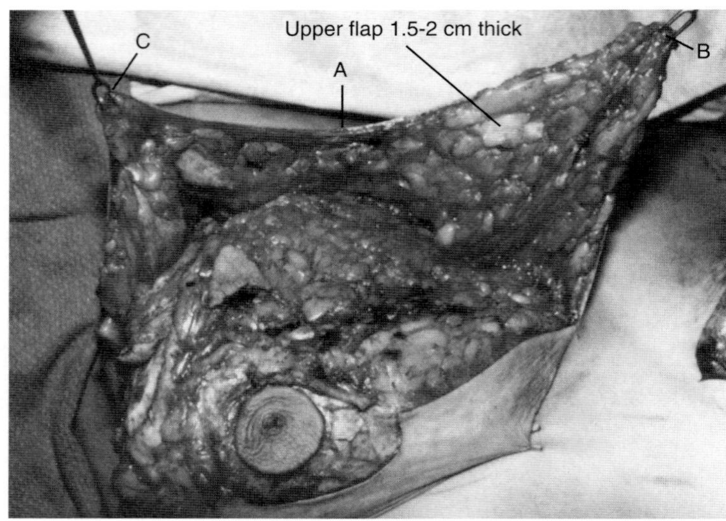

The upper breast flap is mobilized upward centrally, medially, and laterally with at least 1.5 to 2.5 cm thickness. This thickness ensures good blood flow to the flaps, avoids necrosis later, and produces a small postoperative breast contour over the central mound.

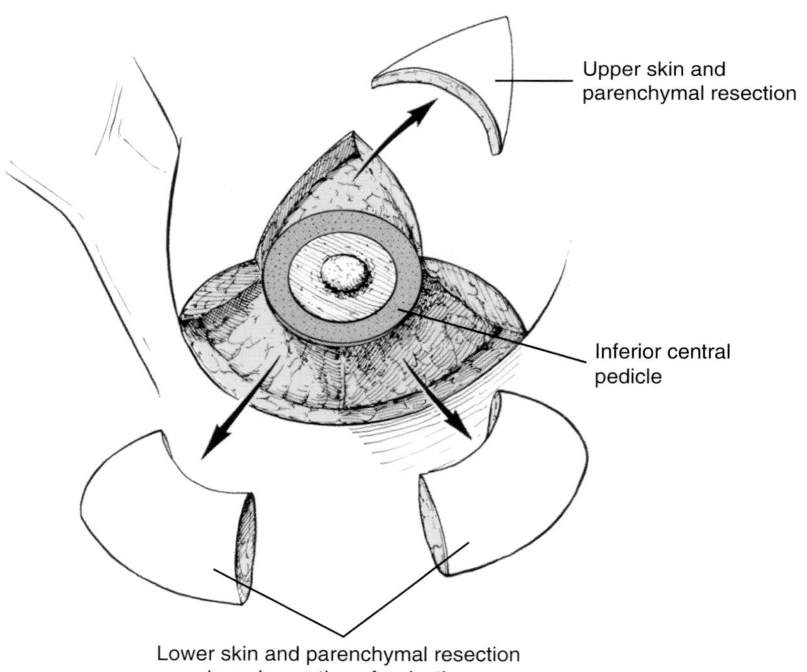

The upper triangle of skin is excised. The inframammary crease incision and future inframammary crease incisions are made. The lower breast skin is resected with 1 to 2 cm of subjacent breast parenchyma.

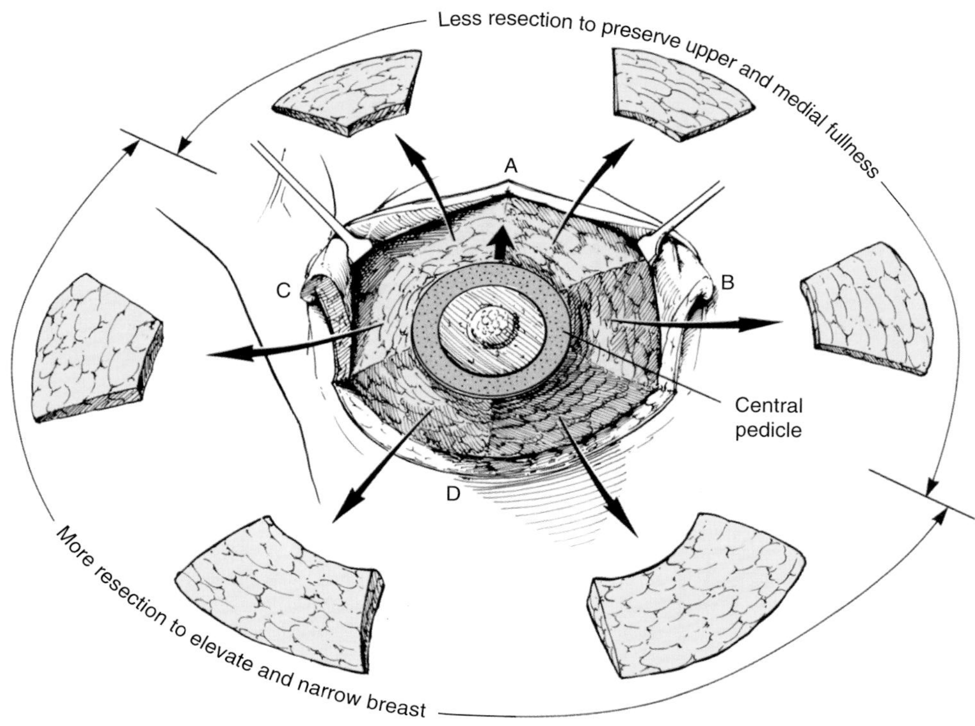

The excess parenchyma is then excised tangentially from the central mound. A conservative resection is done medially and superiorly to avoid deficiency in these areas. More tissue is resected inferiorly and laterally in the primary areas of breast hypertrophy. This excess tissue must be removed to establish a new contour.

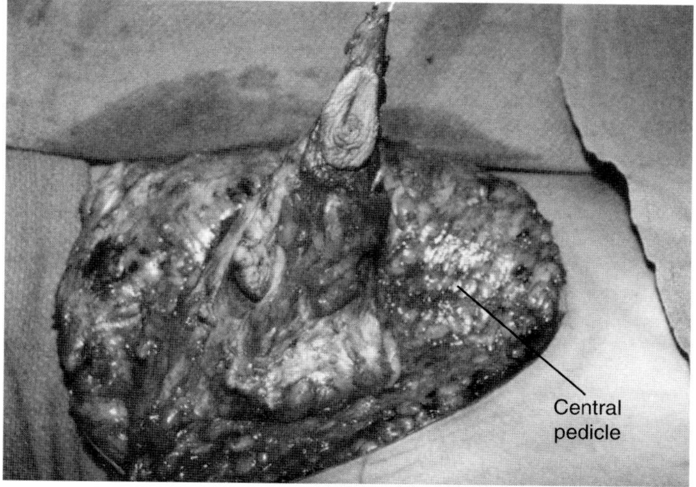

The resection stops short of the deep fascia to preserve additional blood supply to the central breast tissue that enters from the periphery and the lateral and medial intercostal and internal mammary artery perforators.

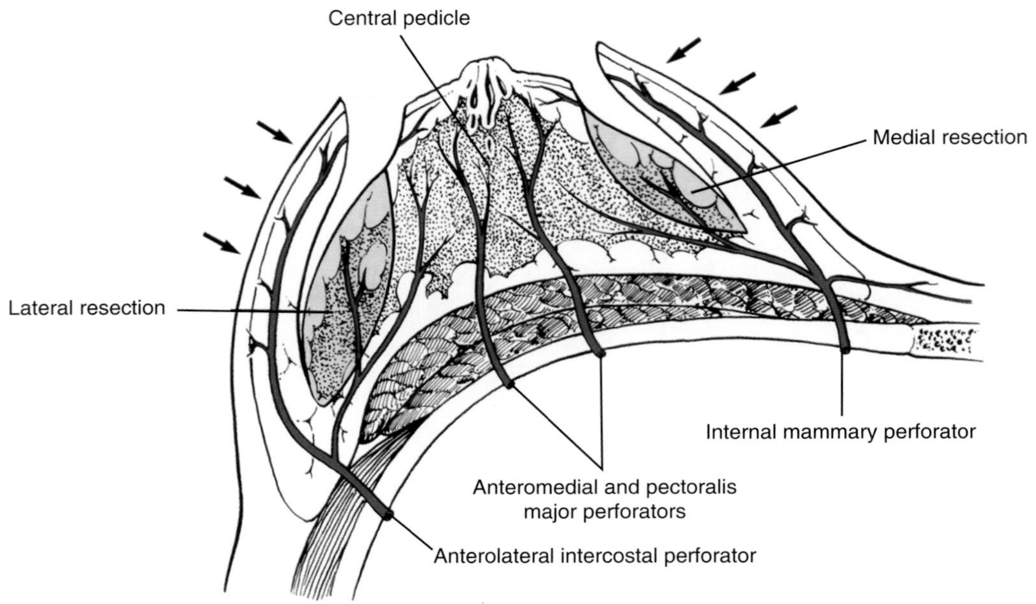

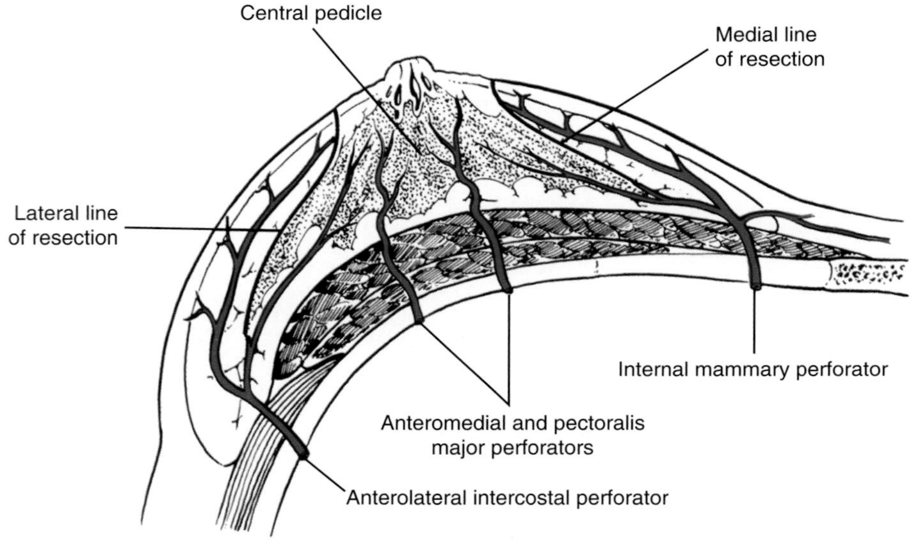

Medial and lateral resections narrow the breast. Central pedicle vascularity is preserved by the central and peripheral vessels.

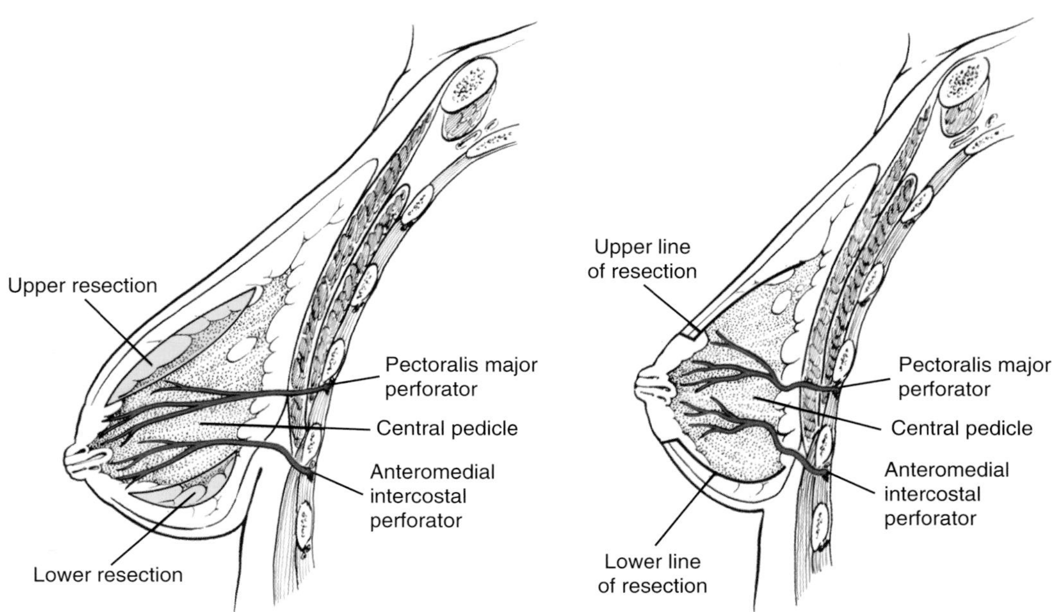

Superior and inferior resections permit lifting the breast and removing ptotic tissue while shifting the breast parenchyma upward. The central pedicle is nourished by musculofascial perforators and also by flow coming from the periphery via the medial and lateral intercostal perforators and external mammary arteries. ***The central mound must not be resected to such a degree that the underlying perforating vessels coursing into it and into the areola are compromised.***

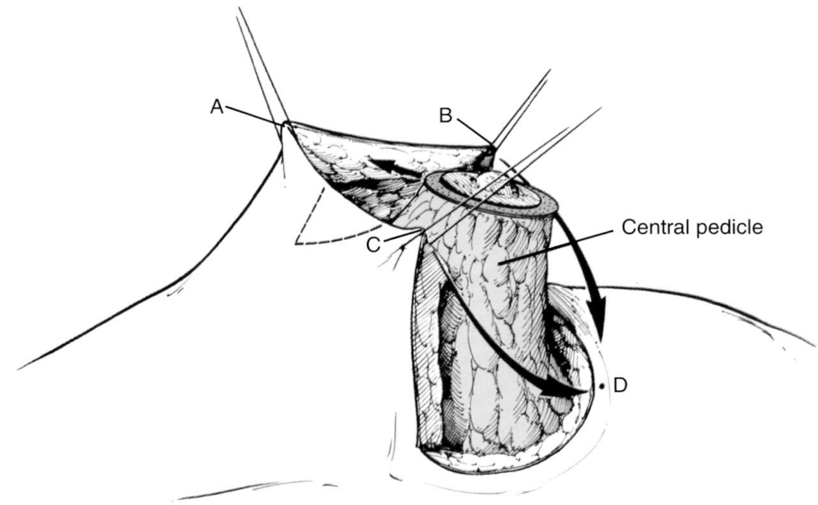

The central pedicle surmounted by the nipple-areola is moved to its new position, and the incisions are closed from lateral to medial. The excellent mobility of the pedicle and the nipple-areola make this technique especially good for larger ptotic breasts.

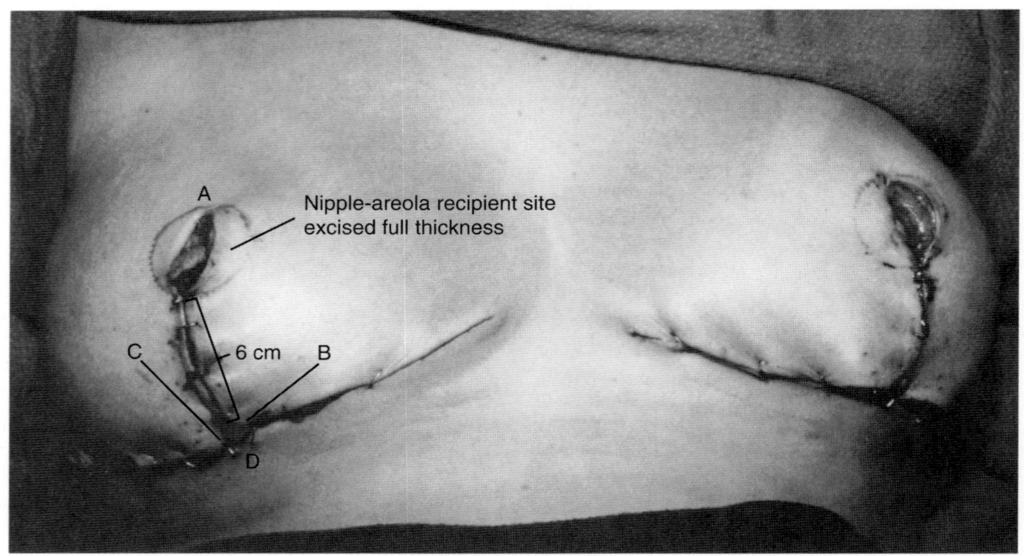

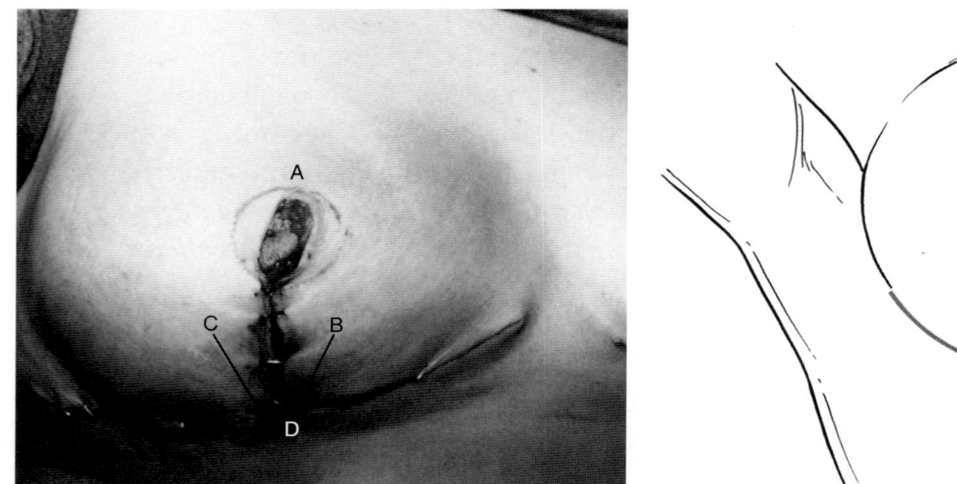

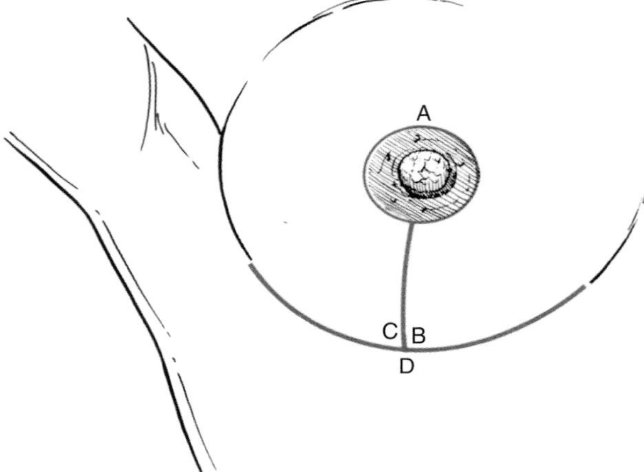

The areola is secured to point A and the lower vertical transverse incisions closed. Excess medial skin is removed centrally along lines A to D, and the vertical limb is closed up to 5 cm above the inframammary crease.

With the patient upright and after adjusting the skin and parenchymal resections for symmetry, the nipple-areolar location is identified, checked for symmetry, and marked. The areola skin site is excised full thickness. Then the nipple-areola is elevated to its new position and the incision closed with deep and intracuticular sutures.

Results

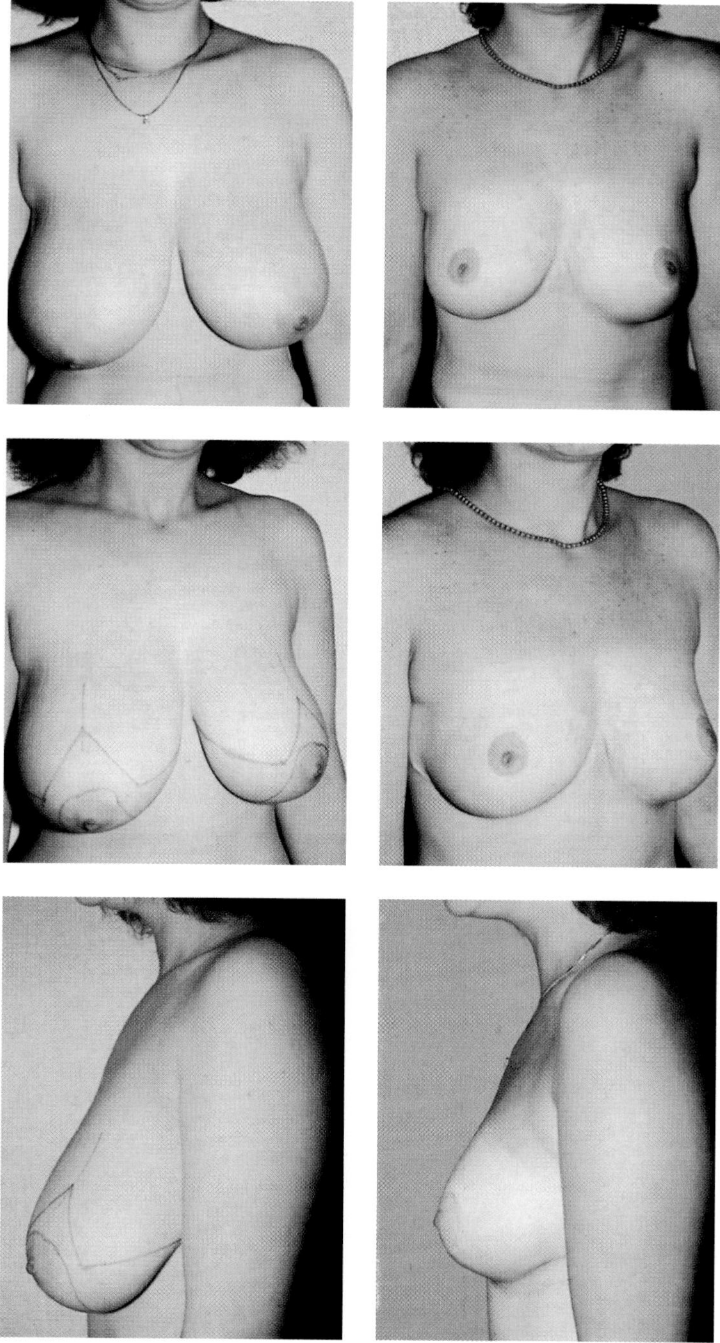

The oblique and lateral views of this 23-year-old woman show the preoperative marks used to plan the procedure. The patient, who formerly wore a 36DD brassiere, now fits into a 36C. Although somewhat more complex and technically demanding, the inferior central pedicle technique offers increased versatility and can produce a superior final result.

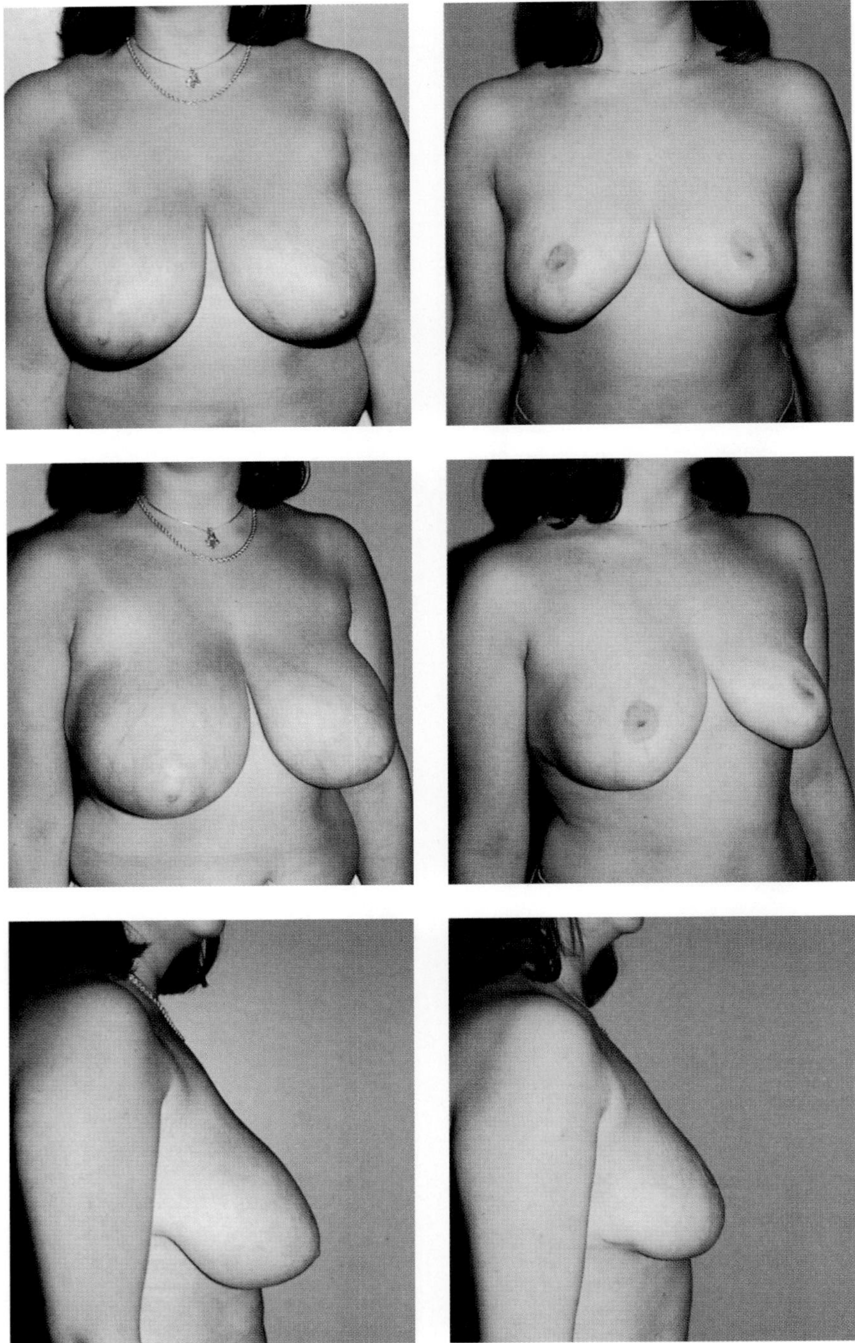

The patient is shown 2 years following the procedure. Her brassiere size has changed from 38D to 38B. She is more comfortable and feels she looks better in clothes. She is also able to participate in a greater range of athletic activities. The inferior central pedicle technique is successful for this type of patient since it permits a major reduction while preserving function and sensation. The volume of the central pedicle, however, contributes to some descent or bottoming out of the lower breast.

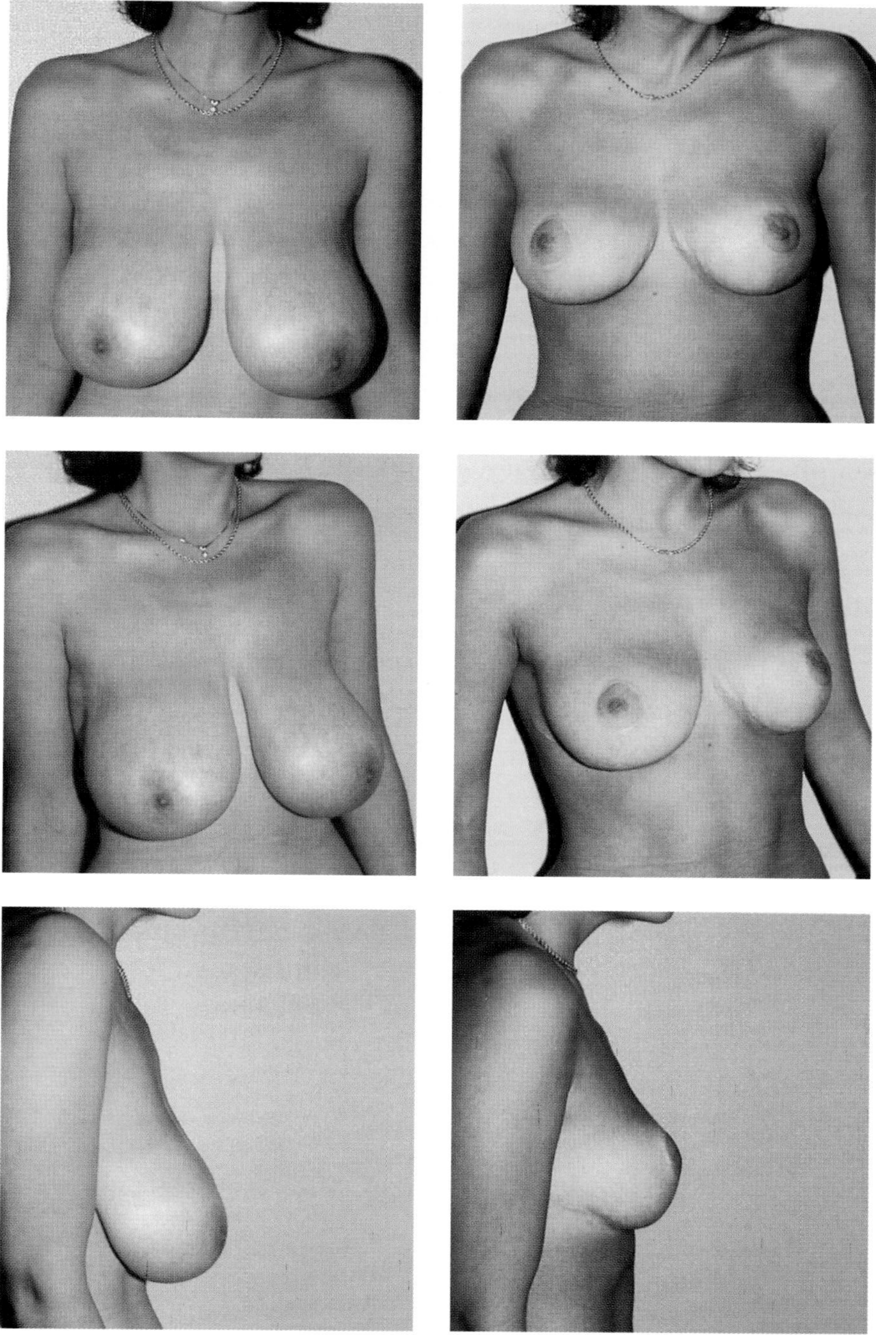

This 22-year-old woman wore a 36D brassiere. Her breasts were very uncomfortable and limited physical activities and choice of clothing. She was not overweight. Because significant elevation of the nipple-areola complex was required, an inferior central pedicle technique was selected. Breast reduction with the inferior central pedicle technique successfully reduced her breasts to a size 36B. She is shown 2 years following breast reduction. The inferior central pedicle permits a major reduction with satisfactory breast shape.

FREE NIPPLE GRAFT

A simple lower and lateral breast resection (as described in the inverted T pedicle technique) combined with a free nipple-areola graft produces fewer breast parenchyma incisions with less internal scarring, making it easier to perform postoperative breast examinations for breast lumps and tumors. The desired breast size can be obtained with this method without requiring excess tissue to "carry" the nipple-areola. Nipple-areolar survival approaches 100% when this technique is used and minimizes the fat necrosis and nipple-areolar devascularization that can occur following complex resections and when large pedicles are developed for women with very large breasts who may have compromised microcirculation, high blood pressure, or obesity. Liposuction can be useful to reduce the lateral breast and axillary fullness and also allow additional resection.

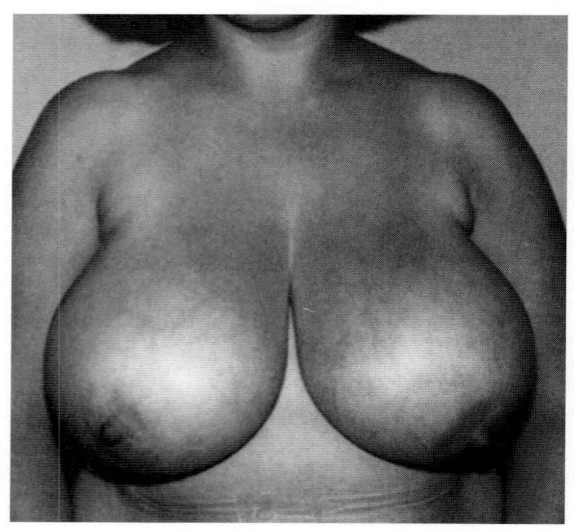

This woman with size 40DD breasts requested reduction to a more comfortable size to relieve the pain in her back, bra strap grooving, and constant moisture beneath her breasts. She has two teenagers and does not plan to have any more children. She has smoked two packs of cigarettes a day for 20 years. Because of the large breast reduction, heavy cigarette smoking, functional considerations, and distance required for pedicle transfer, a free nipple graft technique was selected.

Surgical plan

- Preoperative markings to delineate future site of nipple as well as areas of central breast resection
- Projected amount of horizontal and inferior breast resection
- Liposuction laterally if necessary to reduce lateral fullness
- Harvesting of nipple-areola as full-thickness graft approximately 40 mm in diameter
- Resection of breast parenchyma inferiorly and laterally
- Closure of breast medially and laterally toward center
- Epithelialization of areolar site at appropriate position and suture of areolar graft, which is secured with tie or dressing

Markings and Technique

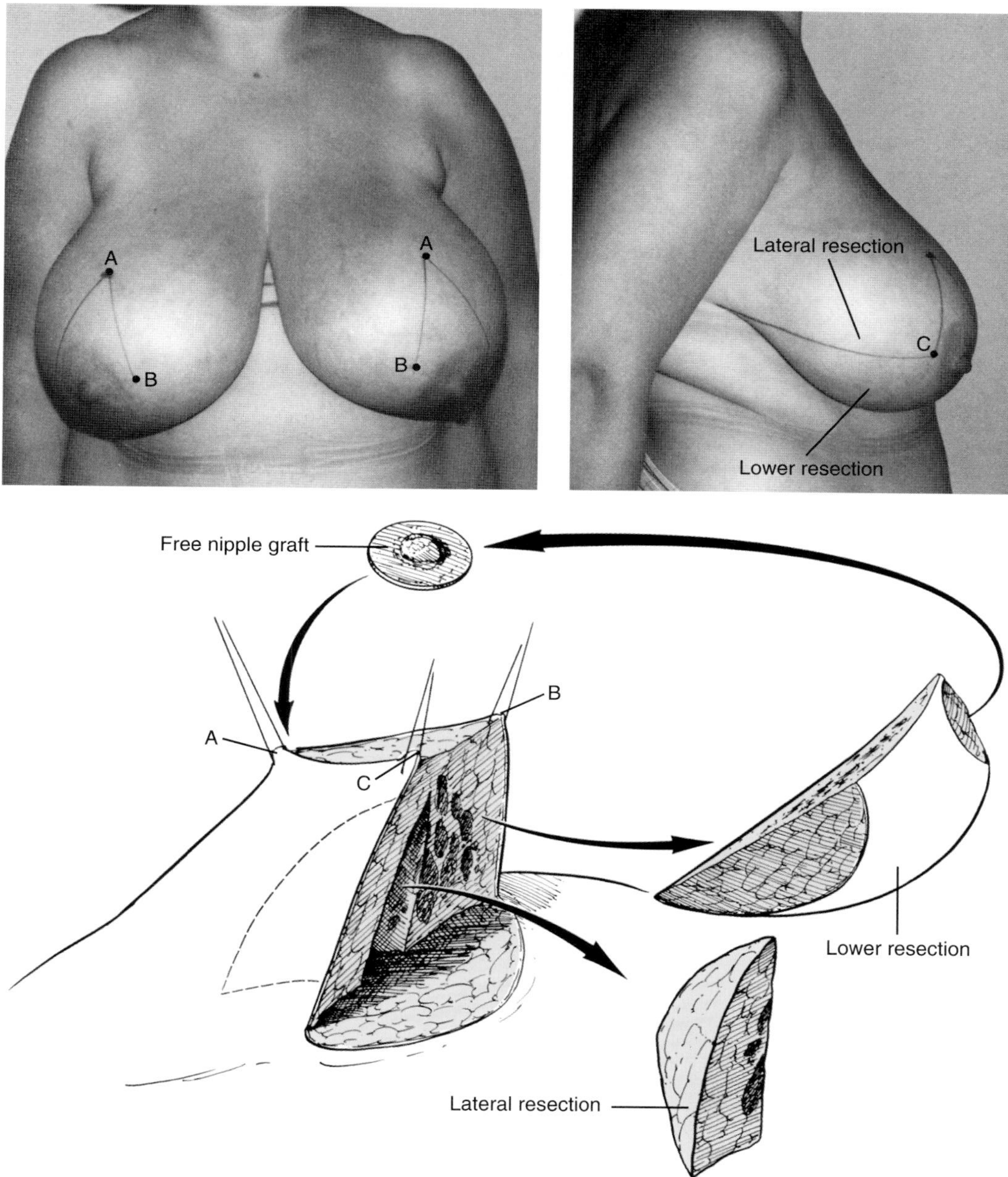

Preoperative markings identify the point of the areola apex (point A), the diameter of the future areola, and the position of the future inframammary crease. This is determined with the weight of the breast supported to prevent point A moving upward after the resection, thus displacing the nipple upward. ***The larger the breasts the more likelihood the remaining breast will spring upward after the resection, leaving the nipple-areola too high.***

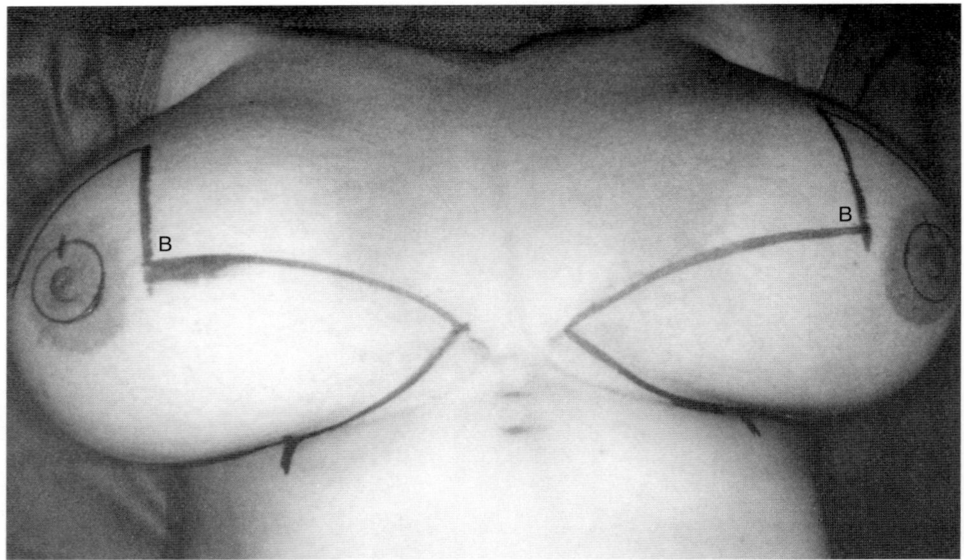

The final inframammary crease incision is marked with the patient supine.

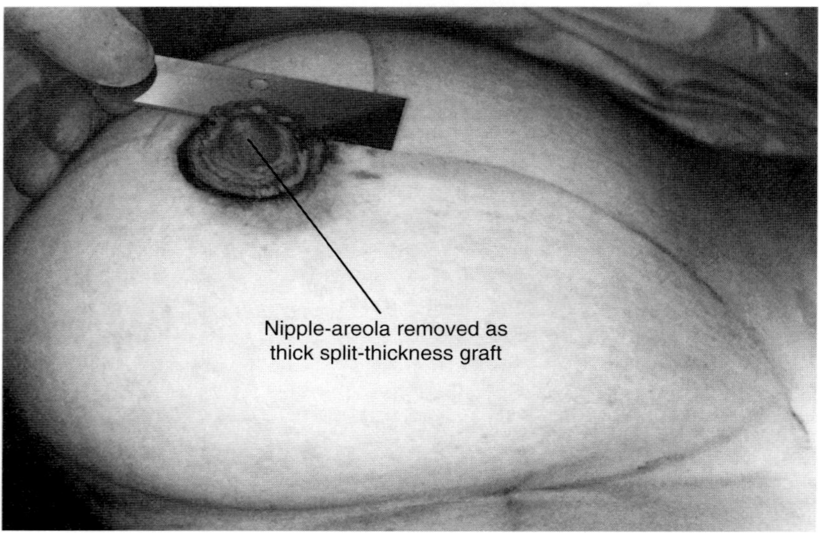

An incision is made around the areola, and the nipple-areola is removed as a thick split-thickness skin graft. The nipple is preserved in a saline sponge for grafting at the end of the procedure.

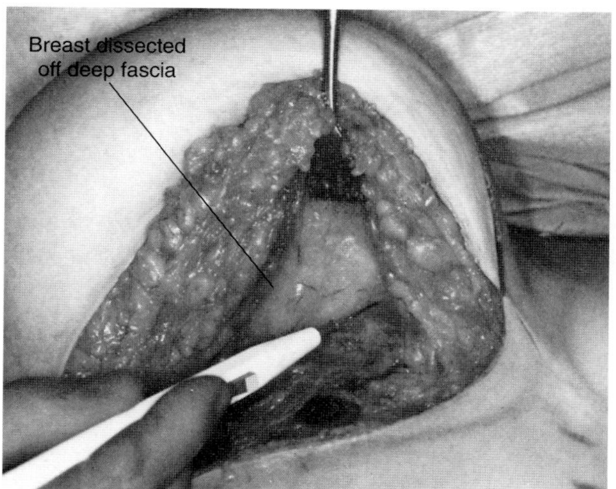

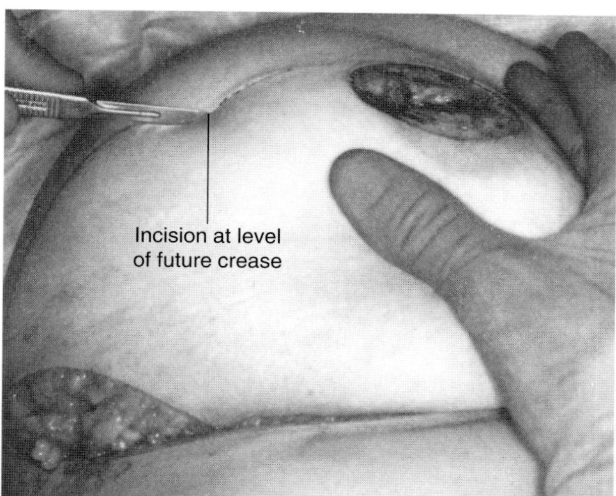

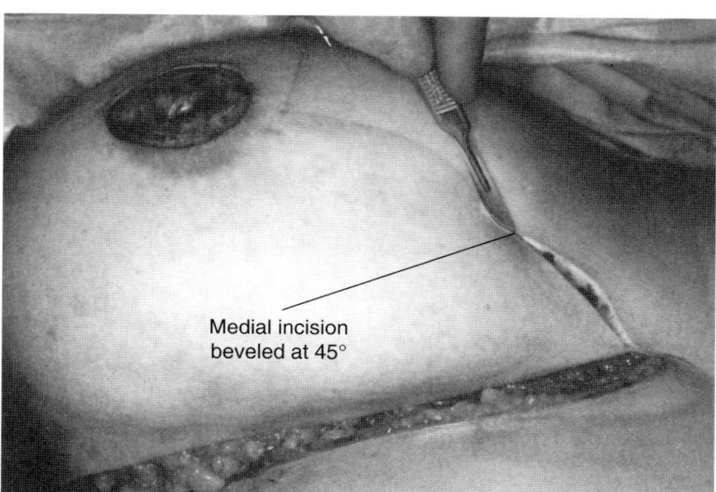

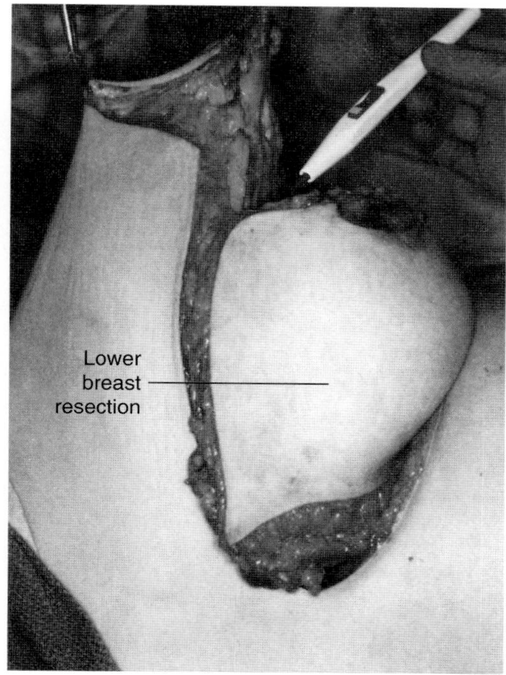

The inframammary incision is made, and the breast is lifted off the deep layer of superficial fascia up to the level of the nipple. The medial and lateral future inframammary crease incisions are made and the incisions beveled upward. The breast is lifted perpendicular to the chest wall, and lower breast tissue is resected below the future inframammary crease.

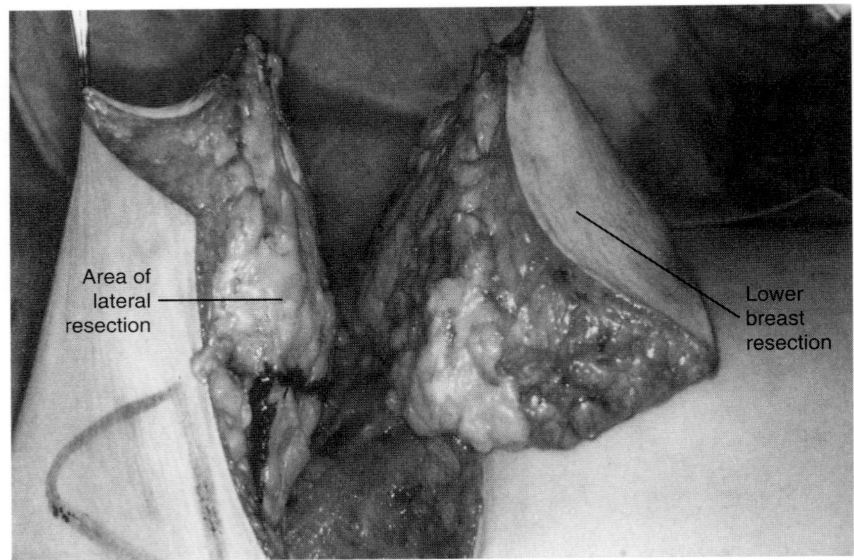

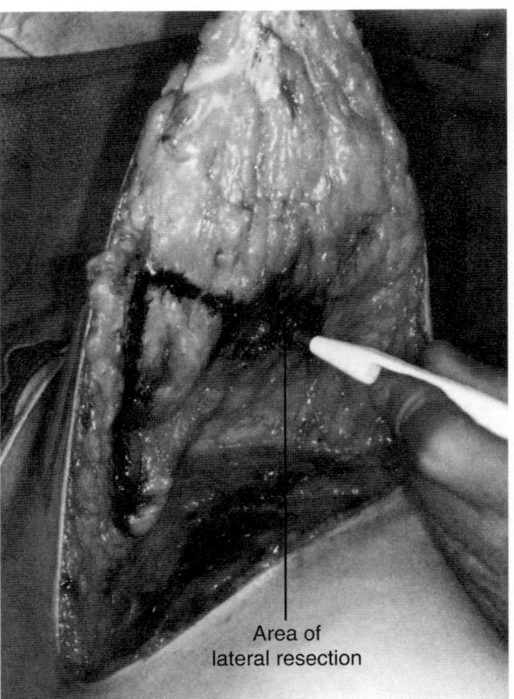

After the portion of breast below the inframammary crease has been removed, it is sent for pathologic and frozen section evaluation of any questionable areas. With the breast lifted from the chest wall, marks are made laterally to identify the lateral parenchyma for additional deep lateral excision.

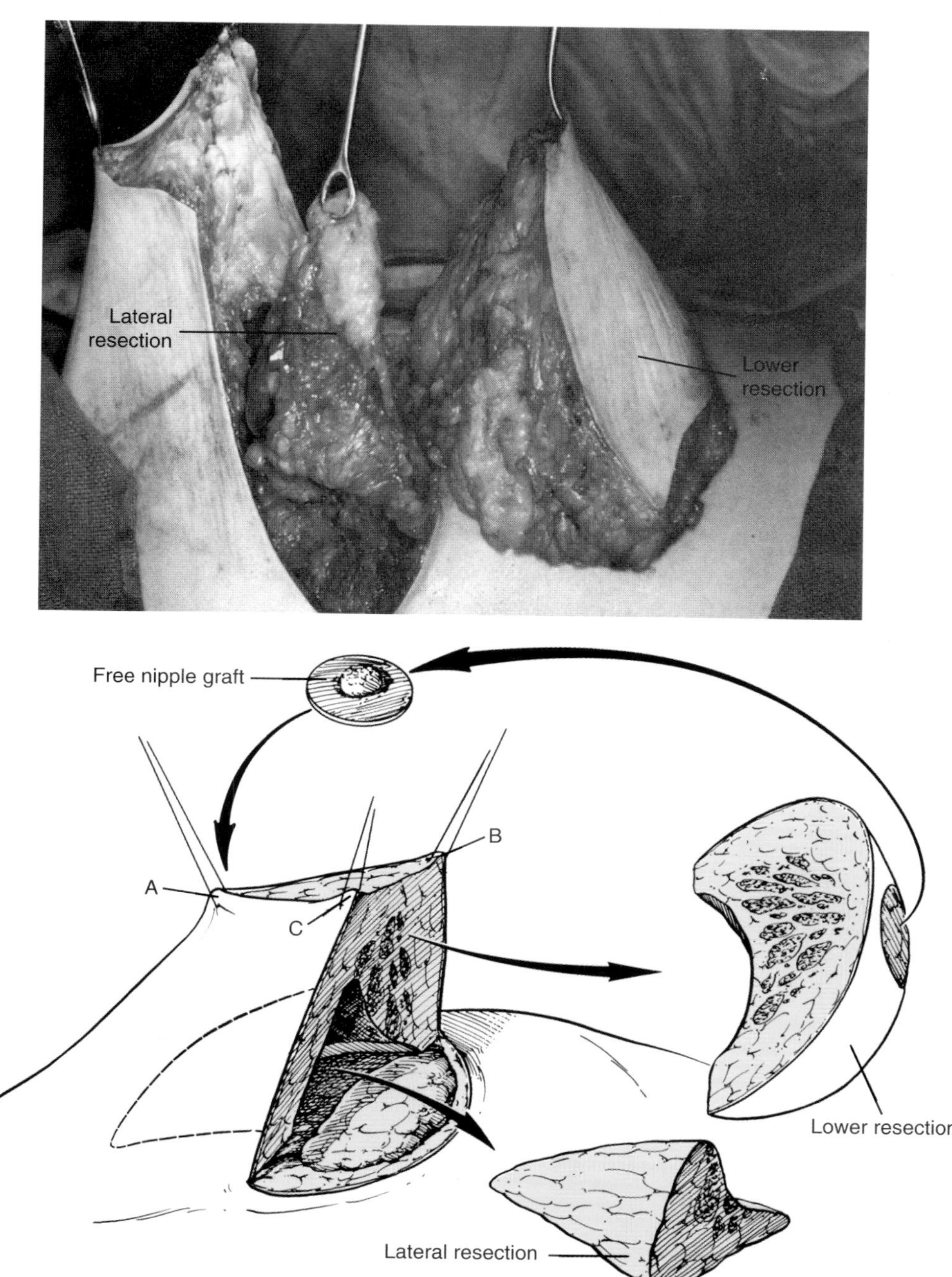

This resection will permit some narrowing of the breasts during closure. The inferior and lateral resected portions of the breast parenchyma are shown.

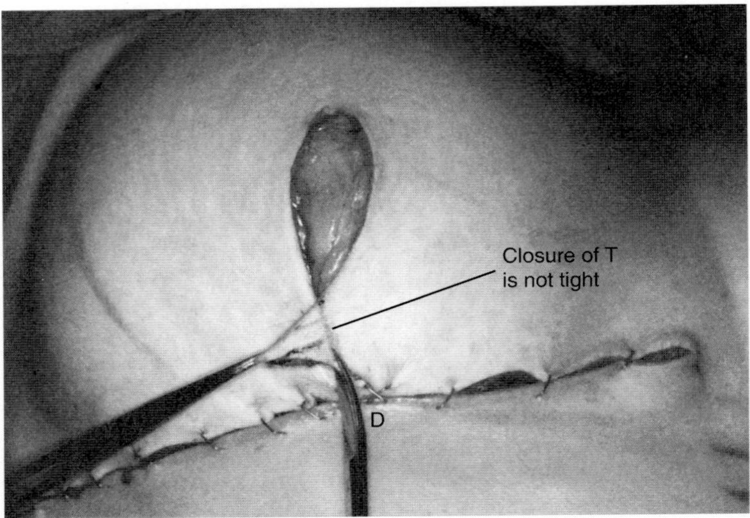

The breast is closed medially and laterally toward the center; excess breast skin is excised centrally to prevent medial and lateral dog ears and to avoid a skin T closure that is too tight.

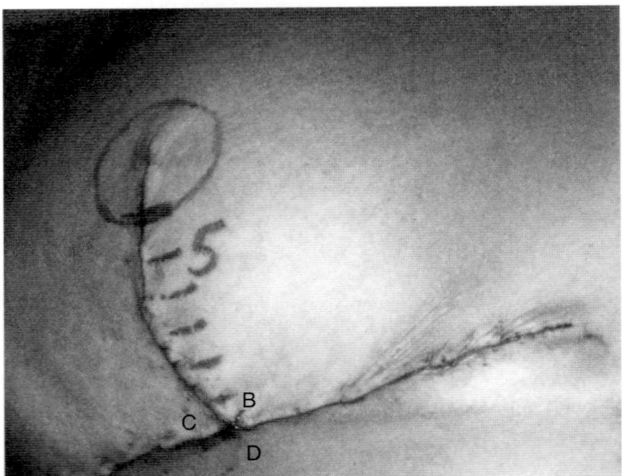

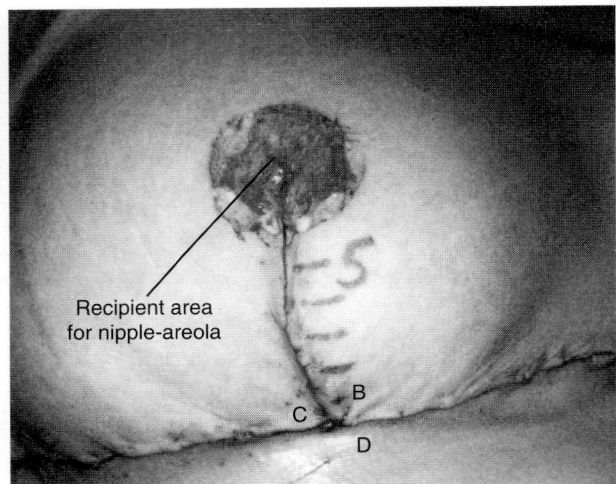

The site for the new areola is determined with the patient in the sitting position and deepithelialized thinly to receive the nipple-areola graft.

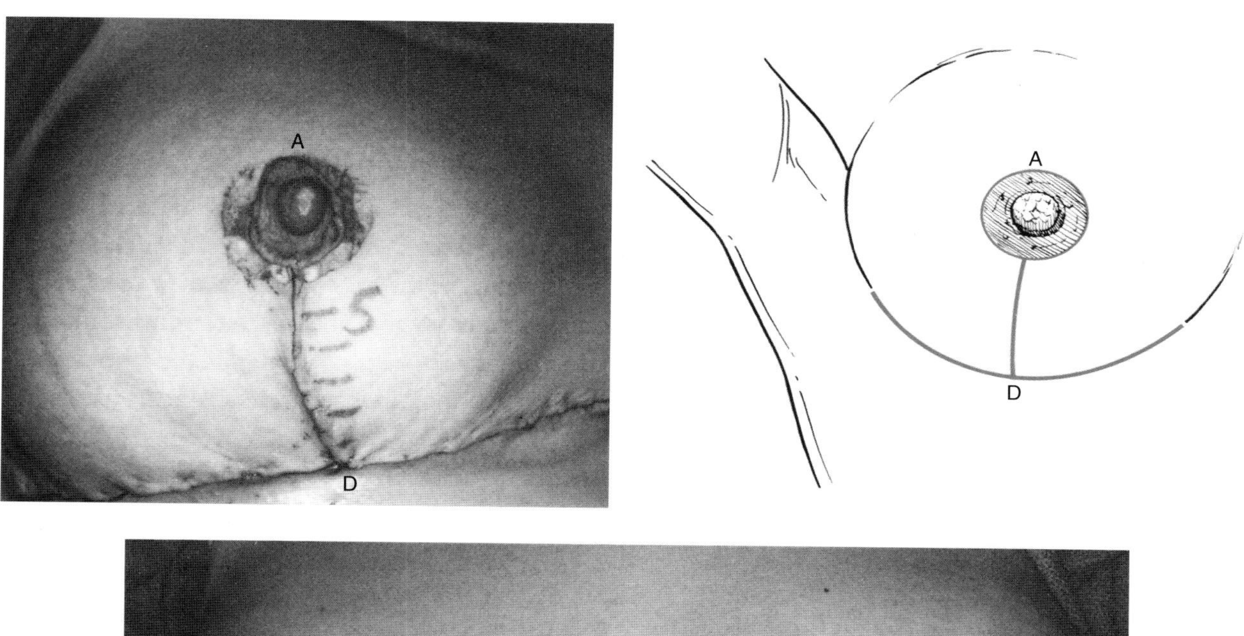

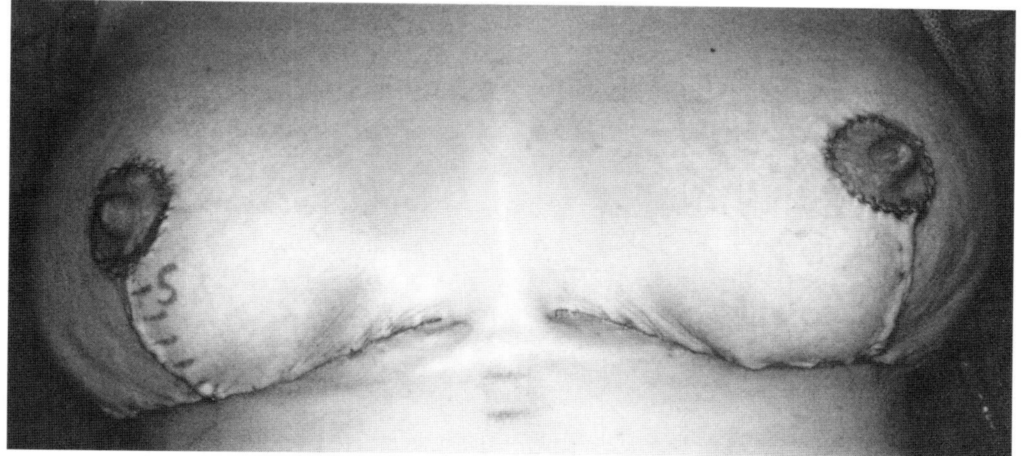

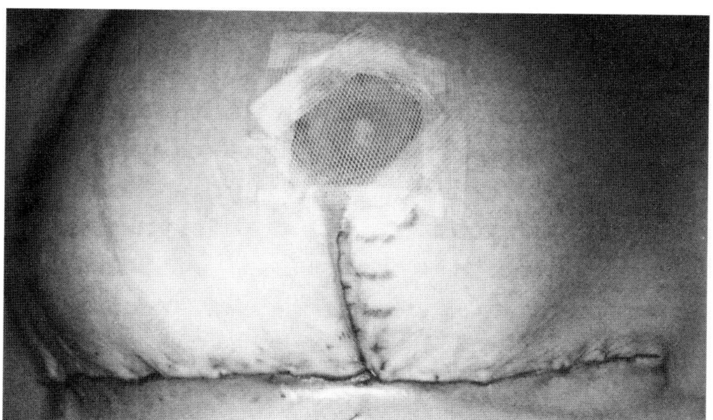

The full-thickness nipple-areola graft is sutured circumferentially with fine absorbable plain catgut sutures. A silicone stent is placed over the graft. Steri-Strips are used to secure the stent and also are placed longitudinally along the incisions. A 7 mm wide siliconized drain is inserted laterally; it will be removed the following day.

Results

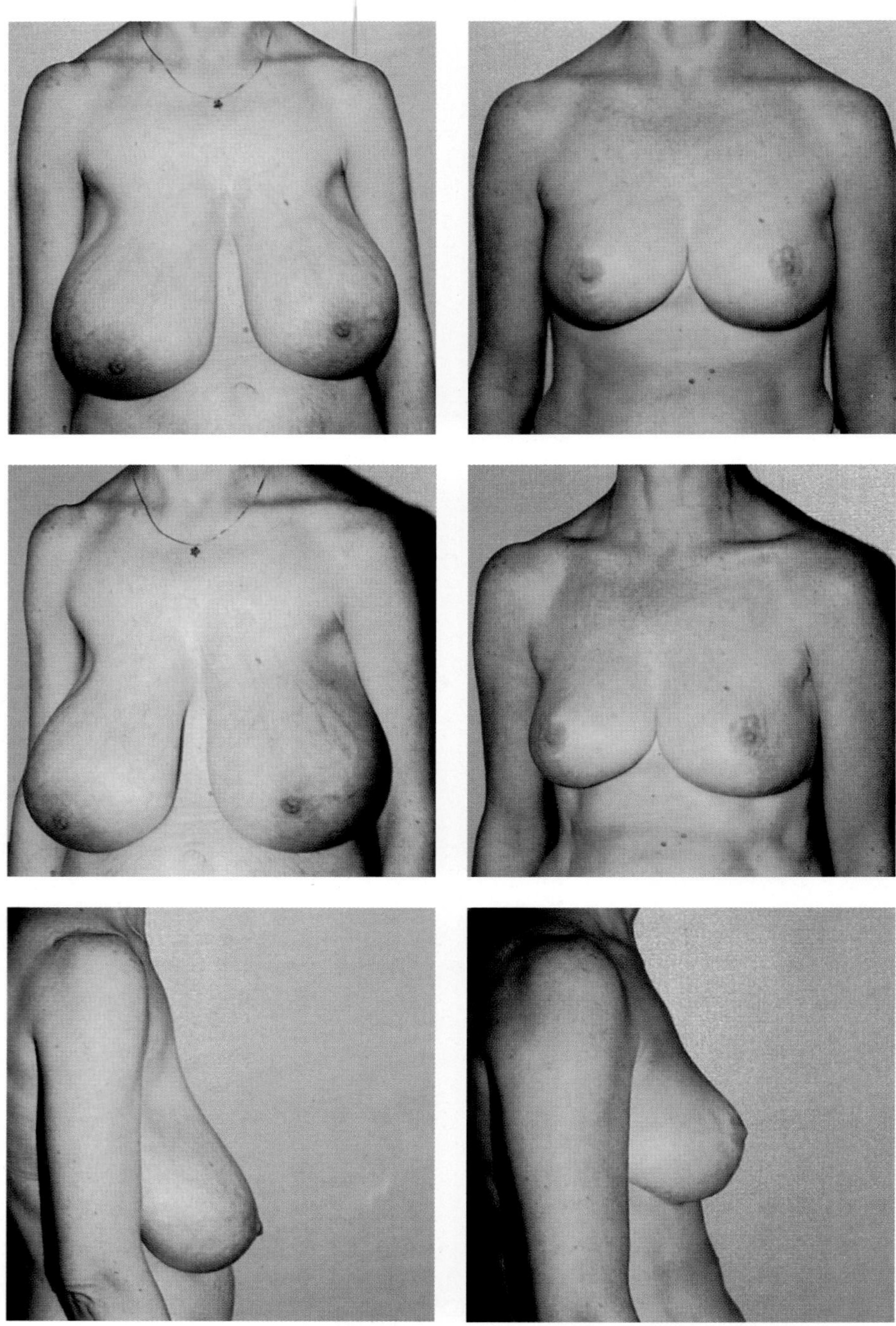

This 62-year-old woman is shown 2 years following breast reduction. Because she was a cigarette smoker with a 60+ pack-year history, she was at high risk for nipple-areolar and fat necrosis with a traditional technique. Mammograms revealed no negative findings and no dominant masses, but her breasts were quite lumpy and firm. She requested a significant breast reduction with more uplifted breasts. A free nipple graft technique was chosen.

A smaller diameter nipple-areola was planned to reduce the chance of distortion if the nipple-areola graft was lost. Although nipple-areolar pigmentation was diminished, sensation returned after approximately 6 months. She is delighted with the new size and appearance of her breasts and the relief of symptoms.

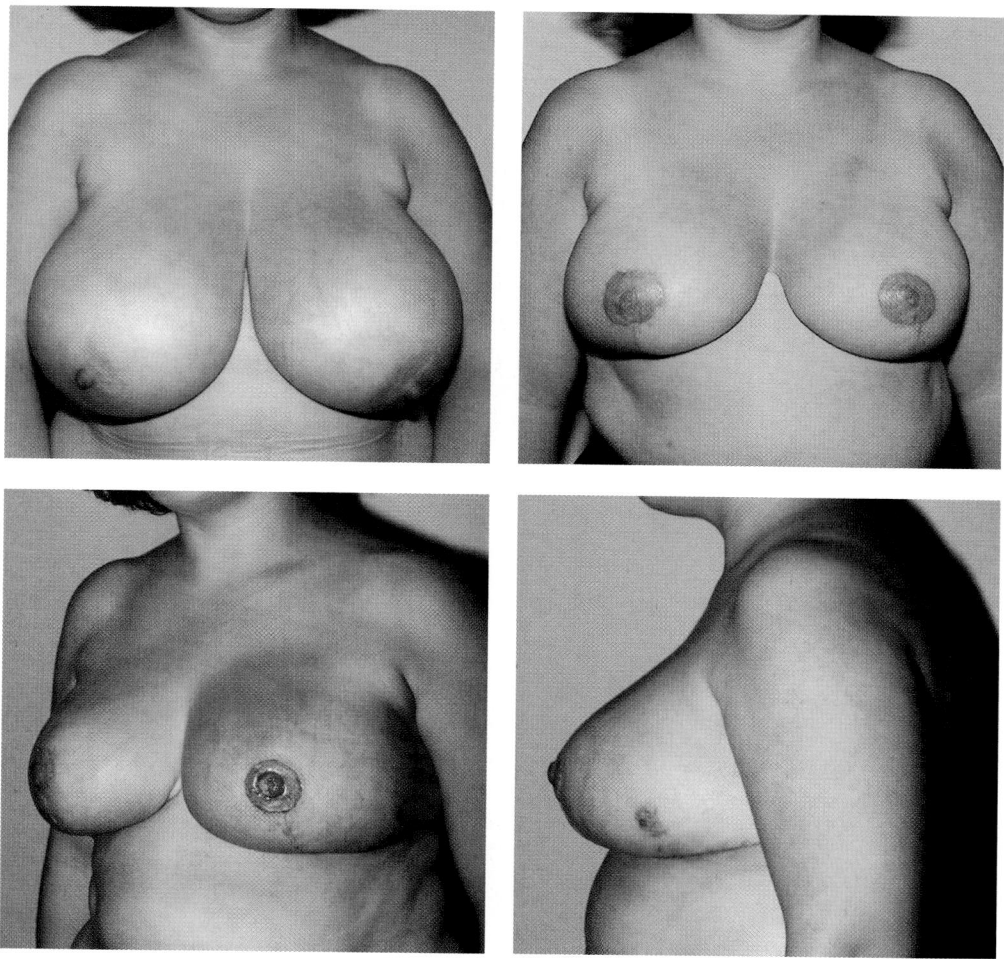

Although 1700 gm of tissue was removed from each breast, they were not overreduced. The patient is shown 1 month following the procedure. Liposuction of the lateral area and axillary region would probably have improved breast contour. The nipple-areola grafts healed well, although some superficial desquamation of the areola skin is evident. Pigmentation will probably diminish over time. This would be more noticeable if she had a more pigmented nipple-areola. No lactation potential remains and return of sensation will usually be determined by the amount of skin preserved.

Ancillary Procedures

REDUCTION-AUGMENTATION FOR UPPER BREAST FULLNESS

Some patients want smaller breasts but still desire a youthful fullness in the upper aspect. If significant ptosis accompanies the hypertrophy and practically all the breast tissue is below the inframammary crease, reduction mammaplasty with any of the techniques described earlier will not permanently restore upper fullness.

I have been able to achieve a good, long-lasting correction by placing an implant subpectorally in the upper breast region and subglandularly in the lower part of the breast. This strategy also permits additional lower breast resection and is particularly helpful in providing more permanent corrections for women with stretched, inelastic breast skin. Before this approach is chosen, it must be discussed in detail with the patient. Third-party providers and managed care companies will probably not reimburse for this procedure because the amount of breast resected is often less than 500 gm. However, this approach merits consideration in the patient group described to ensure satisfaction.

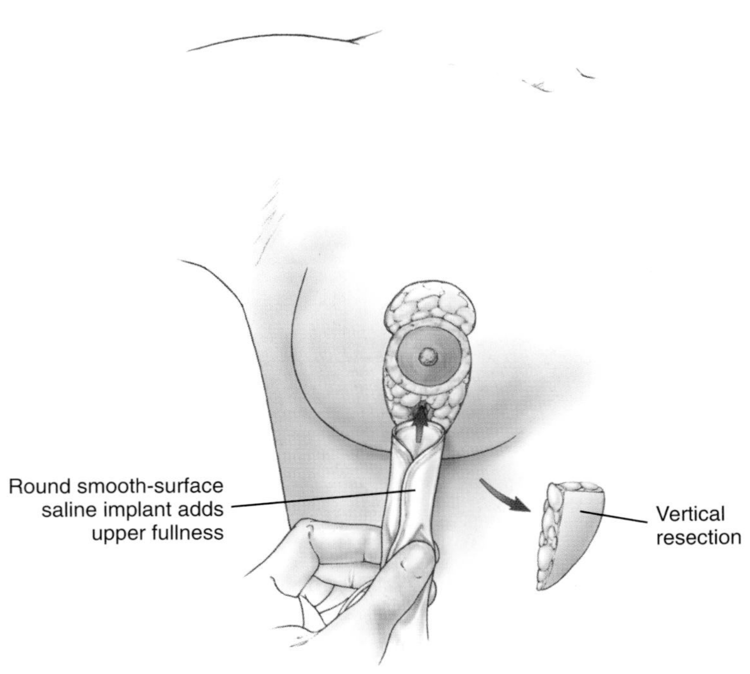

When combining breast reduction with an implant insertion, I prefer to move the nipple-areola up on an upper or superior medial pedicle, not an inferior pedicle. This ensures the best blood supply for the nipple-areola. The elevation of the pocket for the breast implant could detach the perforators when the area to be augmented is elevated beneath the inferior pedicle. There should be no skin tension or delayed healing of the T. ***The final form is dependent on the implant and preserved parenchyma, not on a tight skin closure.***

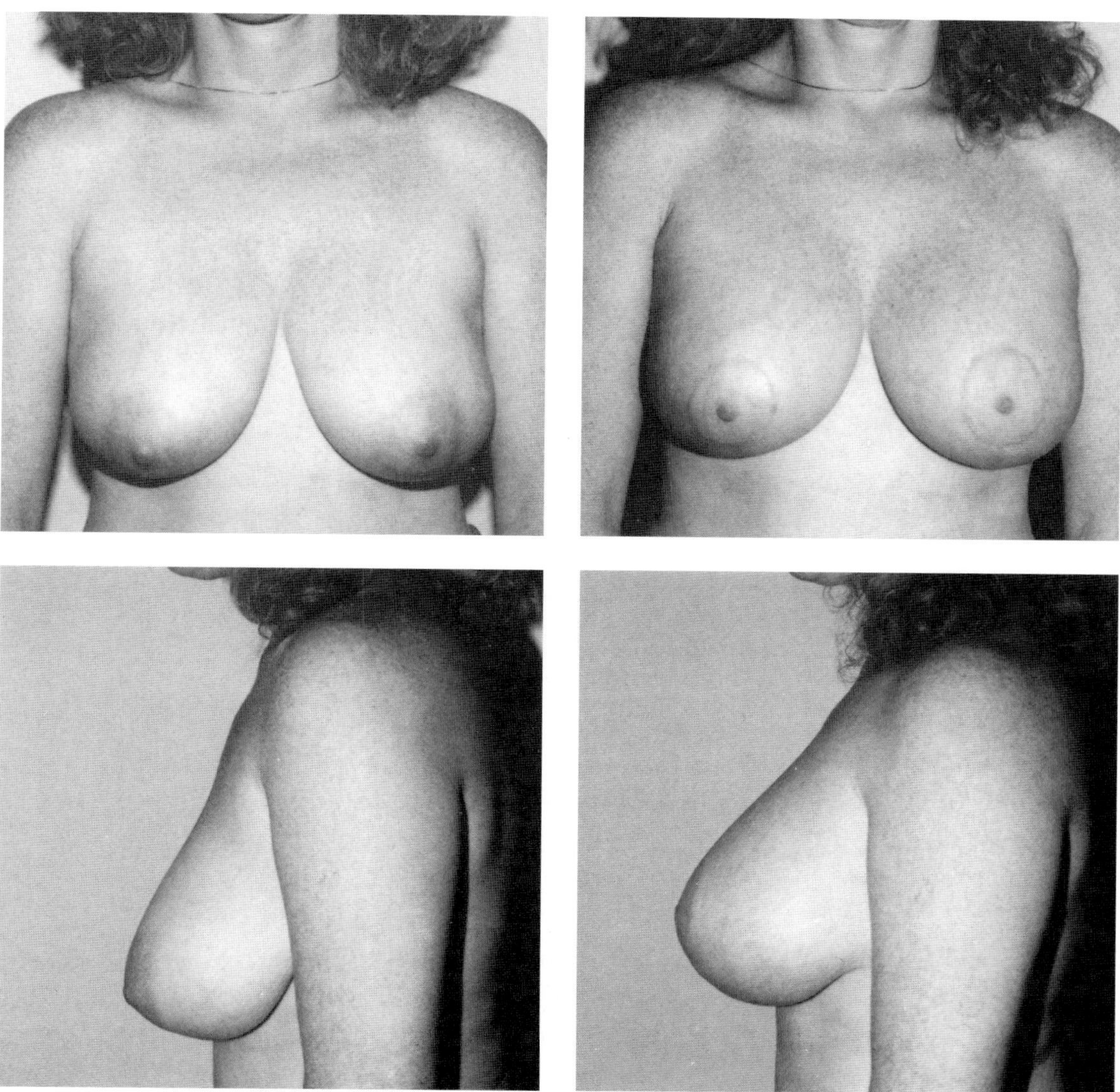

This technique can be used to obtain symmetry with an opposite breast reconstruction in which an implant or an expander implant has been placed. Bilateral implants usually provide better long-term symmetry. When final size is not fully defined, an adjustable implant can be used beneath both breasts to permit the patient to more accurately determine the desired final size and the surgeon to have more versatility in creating a symmetric result.

LIPOSUCTION AND SURGICAL EXCISION TO TREAT LATERAL, AXILLARY, AND PRESTERNAL FULLNESS

When the inframammary fold extends beyond the breast laterally toward the back, this condition should be pointed out to the patient before the initial procedure and addressed at the time of the reduction mammaplasty. If extra lateral tissue is not removed, considerable fullness will persist in this region and the lateral breast fold will be poorly defined. ***The lateral tissue should be removed low and at the level of the inframammary fold with liposuction (my preference) or by excision.***

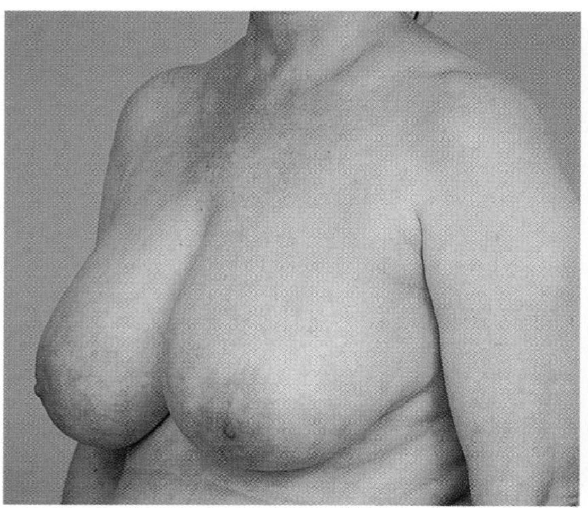

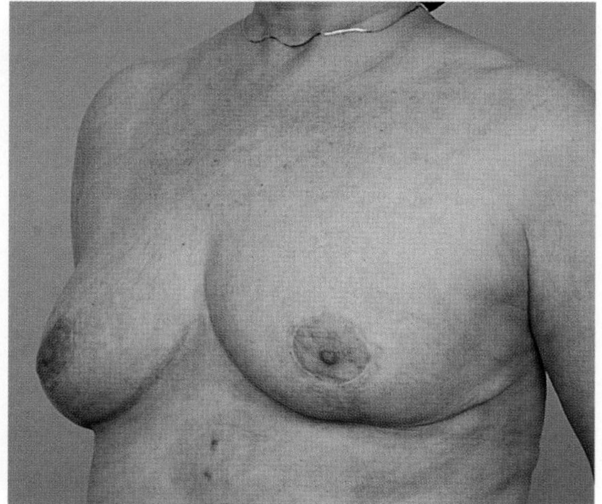

Liposuction is a useful method for contouring the peripheral and lateral chest areas to create a thinner contour and provide better breast definition laterally with the chest wall. I infiltrate wetting solution into the proposed areas to be suctioned to reduce blood loss and provide postoperative anesthesia.

Axillary and presternal fullness are also successfully managed with standard liposuction because it provides better medial breast definition after treatment of gynecomastia. Ultrasound-assisted liposuction is even better for cavitating and liquefying the fibrous parenchyma associated with gynecomastia; however, it is not recommended for reducing the female breast until further data on its safety for this application are evaluated. Smaller degrees of deformity are reduced by standard liposuction through the reduction incision. Any thickening or mass remaining postoperatively is easily approached and excised.

Before liposuction was available for reducing this lateral fullness, it was necessary to make a lateral extension of the horizontal inframammary fold excision and then to excise the excess ptotic skin and underlying fat directly. When the tissue is excised, the scar should not extend upward toward the axilla, for incisions in this region are more difficult to cover with sportswear and will extend beyond the edge of a brassiere.

LIPOSUCTION FOR ABDOMINAL CONTOURING

A distinct fatty roll in the upper abdomen is often accentuated and may actually appear larger than it is if reduction mammaplasty is performed on a pendulous breast. Patients with this problem have been pleased with upper abdominal and low chest liposuction. If additional suctioning in the abdomen or other areas is contemplated, the patient is assessed for her suitability as a candidate and health status. The use of wetting solution in the breast and lateral areas prior to the procedure reduces blood loss and provides for postoperative pain relief.

The patient should understand that liposuction is followed by discoloration and bruising for about 4 to 6 weeks. Lumpiness can persist for many months. I ask my patients to massage the suctioned areas several times a day after the first 2 postoperative weeks. Patience is necessary since it may take many months before the final result is realized. The lateral suctioned area is often more painful than the reduced region.

Postoperative Considerations

Following breast reduction the incisions are covered with Steri-Strips, gauze, and a soft brassiere. Often a drain from the operative site will extend laterally to the suctioned lateral region. The following day the patient can remove the dressing down to the Steri-Strips and shower without massaging or disturbing the breast area. If a drain has been placed, I remove it the day after the operation. Activities requiring raising the arms overhead are avoided for 4 to 6 weeks to avoid strain and pull on the incisions, which could result in widened scars. Aspirin and aspirin-related products are avoided for about 3 weeks to reduce the possibility of late bleeding and hematomas.

Cigarettes should not be used and environmental smoke should be avoided for 2 weeks postoperatively. They can have a deleterious effect on nipple-areolar vascularity and skin graft survival and can contribute to fat necrosis within the breast.

Breast sensation predictably is diminished for the first weeks to months after breast reduction. The patient is alerted to this condition and cautioned not to be alarmed by it. Sensory return and reinnervation can be accompanied by dysesthesias and paresthesias. To minimize these sensations I ask the patient to desensitize the breasts with massage and to use different temperatures of water and textured washcloths during bathing to desensitize and reeducate her breasts.

Special Problems

THE ELDERLY PATIENT

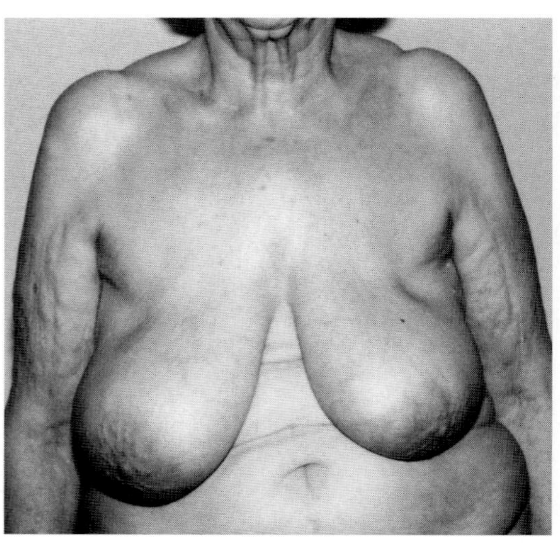

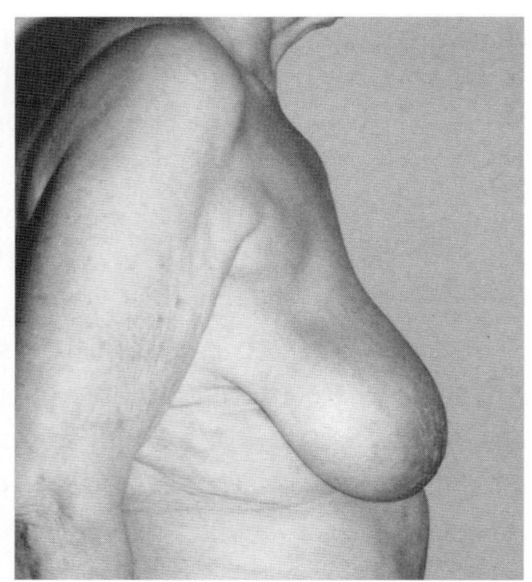

I do not recommend breast reduction in women 65 years of age or older unless, after a history and physical examination and consultation with their personal physician, I am assured of their good health and their strong motivations and compelling physical findings and symptoms. These women generally want sufficient reduction to alleviate heaviness and the pull on their brassiere straps and to eliminate skin-to-skin contact underneath the breast, which often causes a rash or irritation of the skin. Sensory changes often occur in the hands and upper extremities. If the nipple-areola needs to be moved a considerable distance, I prefer the free nipple graft. This technique is safer from the standpoint of nipple-areola survival and avoids the very real risk of loss of the nipple-areola from transposition and fat necrosis.

Because women in this age group are prone to fat necrosis (it can sometimes even occur spontaneously), I try to reduce their breasts with a simple transverse excision and avoid complex techniques associated with an inferior or superior medial pedicle.

WOMEN AT RISK FOR BREAST CANCER

When a woman is at high risk for breast cancer or has had breast cancer in one breast, breast reduction poses special concerns in that residual parenchymal scarring can make it difficult to differentiate breast cancer. I recommend preoperative mammograms for all of my patients at high risk and all those over 30 years of age. Questionable areas should be evaluated, consultation with a surgical oncologist considered, and biopsies performed.

Breast reduction operations, particularly in women at risk, should be planned to produce minimal intraparenchymal incisions and thereby reduce the potential for fat necrosis and folded pedicles that can complicate mammographic interpretation. When fat necroses, it becomes firm and can mimic a malignancy or develop later calcifications visible on a mammogram, presenting problems in monitoring for the woman and her physicians.

I prefer the simpler breast resection techniques in higher risk patients. The line of resection is brought down to the inframammary crease. Any postoperative mass in the upper nonoperated breast tissue is unlikely to be surgically induced and can be visualized with conventional imaging techniques or evaluated by fine-needle biopsy.

Intraoperatively the surgeon needs to be alert to possible masses or suspicious areas; these are sent for pathologic evaluation. A protocol for responding to a cancer detected during surgery is essential. A surgical oncologist should be available for consultation. ***Care should always be taken to separate the right and left sides of any breast resection to avoid confusing them. Major portions of the specific breast resection should be labeled "medial," "lateral," etc. to facilitate the identification and location of a tumor if discovered.***

Occasionally a cancer may be entirely removed in the specimen of the reduction mammaplasty, and the resection is thus considered a therapeutic lumpectomy. At this time the woman should have an evaluation by a surgical oncologist. He may recommend that she have an axillary dissection or sentinel node evaluation and pathologic evaluation to determine if the cancer has spread. A course of adjunctive radiation therapy may be advised following the lumpectomy for infiltrating carcinoma. Another alternative when a tumor is removed and after the woman has had time to evaluate the situation is a total mastectomy followed by immediate or delayed reconstruction; however, breast conservation is usually the approach selected. (Chapter 17 describes how breast reduction can be used as a strategy for conservative surgery.)

The woman and surgeon should become familiar with the feel of her breast after the reduction. Any change or "new" lump must be explained. Mammography is performed 6 months postoperatively for women over 30 years of age and then at yearly intervals along with breast self-examination and yearly physician evaluation. The radiologist should be familiar and comfortable with interpreting mammograms for patients who have had aesthetic breast surgery.

Breast reconstruction in patients who have had a previous breast reduction is a difficult problem. Their breast skin is often thin. The lower flaps at the T are thin and are subject to necrosis and delayed healing. Usually a flap is needed to protect and cover an implant or expander implant. As an alternative, autologous breast reconstruction using a deepithelialized TRAM flap can provide a good breast reconstruction without risking implant exposure.

Problems and Complications

The complications of breast reduction fall into two broad categories: aesthetic and operative. Most complications can be avoided by careful patient selection and preoperative planning. The most common aesthetic shortcomings of reduction mammaplasty are failure to sufficiently reduce the breast, asymmetries, dog ears, unattractive scars, nipple-areolar problems relating to malposition and diminished vascularity, and overreduction. Frequently secondary procedures are required for correction of these conditions. These are usually delayed for 1 year after the initial operation to allow sufficient time for the breasts to heal and settle and a plan to be formulated.

HEMATOMA

Hematoma caused by bleeding usually occurs in the first few postoperative hours from insufficient intraoperative hemostasis, a bleeding tendency, or postoperative hypertension. I use wetting solution liberally in the region of resection to minimize bleeding, decrease the risk of postoperative hematomas, and reduce postoperative pain. Bleeders coming from the breast base, the chest wall through the fascia, and especially the lateral and medial vessels must be completely and securely controlled prior to closure. A drain is no substitute for hemostasis. If the patient develops a bilateral fullness (usually serosanguineous accumulation) after the operation, I aspirate the fluid.

Aspirin, aspirin-related products, and nonsteroidal analgesics taken before surgery can cause prolonged intraoperative bleeding and should be avoided. Patients are given a "bleed sheet" preoperatively to alert them to which medications must be discontinued preoperatively and postoperatively.

INFECTION

Infection in plastic surgery patients is usually related to decreased blood supply and nonviable tissue. It is remarkable that the infection rate after breast reduction is so low in view of the fact that there are bacterial flora within the breast ducts, especially *Staphylococcus.* These ducts are always divided during breast reduction. This source should be checked if an infection develops. Initially I generally use a cephalosporin antibiotic intraoperatively and then ask the patient to take the oral form for 2 to 3 days postoperatively. A seroma or hematoma can become secondarily infected; therefore drainage is an important component of management.

DELAYED HEALING OF THE T

This condition is usually caused by excessive tension and is best avoided by making the preoperative markings such that excess skin is left in this medial area during closure. The vertical approach avoids this T closure and generally is characterized by excellent healing. Any tightness is taken up laterally, the skin is closed from the periphery to the T, and the skin of the T is cut so it is not tight but literally falls together. I often use three clips in addition to deep sutures and the intracuticular closure to further support this area for 1 to 2 weeks.

Decreased microcirculation can contribute to this problem, especially with a tight closure. When it develops, patience and judicious debridement represent the preferred approach. Reexcision and closure will require increased tension and often fail to correct the problem.

DOG EARS

Dog ears can occur if insufficient medial or lateral skin or parenchyma is removed or if some breast parenchyma is left beneath this area. Medial and lateral dog ears are particularly disconcerting to the patient; they seem more prominent when she views them from above than from a distance. When this problem exists, the patient is advised to massage the area to soften the skin and allow it to smooth out without the need for additional correction. If this strategy is unsuccessful, the excision of skin along with the extra subcutaneous tissue will correct the prominence.

INADEQUATE REDUCTION

Inadequate reduction during the primary procedure or breast regrowth or weight gain and consequent breast enlargement is the most frequent reason patients request reoperation. Other patients, while initially satisfied, find that after weight gain, pregnancy, or lactation their breasts enlarge and do not involute to their smaller reduced size. Young patients who have a reduction mammaplasty before the completion of breast growth also may need a secondary reduction mammaplasty. (See Chapter 9 for details on reoperative surgery.)

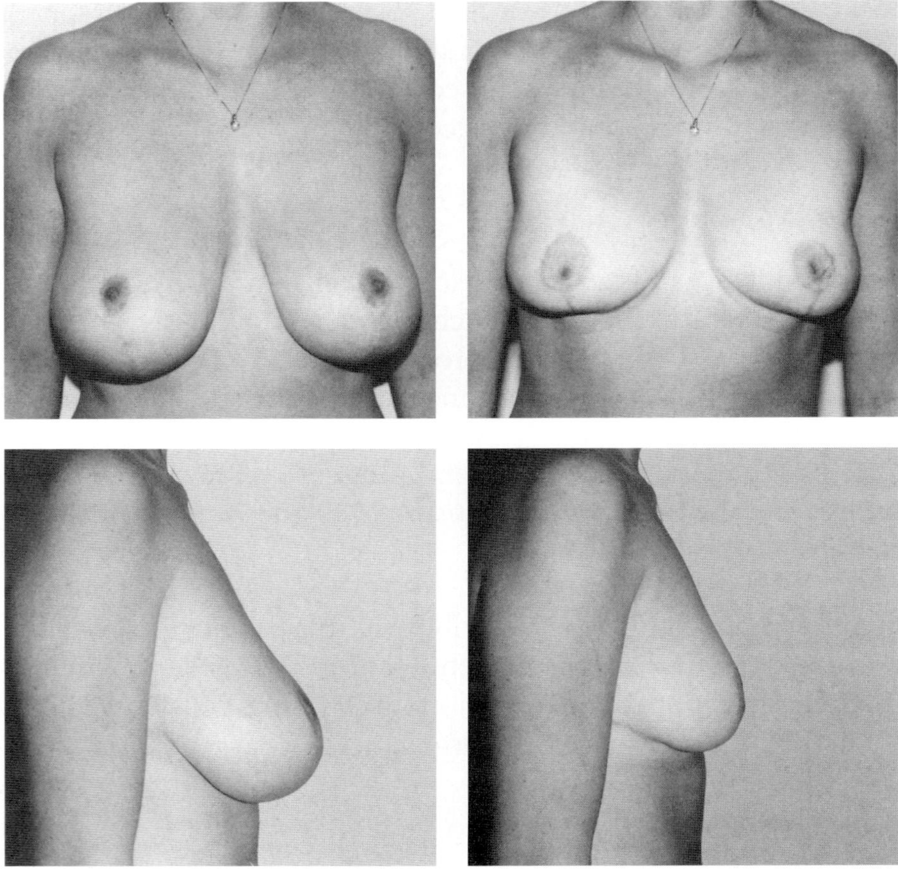

This 25-year-old patient had reduction mammaplasty 5 years before her consultation for a second reduction procedure. Immediately postoperatively she felt that her breasts had not been reduced enough. The original operative note showed that a superior pedicle reduction technique was used. A similar technique was used for her second reduction mammaplasty. Additional tissue was removed inferiorly and from the deep and lateral portions of the breast to further reduce the breast. The nipple-areola was elevated, as is done with the superior pedicle technique. The patient is shown 1 year after her second reduction mammaplasty.

NIPPLE-AREOLAR PROBLEMS

Avoiding procedures that compromise nipple-areola blood supply is important in preventing the dreaded complication of necrosis. ***If there is any question about nipple-areola viability intraoperatively (e.g., no blood flow in the surrounding dermis or no blood return when tested), the nipple-areola can be harvested as a split-skin graft and grafted rather than pedicled to its new position.*** If the nipple-areola seems tight, simply releasing a few sutures sometimes can reestablish flow; these sutures can be replaced a few days later.

Unfortunately the vascularity of the underlying breast parenchyma using the parenchymal techniques described can also be compromised and either a fat necrosis or frank ischemia may develop. The assessment is made more difficult if epinephrine solution has been injected into the nipple-areola area.

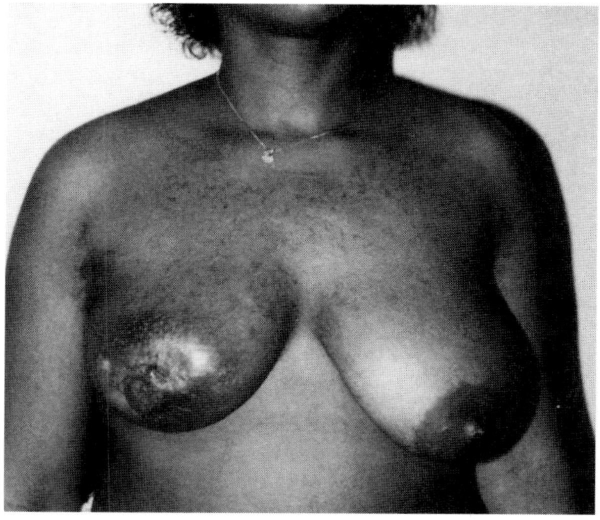

When partial nipple-areola necrosis develops, the superficial tissue should be allowed to heal and debrided judiciously as needed. Accompanying necrosis of the underlying breast parenchyma may be present, especially when the central pedicle technique is used.

After healing by secondary intention, nipple-areola reconstruction is completed with the techniques described in Chapter 20.

Loss of pigmentation can occur in the heavily pigmented areola when transferred as a skin graft; tattooing is useful for improving the coloration. Adjustments in areolar diameter may also need to be made (see Chapter 20).

When the nipple-areola is positioned too high, it may be moved by excising skin and repositioning it lower on the breast. With this maneuver another breast scar may be created above the areola. Although there have been a number of suggestions for nipple-areola transposition without a scar, none has been particularly successful in achieving significant lowering. Possibly tissue expansion will be of help in the future.

Sometimes ptotic breast parenchyma below the inframammary fold may give the nipple-areola the appearance of being too high when it actually is properly positioned. This condition is treated by resecting this ptotic breast parenchyma; sometimes a breast implant is requested to replace the removed bulk and provide some upper breast fullness. (See Chapter 20 for more information on correction of nipple-areolar problems.)

WIDE AND HYPERTROPHIC BREAST SCARS

As with all complications, avoidance or prevention is the best solution. Patients with an obvious tendency to hypertrophic scarring should give serious consideration to not having reduction mammaplasty in view of the inevitable scars. The vertical approach avoids the horizontal scar and is a good strategy for these patients.

There are a number of things that the surgeon can do, however, at the time of reduction mammaplasty to improve the quality of the resulting scars.

Strategies for improving scar quality

- Use vertical or reduced scar techniques.
- Tight skin should not be relied on to form the new breast.
- Tight closure of the horizontal limb of the T contributes to hypertrophic scar formation and should be avoided.
- Breast parenchyma should be positioned so that it can be molded to form the new breast rather than relying on tight skin to accomplish this goal.
- The breast should not be shaped by excising extra skin laterally in an S configuration. This extra excision simply adds to scar tension and produces wider, often hypertrophic scars.
- Medial and lateral incisions should not curve upward to create a tight closure; this orientation of the incisions will increase the coning of typical reduction mammaplasty and cause tight, thickened hypertrophic scars.
- Preoperative markings that provide for final skin excision at the end of the procedure permit more flexibility for tailoring the skin without creating undue tightness.

- The nipple-areola is cut to a larger diameter than the recipient circle so that tension is avoided during closure.
- The wound is closed in layers—most of the wound strength is in the dermal and superficial fascial closure.
- Steri-Strips provide pressure on the incisions to resist spreading of the incisions; they are used for 2 months after the operation.
- The patient is advised not to extend her arm overhead for about 2 months to avoid stretching the lateral scars.
- Silicone sheeting can flatten scars when they begin to thicken.

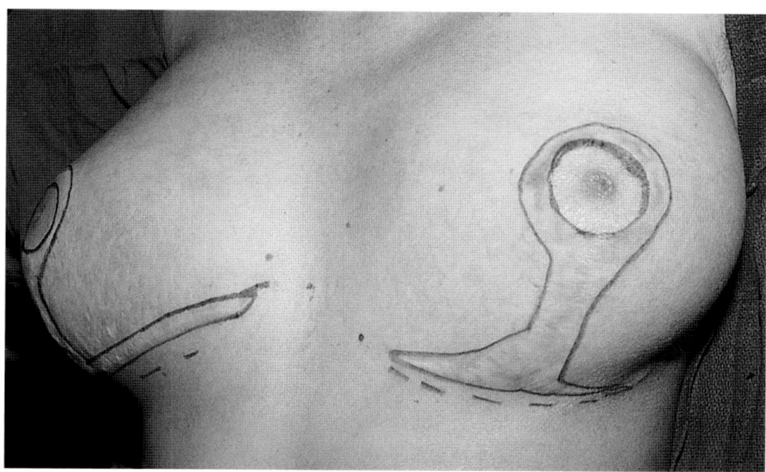

When hypertrophic or wide scars do occur, time and the application of intralesional triamcinolone, 10 mg/ml, are the first treatment strategies. The patient is encouraged to wait as long as possible for secondary corrections because these scars invariably fade and are less noticeable with time. When the scars need to be revised, I wait at least 1 year and preferably longer before planning a revision. (See Chapter 9 for details on scar revision.)

BREAST ASYMMETRY

Although optimal symmetry is the goal, realistically most breasts are not symmetric before reduction mammaplasty and discrepancies in size or shape may sometimes be magnified when the breasts are smaller. ***Immediate reoperation to correct any but gross asymmetries is discouraged.*** The asymmetry in the early postoperative period may stem from variations in swelling, hematoma, or seroma. Much of the initial appearance of asymmetry often disappears with the stretching of the skin and the settling of the breast parenchyma. Remaining problems can then be addressed at a later date. (See Chapter 9 for details on treating breast asymmetry.)

FAT NECROSIS

Fat necrosis can occur spontaneously after trauma or after a breast reduction. It is caused by decreased blood flow or trauma to a portion of the breast. It usually occurs in patients with decreased vascularity to a portion of fat and in women with predominantly fatty breasts who have poor microcirculation. The area at first is thickened. A central portion of the area can actually become necrotic and liquefy. After a few months and up to 1 to 2 years after the occurrence, the fat necrosis area can develop actual microcalcifications, resulting in atrophy and reduced volume of the affected breast. They have a characteristic appearance on mammography. A thickened area in the breast should be explored. Usually fine-needle aspiration biopsy is necessary for evaluation. Aspiration sometimes removes the fluid and reduces breast size.

OVERREDUCTION AND UPPER BREAST FLATTENING

Sometimes the breasts are reduced too much for the patient's taste despite her original request. The patient who has lost weight after the reduction and consequently experienced breast volume loss may feel that her reduced breasts are now too small. Patients with considerable preoperative ptosis combined with breast hypertrophy may be disappointed if their breasts do not exhibit some upper fullness, which is hard to obtain with a reduction mammaplasty alone. Transposition of lower breast parenchyma to the upper breast is one strategy that may be considered in this situation. Correction of these problems generally requires the insertion of a breast implant. In rare instances autologous tissue such as a latissimus dorsi back flap is transposed for this purpose. (See discussion of augmentation and reduction in Chapter 9.)

Long-Term Results

When a reduction mammaplasty removes enough breast parenchyma to satisfy the patient and the breasts have been restored to a natural appearance, the long-term results are usually highly satisfactory. However, certain situations and conditions can affect appearance over time. Weight gain can cause additional enlargement of the breast and bring the patient back for further breast reduction. Weight loss or involution of the breast following pregnancy can result in even smaller breasts, and the patient may request breast implants. Involution of the breasts, particularly when the skin is inelastic, can result in breast ptosis and necessitate additional breast excision, sometimes accompanied by insertion of a breast implant. The best long-term results are usually achieved when the breasts are reduced to a normal, small size. When the breasts remain heavy after reduction mammaplasty, they may become ptotic and the effects of gravity on the large mass may leave preoperative symptoms unabated. Following reduction, breasts can be monitored for breast cancer by regular breast self-examination, physician examination, and serial mammography.

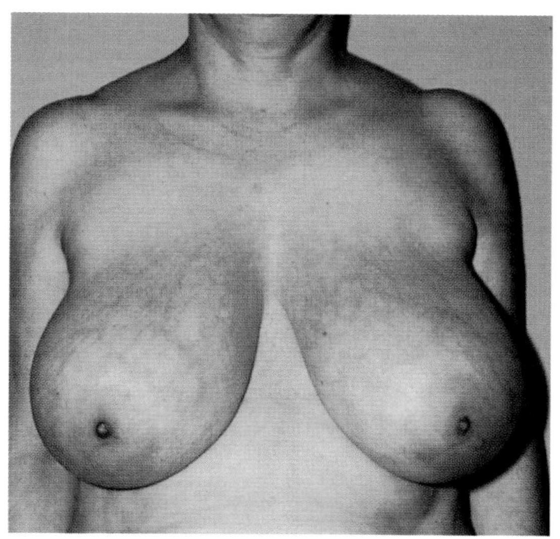

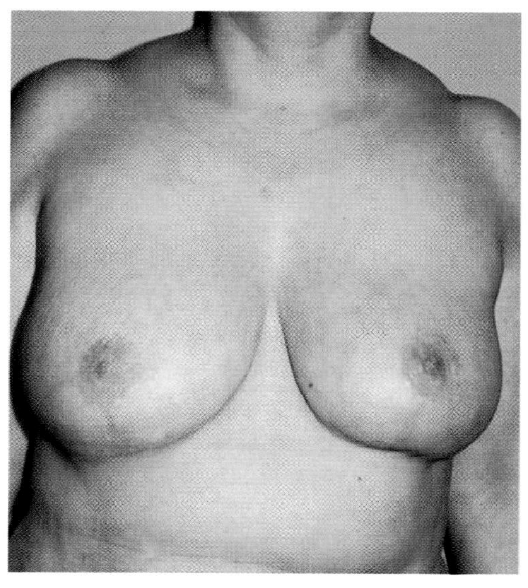

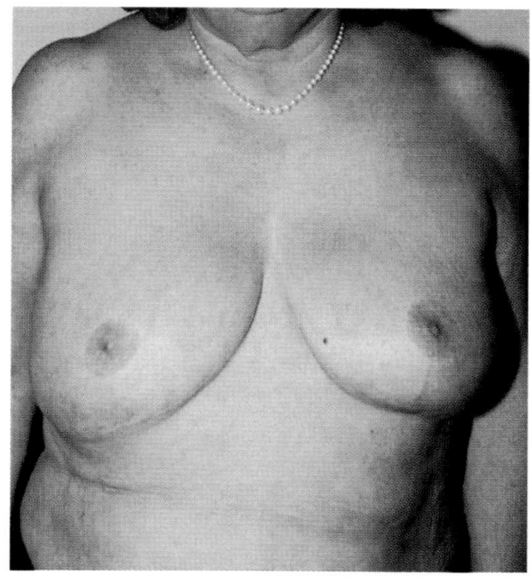

This 56-year-old woman's size DD breasts were disabling and uncomfortable. She was developing numbness in her hands in the distribution of C8-T1. The free nipple graft technique was selected because of the considerable degree of ptosis and her postmenopausal status. A total of 1600 gm was removed. The patient is shown 2 and 14 years following the operation. Her breast contour is greatly improved, and her neurologic symptoms have disappeared. The early ptosis of the right inframammary crease has become accentuated over the years.

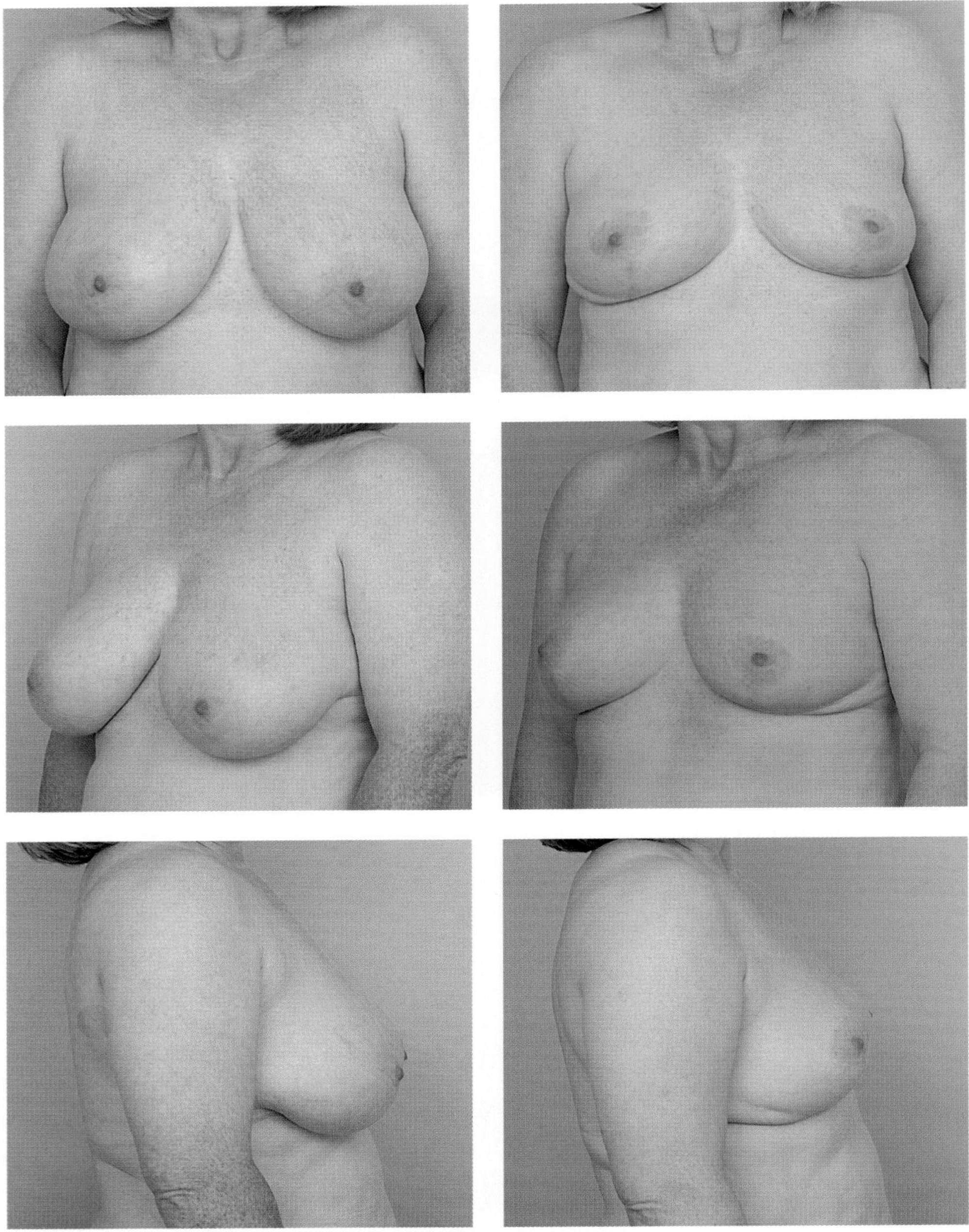

This 38-year-old woman had difficulty with her large breasts for many years. She had symptoms related to heaviness of her breast as well as back and shoulder pain and requested breast reduction, preferably with minimal scars. She had breast reduction with the vertical approach, which included liposuction of the breast parenchyma, the anterior axillary region, and the lateral breast region. Her total breast reduction was 1800 gm. She is shown 2 years postoperatively. The symptoms of macromastia are relieved and she likes her changed appearance. Her scars have healed well without hypertrophy. She also appreciates the reduced fullness laterally as well as in the axillary region. Since the lower breast parenchyma was resected, the postoperative appearance has remained satisfactory without ptosis of the lower breast segment.

PREGNANCY AND LACTATION

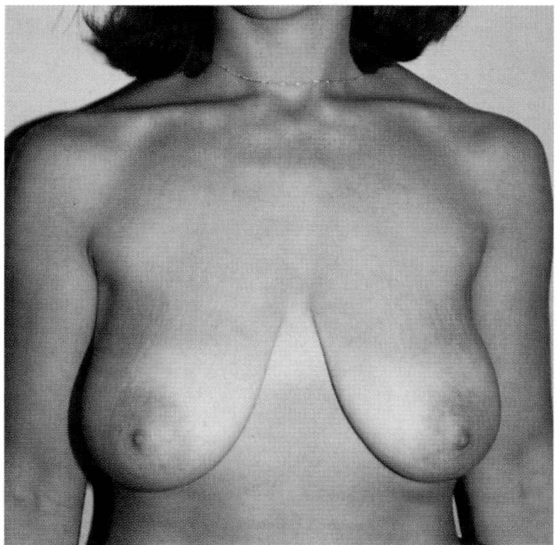
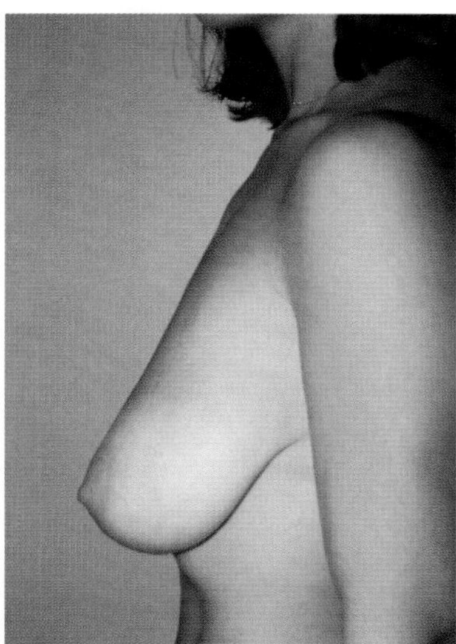

This 25-year-old patient had a reduction mammaplasty with the superior pedicle technique; she was pleased with the initial result.

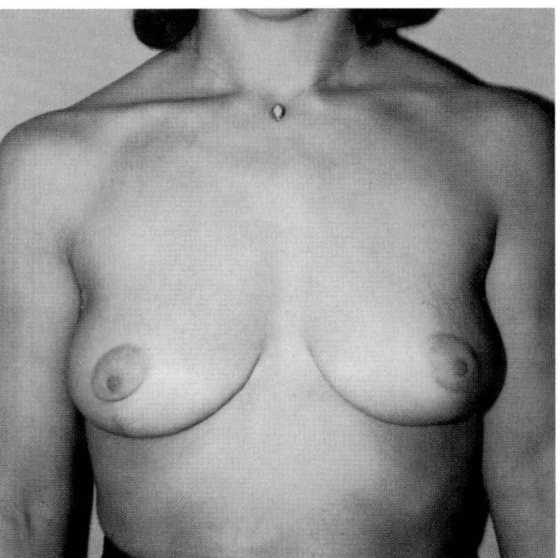
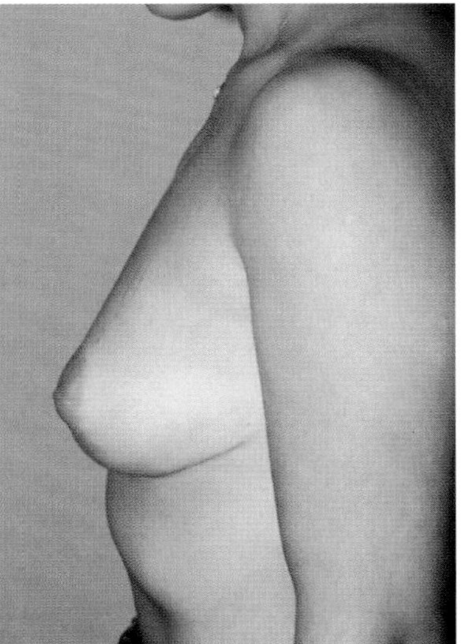

She is shown 1 year after the initial reduction mammaplasty; her scars are healing well.

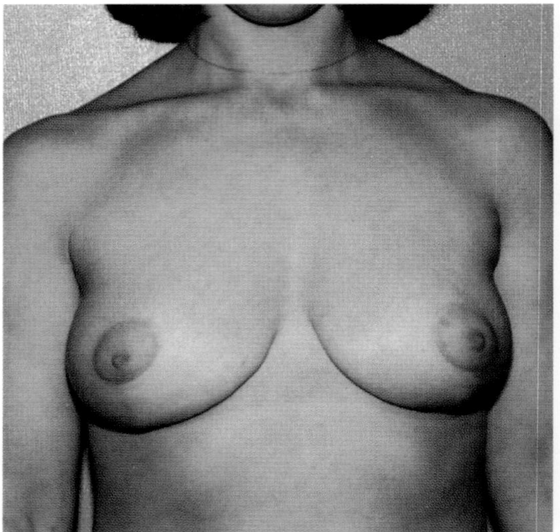
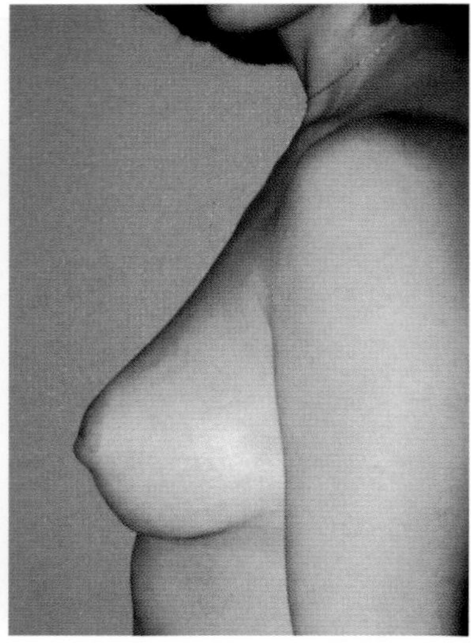

She is shown 8 months later when she is 3 months pregnant. She had a normal delivery and breast-fed her son for 4 months.

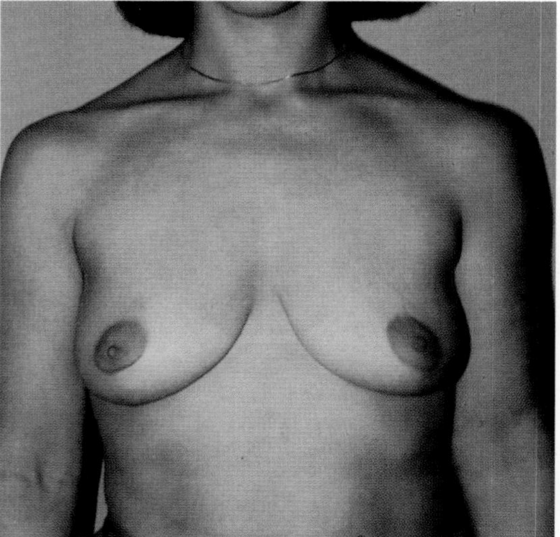
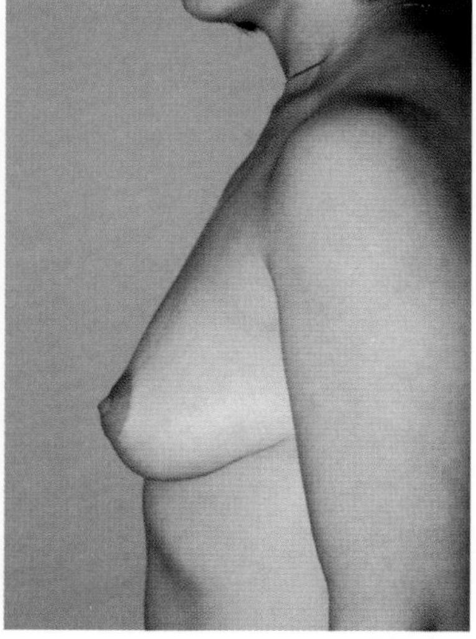

Five years after the initial reduction and 2 years after her pregnancy, her breasts are involuted and are smaller than before she became pregnant. This patient has good skin with excellent elasticity. She also had a breast reduction to a relatively small size. These factors contribute to a lasting long-term result. Often some change in breast volume can be expected after pregnancy and lactation. Despite some involution of her breast parenchyma, this patient still finds her breast appearance and size acceptable.

WEIGHT FLUCTUATION

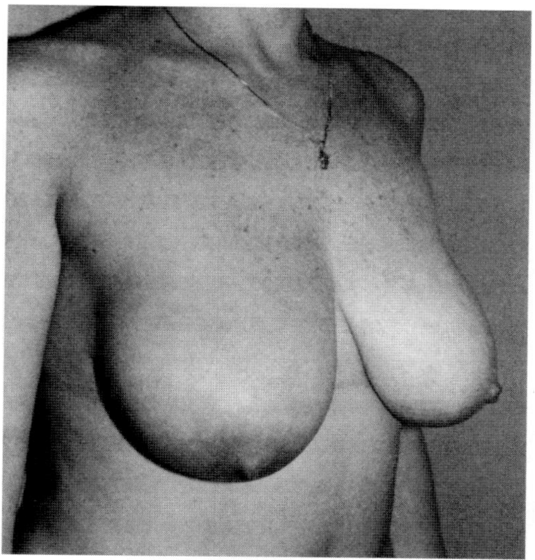

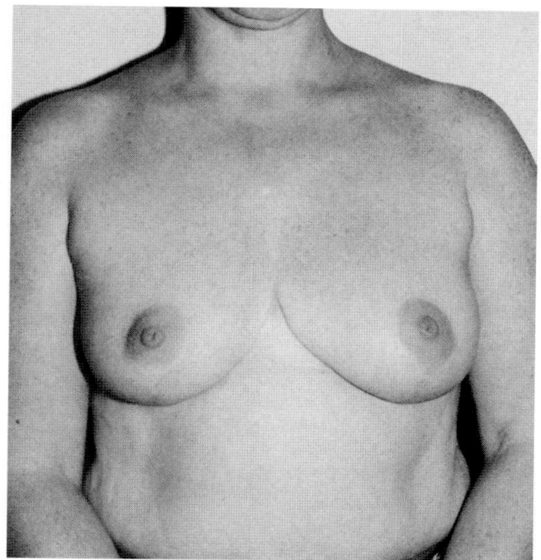

This 36-year-old patient requested a reduction mammaplasty. The inferior pedicle technique was selected. The patient is shown 3 years later; she has begun to gain weight, but remains pleased with her breast proportions.

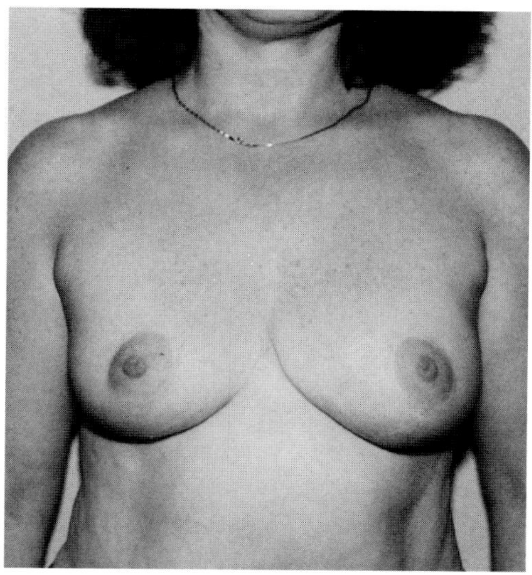

One year later she has gained an additional 15 pounds and finds that her breasts are larger than she desires. She is told that they are in proportion to her body habitus and advised not to have a second reduction mammaplasty.

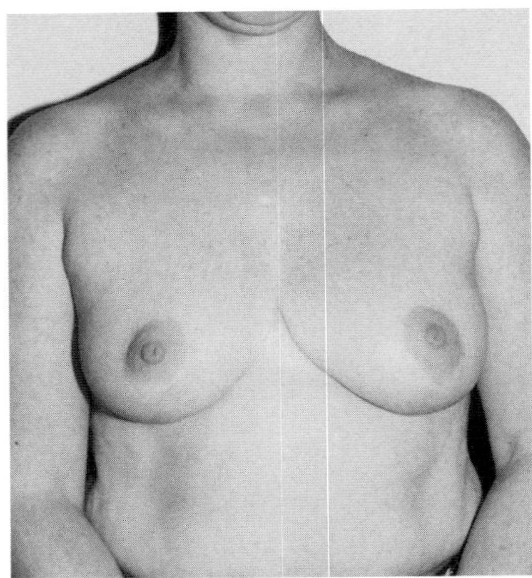

After another year she has gained an additional 10 pounds and her breasts are still larger than she desires.

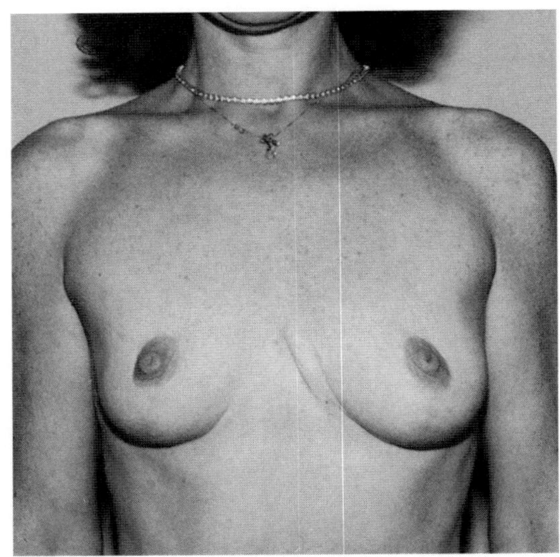

She returns 3 years later (8 years after the initial reduction mammaplasty) after having lost a large amount of weight. Her breasts are now smaller than she desires! She is told to return when her weight has stabilized.

This long-term study of a woman whose weight has fluctuated shows the multiple changes that can occur in aesthetic breast patients. The body fat content and the patient's breast response to this are all individual factors and impossible to predict. It is important for the patient's weight to have stabilized before reduction mammaplasty if this type of problem is to be avoided.

REFERENCES

Abboud M, Vadoud-Seyedi J, De Mey A, Cukierfajn M, Lejour M. Incidence of calcifications in the breast after surgical reduction and liposuction. Plast Reconstr Surg 96:620, 1995.

Aboudib JH Jr, Cardoso de Castro C. Mammaplasty utilizing the periareolar approach. Aesthetic Plast Surg 22:51, 1998.

Aldo Mottura A. Breast reduction under intravenous sedation: A review of 50 cases. Plast Reconstr Surg 99:2113, 1997.

Ariyan S. Reduction mammaplasty with the nipple-areola carried on a single, narrow inferior pedicle. Ann Plast Surg 5:167, 1980.

Arons MS. Reduction of very large breasts: The inferior flap technique of Robbins. Br J Plast Surg 29:137, 1976.

Aufricht G. Mammaplasty for pendulous breasts: Empiric and geometric planning. Plast Reconstr Surg 4:13, 1949.

Baasch M, Nielsen SF, Engholm G, Lund K. Breast cancer incidence subsequent to surgical reduction of the female breast. Br J Cancer 73:961, 1996.

Berg A, Palmer B. Quality assurance in plastic surgery: Reduction mammaplasty. Scand J Plast Reconstr Surg Hand Surg 31:327, 1997.

Berrino P, Galli A, Rainero ML, Santi P. Unilateral reduction mammaplasty: Sculpturing the breast from the undersurface. Plast Reconstr Surg 82:88, 1988.

Boschert MT, Barone CM, Puckett CL. Outcome analysis of reduction mammaplasty. Plast Reconstr Surg 98:451, 1996.

Brinton LA, Malone KE, Coates RJ, Schoenberg JB, Swanson CA, Daling JR, Stanford JL. Breast enlargement and reduction: Results from a breast cancer case-control study. Plast Reconstr Surg 97:269, 1996.

Brown MH, Weinberg M, Chong N, Levine R, Holowaty E. A cohort study of breast cancer risk in breast reduction patients. Plast Reconstr Surg 103:1674, 1999.

Bruhlmann Y, Tschopp H. Breast reduction improves symptoms of macromastia and has a long-lasting effect. Ann Plast Surg 41:240, 1998.

Climo MS, Alexander JE. Intercostothelial circulation: Nipple survival in reduction mammaplasty in the absence of a dermal pedicle. Ann Plast Surg 4:128, 1980.

Cole RP, Shakespeare V. Measuring patient-based outcomes in a plastic surgery service: Breast reduction surgical patients. Br J Plast Surg 51:79, 1998.

Conroy WC. Reduction mammaplasty with maximum superior subdermal vascular pedicle. Ann Plast Surg 2:189, 1979.

Courtiss EH. Reduction mammaplasty by suction alone. Plast Reconstr Surg 92:1276, 1993.

Courtiss EH, Goldwyn RM. Reduction mammaplasty by the inferior pedicle technique: An alternative to free nipple and areola grafting for severe macromastia or extreme ptosis. Plast Reconstr Surg 59:500, 1977; Update, 66:646, 1980.

Crosby ET, Murphy P, Benoit PR. Routine predeposit of autologous blood is not warranted before breast reduction surgery. Can J Surg 38:309, 1995.

Cruz NI, Guerro A, Gonzalez CI. Current findings in the pathologic evaluation of breast reduction specimens. Bol Assoc Med P R 81:387, 1989.

Cruz-Korchin NI. Effectiveness of silicone sheets in the prevention of hypertrophic breast scars. Ann Plast Surg 37:345, 1996.

Dabbah A, Lehman JA Jr, Parker MG, Tantri D, Wagner DS. Reduction mammaplasty: An outcome analysis. Ann Plast Surg 35:337, 1995.

Davies BW, Lewis RD, Pennington GA. Reduction mammaplasty: A comparison of outpatient and inpatient procedures. Aesthetic Plast Surg 20:77, 1996.

Davis GM, Ringler SL, Short K, Sherrick D, Bengtson BP. Reduction mammaplasty: Long-term efficacy, morbidity, and patient satisfaction. Plast Reconstr Surg 96:1106, 1995.

de Souza Pinto E, Erazo PJ, Muniz AC, Prado Filho FS, Alves MA, Salazar GH. Breast reduction: Shortening scars with liposuction. Aesthetic Plast Surg 20:481, 1996.

DeBono R, Rao GS. Vasoconstrictor infiltration in breast reduction surgery: Is it harmful? Br J Plast Surg 50:260, 1997.

Dinner MI, Artz JS. Carcinoma of the breast occurring in routine reduction mammaplasty. Plast Reconstr Surg 83:1042, 1989.

Emory RE, Bean CW, Bonnecarrere ER, Jorgenson DS. Reevaluating the need for routine drainage in reduction mammaplasty. Plast Reconstr Surg 103:2088, 1999.

Evans GR, Ryan JJ. Reduction mammaplasty for the teenage patient: A critical analysis. Aesthetic Plast Surg 18:291, 1994.

Farina R, Villano JB. Reduction mammoplasty with free grafting of the nipple and areola. Br J Plast Surg 25:393, 1972.

Finger RE, Vasquez B, Drew GS, Given KS. Superomedial pedicle technique of reduction mammaplasty. Plast Reconstr Surg 83:471, 1989.

Gasperoni C, Salgarello M. Preoperative breast marking in reduction mammaplasty. Ann Plast Surg 19:306, 1987.

Georgiade NG, Serafin D, Morris R, Georgiade GS. Reduction mammaplasty utilizing an inferior pedicle nipple-areolar flap. Ann Plast Surg 3:211, 1979.

Georgiade NG, Serafin D, Riefkohl R, Georgiade GS. Is there a reduction mammaplasty for all seasons? Plast Reconstr Surg 63:765, 1979.

Glatt BS, Sarwer DB, O'Hara DE, Hamori C, Bucky LP, LaRossa D. A retrospective study of changes in physical symptoms and body image after reduction mammaplasty. Plast Reconstr Surg 103:76, 1999.

Godwin Y, Wood SH, O'Neill TJ. A comparison of the patient and surgeon opinion on the long-term aesthetic outcome of reduction mammaplasty. Br J Plast Surg 51:444, 1998.

Goin MK, Goin JM, Gianini MH. The psychic consequences of a reduction mammaplasty. Plast Reconstr Surg 59:530, 1977.

Goldwyn RM. Reduction Mammaplasty. Boston: Little, Brown, 1990.

Goldwyn RM. Pulmonary function and bilateral reduction mammaplasty. Plast Reconstr Surg 53:84, 1974.

Gonzalez F, Brown FE, Gold ME, Walton RL, Shafer B. Preoperative and postoperative nipple-areola sensibility in patients undergoing reduction mammaplasty. Plast Reconstr Surg 92:809, 1993.

Gonzalez F, Walton RL, Shafer B, Matory WE Jr, Borah GL. Reduction mammaplasty improves symptoms of macromastia. Plast Reconstr Surg 91:1270, 1993.

Gray LN. Liposuction breast reduction. Aesthetic Plast Surg 22:159, 1998.

Greco RJ, Dascombe WH, Williams SL, Johnson RR, Kelly JL. Two-staged breast reconstruction in patients with symptomatic macromastia requiring mastectomy. Ann Plast Surg 32:572, 1994.

Green AR. "The reason for hating myself": A patient's request for breast reduction. Br J Plast Surg 49:439, 1996.

Hallock GG. Salvage by tattooing of areolar complications following breast reduction. Plast Reconstr Surg 91:942, 1993.

Hauben DJ. Experience and refinements with the supero-medial dermal pedicle for nipple areola transposition in reduction mammaplasty. Aesthetic Plast Surg 8:189, 1985.

Hawtof DB, Levine M, Kapetansky DI, Pieper D. Complications of reduction mammaplasty: Comparison of nipple-areolar graft and pedicle. Ann Plast Surg 23:3, 1989.

Hester TR Jr, Bostwick J III, Miller L, Cunningham SJ. Breast reduction utilizing the maximally vascularized central breast pedicle. Plast Reconstr Surg 76:890, 1985.

Hidalgo DA. Improving safety and aesthetic results in inverted T scar breast reduction. Plast Reconstr Surg 103:874, 1999.

Horlock N, Cole RP, Rossi LF. Rationing breast reduction surgery. Br Med J 314:1045, 1997.

Hugo NE, McClellan RM. Reduction mammaplasty with a single superiorly-based pedicle. Plast Reconstr Surg 63:230, 1979.

Hurst LN, Evans HB, Murray KA. Inferior flap reduction mammaplasty with pedicled nipple. Ann Plast Surg 10:483, 1983.

Jansen DA, Murphy M, Kind GM, Sands K. Breast cancer in reduction mammoplasty: Case reports and a survey of plastic surgeons. Plast Reconstr Surg 101:361, 1998.

Kaplan I. Reduction mammaplasty: Nipple-areola survival on a single breast quadrant. Plast Reconstr Surg 61:27, 1978.

Kayar R. 200-gm reduction of breast should be enough for insurance coverage of reduction mammaplasty. Plast Reconstr Surg 97:1312, 1996.

Koger KE, Sunde D, Press BH, Hovey LM. Reduction mammaplasty for gigantomastia using inferiorly based pedicle and free nipple transplantation. Ann Plast Surg 33:561, 1994.

Kreipe RE, Lewand AG, Dukarm CP, Caldwell EH. Outcome for patients with bulimia and breast hypertrophy after reduction mammaplasty. Arch Pediatr Adolesc Med 151:176, 1997.

Kuzbari R, Deutinger M, Todoroff BP, Schneider B, Freilinger G. Surgical treatment of developmental asymmetry of the breast. Long term results. Scand J Plast Reconstr Surg Hand Surg 27: 203, 1993.

Lalardrie JP. The "dermal vault" technique. Transacta der III Tagen der Vereinigung der deutschen plastischen Chirurgen. Köln, 1973.

Lassus C. A 30-year experience with vertical mammaplasty. Plast Reconstr Surg 97:373, 1996.

Lassus C. An "all-season" mammoplasty. Aesthetic Plast Surg 10:9, 1986.

Lassus C. Breast reduction: Evolution of a technique—A single vertical scar. Aesthetic Plast Surg 11: 107, 1987.

Lejour M. Evaluation of fat in breast tissue removed by vertical mammaplasty. Plast Reconstr Surg 99:386, 1997.

Lejour M. Vertical mammaplasty as secondary surgery after other techniques. Aesthetic Plast Surg 21:403, 1997.

Lejour M. Vertical mammaplasty and liposuction of the breast. Plast Reconstr Surg 94:100, 1994.

Lejour M. Vertical Mammaplasty and Liposuction. St. Louis: Quality Medical Publishing, 1994.

Leone MS, Franchelli S, Berrino P, Santi PL. Vertical mammaplasty: A personal approach. Aesthetic Plast Surg 21:356, 1997.

Lewis JR Jr. Reduction mammaplasty. Borrowing the good points of many techniques. Aesthetic Plast Surg 1:43, 1976.

Losee JE, Serletti JM, Kreipe RE, Caldwell EH. Reduction mammaplasty in patients with bulimia nervosa. Ann Plast Surg 39:443, 1997.

Mandrekas AD, Assimakopoulos GI, Mastorakos DP, Pantzalis K. Fat necrosis following breast reduction. Br J Plast Surg 47:560, 1994.

Marchac D, Sagher U. Mammaplasty with a short horizontal scar. Evaluation and results after 9 years. Clin Plast Surg 15:627, 1988.

Marconi F. The dermal pursestring suture: A new technique for a short inframammary scar in reduction mammaplasty and dermal mastopexy. Ann Plast Surg 22:484, 1989.

Marks F. The hazards of using the inferior pedicle technique for reduction in a patient with a previous submammary augmentation. Plast Reconstr Surg 98:751, 1996.

Marshall DR, Callan PP, Nicholson W. Breastfeeding after reduction mammaplasty. Br J Plast Surg 47:167, 1994.

Matarasso A, Courtiss EH. Suction mammaplasty: The use of suction lipectomy to reduce large breasts. Plast Reconstr Surg 87:709, 1991.

Mathes SJ, Nahai F, Hester TR. Avoiding the flat breast in reduction mammaplasty. Plast Reconstr Surg 66:63, 1980.

McKissock PK. Reduction mammaplasty with a vertical dermal flap. Plast Reconstr Surg 49:245, 1972.

McMahan JD, Wolfe JA, Cromer BA, Ruberg RL. Lasting success in teenage reduction mammaplasty. Ann Plast Surg 35:227, 1995.

Meyer TN. Breast reduction under local anesthesia. Plast Reconstr Surg 101:553, 1998.

Millard RD Jr, Mullin WR, Lesavoy MA. Secondary correction of the too-high areola and nipple after a mammaplasty. Plast Reconstr Surg 58:568, 1976.

Miller AP, Zacher JB, Berggren RB, Falcone RE, Monk J. Breast reduction for symptomatic macromastia: Can objective predictors for operative success be identified? Plast Reconstr Surg 95:77, 1995.

Miller JA, Festa S, Goldstein M. Benign fat necrosis simulating bilateral breast malignancy after reduction mammoplasty. South Med J 91:765, 1998.

Mitnick JS, Vazquez MF, Plesser KP, Pressman PI, Harris MN, Colen SR, Roses DF. Distinction between postsurgical changes and carcinoma by means of stereotaxic fine-needle aspiration biopsy after reduction mammaplasty. Radiology 188:457, 1993.

Oneal RM, Goldstein JA, Rohrich RJ, Izenberg PH, Pollock RA. Reduction mammoplasty with free-nipple transplantations: Indications and technical refinements. Ann Plast Surg 26:117, 1991.

Papay FA, Verghese A, Stanton-Hicks M, Zins J. Complex regional pain syndrome of the breast in a patient after breast reduction. Ann Plast Surg 39:347,1997.

Peixoto G. The infra-areolar longitudinal incision in reduction mammoplasty. Aesthetic Plast Surg 9:1, 1985.

Peixoto G. Reduction mammaplasty: A personal technique. Plast Reconstr Surg 65:217, 1980.

Petit JY, Rietjens M, Contesso G, Bertin F, Gilles R. Contralateral mastoplasty for breast reconstruction: A good opportunity for glandular exploration and occult carcinomas diagnosis. Ann Surg Oncol 4:511, 1997.

Pitanguy I. Breast hypertrophy. In Transactions of the International Society of Plastic Surgeons, Second Congress. Edinburgh: Churchill Livingstone, 1960.

Pitanguy I. Surgical treatment of breast hypertrophy. Br J Plast Surg 10:78, 1967.

Pontes R. Single stage reconstruction of the missing breast. Br J Plast Surg 26:377, 1973.

Raispis T, Zehring RD, Downey DL. Long-term functional results after reduction mammaplasty. Ann Plast Surg 34:113, 1995.

Reus WF, Mathes SJ. Preservation of projection after reduction mammaplasty: Long-term follow-up of the inferior pedicle technique. Plast Reconstr Surg 82:644, 1988.

Robbins LB, Hoffman DK. The superior dermoglandular pedicle approach to breast reduction. Ann Plast Surg 29:211, 1992.

Robbins TH. A reduction mammaplasty with the areola-nipple based on an inferior dermal pedicle. Plast Reconstr Surg 59:64, 1977.

Ryan RF, Pernoll JL. Virginal hypertrophy. Plast Reconstr Surg 75:737, 1985.

Sarwer DB, Bartlett SP, Bucky LP, LaRossa D, Low DW, Pertschuk MJ, Wadden TA, Whitaker LA. Bigger is not always better: Body image dissatisfaction in breast reduction and breast augmentation patients. Plast Reconstr Surg 101:1956, 1998.

Schnur PL, Schnur DP, Petty PM, Hanson TJ, Weaver AL. Reduction mammaplasty: An outcome study. Plast Reconstr Surg 100:875, 1997.

Seitchik MW. Reduction mammaplasty: Criteria for insurance coverage. Plast Reconstr Surg 95: 1029, 1995.

Shakespeare V, Cole RP. Measuring patient-based outcomes in a plastic surgery service: Breast reduction surgical patients. Br J Plast Surg 50:242, 1997.

Short KK, Ringler SL, Bengtson BP, Hunstad JP, Henry E. Reduction mammaplasty: A safe and effective outpatient procedure. Aesthetic Plast Surg 20:513, 1996.

Singer R, Krant SM. Intravenous fluorescein for evaluating the dusky nipple-areola during reduction mammaplasty. Plast Reconstr Surg 67:534, 1981.

Skoog T. Plastic Surgery. Philadelphia: WB Saunders, 1974.

Skoog T. A technique of breast reduction, transposition of the nipple on a cutaneous vascular pedicle. Acta Chir Scand 126:453, 1963.

Slezak S, Dellon AL. Quantitation of sensibility in gigantomastia and alteration following reduction mammaplasty. Plast Reconstr Surg 91:1265, 1993.

Smith JW, Gillen FJ. Repairing errors of nipple-areolar placement following reduction mammoplasty. Aesthetic Plast Surg 4:179, 1980.

Smith ML, Evans GR, Gurlek A, Bouvet M, Singletary SE, Ames FC, Janjan N, McNeese MD. Reduction mammaplasty: Its role in breast conservation surgery for early-stage breast cancer. Ann Plast Surg 41:234, 1998.

Somerville M, Radford G, Hews N. Should breast reduction surgery be rationed? Interventions requested for psychological reasons should be studied. Br Med J 313:1479, 1996.

Spear SL, Burke JB, Forman D, Zuurbier RA, Berg CD. Experience with reduction mammaplasty following breast conservation surgery and radiation therapy. Plast Reconstr Surg 102:1913, 1998.

Steinberg RB, Stueber K. Sympathetically mediated pain after reduction mammoplasty: An unusual complication. J Clin Anesth 10:246, 1998.

Strömbeck JO. Reduction mammoplasty: Some observations and reflections. Aesthetic Plast Surg 7:249, 1983.

Strömbeck JO. Reduction mammaplasty. Surg Clin North Am 51:453, 1971.

Strömbeck JO. Macromastia in women and its surgical treatment. Acta Chir Scand [Suppl] 341:1, 1964.

Strömbeck JO. Mammaplasty: Report of a new technique based on the two pedicle procedure. Br J Plast Surg 13:79, 1960.

Stryker AK. Breast reduction under local anesthesia with intravenous sedation. Plast Reconstr Surg 99:256, 1997.

Tang CL, Brown MH, Levine R, Sloan M, Chong N, Holowaty E. Breast cancer found at the time of breast reduction. Plast Reconstr Surg 103:1682, 1999.

Tapia A, Blanch A, Salvador J, Prat J, Albert I. Evolution of the vertical scar in Lejour's mastopexy technique. Aesthetic Plast Surg 20:377, 1996.

Teimourian B. Suction Lipectomy and Body Sculpturing. St. Louis: CV Mosby, 1987.

Townsend PLG. Nipple sensation following breast reduction and free nipple transplantation. Br J Plast Surg 27:308, 1974.

Uribe Barreto A. Juvenile mammary hypertrophy. Plast Reconstr Surg 87:583, 1991.

van der Meulen JC. Superomedial pedicle technique of reduction mammaplasty. Plast Reconstr Surg 84:1005, 1989.

van der Torre PM, Butzelaar RM. Breast cancer and reduction mammoplasty: The role of routine pre-operative mammography. Eur J Surg Oncol 23:341, 1997.

Villafane O, Stanley P, Venkataramakrishnan V. Breast reduction and carcinoma-in-situ. Br J Plast Surg 49:499, 1996.

Wallace MS, Wallace AM, Lee J, Dobke MK. Pain after breast surgery: A survey of 282 women. Pain 66:195, 1996.

Wallace WH, Thompson WO, Smith RA, Barraza KR, Davidson SF, Thompson JT II. Reduction mammaplasty using the inferior pedicle technique. Ann Plast Surg 40:235, 1998.

Weiner DL, Aiache AE, Silver L, Tittiranonda T. A single dermal pedicle for nipple transposition in subcutaneous mastectomy, reduction mammaplasty, or mastopexy. Plast Reconstr Surg 51:115, 1973.

Weiner DL, Dolich BH, Miclay MI Jr. Reduction mammoplasty utilizing the superior pedicle technique: A six-year retrospective. Aesthetic Plast Surg 6:6, 1982.

Westreich M. Anthropomorphic breast measurement: Protocol and results in 50 women with aesthetically perfect breasts and clinical application. Plast Reconstr Surg 100:468, 1997.

White RR IV. Incidence of breast carcinoma in patients having reduction mammaplasty. Plast Reconstr Surg 102:1774, 1998.

Widdice L. The effects of breast reduction and breast augmentation surgery on lactation: An annotated bibliography. J Hum Lact 9:161, 1993.

Wilmink H, Spauwen PH, Hartman EH, Hendriks JC, Koeijers VF. Preoperative injection using a diluted anesthetic/adrenaline solution significantly reduces blood loss in reduction mammaplasty. Plast Reconstr Surg 102:373, 1998.

Wise RJ. A preliminary report on a method of planning the mammaplasty. Plast Reconstr Surg 17: 367, 1956.

Wise RJ. Treatment of breast hypertrophy. Clin Plast Surg 3:289, 1976.

Wuringer E. Refinement of the central pedicle breast reduction by application of the ligamentous suspension. Plast Reconstr Surg 103:1400, 1999.

Yamamoto Y, Sugihara T. Application of reduction mammaplasty in treatment of giant breast tumour. Br J Plast Surg 51:109, 1998.

Zukowski ML, Ash K, Klink B, Reid D, Messa A. Breast reduction under intravenous sedation: A review of 50 cases. Plast Reconstr Surg 97:952, 1996.

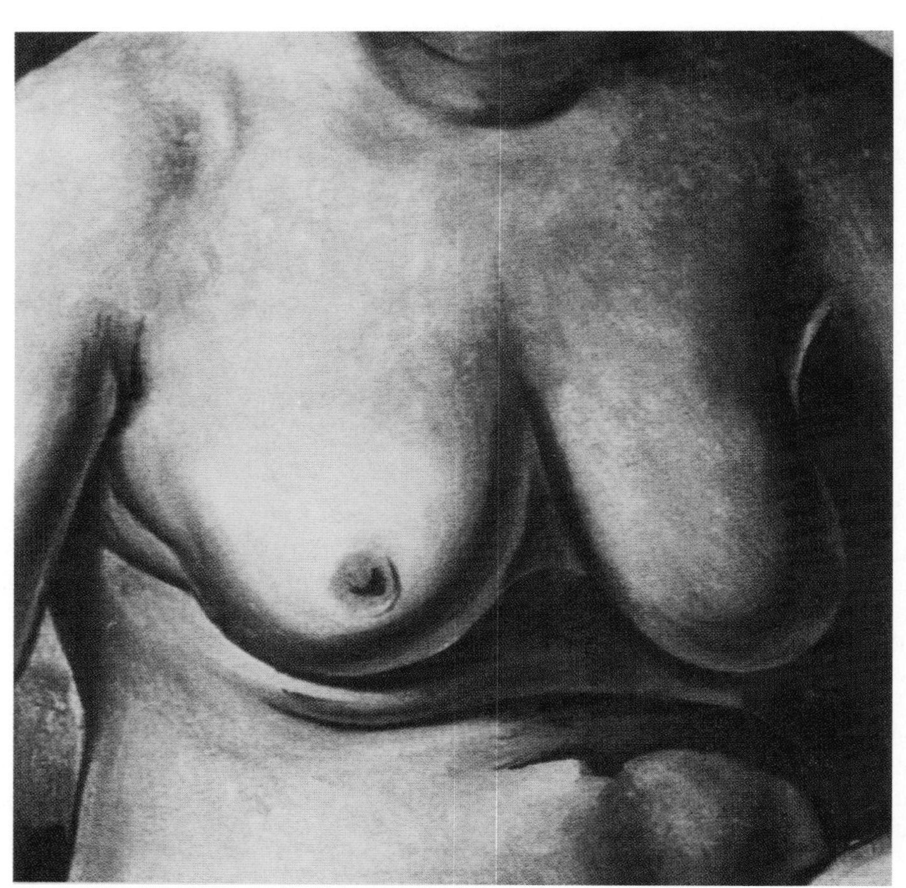

8 *Mastopexy*

Key Topics

Ptosis Classification

Options for Ptosis Correction

Augmentation

Periareolar Scar Technique

Circumareolar Scar Technique With Periareolar Purse-String Closure

Vertical Mastopexy

- Vertical and Short Horizontal Scar Technique
- Vertical and Horizontal Scar Technique (Inverted T)

Problems and Complications

Long-Term Results

Observations

Mastopexy is an operation of temporal value meant to restore a youthful, uplifted appearance to aging breasts that have sagged and lost their shape. The improvement effected is usually not a lasting one. Time and the forces of gravity can eventually undo some of the tightening and uplifting produced by the surgeon's scalpel. Furthermore, this operation exacts a price. The payment for more uplifted breasts is the scars that remain. Even though vertical and periareolar purse-string mastopexy techniques have reduced the length of these scars, they have not eliminated them. When the breasts once again begin to sag, as they usually do, obliterating the effects of early surgery, the scars will be a permanent reminder of the surgical intervention.

I consider mastopexy to be one of the more problematic aesthetic breast procedures: it is fraught with trade-offs and none of the solutions is permanent or trouble-free. Mastopexy alone can leave significant visible scars, particularly when there is major ptosis and minimal skin elasticity. Additionally, the patients are not always clear about the breast alteration they seek nor do they understand the limitations of the procedure itself, especially in addressing upper breast fullness. All they know is that their breasts hang lower than previously and are flattened above, producing an aged appearance. Frequently I find that they are discontented with more than the low breast position. The altered breast shape that has lost much of its upper breast fullness may be the real source of discontent. If I were only to tighten the lower portion of breasts and elevate the nipple-areolae, the result would not be pleasing to most patients because the upper breast flatness would be unaffected. They really want and need more volume in addition to the lift to fill out the breasts and give them an attractive appearance. I often suggest a breast implant to improve the shape of the ptotic breast, to give a more youthful upper pole breast fullness, and to add an element of permanence to the correction while minimizing the length of the mastopexy scars. This solution, however, introduces the possible concerns, objections, and complications associated with breast implants (see Chapters 5 and 6).

My primary concern, then, is whether this patient should have an operation to correct ptosis or whether her expectations are too vague or unattainable. Many women have confused expectations of this operation. They want lovely, uplifted breasts without visible scars or a breast implant. Frequently this type of result is just not possible, and it is important to explain this to the patient before a decision is made to perform mastopexy. Breast implants can provide upper fill and enlarge some breasts with minimal early ptosis. The risk-benefit ratio of this procedure must be carefully discussed with the patient. Several basic questions must be addressed: Does the breast lift justify the resulting scars? Would placement of an implant be the best strategy? Will insertion of an implant provide additional breast fullness and permit shortening of the scars sufficiently to justify the increased concern associated with these devices?

Patient Assessment and Selection

Women with breast ptosis have an excess of breast skin in comparison to the amount of underlying mobile breast tissue. The volume of breast parenchyma is highly variable. This skin is usually lax, has poor elasticity, and does not support and shape the breast. Furthermore, the skin is often thin with reduced strength and elasticity, and striae reflect actual tears and weakness in the deep dermis. The striae are covered with epidermis but retain little if any underlying dermis to contribute strength and elastic support. The glandular tissue is quite mobile over the chest wall because of attenuation of the fascial supports and Cooper's ligaments. When the woman with ptosis stands, her breasts assume a lower than normal position, and a varying percentage of breast tissue rotates or droops over a fixed inframammary crease. The nipple-areolae are also low relative to normal breast position, located at or below the inframammary crease. Upper pole flattening occurs because of the descent of the breast parenchyma and deficiency or atrophy of upper breast parenchyma.

Many women with ptosis recall when their breasts (either during puberty or pregnancy and lactation) were full, youthful, and uplifted. Others mention that their breasts were always poorly shaped and ptotic even when they were teenagers; they say their breasts never had an attractive, full, youthful appearance. Ptosis is disturbing—drooping breasts symbolize the aging process.

PATIENT PROFILES
Young Women With Large, Full Breasts and Thin Skin

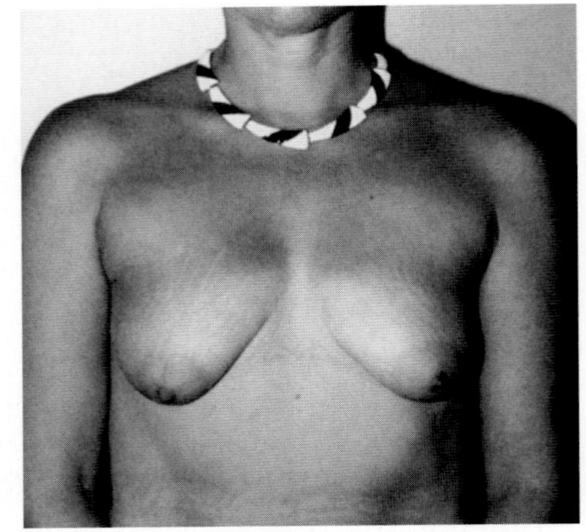

Ptosis develops relatively early in some women—during puberty or the late teens. They tend to have somewhat larger breasts, but unlike the teenage patients described previously, they also have thinner inelastic skin and increased breast mobility over the musculofascial layer of the chest wall. The inframammary fold may be higher or constricted. Frequently they have previously experienced episodes of weight gain and loss, and their breasts have not returned to the condition before the weight variation. Their breasts are characteristically soft and loosely attached to the fascia, with attenuation of the internal support and laxity of Cooper's ligaments. The nipple-areola complex is positioned low on the gland. Sometimes the inframammary crease is constricted and a tubular breast deformity is evident. (For more detailed information on this problem, see Chapter 9.)

Women With Ptosis Associated With Obesity, Pregnancy, or Lactation

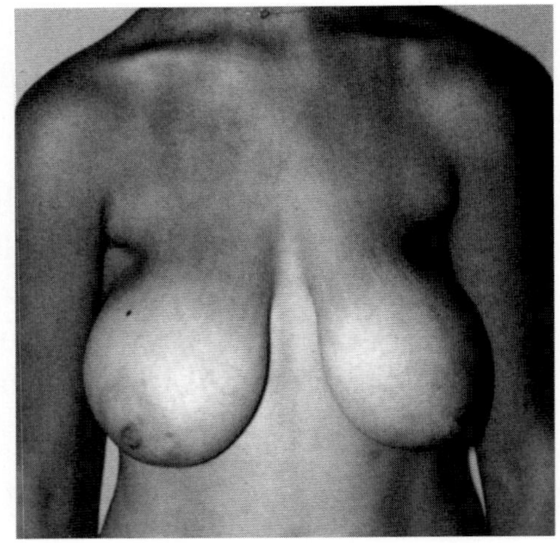

Most obese women have a large percentage of fatty tissue within their breasts. Their breasts, by their very weight, are stretched and heavy and actually rotate over the inframammary crease. Weight loss with decreased breast volume can result in additional ptosis, especially when the skin does not contract to its original volume and the internal breast support does not retighten—the larger the breasts, the more likely this will occur.

Breast ptosis often develops after pregnancy and lactation. After the skin has been stretched, tears occur in the thinned dermis and striae develop. Breasts with striae are less likely to tighten and firm up to their former shape after lactation. The ptosis seems to increase with every pregnancy and is not entirely related to the increase in breast size or the duration of lactation. After lactation the breasts can develop involutional hypoplasia, and in the presence of the more inelastic skin, ptosis or pseudoptosis develops.

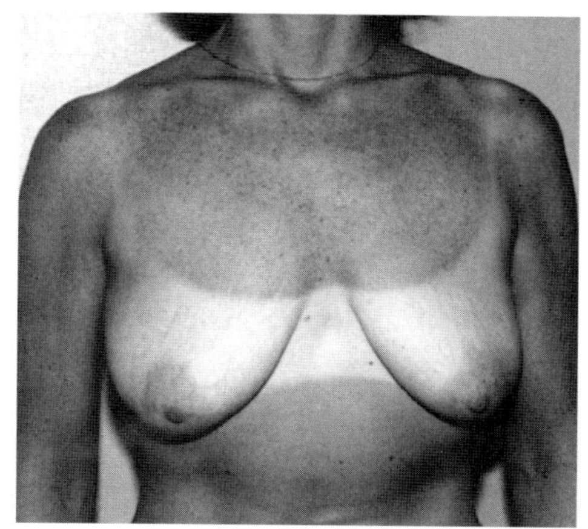

Women After Menopause

These women usually have ptosis secondary to involution after pregnancy and lactation; this condition is further aggravated by the involution and loss of skin elasticity that follows menopause. Because the blood flow to the breast skin and breast parenchyma is diminished after menopause, they often have thin, inelastic skin that is poorly vascularized. ***When the patient is thin and the breast parenchyma is mobile underneath the skin, skin flaps should be elevated carefully so as not to damage the subdermal plexus.***

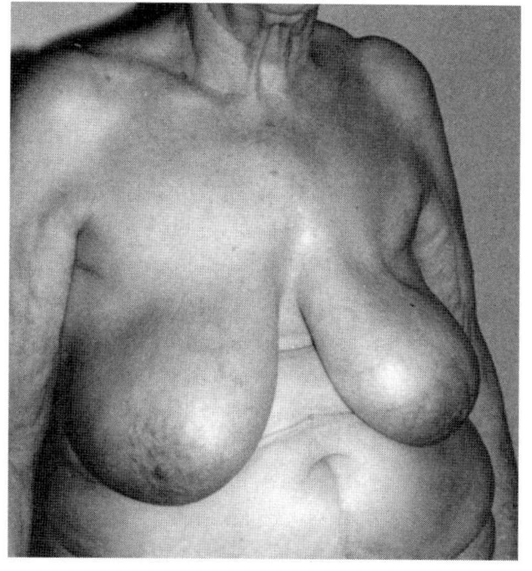

These women's scars usually heal without hypertrophy. Since women in this age group are at higher risk for breast cancer, preoperative mammography and evaluation of removed glandular tissue are recommended. Internal flaps of breast parenchyma can become devascularized and develop fat necrosis or calcifications that will later be seen on mammograms. These changes can mimic breast cancer and confuse future breast surveillance.

Concerns of Patient and Surgeon

BREAST POSITION AND CONTOUR

Most patients are concerned about how their breasts will look, how they will be shaped and contoured, how big they will be, and where the scars will be located. ***They usually want their breasts uplifted, with some fullness centrally and in the upper pole.*** They want to avoid "sagging" of the breast below the inframammary crease and would prefer a correction that would not require them to wear a brassiere to give this elevated appearance. They also want the shortest, least obvious scars possible.

BREAST SIZE

Most patients who request a mastopexy do not want their breasts to look "smaller" after their breast lift. Many actually prefer an enlargement, especially one that creates fullness of the upper pole. Simply tightening the lax skin can make their breasts appear even smaller. Before a mastopexy, the loose ptotic breast is observed to flow and project outward when the patient looks down. This gives the appearance of breast projection. ***During the preoperative evaluation it is important to tighten the breast skin while the patient is looking down as well as in a mirror to preview how she will look after mastopexy without using an implant.*** During this preoperative visualization the breast parenchyma should not be pushed up because mastopexy does not deliver a permanent lift that significantly fills a flattened upper breast region. The tightened breast does not project as much as the untightened breast, and it will not look as big to the patient when she views it from above. The woman can usually tell whether she likes this look; a frequent patient reaction is that it now "looks smaller" and there is still not enough upper breast fill. In that case an implant is discussed to provide increased projection and upper pole fullness. ***It is explained that tightening of the lower pole can lift the breast parenchyma above the inframammary fold but often will not be sufficient to permanently restore the fullness in the upper pole. A breast implant is usually necessary to achieve this full upper look.***

SCARS

It is relatively easy to lift the breasts to a new position before the operation; manual repositioning does not produce scars. Mastopexy, however, is not so kind. Many women are alarmed when the surgeon describes the scars that will be necessary to produce a more youthful breast appearance. Although the vertical mastopexy and periareolar purse-string mastopexy reduce the length of the scars, they are still located centrally and are quite visible. The patient must determine if the improved shape and position justify the scars. If she decides to proceed, she wants the scars to be minimal, inconspicuous, and thin.

IMPLANTS

Many women do not like the idea of breast implants and think that they only need their breasts to be tightened and raised. Implants alone, however, can often fill the lax skin, producing a better upper breast contour while reducing the scar length to that required for breast augmentation. An implant may sometimes provide a satisfactory solution in itself without incurring mastopexy incisions. The mastopexy can then be postponed for a few years. When an augmentation is to be combined with the mastopexy, the potential problems associated with implants must be fully explained to the woman.

PERMANENCE

Mastopexy alone is usually not a permanent procedure. The conditions that caused the initial drooping are often unabated and continue to progress. Inelastic skin and breast parenchyma with weak fascial attachments indicate that simple skin tightening will not create a lasting correction. The patient requesting this procedure must understand that mastopexy correction is a long-term, ongoing problem, and after appropriate counseling, she can decide the timing for the longer incisions. Patients are most pleased when they have a marked degree of breast ptosis and a good correction is obtained with mastopexy. Again, implants may be inserted for correction of upper breast flattening and more permanent fullness. ***Resection of the lower ptotic breast parenchyma can also reduce the lower breast parenchyma subject to ptosis and add an element of permanence to the result.***

SYMMETRY

The patient should be informed during the preoperative discussion that her breasts will not be perfectly symmetric after a mastopexy, especially when there is asymmetry preoperatively. ***Breast asymmetry with ptosis is best corrected at the first procedure by retaining similar amounts of breast parenchyma so that the breasts will age and descend symmetrically over the long term.*** To achieve this goal an asymmetric breast parenchymal excision may be required at the time of the initial procedure (see Chapter 9).

ONCOLOGIC CONSIDERATIONS

Concerns about cancer are similar to those expressed about augmentation and reduction (see Chapters 6, 7, and 10).

Planning

Key anatomic reference points must be considered when evaluating the ptotic breast and planning a mastopexy. ***The first consideration is the degree of ptosis and the nipple-areolar position. Other areas for evaluation include breast volume and breast parenchymal distribution, the inframammary crease and possible constrictions, the fascial attachments, skin and tissue quality, the lateral folds, and sites for skin excision and incision placement.***

CLASSIFICATION OF PTOSIS

Regnault's classification defines the different degrees of breast ptosis and facilitates evaluating the problem and planning therapy.

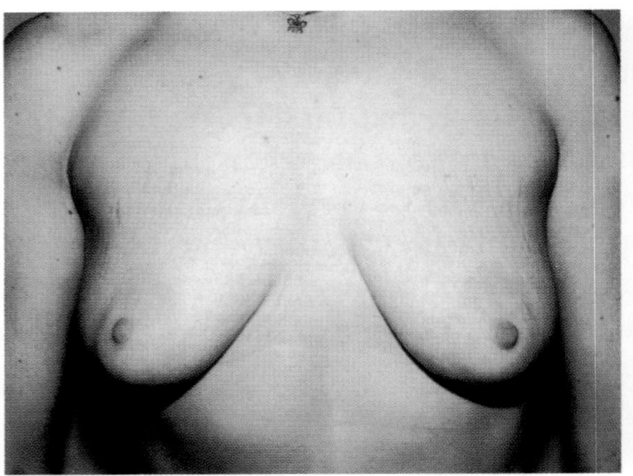
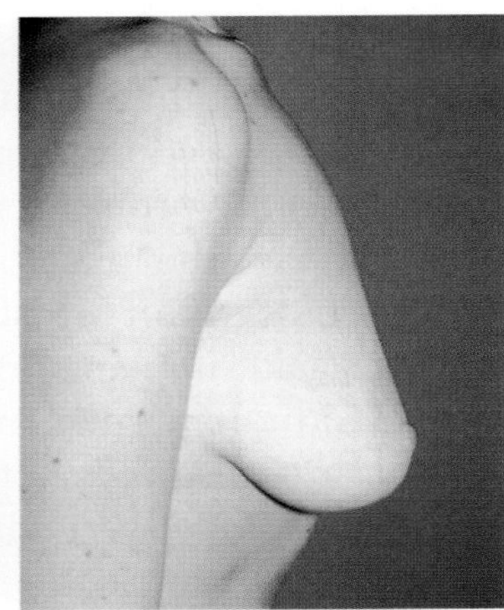

Minor ptosis
Nipple at level of inframammary fold

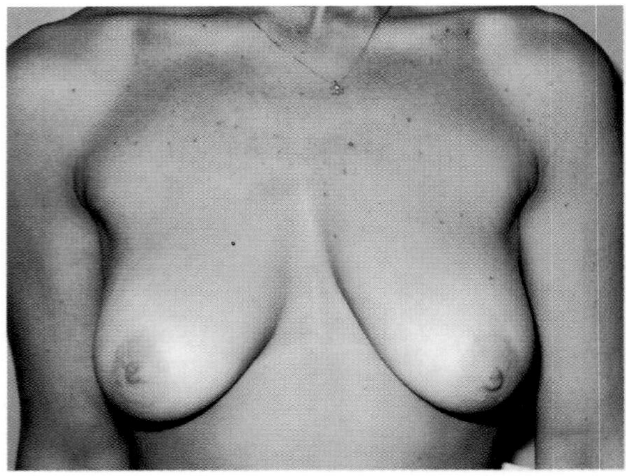
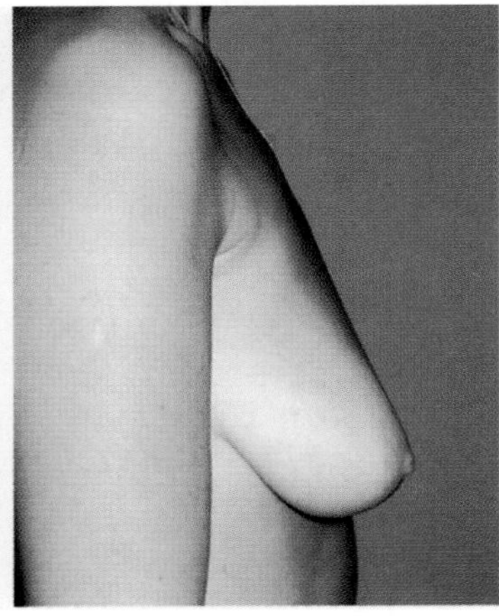

Moderate ptosis
Nipple below inframammary fold, but above lower breast contour

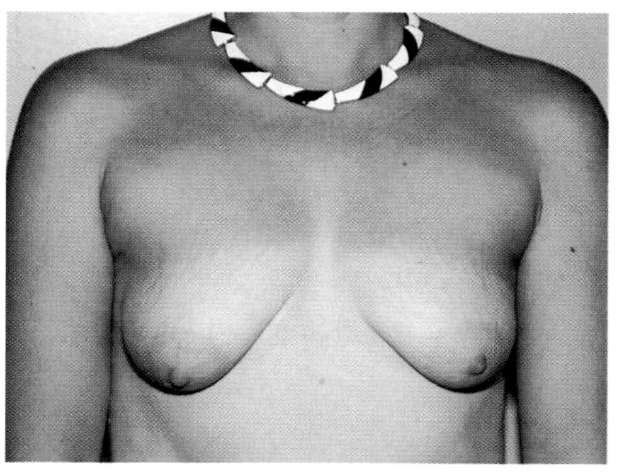
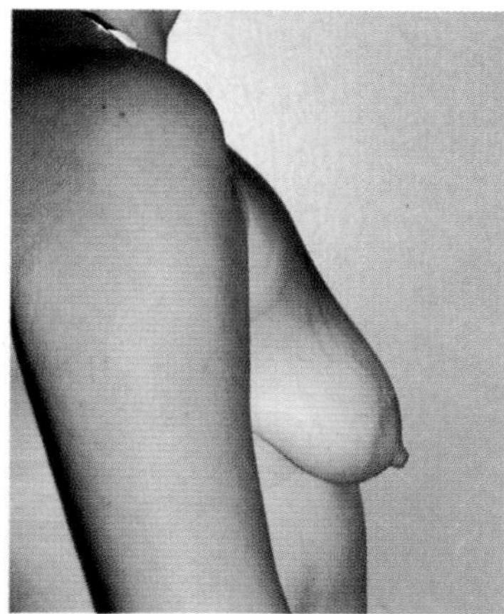

Major ptosis
Nipple at lower breast contour; breast below inframammary fold

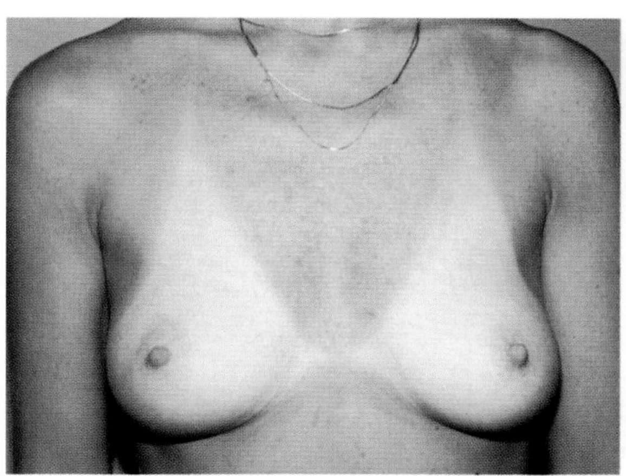
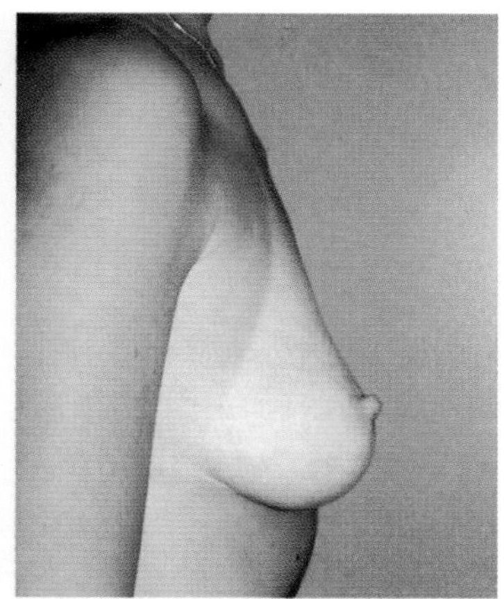

Glandular ptosis
Nipple above fold; breast descended below fold

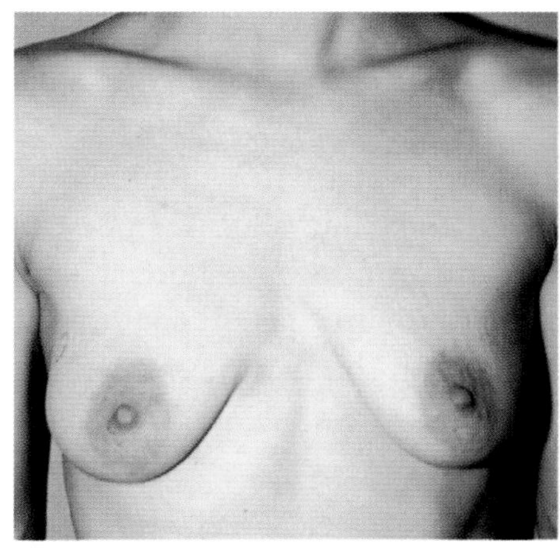
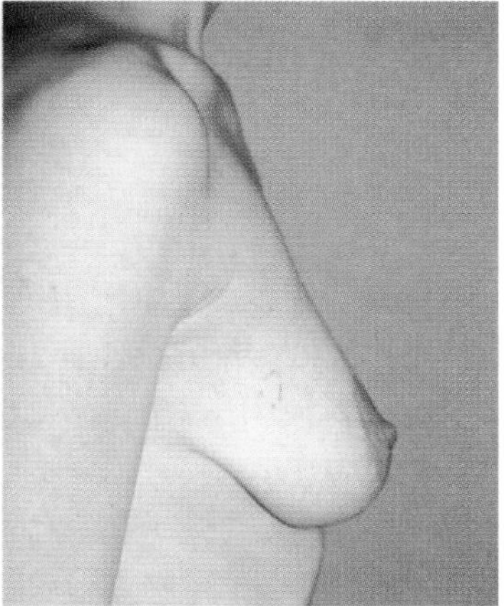

Pseudoptosis
Nipple higher above fold; gland hypoplastic with some breast descended below fold

BREAST VOLUME

When planning a mastopexy I always consider reducing or elevating the portion of the breast parenchyma that falls below the inframammary crease when the patient is upright, particularly in women with very large breasts. I explain to these patients that this lower breast tissue is likely to cause recurrence of ptosis, and a reduction of breast volume will lessen the effects of gravity and produce a more long-lasting result.

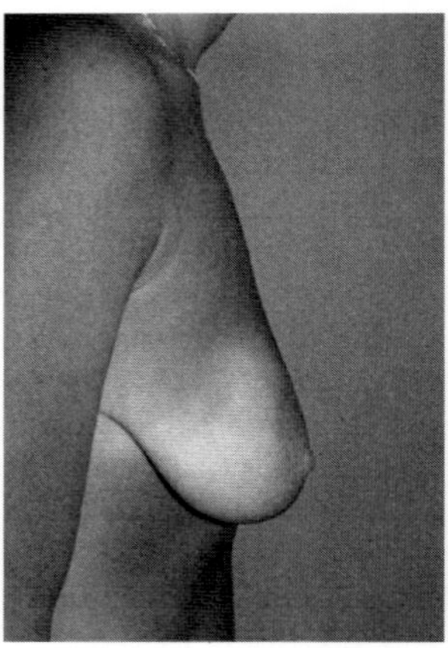
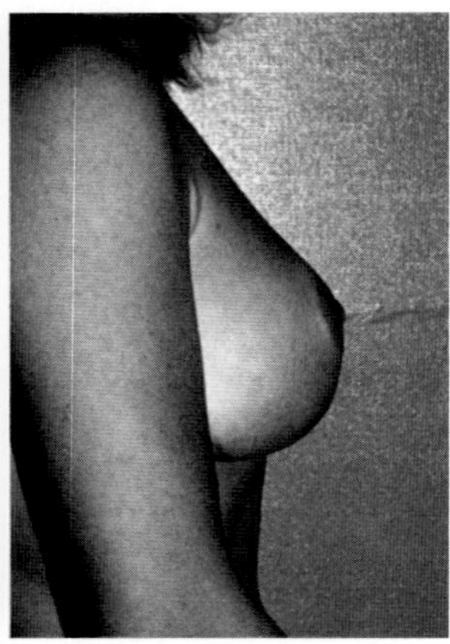

For smaller breasted women and those with upper pole flatness who indicate that they want more fullness in the upper breast, augmentation mammaplasty is often the best option. Using this approach I can fill out the skin envelope and elevate the nipple, thereby permitting shorter vertical mastopexy incisions with horizontal extensions. The additional volume obtained by augmentation does not have the same tendency to sag as the natural breast tissue if it is held in the dissected pocket. ***I use subpectoral saline implants for these operations.*** Alternatively, the use of the lower central tissue from a vertical mastopexy, similar to that resected in a vertical breast reduction, can also produce more projection and upper fullness by rotating it upward and suturing it behind the upper breast parenchyma.

Some surgeons have advocated transposition of the lower breast to the upper breast via flaps to add fill for the supra-areolar region. I personally have had little lasting success with these procedures and have had several patients in whom firmness developed from fat necrosis in these flaps, creating oncologic concerns and difficulty in distinguishing the firmness from breast cancer without a biopsy.

The use of internal sutures to tack breast tissues up higher is also somewhat suspect because of the increased breast mobility and the inability of sutures to counteract the forces of gravity over time. I prefer to use a breast implant to give upper pole fullness. It is predictable and its volume can be controlled.

INFRAMAMMARY CREASE

The position, length, and definition of the inframammary crease are evaluated when planning a ptosis correction. When the inframammary crease is positioned normally and extends the full width of the lower breast area, the operative plan includes its position and extent as the future inframammary crease after the ptosis correction.

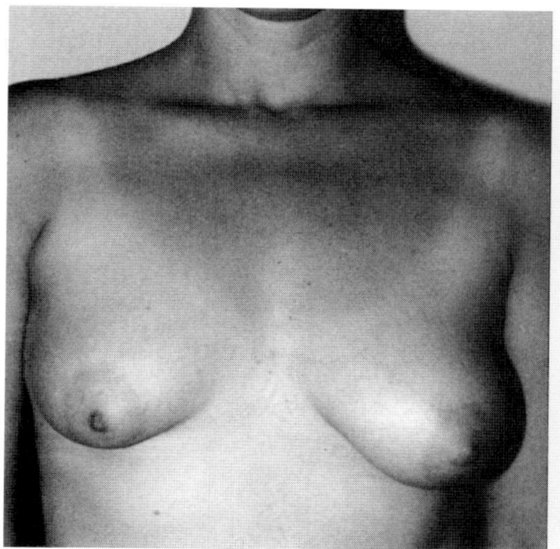

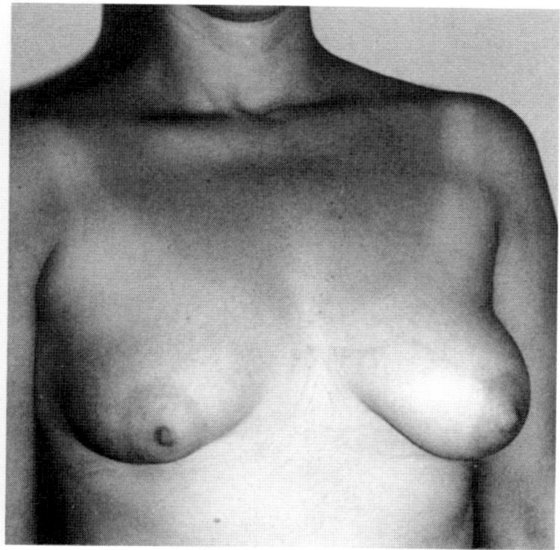

This patient with breast ptosis has asymmetric breasts. One breast has a normal inframammary crease, whereas the other is constricted and has a lower pole deficiency and an elevated inframammary crease.

When the breast is constricted, it is more likely that the upper breast parenchyma will rotate over the high, tight inframammary crease and deficient lower breast. In these situations the proper position of the inframammary crease is determined preoperatively and plans are made to reposition it during the mastopexy. ***When the inframammary crease is well defined, the dermis at the crease is usually attached to the underlying fascia. These attachments must be divided during mastopexy.*** Since there is no breast parenchyma below the inframammary crease and the upper breast parenchyma may be tight and constricted, some radial releases of the lower breast parenchyma may also be necessary to accommodate the proposed change in breast width with a breast implant. When mastopexy is to be combined with augmentation mammaplasty, a saline breast implant is used to provide and retain the new definition of the inframammary crease. Intraoperative expansion facilitates stretching of the lower pole region to accommodate a wider and lower pocket for the breast implant.

FASCIAL ATTACHMENTS

The firmness of the glandular attachments and the degree of mobility on the underlying deep fascia are also key to effective planning. When the breasts move easily, dissection in the retromammary area with subsequent upward positioning and suturing of the posterior layer of the superficial fascia to the deep fascia may provide more support for the breast gland by developing a fibrous adherence, thereby delaying recurrence.

SKIN AND TISSUE QUALITY

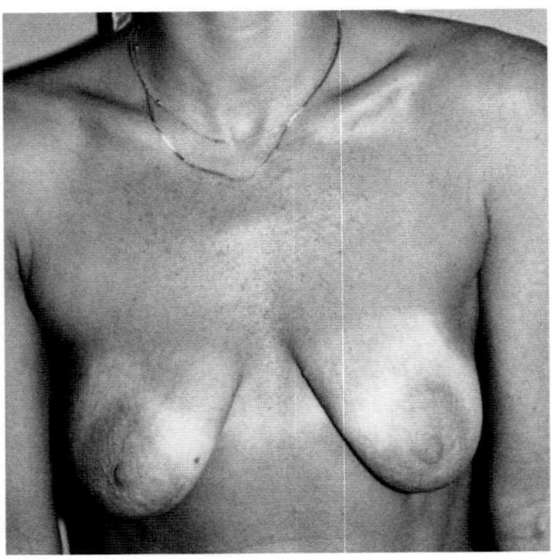

Skin tightening in patients with inelastic, striated skin provides minimal lasting breast support. Recurrence of ptosis is predictable. The skin below the areola, the point of maximum stress because the weight of the breast is concentrated here, stretches and the breast "bottoms out." An unnatural proportion of the breast is rotated below the inframammary crease and seems to sink below the nipple-areola, giving it an unnaturally elevated appearance. Attempts to create the illusion of ptosis correction with overelevation of the nipple will soon result in a nipple that is too high and the appearance of glandular ptosis. The real problem, however, is attributed to the stretched skin extending from the lower areola to the inframammary crease. This thin skin with reduced dermal components is also susceptible to slow healing, particularly when the patient is a cigarette smoker or microcirculation is otherwise compromised. Whenever possible, I try to avoid a T incision in these patients. Problems tend to occur at the point of the T when thin skin flaps have been elevated and the skin is closed under tension; vertical incisions are safer.

LATERAL FOLDS

If the woman has had significant weight loss, a fold of skin may be found extending laterally around to her back. The presence of such a fold must be identified preoperatively and a strategy for its correction incorporated into the operative plan. ***If not managed at the time of the mastopexy, any lateral skin and tissue excess will seem more obvious and disproportionate after the operation.*** A long secondary excision with a resulting scar will then be required to correct this problem. Liposuction can help reduce the lateral and subaxillary fullness (see Chapter 7).

SKIN REMOVAL AND INCISION PLACEMENT

Similar to excisions for reduction mammaplasty, skin removal for mastopexy is planned to permit circumareolar, vertical, and when necessary horizontal excisions and remolding of the breast to a more natural, uplifted conical shape. This skin removal should also allow repositioning of the nipple-areola and, if ptosis recurs, additional corrections through the initial incisions. ***The incisions and skin excisions are planned on a continuum from periareolar to circumareolar to vertical scars and then to horizontal scars. With this approach, additional breast tissue can be excised later.*** I sometimes remove only skin vertically but resect some horizontal breast parenchyma at the inframammary crease similar to the vertical mammaplasty reduction technique (see Chapter 7).

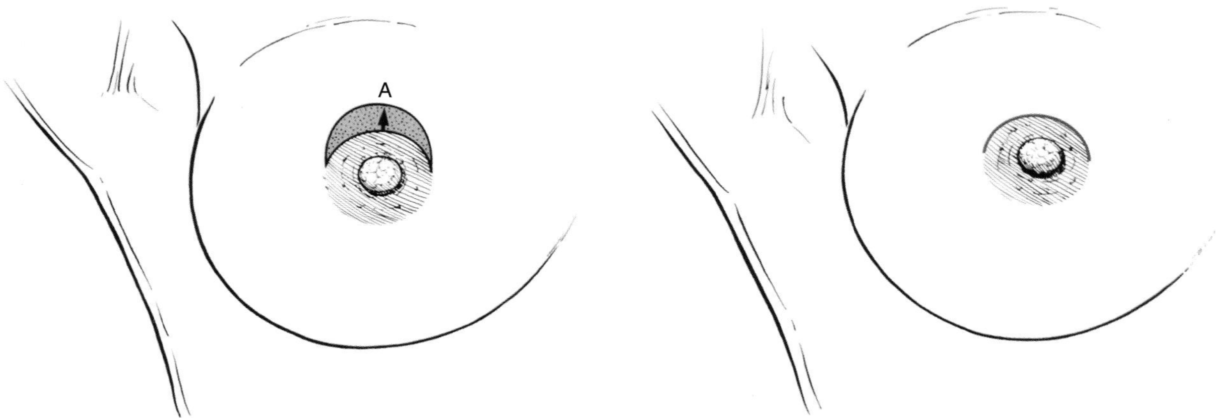

When the nipple-areola is low and needs a small degree of elevation of 1 to 2 cm, an upper periareolar crescentric ellipse can be excised to elevate it. An augmentation mammaplasty is usually done through this incision; the breast implant volume helps to produce an elevated nipple-areola appearance.

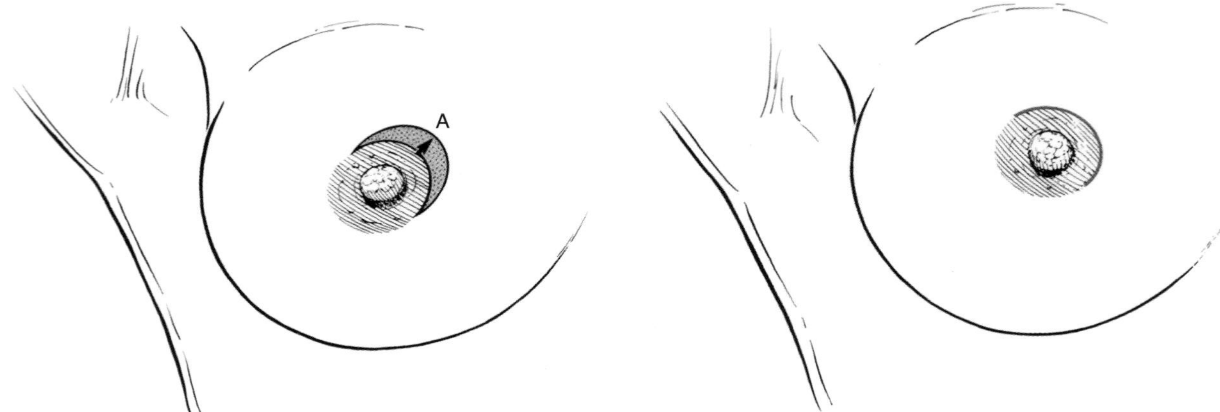

This upper periareolar ellipse can be rotated when specific positioning of the nipple-areola is necessary to move it to a more aesthetic position on the breast.

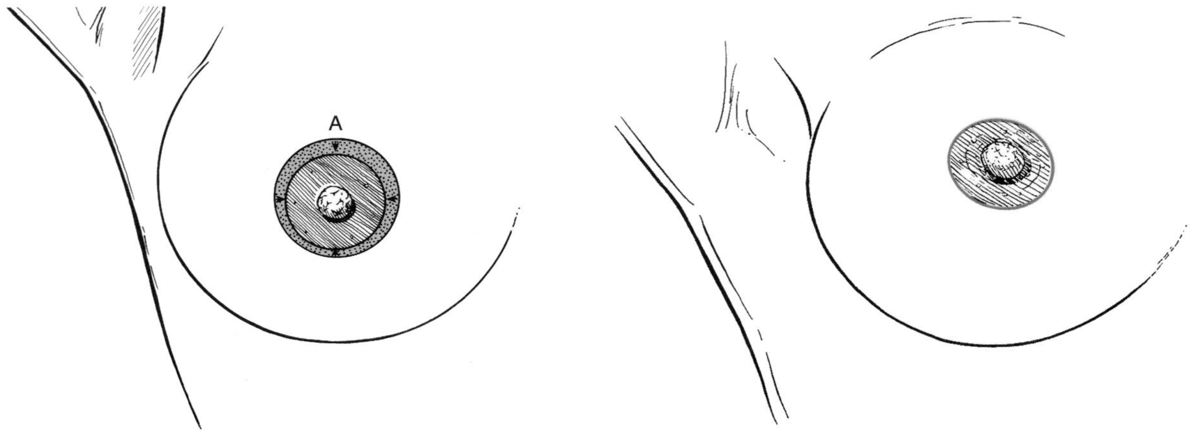

A circumareolar skin excision with periareolar purse-string closure tightens the skin minimally without elevating the areola. It is effective for patients with tubular breasts with protuberant areolae and for patients with very large areolae and pseudoptosis who are to have augmentation mammaplasty. Removal of breast skin leaves only a central circular scar. The scar, however, tends to widen and the nipple position is minimally elevated. It can also result in unnatural central breast flatness and loss of attractive central projection; however, an implant can minimize this flatness. ***A permanent circular suture in the skin periphery, the periareolar purse-string approach, can reduce final skin tension and produce a finer scar; this approach extends the application of this technique to some patients with moderate ptosis. This strategy is helpful in avoiding a tight point beneath the areolar closure of a vertical mastopexy.***

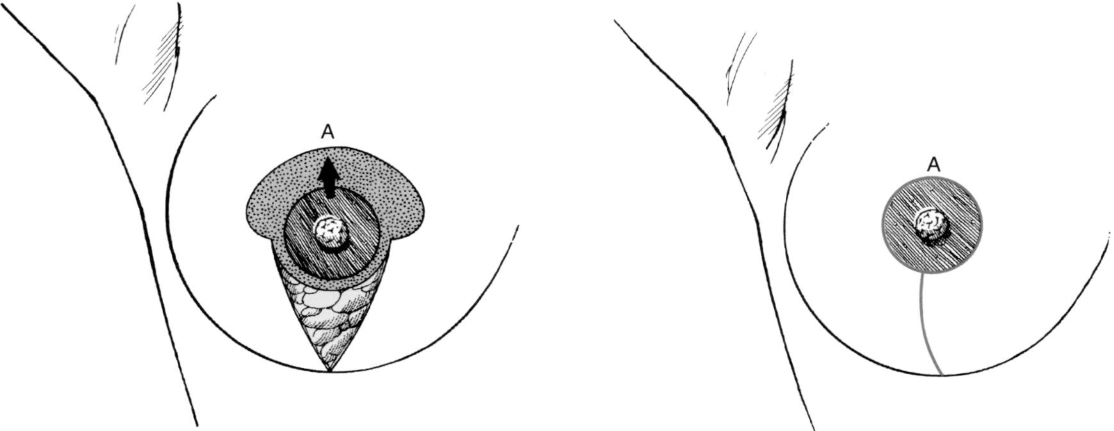

In patients with glandular and minor ptosis the circumareolar excision with a short vertical ellipse tightens the skin and elevates the nipple-areola. Care must be taken to avoid too much tightness below the areola.

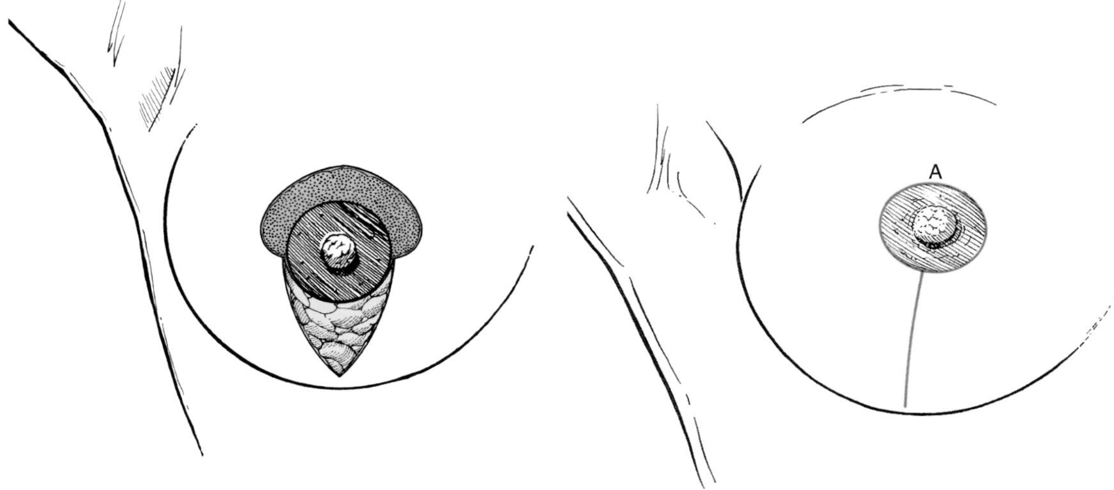

For minor ptosis the circumareolar excision with a vertical ellipse tightens the skin and lifts the nipple without the necessity for an inframammary incision. This incision can be shortened because the vertical component is used primarily to close the defect from the transposed nipple-areola. It also tends to shorten in the postoperative period with scar contraction.

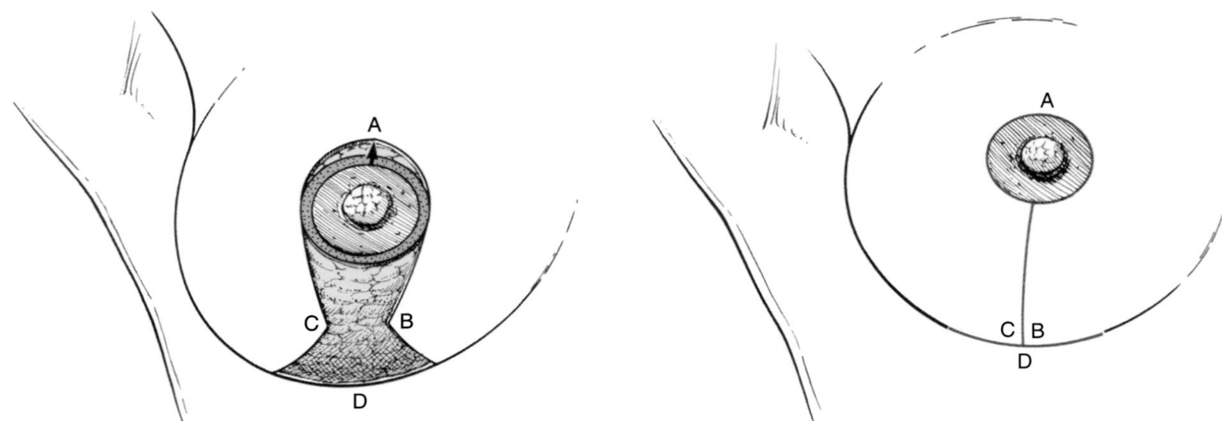

For moderate ptosis the circumareolar excision with a vertical and occasionally a short horizontal ellipse produces a short inframammary scar and tightens the breast while shortening the inframammary distance. This approach is used only when there is excess skin after vertical mammaplasty.

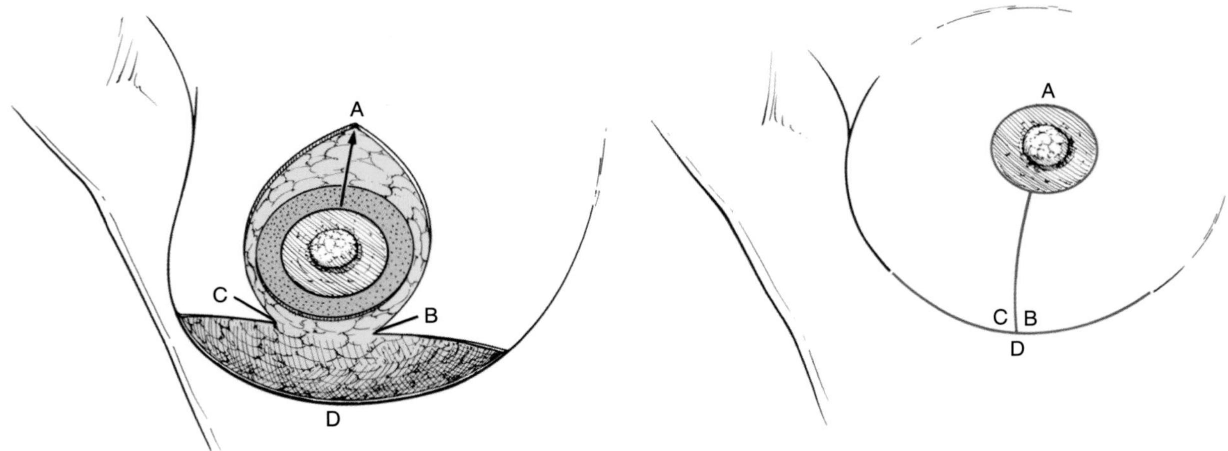

For patients with major ptosis who need maximal breast elevation a vertical and horizontal excision provides effective breast elevation even though this approach produces a longer inframammary scar than procedures for patients with less advanced ptosis. For these patients it is more often necessary to have longer inverted T pattern scars. In the past few years I have primarily used the vertical approach, even for most cases of major ptosis, and try to avoid the inverted T scars in most women.

Surgical Approach: Matching the Technique to the Problem

Degrees of ptosis vary with each patient. Effective surgical treatment draws from a spectrum of techniques focused primarily on altering the nipple-areolar position and size, removing excess breast skin, and changing breast volume and contour. Versatility is essential. Sometimes procedures are combined to produce more attractive breasts for a particular patient. For instance, breast augmentation or resection and reduction of breast parenchyma may be combined with mastopexy. Clinical judgment guides this decision-making process in selecting the techniques that most effectively solve each patient's problem, providing optimal ptosis correction in a specific case.

Options for ptosis correction

- Augmentation only or with a mastopexy technique
- Periareolar scar technique
- Circumareolar scar technique with periareolar purse-string closure
- Vertical mastopexy
  - Vertical and short horizontal scar technique
  - Vertical and horizontal scar technique (inverted T)

When the upper breast is flattened, augmentation mammaplasty is usually the technique of choice, particularly if the patient's breasts are also hypoplastic and involuted. These patients often have pseudoptosis with breast parenchyma below the inframammary crease. Implants can take up some of the loose skin and allow shorter incisions than those required for a standard mastopexy; often a short inframammary fold incision using an endoscopic technique and a breast implant can reduce the mastopexy incision to 5 cm. Patients appropriate for this procedure should not require nipple-areolar elevation because their nipple-areolae are already positioned at or above the inframammary crease. Although there is usually some apparent nipple-areolar elevation, I always explain that the patient should not expect a major ptosis correction (i.e., nipple elevation) with this technique; rather she should expect larger, fuller breasts with more upper breast fullness.

MASTOPEXY WORKSHEET

PATIENT DATA
Name: ______
Age: ______ Height: ______ Weight: ______
Married: ______ Single: ______
Nulliparous: ______ Pregnancies: ______
Children: ______ Nursing: ______

ONCOLOGIC INFORMATION
Family history of breast CA: ______
Prev. breast cancer: ______
Prev. breast surg.: ______
Mastodynia: ______
Fibrocystic chg.: ______
Breast disease: ______
Mammogram: ______
Masses: R ______ L ______
Biopsies: R ______ L ______

MEDICAL INFORMATION
Systemic disease: ______
Diabetes: ______
Bleeding problems: ______
Allergies: ______
Medications: ______
Smoking (pk-yr): ______
Alcohol/wk: ______
Other: ______

PHYSICAL EXAMINATION
Chest wall:
Pectus defor.: ______ Scoliosis: ______
Asymmetries: R ______ L ______
Constriction: R ______ L ______
Tubular: R ______ L ______
Breast scars: ______
Neurologic exam.:
Normal: ______ Problem: ______

INFORMED CONSENT
Verbal explan.: ______ Signed form: ______
Bleed sheet: ______ Preop. mamm.: ______
FDA info.: ______ Mfg. info.: ______

EXPECTATIONS ______

SPECIFIC DESIRES
To achieve: ______
To avoid: ______

SYMPTOMS ______

MEASUREMENTS AND PLAN
Chest circum.: ______
Bra size: ______
Breast width:
R ____ cm L ____ cm
N → infr. cr.:
R ____ cm L ____ cm
SN → N:
R ____ cm L ____ cm
Vol.: R ______
L ______

Ptosis: Pseudo: ____ Mild: ____ Mod.: ____ Major: ____
Striae: R ______ L ______
Upper breast fullness: ______
Areolar diameter: R ______ L ______

PLANNED CHANGE TECHNIQUE
Right:
Aug. ____ Per. ____ Circ. ____ V ____ V&H+ ____
Left:
Aug. ____ Per. ____ Circ. ____ V ____ V&H+ ____
Implant type: Vol. R ______ L ______
Skin removal: ______
Incisions: ______
Lateral tissue to remove: ______
Inferior tissue to remove: ______
Abdominal excess: ______
In. crease change: R ______ L ______

IMPRESSIONS AND NOTES ______

PLAN ______

SURGICAL OPTIONS FOR PTOSIS CORRECTION

AUGMENTATION ONLY

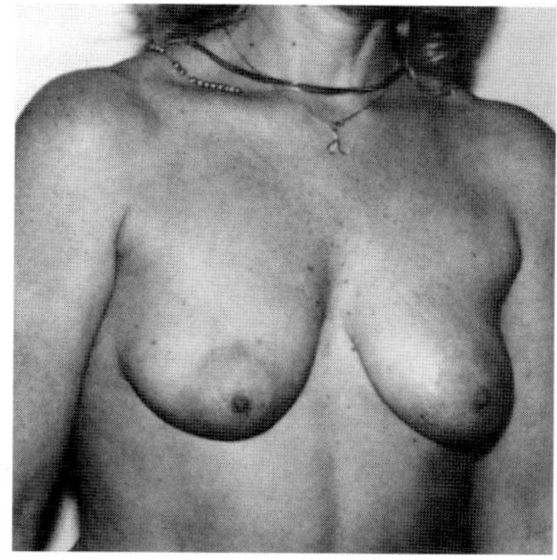

Type: Glandular, pseudoptosis, minor ptosis
Skin quality: Fair to good
Nipple elevation: 0-1 cm
Breast resection: 0

PERIAREOLAR SCAR TECHNIQUE WITH IMPLANT

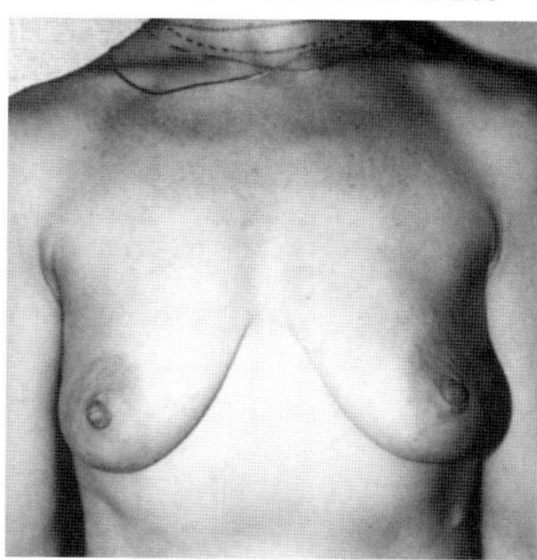

Type: Glandular or tubular
Skin quality: Elastic
Nipple elevation: 0-1 cm
Breast resection: 0
Areola: Large

CIRCUMAREOLAR SCAR TECHNIQUE WITH PERIAREOLAR PURSE-STRING CLOSURE

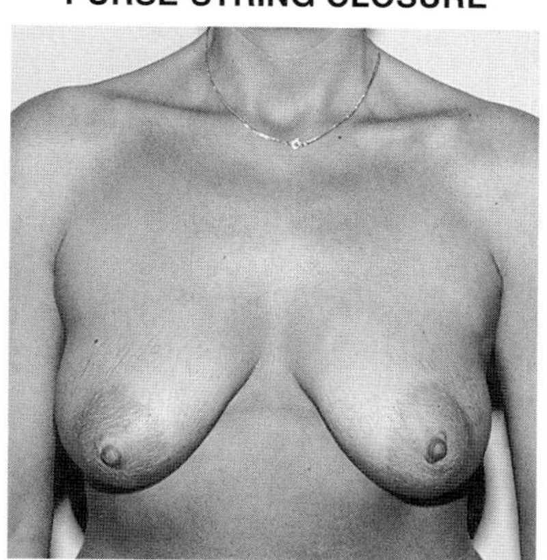

Type: Minimal
Skin quality: Fair
Nipple elevation: 2-4 cm
Breast resection: 0
Areola: Reduce

VERTICAL SCAR TECHNIQUE WITH IMPLANT

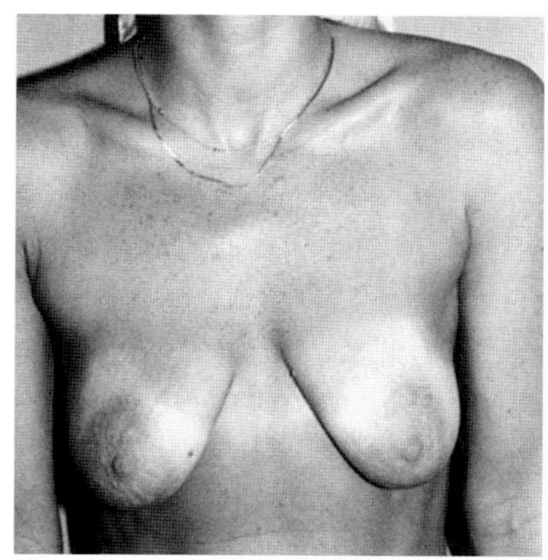

Type: Moderate
Skin quality: Poor to fair
Nipple elevation: 5-7 cm
Breast resection: 0-200 gm

VERTICAL SCAR TECHNIQUE WITH IMPLANT

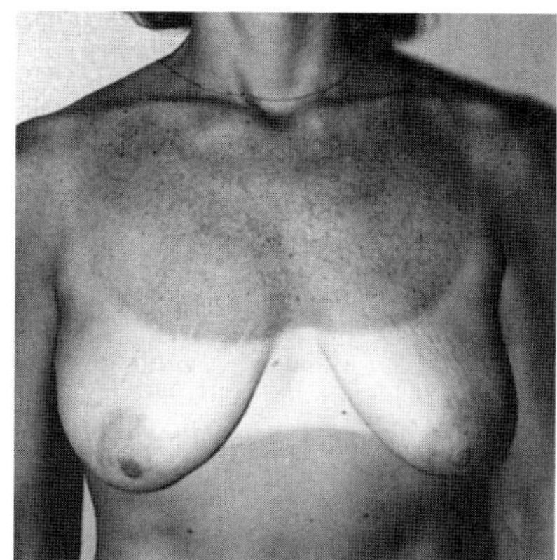

Type: Minimal to moderate
Skin quality: Fair
Nipple elevation: 3-5 cm
Breast resection: 0-100 gm

VERTICAL AND HORIZONTAL SCAR TECHNIQUE (INVERTED T)

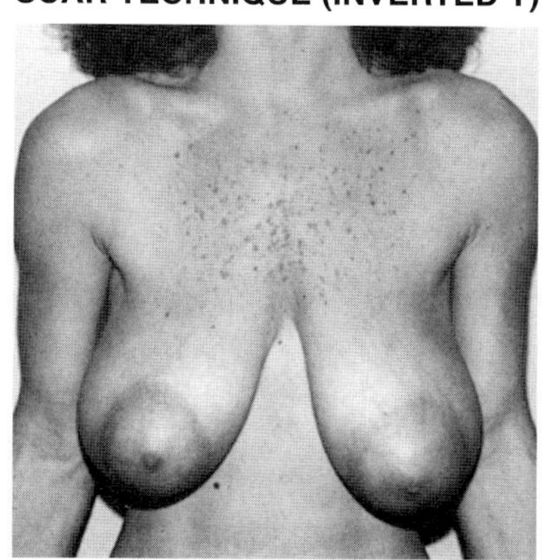

Type: Moderate to major
Skin quality: Poor
Nipple elevation: 7+ cm
Breast resection: 0-300 gm

For women with tubular breasts or with minor ptosis and areolae larger than 4 cm in diameter, the circumareolar excision with a periareolar purse-string closure removes a portion of the areolar skin, a peripheral "doughnut," to tighten the breast and reduce the areolar diameter. In patients with upper breast flatness, subpectoral breast augmentation is sometimes combined with this procedure to avoid central breast flattening.

Candidates for the vertical skin ellipse with nipple-areolar elevation should have a preoperative nipple to inframammary crease distance no greater than 10 to 12 cm. When the distance exceeds this amount, the newly positioned nipple may accentuate the appearance of glandular ptosis.

Patients with minor and moderate degrees of ptosis but not the severe sagging observed in patients with major ptosis are appropriate candidates for the vertical and short horizontal ellipse. In these women the lower areola to inframammary crease distance is greater than 7 to 8 cm. This procedure can reduce the distance to 6 to 7 cm. The resulting reduced requirements for skin excision allow this lower horizontal ellipse to extend only 3 to 4 cm on either side of the inframammary line at the midnipple line.

For patients with moderate or major ptosis the vertical and horizontal scar allows removal of excess skin and shortening and proper positioning of the final areola to inframammary crease distance. The resulting inframammary scars are kept as short as possible and are not visible from above. They are placed in the inframammary crease and do not extend beyond the natural breast lines and shadows. I use the vertical mammaplasty technique without the horizontal extension for most of these patients.

AUGMENTATION MAMMAPLASTY

Augmentation is reserved for pseudoptosis and minor ptosis, and in selected patients a mastopexy can often be avoided. Further skin excision may be necessary at a later date. The patient should understand that an implant restores some upper pole fullness and gives the appearance of tighter skin, but it does not significantly elevate the nipple-areola. (There is often an apparent small elevation as the skin is redraped over the implant.) If she desires a more elevated nipple-areola, then circumareolar incisions may be necessary. If the nipple-areola is below the inframammary crease, a breast implant positioned above the fold may actually accentuate the deformity.

Markings and Technique

The technique for augmentation is described in Chapter 6. I usually prefer inframammary or periareolar incisions because they provide greater flexibility and can be used if future excisions are needed to tighten the patient's breasts. The periareolar incision can be used with a small horizontal extension to modify nipple-areolar shape or position. When the augmentation is intended to correct breast ptosis, the breast implant is usually positioned in the subpectoral position in the upper portion of the breast but in a subglandular position in the lower part of the breast. This positioning permits the breast implant to better define the inframammary crease and to descend along with the breast parenchyma postoperatively. A tight lower submusculofascial pocket can restrict the proper descent of the breast implant and the breast parenchyma may rotate over it, thus creating a "double-bubble" deformity.

Results

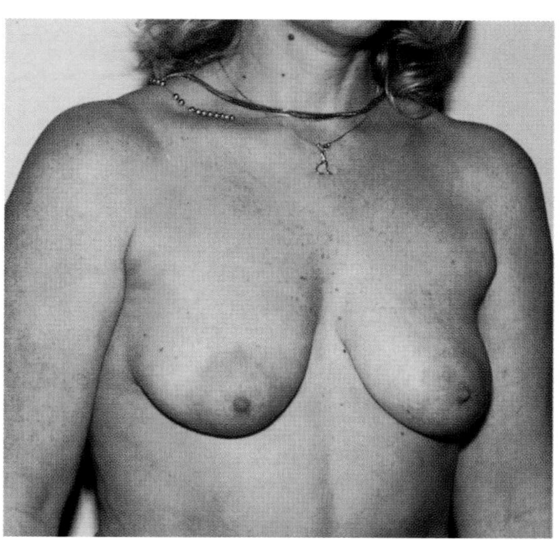

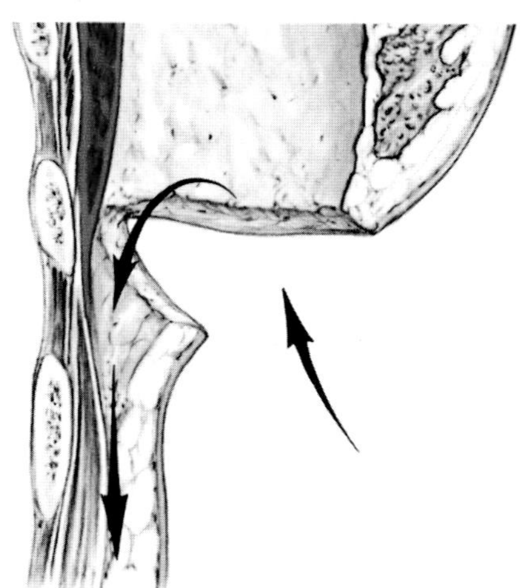

This 35-year-old woman developed some breast involution with subsequent ptosis after each of her two pregnancies. Although her nipples were low, her primary complaint was the upper pole flattening. Wanting to avoid any long or periareolar incisions at this time, she requested a breast lift and augmentation with minimal scars. Physical examination revealed wide, full breasts with minor ptosis, wide areolae, and significant upper pole flattening. The distance from the lower areola to the inframammary crease was 8 cm.

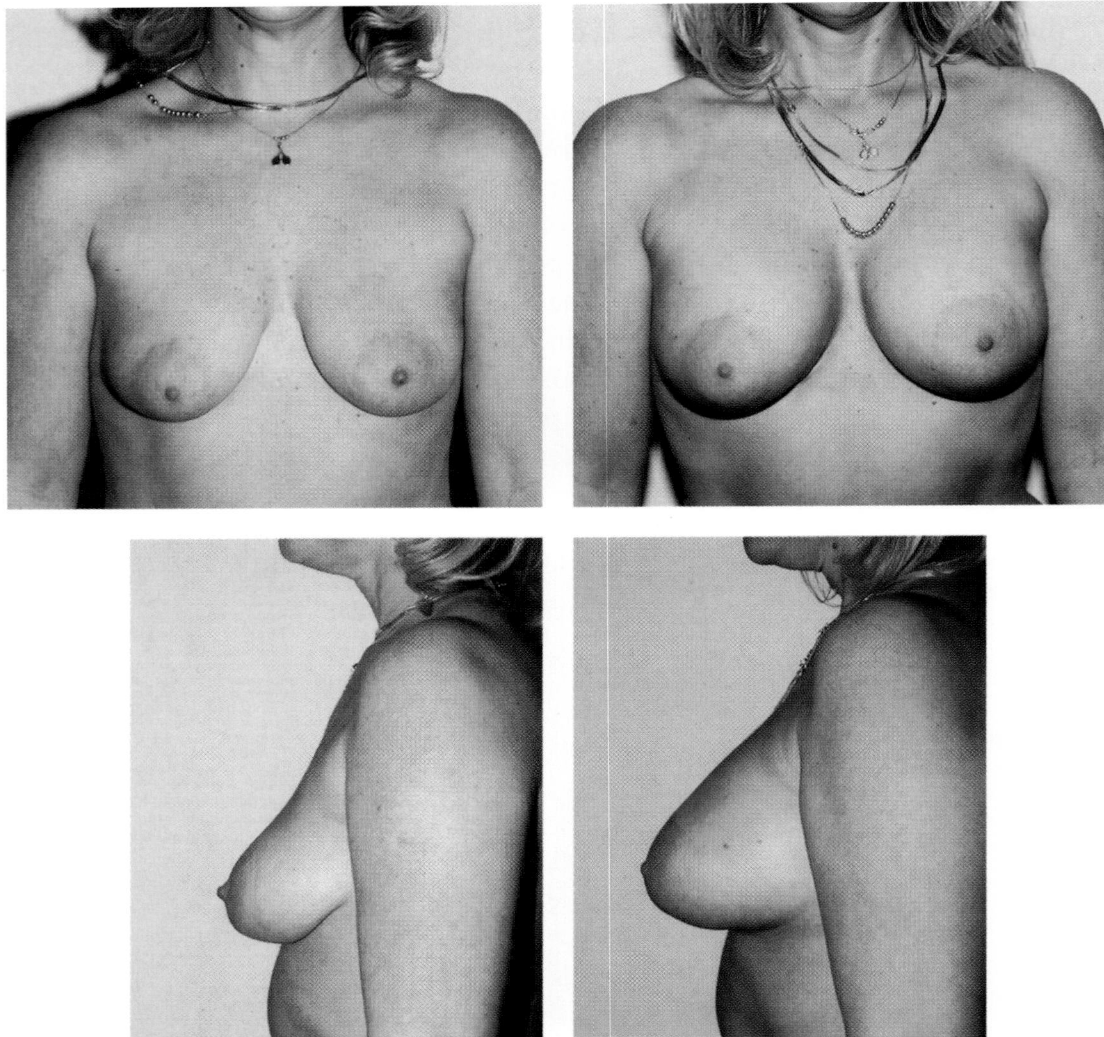

The inframammary crease was modified by lowering it 2 cm to allow the breast implant to be positioned low enough so that there was not too much upper pole fullness and to avoid the double-bubble deformity. Lowering of the crease was accomplished by dividing its dermal and deeper attachments from the skin to the subcutaneous tissue. The augmentation was done through an inframammary incision 4 cm in length. The patient is shown 1 year following the procedure.

PERIAREOLAR SCAR TECHNIQUE

The upper periareolar excision can elevate the areola about 1 cm and incline it upward. It is also useful for correcting a unilateral malposition of the areola. This approach provides a subtle ptosis correction; however, it exacts a price—an upper areolar incision. When more areolar elevation is needed, another technique should be selected. ***More than a modest upper areolar skin excision can noticeably deform the areola circle.*** This excision is sometimes accompanied by a lateral skin excision when ptosis correction of the opposite breast is combined with a total mastectomy.

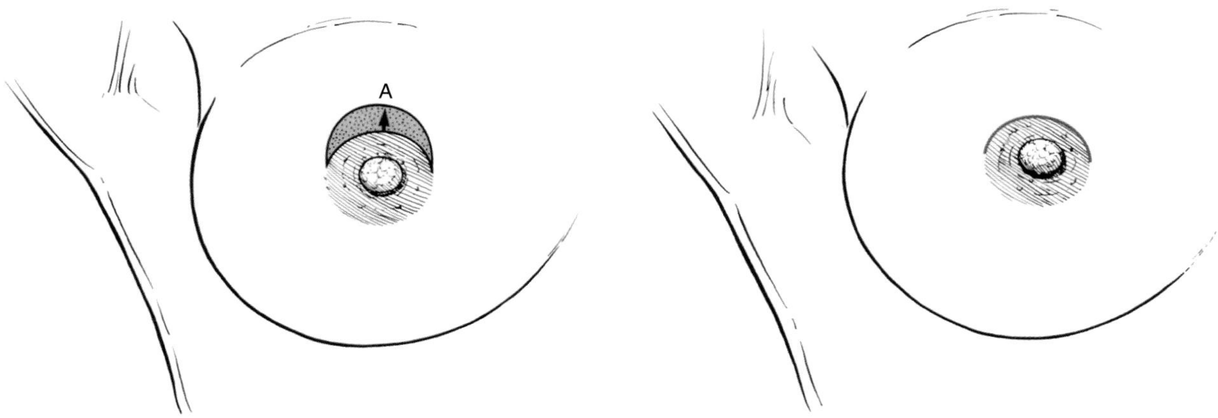

When using this approach for breast augmentation, I prefer to dissect subcutaneously and medially to enter the subglandular space in the medial portion of the breast. The implant can be placed in either the subpectoral position or the subglandular position via this incision. I generally elect to place it subpectorally when the upper breast parenchyma is especially thin. The pectoralis major muscle can be divided in the direction of its fibers in this region and a blunt subpectoral dissection accomplished. I use a smooth-surface implant placed in the subpectoral position above and the subglandular position below.

Result

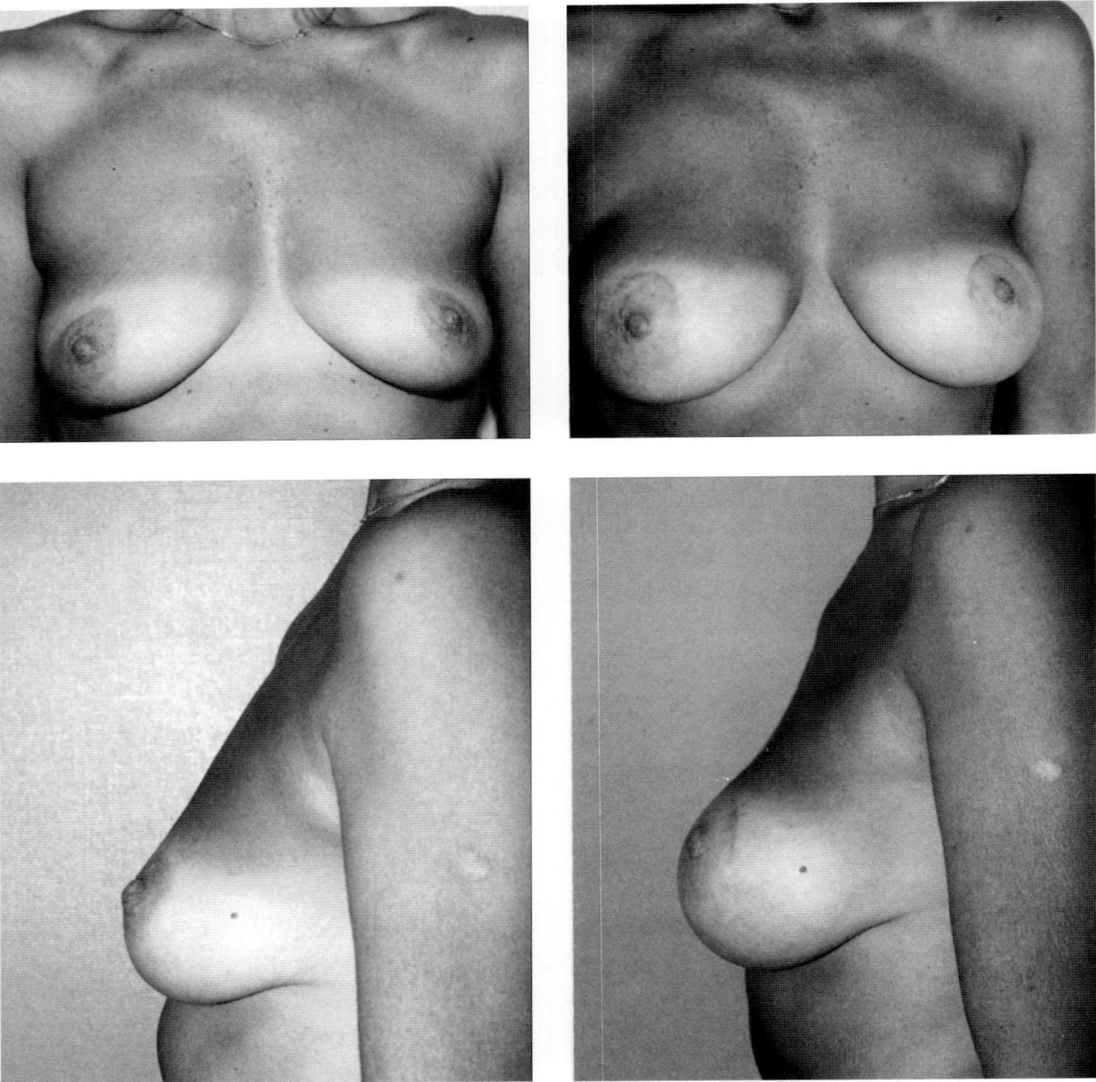

This 38-year-old woman has mild pseudoptosis. She requested that her areolae be as elevated as possible. A subglandular implant was placed via a supra-areolar incision. An ellipse of skin just above the areola was excised to elevate the areolae somewhat and to provide access for implant placement. I personally do not prefer this approach. For most patients with this type of breast who request an augmentation and some elevation, I prefer an inframammary or lower periareolar incision.

CIRCUMAREOLAR SCAR TECHNIQUE WITH PERIAREOLAR PURSE-STRING CLOSURE

In my experience, a circumareolar excision, by itself, does not produce an adequate mastopexy correction. It does not elevate the nipple-areolae and has obvious drawbacks, including the circumareolar scar and central flattening of the breast that compromises normal breast flow and projection. I limit its use to patients who have unusually large areolae and do not want them enlarged further by breast augmentation. I also use it for reducing the central protrusion of a tubular breast in combination with a breast implant to improve some of the upper pole flatness and enhance projection. ***The circumareolar technique used alone without an implant can flatten the breast centrally. Therefore, in the majority of cases, I prefer to use a periareolar purse-string technique that extends this approach and allows upward nipple-areolar positioning.*** The suture controls the diameter of the areola and minimizes postoperative changes or widening of the areola.

Surgical plan

- Elevation of nipple-areola to higher position, tightening of breast skin, and reduction of areolar diameter
- Preoperative markings for future areolar diameter with outer circle designating central skin excision
- Excision of peripheral skin
- Placement of implant in subpectoral position if needed
- Placement of periareolar purse-string suture on each side to control areolar diameter
- Suturing of new areola in layers with interrupted deep sutures and final intracuticular suture for closure

Markings and Technique

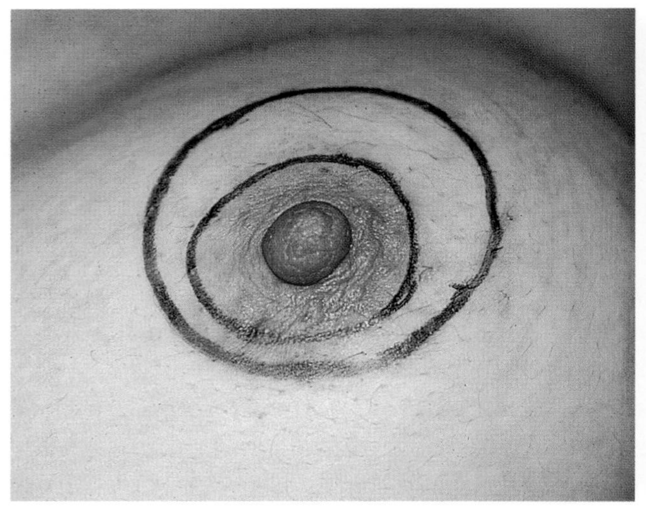

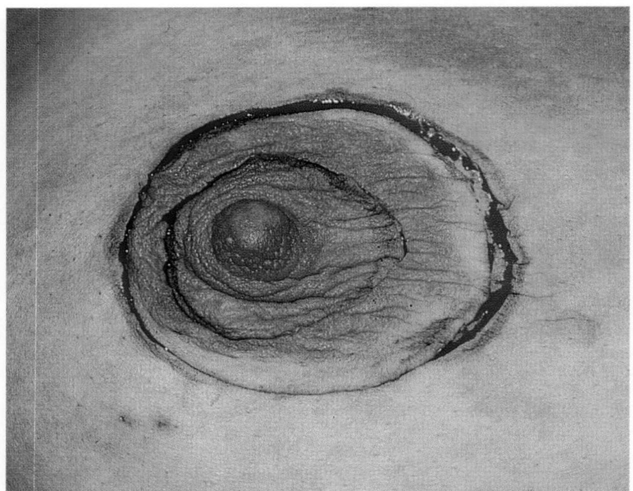

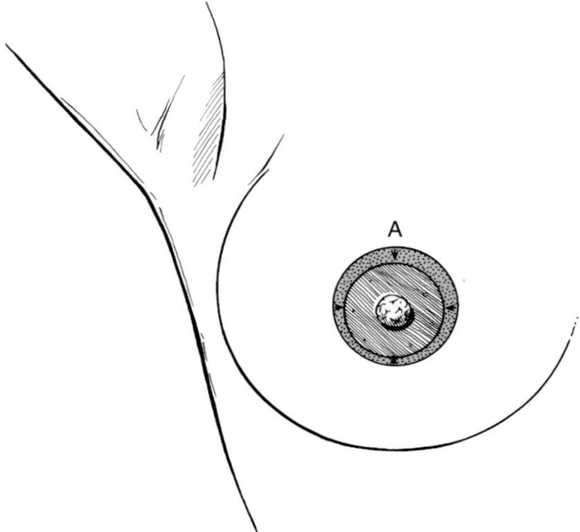

The circle for the future areola is marked 40 to 45 mm in diameter. A second outer circular ellipse is drawn around the periphery of the areola and upward. The top is at the site of the ellipse of the future areola and the bottom is just below the present areola. The widths are minimal to permit the volume increase with an implant.

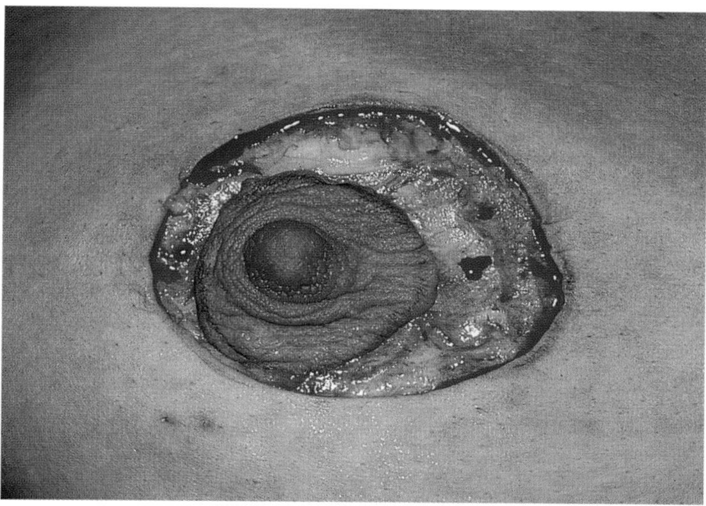

The intervening strip of areola skin is deepithelialized.

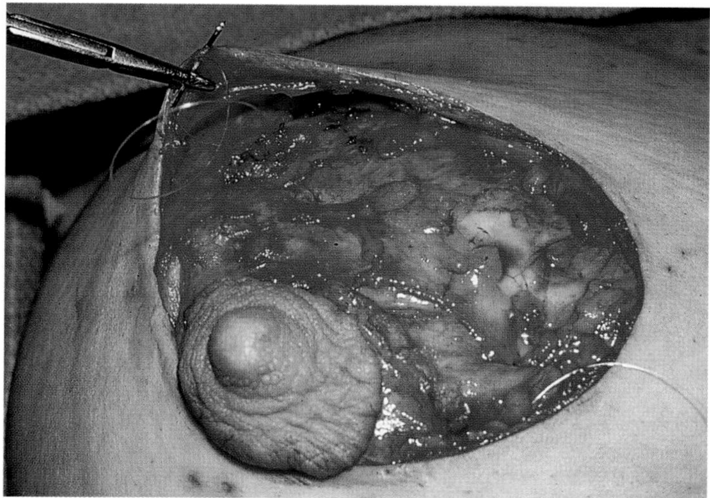

A subcutaneous dissection down to the inframammary crease, beginning at the lower areola and continuing around the lower pole of the breast, gains access to the subglandular space. At this level the dissection elevates the breast from the deeper fascia and is carried up to the lower margin of the pectoralis major muscle for an upper subpectoral dissection. The lower pectoralis major fibers are released to permit proper positioning of the implant. ***When there is some constriction of the lower breast, radial incisions can be made in the breast parenchyma to permit it to expand.*** When the inframammary crease needs to be modified, particularly lowered, the subcutaneous dissection is extended down to the future level of the inframammary crease.

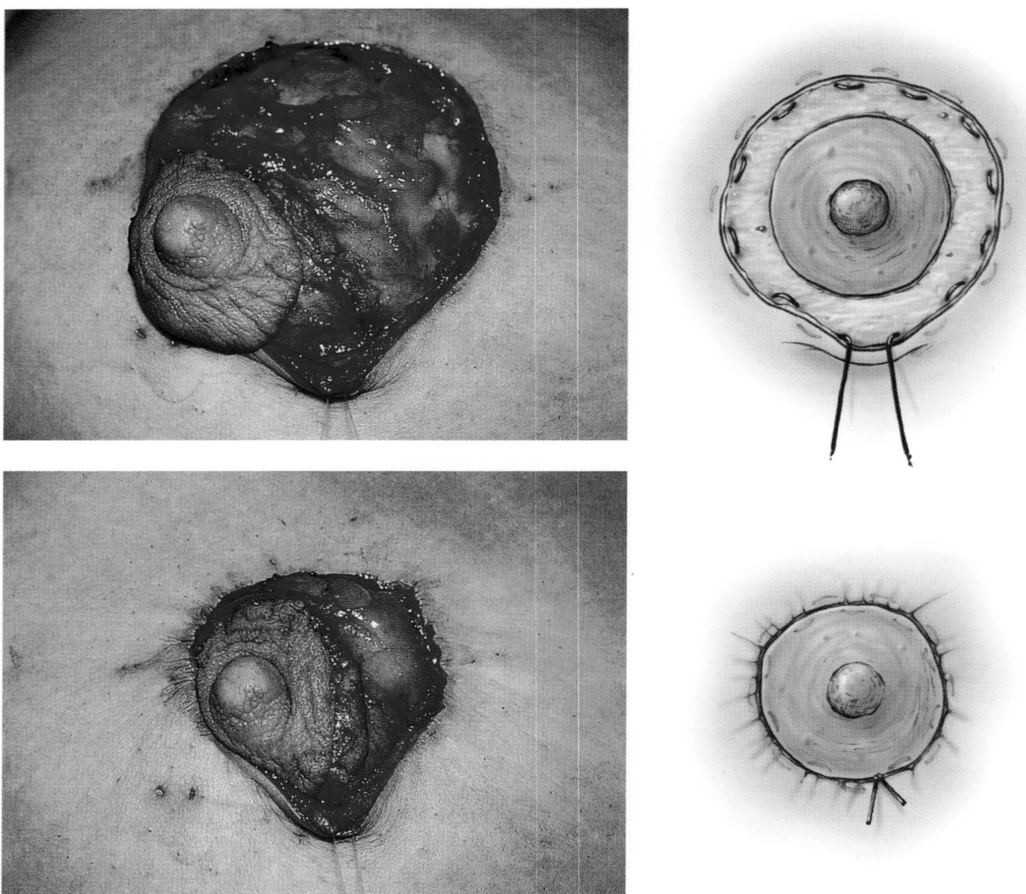

The nipple-areola is closed by first placing a purse-string suture around the periphery of the breast skin and then placing sutures at each quadrant and filling in the spaces between each quadrant with interrupted deep sutures.

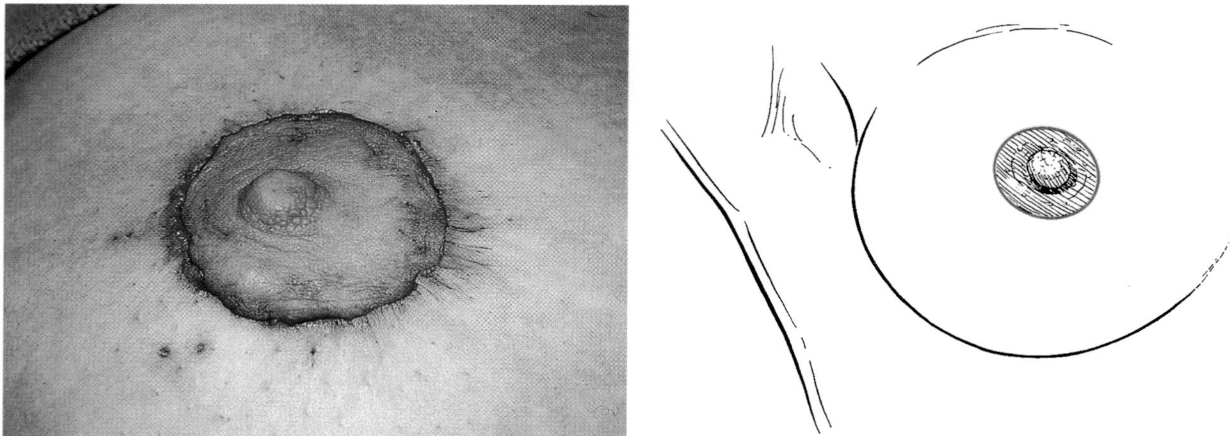

A final intracuticular suture closure leaves the most acceptable areolar scar.

Results

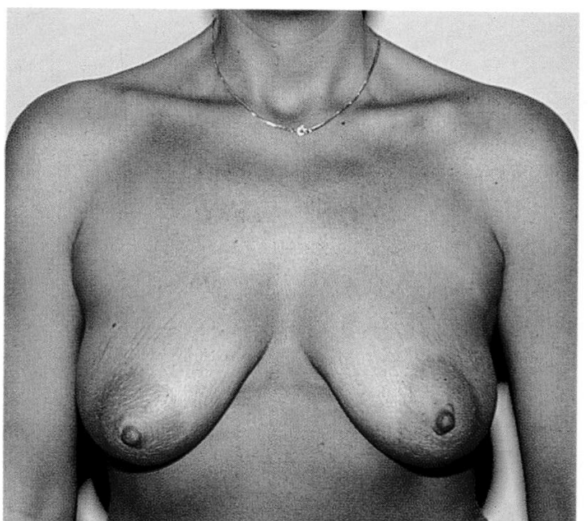
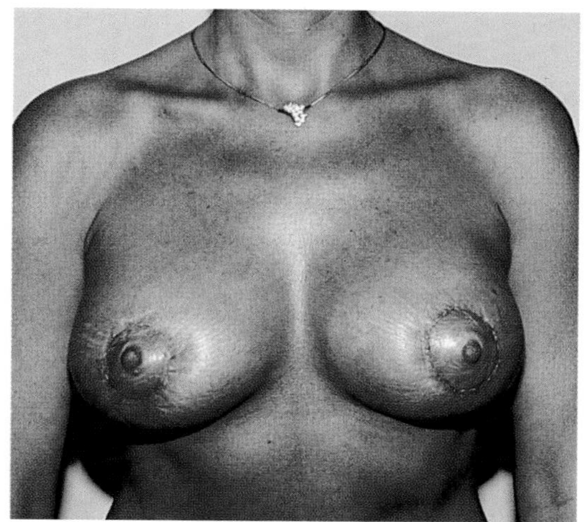

This 36-year-old woman has children ages 13 and 7. With each passing year she noted that her breasts seemed to sag lower with increasing upper pole flattening. She also disliked the large size of her areolae. She was active physically and concerned about her appearance; she felt that her breasts were aging and unattractive. She has enjoyed good health and had no dominant breast masses or positive findings on mammography. Breast examination showed upper pole flattening with large areolae and moderate ptosis. A vertical mastopexy without implants was discussed, but the patient did not think this approach would provide the upper breast improvement that she desired. Therefore a periareolar purse-string mastopexy with placement of subpectoral implants was planned. This operation permits narrowing of the diameter of her areolae while allowing the breast implants to widen the breast base and contribute upper pole fullness and areolar elevation. Bilateral 325 cc smooth-surface saline implants were placed under the pectoral muscle, which was released superiorly from the level of the top of the areola downward so that the implant was in a subglandular position below and was not constricted or elevated by a contracting pectoral muscle. The patient is satisfied with the improvement in breast size and breast position. Her areolae have been reduced from a diameter of 55 to 40 mm.

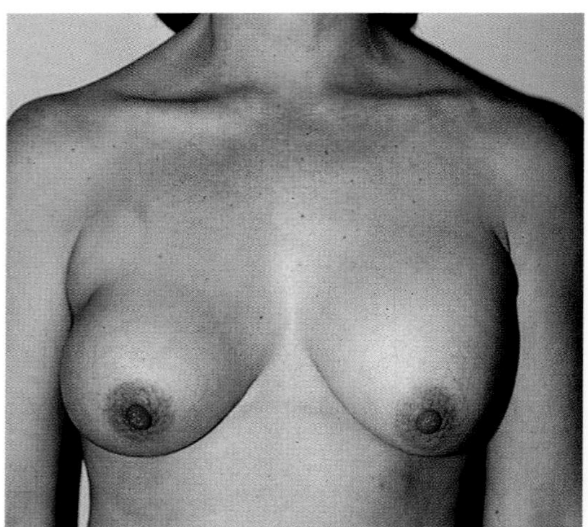

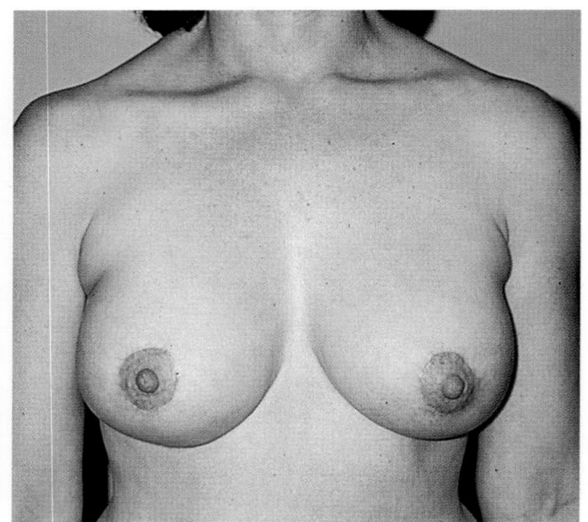

This 42-year-old woman had breast implants placed in the subglandular position to improve minor breast ptosis. She developed capsular contracture with elevation of the implants, which accentuated the appearance of ptosis in addition to the firmness of the breast implants. She requested elevation of the nipple-areolae and softer breast implants because she felt that her breast deformity and breast hardness were increasing over time. She had firm capsular contractures and her left breast was more ptotic than her right. A bilateral periareolar purse-string approach was planned. This permitted elevation of the nipple-areolae without a vertical incision, which would narrow the lower portion of the breast. More skin was to be removed on the left than on the right to elevate the left nipple to a more symmetric position. The inframammary fold was lowered about 1 cm on each side, and capsulectomies were performed bilaterally followed by placement of 300 cc smooth-surface saline implants through the lower portion of the periareolar incisions. The periareolar incisions were then closed. Following this operation the patient's breasts have remained soft and she is pleased with the improved contour, feel, and elevation.

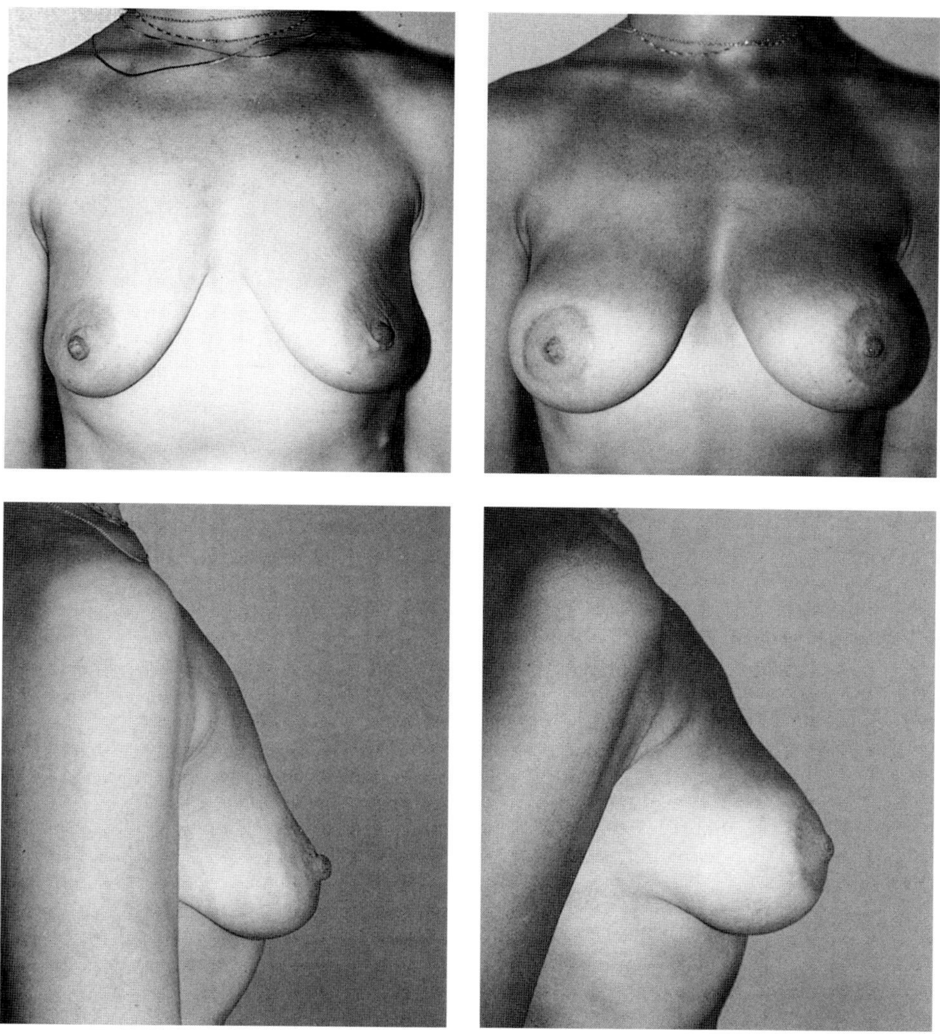

This 32-year-old patient had minor ptosis with upper pole flattening and rather large areolae. She requested breast augmentation to improve the upper pole fullness. She also was concerned with the large areolar diameter. The nipple skin was excised through a periareolar incision, through which 280 cc breast implants were placed subpectorally. The concentric mastopexy was then closed directly with intracuticular sutures. Although upper pole fullness was enhanced, some truncation of the breast and firmness as a result of capsular contracture of the smooth-surface implant limited the postoperative result.

VERTICAL MASTOPEXY

A major improvement of moderate and major degrees of ptosis is unusual with only the basic vertical mastopexy. ***The combination of nipple-areolar elevation, subpectoral breast implant placement (or a flap of lower parenchymal tissue for the woman who does not want an implant), and vertical breast closure, however, provides sufficient nipple-areolar elevation to disguise the breast ptosis.*** The implant or flap contributes the necessary upper breast fullness, which is a primary complaint and concern of these patients. These are the procedures I perform most often for ptosis correction.

VERTICAL SCAR TECHNIQUE WITH IMPLANT PLACEMENT

With the vertical scar technique, excess skin is excised through a vertical ellipse extending from the inframammary crease to the upper portion of the new areola. A horizontal incision is avoided. This vertical incision usually heals with an acceptable, nonhypertrophied scar. This technique seems to limit further distortion of areolar shape and reduces the chance of postoperative areolar diameter asymmetry that is more common with the periareolar purse-string approach. Breast augmentation provides additional breast fullness, especially centrally and in the upper breast, and limits the length of the mastopexy incisions.

Surgical plan

- Preoperative markings to designate new nipple position and circumference of future areola
- Displacement of breast medially and laterally before drawing vertical line from lower portion of new areola to point 1 cm above inframammary fold
- Areola left in situ and upper and lower areas deepithelialized
- Excision of lower breast tissue in V and transposition upward
- Placement of implant under pectoralis major muscle above and subglandular tissue below with parenchymal closure
- Transposition and inset of nipple-areola to new position
- Placement of intracuticular or slowly absorbable sutures for vertical scar shortening

Markings and Technique

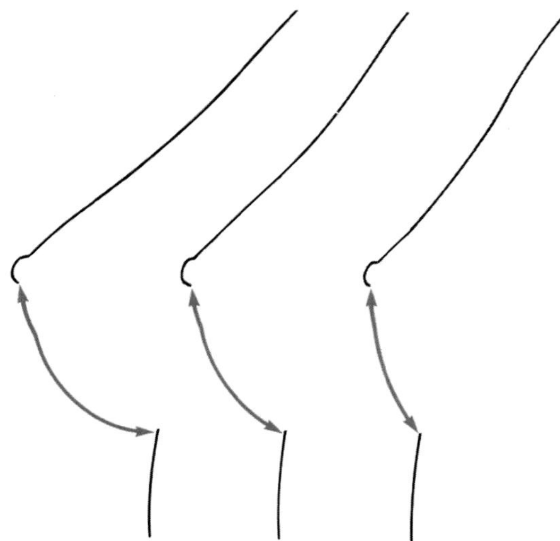

Determining the approximate new position of the nipple is the starting point for this procedure. The nipple-areola is located on the mid-breast line 1 to 2 cm above the projection of the inframammary crease in patients with breast volumes of 150 to 250 cc. This distance will vary with larger or smaller breast volumes: for smaller breasts of 100 to 150 cc it is slightly more than 2 cm; for breasts with volumes of 250 to 350 cc it is 1 cm; for larger breasts it is positioned at the inframammary crease. ***As breasts become larger, the distance from the inframammary fold to the nipple is progressively longer.***

Another method for determining the new position of the nipple is to physically move it to a new position that looks correct. This position is then marked on the sternum and the nipple level transferred to its new position on the nipple line. ***When the nipple is repositioned, it should be elevated along the nipple line, that is, a bit more medial with each degree of elevation.***

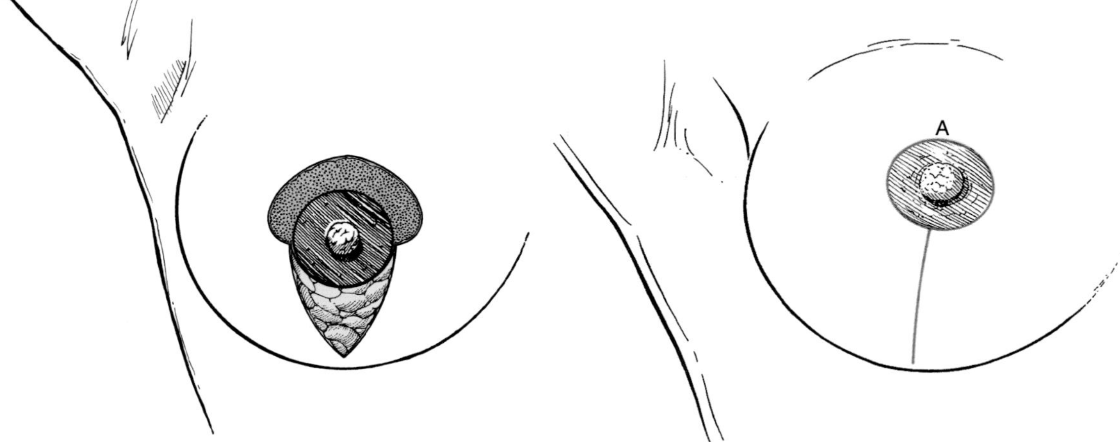

Preoperative markings are made with the patient sitting or standing upright. The apex of the new areolar site and the diameter of the new areola are marked. An outer line slightly shorter than the circumference of the areola is chosen. A vertical ellipse is then drawn from the top of the new areola, around the areola, and downward to complete the ellipse. The width of the ellipse is determined by displacing the breast medially and laterally and drawing vertical lines from the lower areolar site to a point on the breast line 1 to 2 cm above the inframammary fold. If an augmentation is part of the surgical plan, I remove only the minimal amount of skin initially to allow upward nipple-areolar positioning and to complete the ellipse. Then I use the tailor-tack method to determine the remainder of skin excision after the breast implant is positioned. ***When a wide nipple-areola is transposed upward, tight closure at the lower pole of the areola can result.*** This problem will be accentuated by breast constriction or placement of a large implant. For these patients the periareolar purse-string technique may be a better choice. ***The vertical mastopexy narrows the breast. The periareolar purse-string mastopexy does not.*** Preservation of some pigmented skin below the transposed nipple-areola, with later excision after the skin has settled and stretched, is one strategy to alleviate a vertical excision that proves too tight.

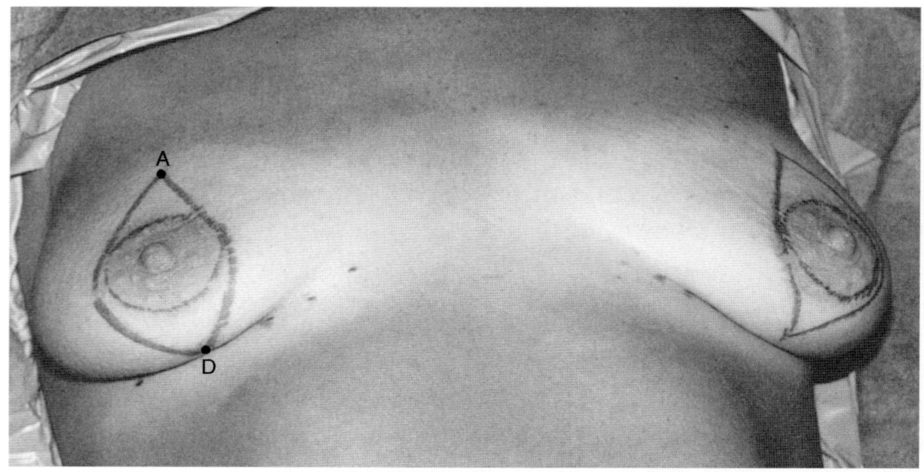

Moderate ptosis in this 38-year-old woman developed after the delivery of her two children. She was particularly concerned about the upper pole flattening, the general breast involution, and the low position of her nipple-areolae. She requested fuller, more elevated breasts.

The patient is checked for symmetry bilaterally. If there is asymmetry with breast constriction or vertical nipple-areolar asymmetry, this should be noted preoperatively and markings made to correct these asymmetries.

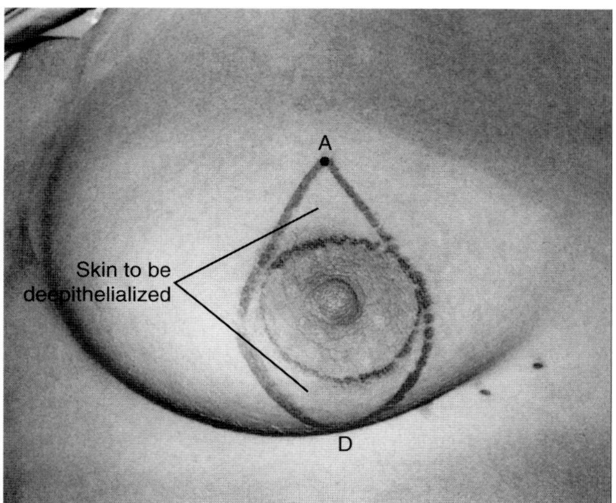

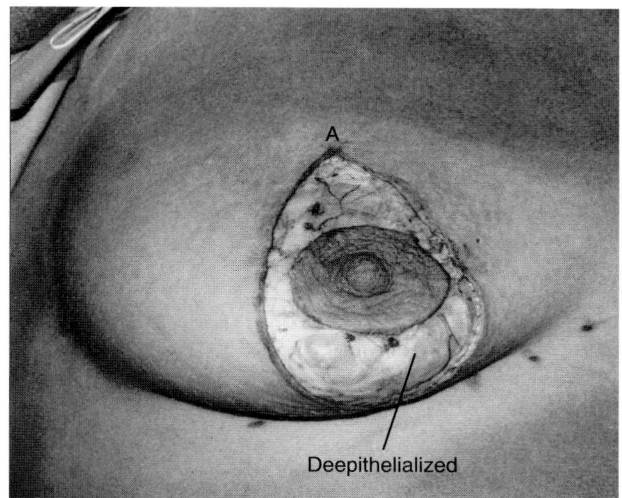

An incision is made around the areola and then along the marks of the ellipse. The skin is deepithelialized within the ellipse, preserving the nipple-areolar vascularity on a parenchymal base.

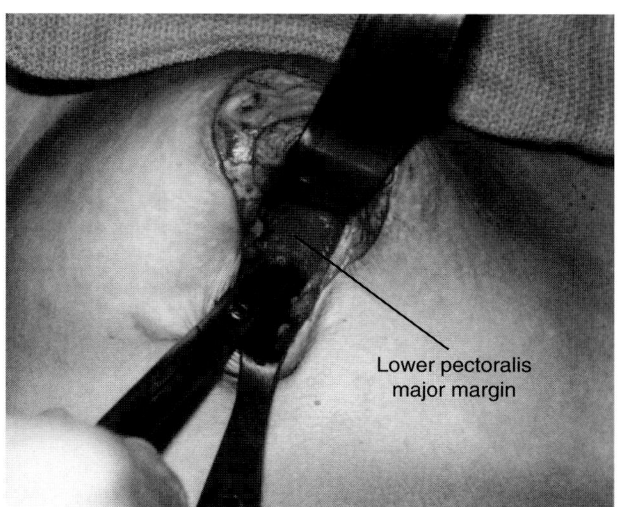

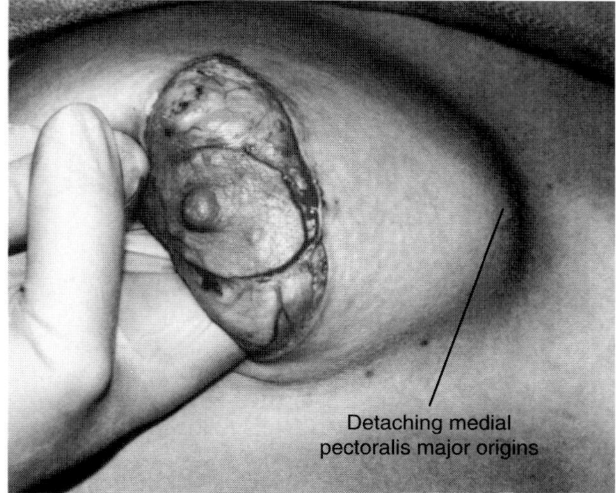

Dissection is then carried around the lower pole of the breast and beneath the deep portions of the breast to the lower margin of the pectoralis major muscle. When the lower margin of the pectoralis major muscle is identified, the upper subpectoral space is entered with blunt scissors dissection. The subpectoral pocket is developed medially with finger dissection. The fibers of the pectoralis major muscle are stretched and elevated to allow anterior expansion and projection of the breast implant. The lower fibers of the pectoralis major muscle are divided either bluntly or under direct vision with a lighted retractor and the electrocautery unit.

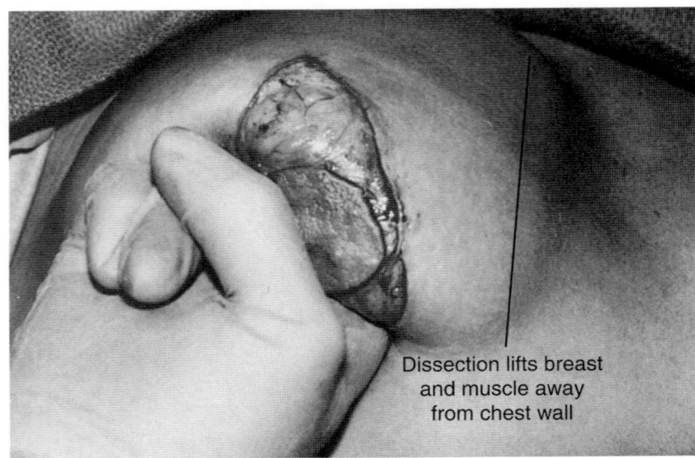

The dissection then continues superiorly up to the level of the second rib to create an adequate upper breast pocket.

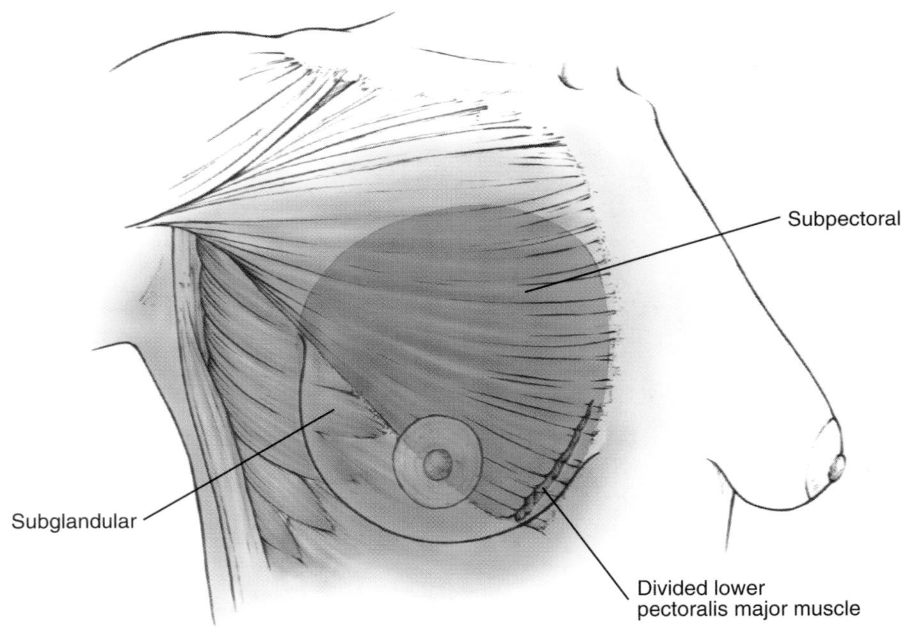

The dissection continues laterally to widen the pocket to accommodate the breast implant. The anterolateral intercostal neurovascular bundles preserve sensation to the nipple-areola and breast. The pocket is checked for symmetry and for adequate hemostasis. Because of the blunt dissection, electrocautery is usually not required for hemostasis after the customary 5-minute wait.

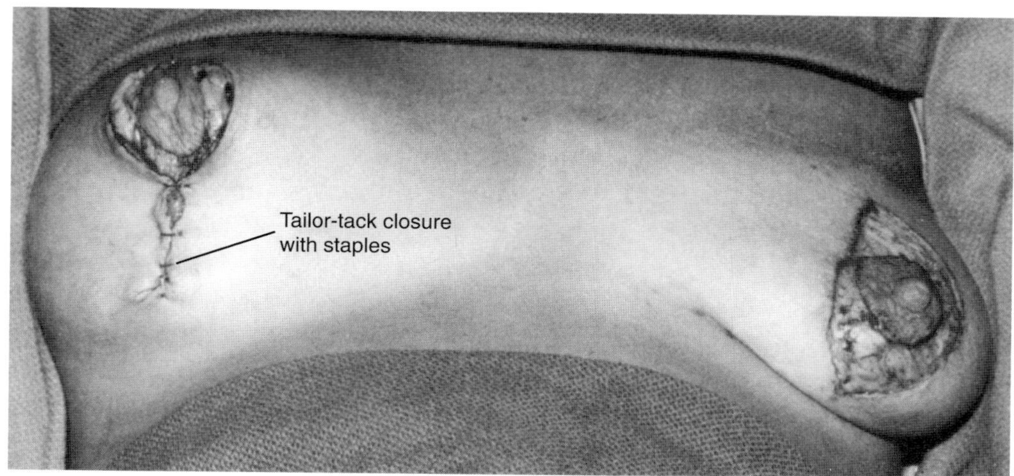

The implant is selected and positioned through the lower incision into the subpectoral space above and the subglandular space below. This positioning allows the implant to settle postoperatively. Either smooth-surface or textured-surface saline implants may be used.

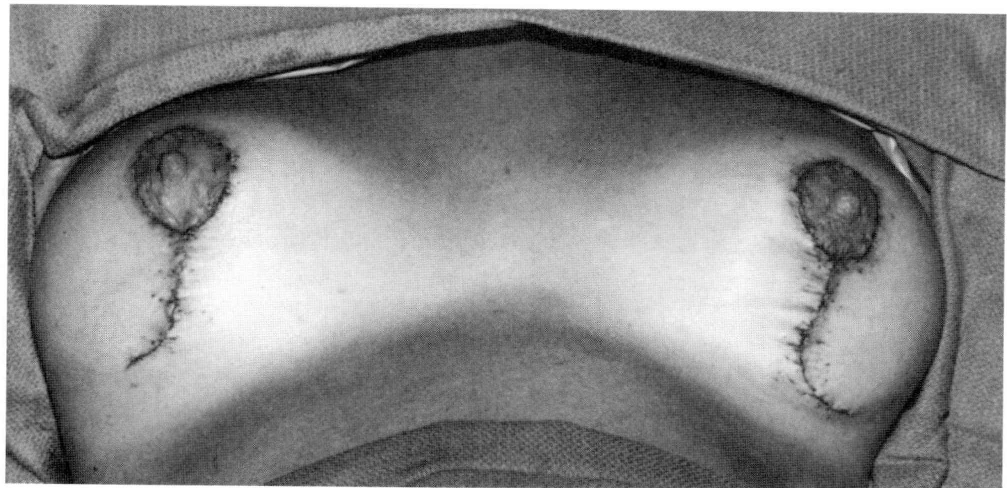

The breast is then closed temporarily up to the lower border of the future areola. At this point, if extra lower breast parenchyma is prominent through the lower open incision, it can be excised just under the subcutaneous region. If there is tightness below the areola, additional intraoperative expansion can be done manually and with the tissue expander.

When the distance from the lower areola to the inframammary crease is greater than 8 cm, then a lower transverse ellipse is made, converting the incision to a short horizontal T.

The site for the nipple-areola is cut out as a circle with a diameter a few millimeters smaller than the original areola, and the remainder of the incision is closed with subcuticular and interrupted buried absorbable polyglycolic sutures. The incisions are covered with Steri-Strips for 2 to 3 months to improve the scar appearance. When smooth-surface implants are used, postoperative displacement exercises are begun within the first week.

Results

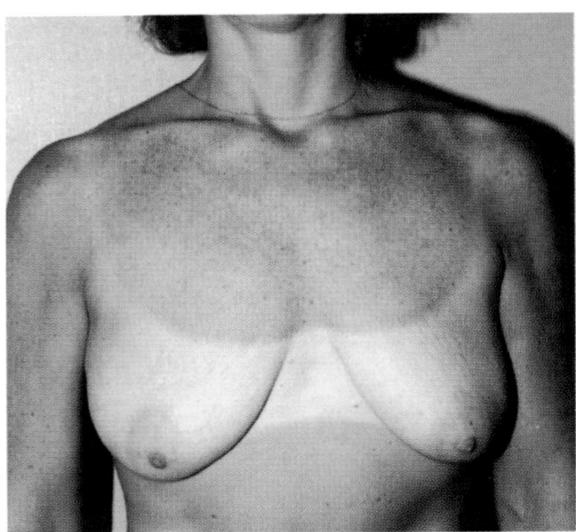

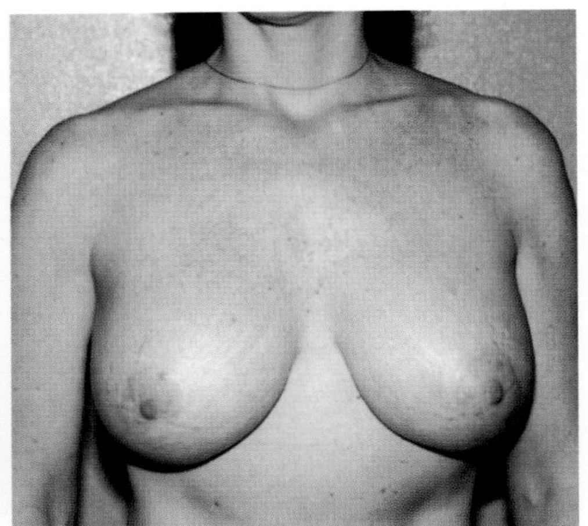

This woman requested mastopexy with increased breast fullness without extensive scars. The vertical mastopexy elevated her nipple-areolae. The inframammary crease was lowered approximately 2 cm, and 325 cc implants were selected to give additional breast fullness. Since these implants also took up some of the excess skin, only a vertical incision was necessary for adequate closure and to achieve the desired postoperative appearance. The patient is shown 1 year following the procedure. This patient had some preoperative asymmetry that has persisted following the mastopexy. Even though a narrow skin resection was done below, she still has some tightness of the right areola.

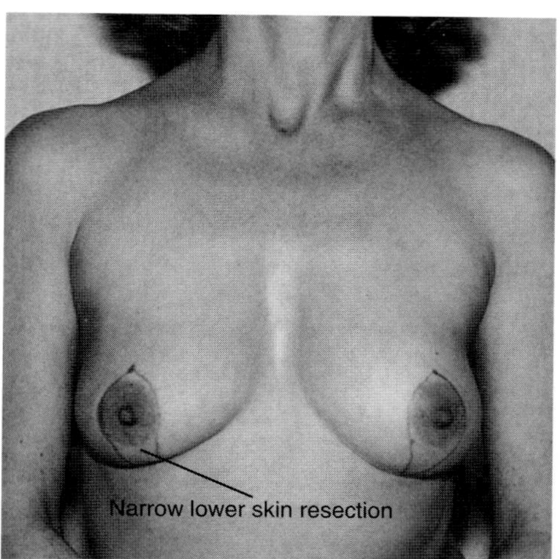

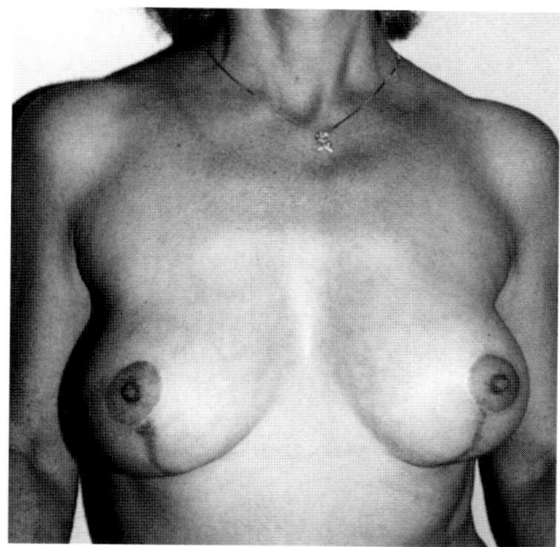

This 38-year-old patient was concerned about breast hypoplasia and involution, upper pole flattening, a low nipple, pseudoptosis, and breast asymmetry. She requested nipple-areolar elevation and a breast augmentation. The nipple-areolae were elevated with a periareolar incision and a vertical incision. The 240 cc smooth-surface implants were placed in a subpectoral position above and a subglandular position below.

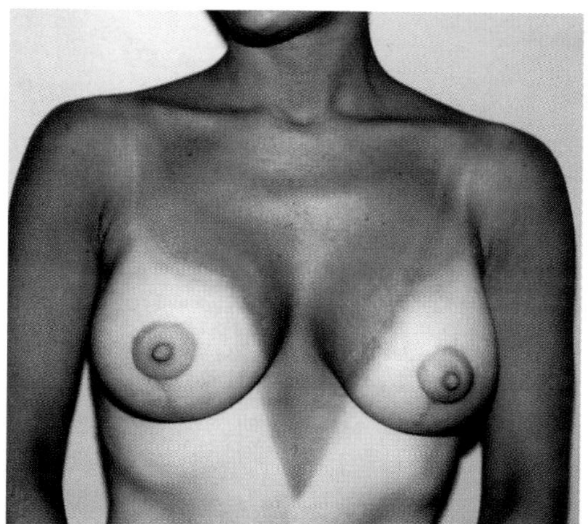

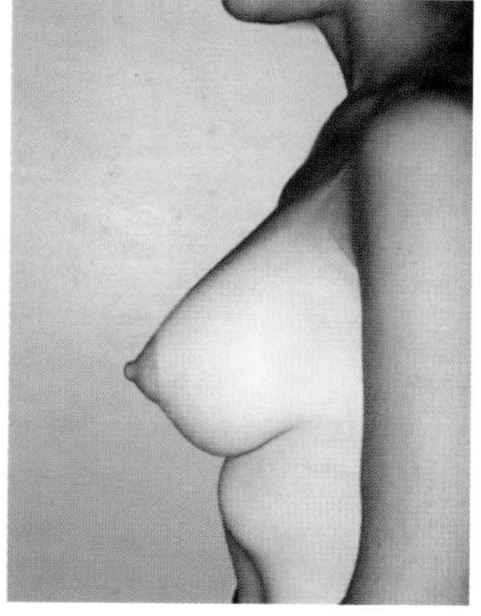

This 28-year-old woman had moderate ptosis with significant flattening and atrophy in the upper portion of her breast after a 20-pound weight loss following the birth of her child. She requested elevation of her nipple-areolae as well as correction of the upper pole fullness. She had a vertical mastopexy with 250 cc saline implants placed in the subpectoral position above and in the subglandular position below. She is very pleased with the elevation of the nipple-areola as well as the upper breast fullness. The vertical incision has healed satisfactorily and her breasts have been elevated to a more youthful position. The position and appearance of the vertical scars are demonstrated.

VERTICAL SCAR TECHNIQUE WITH IMPLANT EXCHANGE

Some patients with moderate to major ptosis have had breast implants placed in hopes of improving the ptosis and avoiding the mastopexy incision. Sometimes the patient gains additional weight after this procedure, the implants assume a lower position, and the breasts appear too large without enough upper breast fill. One solution for this problem is to replace the breast implants with smaller implants, to resect the lower ptotic tissue, and to perform vertical mastopexies to remove the central breast parenchyma, narrow the breast, and reduce the lower breast ptosis.

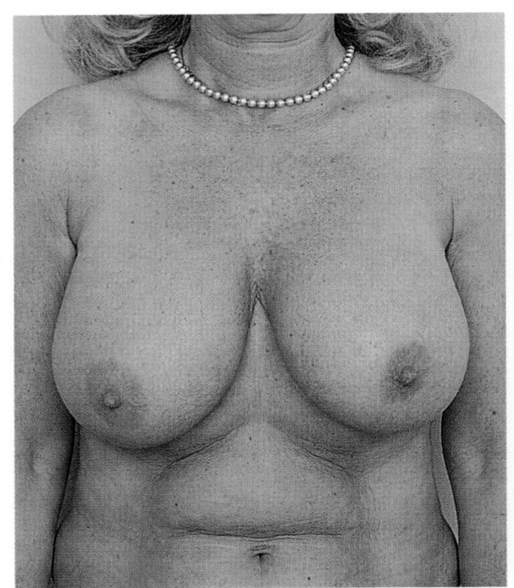

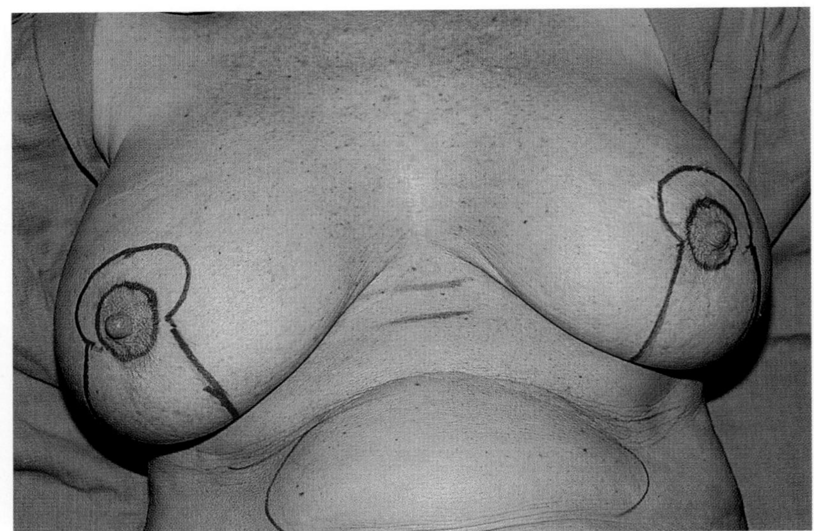

This 47-year-old woman had breast implants placed 10 years prior to this procedure. She gained 20 pounds over the years and became increasingly dissatisfied with her larger, sagging breasts. She requested smaller, more uplifted breasts but still wanted upper breast fullness and less lower breast ptosis. She is shown on the operating table with the preoperative markings to detail the plan for reducing the areolar diameter, elevating the nipple-areolae, and removing the lower excess skin and breast parenchyma. Access to the implant pocket for implant exchange is also provided.

Surgical plan

- Reduction of ptotic breast tissue, elevation of nipple-areola, and exchange of underlying breast implant
- Preoperative markings to indicate top of areola
- Displacement of breast medially and laterally before marking vertical lines
- Vertical excision extending 1 to 2 cm above inframammary fold
- Incision of vertical lines and excision of ptotic breast parenchyma
- Removal of underlying breast implant and capsulectomy
- Placement of implant and approximation of breast pillars over implant
- Transfer and inset of nipple-areola to new position
- Approximation of vertical skin limbs and closure with intracuticular suture to shorten vertical line

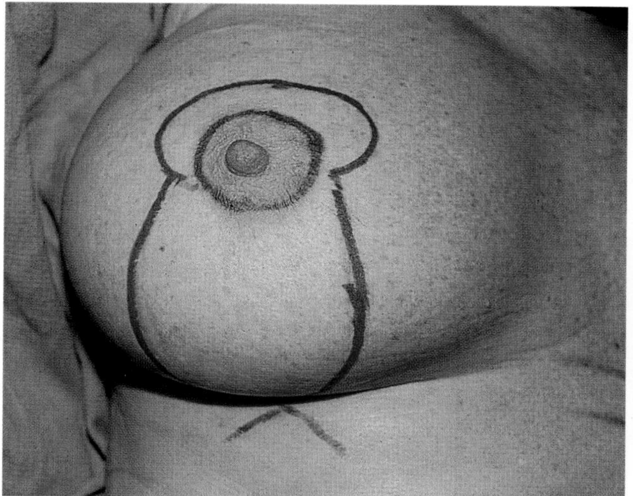

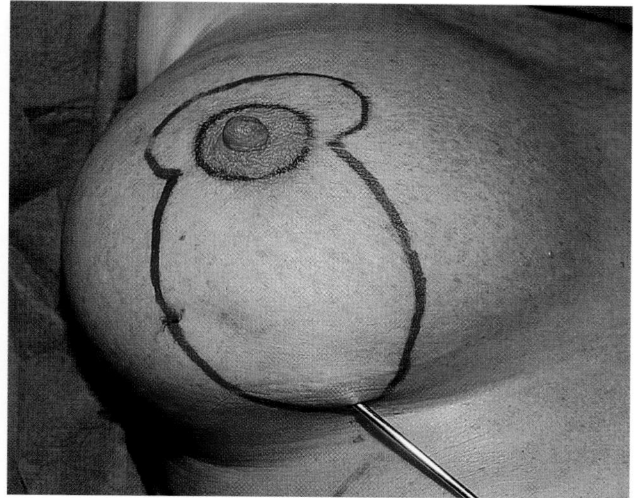

The preoperative markings illustrate the vertical approach and the size of the areola, which is usually 40 to 45 mm in diameter. The upper ellipse is the circumference of the future areola. The breasts are displaced medially and laterally before marking the vertical limbs. If some parenchyma is to be removed, the vertical lines are marked to accommodate this additional skin excision. The implant will be exchanged through the lower breast incision.

Wetting solution containing 1000 ml of Ringer's lactate, 1 ml of 1:1000 epinephrine, and 25 ml of lidocaine is infiltrated in the area of the resection. This solution contains lidocaine to decrease postoperative pain as well as epinephrine to reduce intraoperative bleeding.

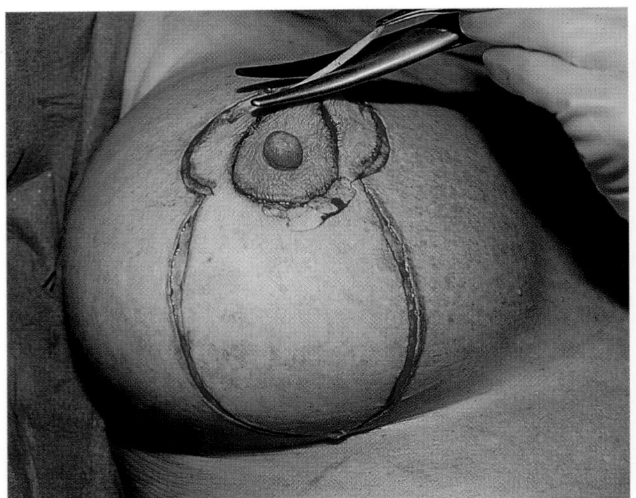

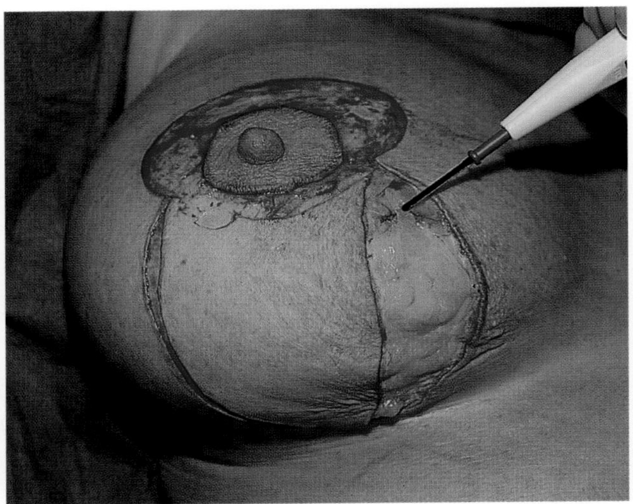

After the incisions are made, the upper circle is deepithelialized. Next vertical incisions are made to create medial and lateral breast pillars and to define the amount of central breast skin and parenchyma to be excised in the V.

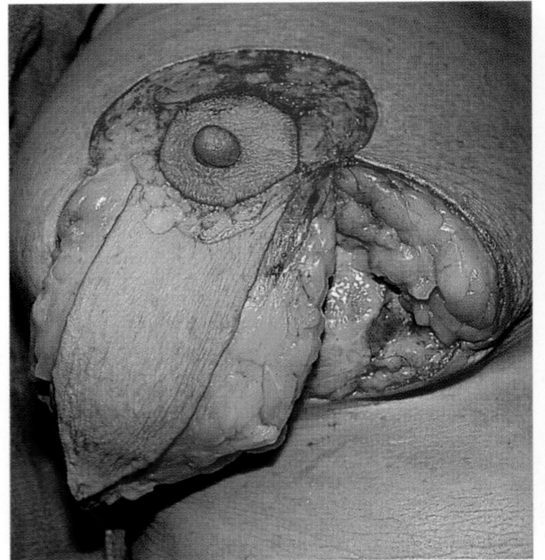

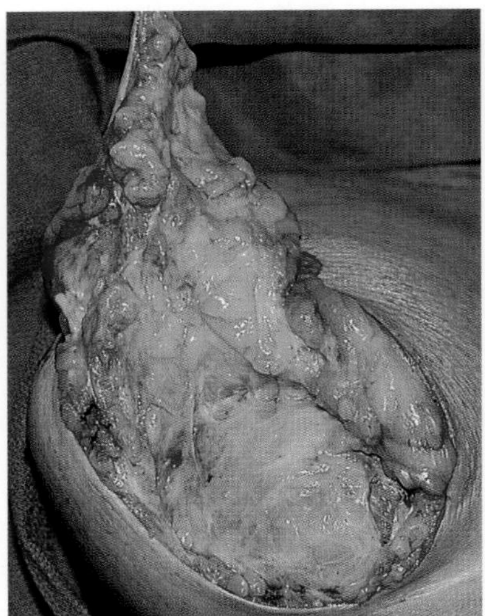

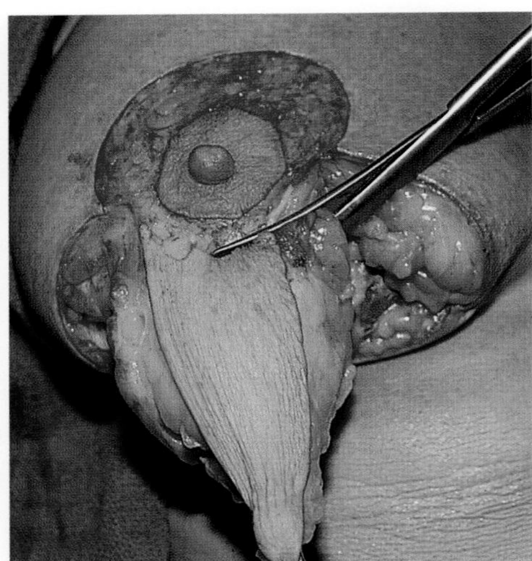

The central breast parenchyma is elevated off the breast capsule and resected. This parenchyma contributes to both breast heaviness and width.

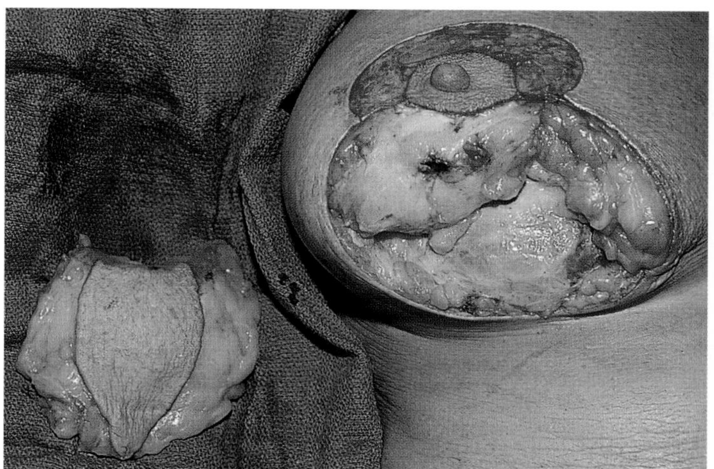

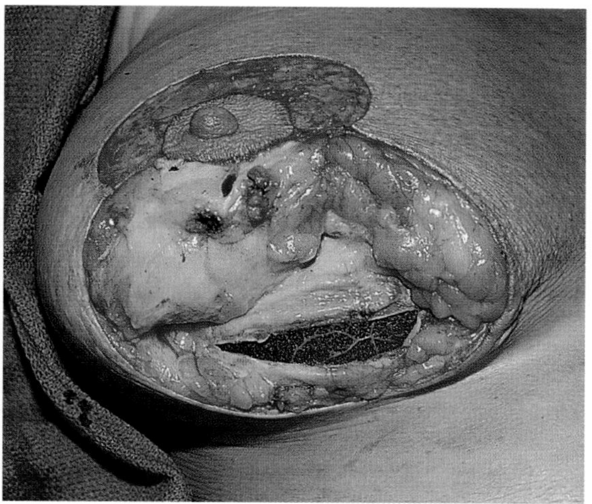

Following resection of the central breast parenchyma, open capsulectomy is done to expose the textured-surface breast implant.

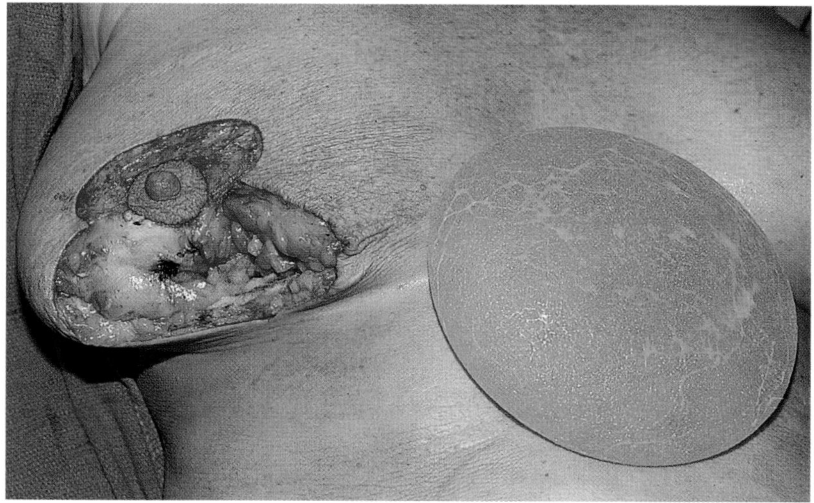

The implant is removed. Capsular contracture is not significant and only a partial lower breast capsulectomy is done.

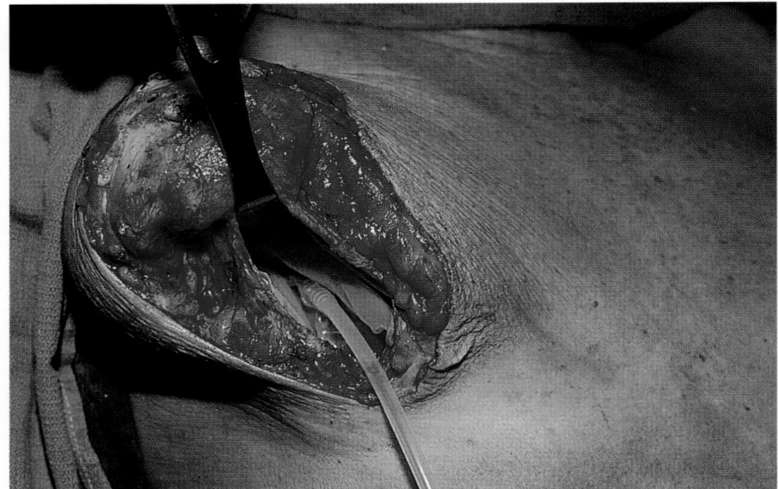

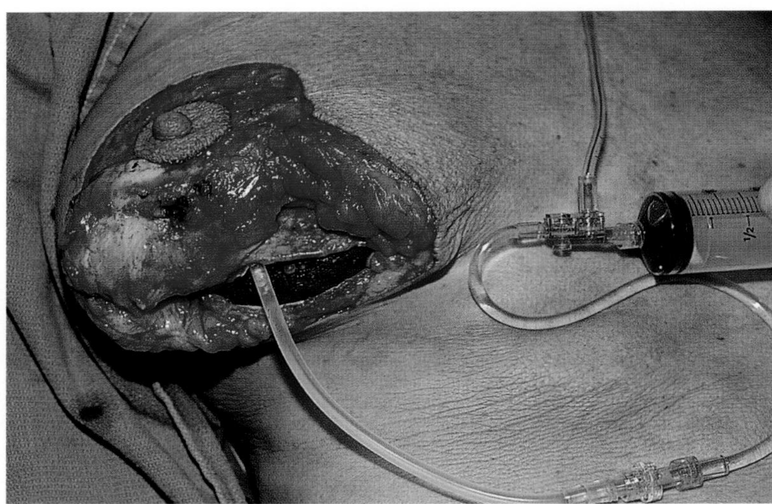

A smooth-surface saline implant with a 2 cm narrower diameter is positioned to accommodate the smaller size of her breast. This saline implant is then inflated to 320 cc, 20 cc larger than its preoperative size of 300 cc. The nipple is moved to its new position and the pillars of the breast are reestablished with interrupted 2.0 absorbable sutures.

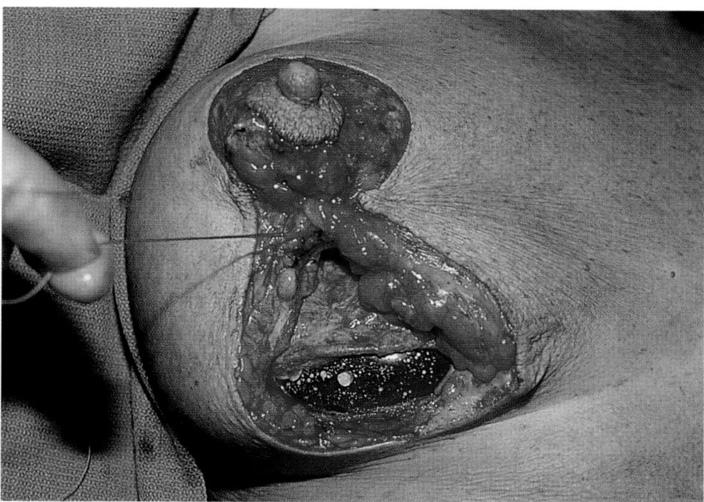

The circle for the areola is reestablished by bringing the upper breast pillars together.

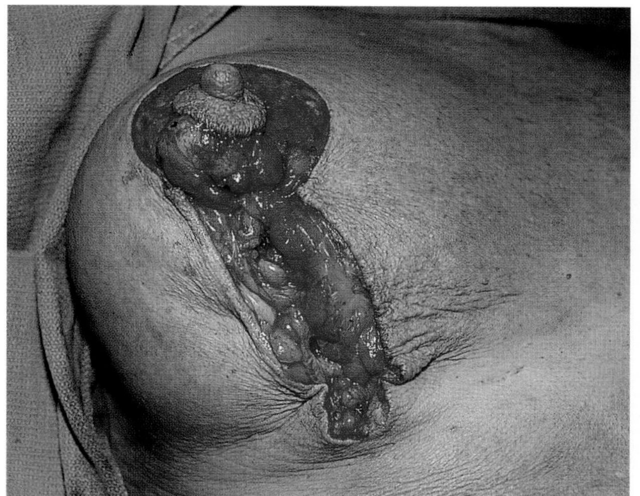

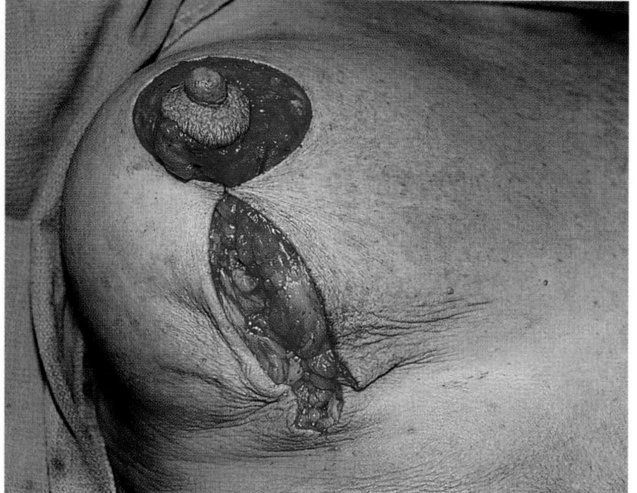

The pillars of the breast are then reapproximated using 2.0 absorbable sutures.

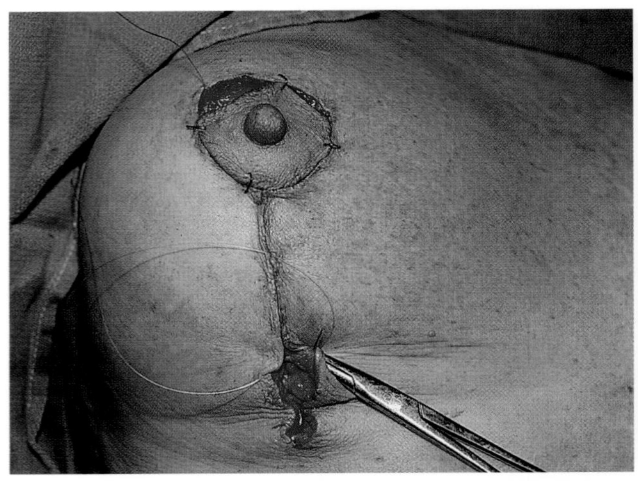
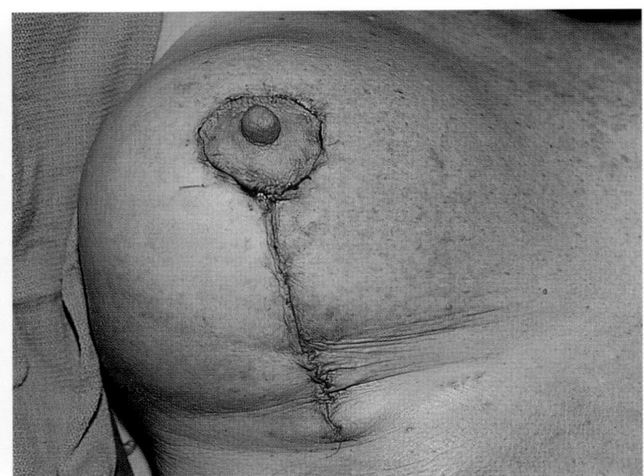
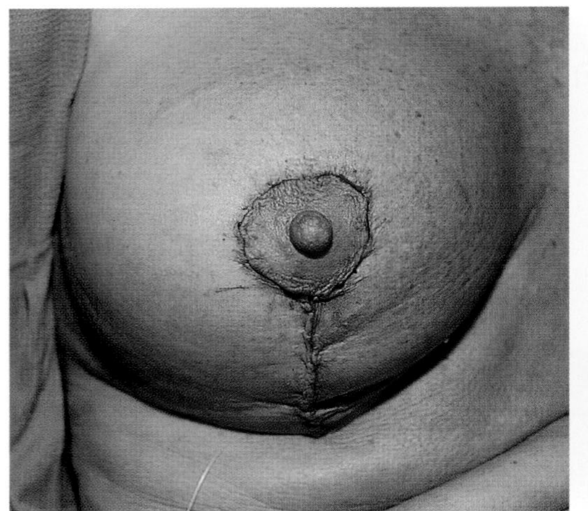
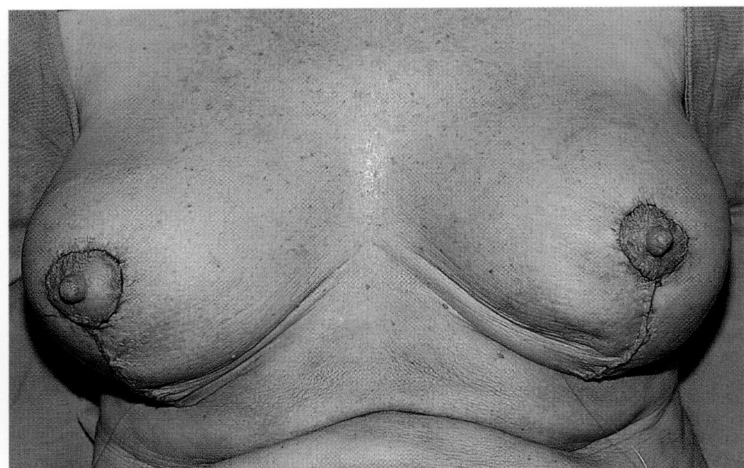
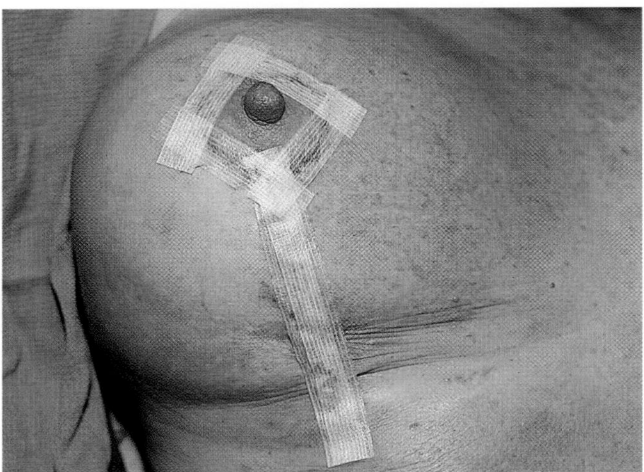

Closure is accomplished with additional deep 3.0 absorbable sutures and running intracuticular 3.0 clear PDS sutures, which can be tightened to shorten the length of the vertical scar. Note the narrower breast and the reduction of lower breast fullness. The saline implant continues to give some central and upper breast fullness.

Results

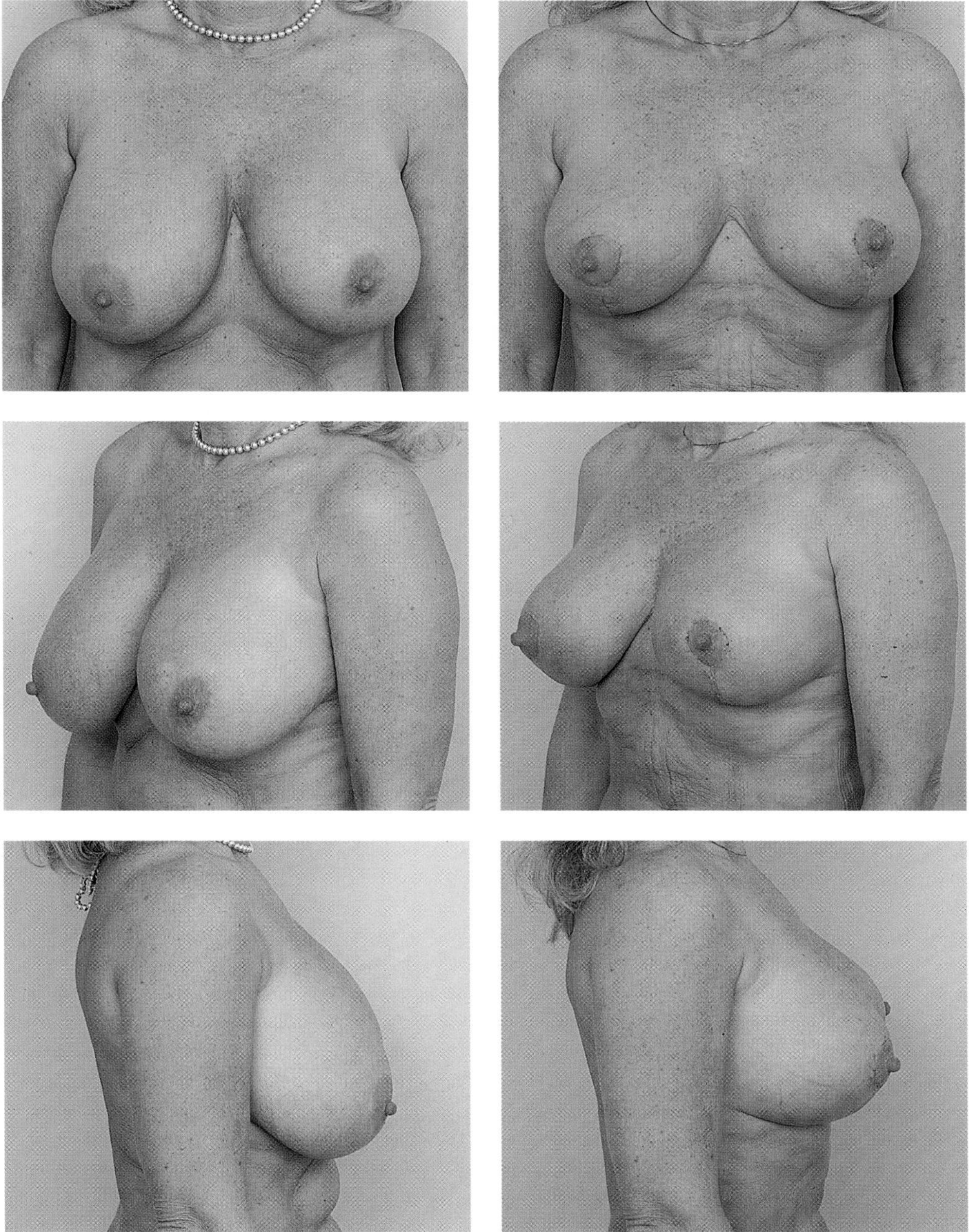

The patient is shown before and 3 months following the operation. She is particularly satisfied with the reduced breast ptosis as well as the breast volume. She appreciates the fullness in her upper breast region and feels that her breasts are more attractive, softer, and better proportioned. There is no evidence of capsular contracture, and while some asymmetry exists it is acceptable. The irregularities of the vertical incision in the inframammary fold skin have smoothed out, and the vertical scar is healing without hypertrophy.

VERTICAL SCAR TECHNIQUE WITH LOWER PARENCHYMAL FLAP FOR UPPER BREAST FULLNESS

Some patients with breast ptosis and upper breast flattening request a mastopexy that will fill in the upper breast area without using implants. One strategy for these individuals is to move some of the lower breast parenchyma to the central and upper breast region. This lower parenchymal tissue is based on the upper parenchyma; it is turned underneath the nipple-areola and sutured beneath the upper pole of the breast. With this approach the central ptotic breast parenchyma is removed and the upper breast area is filled in. Improvement generally is not as significant as that observed after implant placement, but it is usually satisfactory for patients who object to implants.

Surgical plan

- Preoperative markings to designate new areolar position and central breast excision
- Deepithelialization of upper areola site with lower triangle rotated to central and upper breast region
- Resection of lower central portion of breast parenchyma with preservation of pillars on medial and lateral flaps
- Amount of parenchymal excision based on degree of breast elevation and parenchymal reduction needed
- Removal of subcutaneous tissue medially and laterally to reduce length of pillars
- Suturing of tip of V to pectoralis muscle fascia to rotate flap underneath breast for upper breast fill
- Closure of areola site
- Closure of vertical incision to shorten scar

Markings and Technique

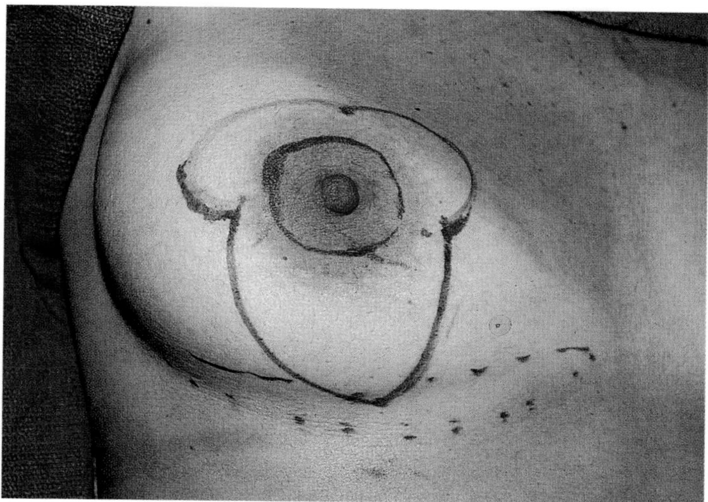

This patient with moderate breast ptosis requested mastopexy with improved upper breast fullness and no breast implants. The operative markings show the proposed circle for the new areola as well as the central breast excision. The areolar diameter is left at 45 mm.

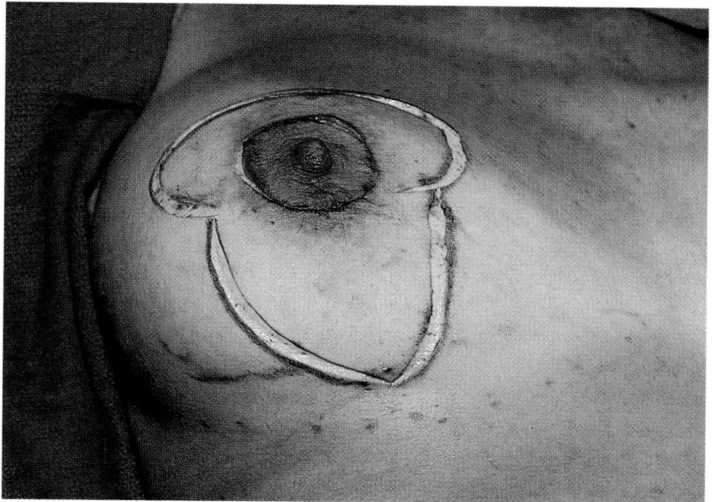

The incisions go around the areola and the proposed skin excision. The upper area is deepithelialized, and the lower triangle will be used for rotation to the central and upper breast region. The two incisions are made for the V.

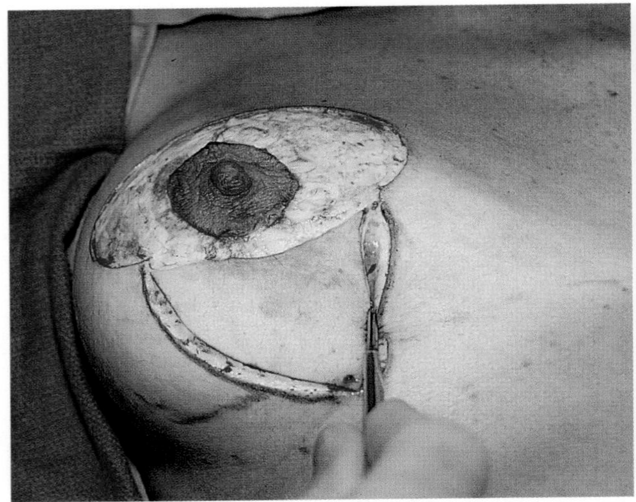

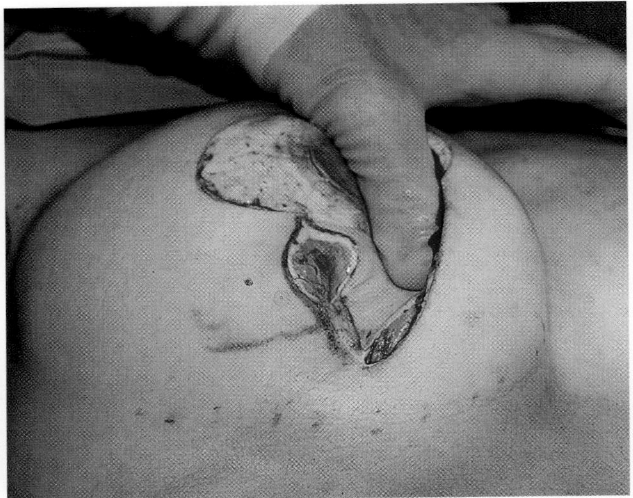

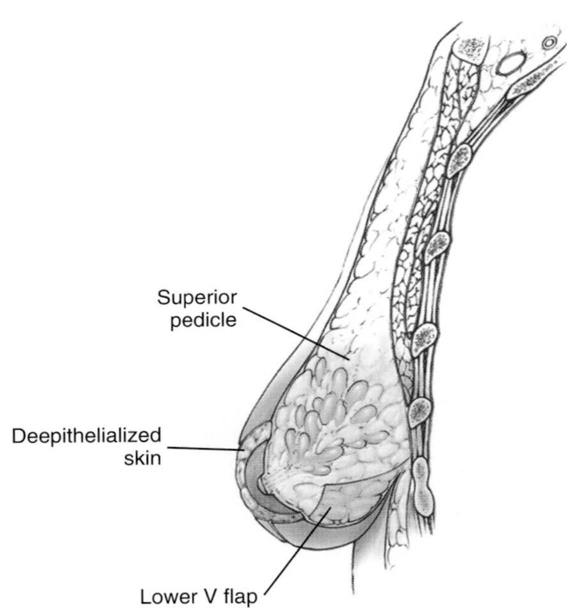

The incisions are made to remove the lower central portion of the breast parenchyma, preserving the breast pillars on the medial and lateral flaps. The pillars will be resutured at final closure. ***The amount of parenchymal excision is determined by the proposed amount of breast elevation and breast parenchymal reduction.*** The incisions are taken down to the external fascia and the muscles of the chest wall.

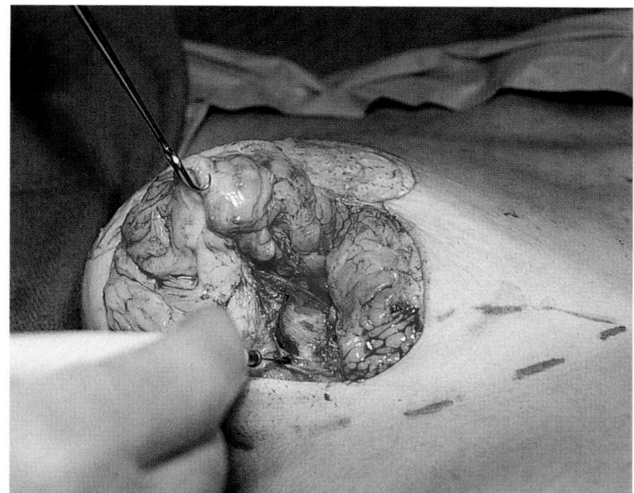

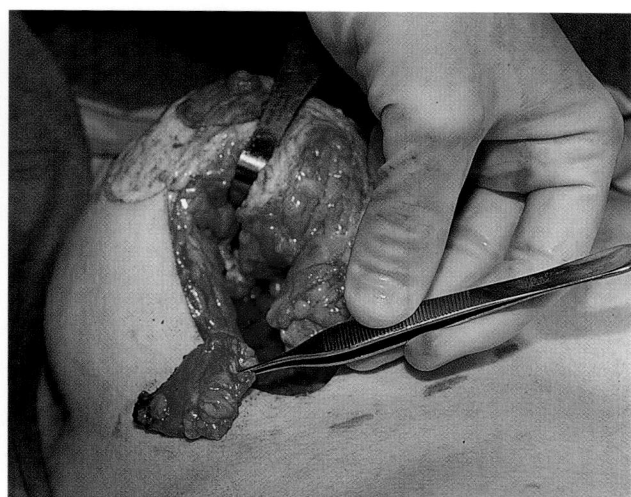

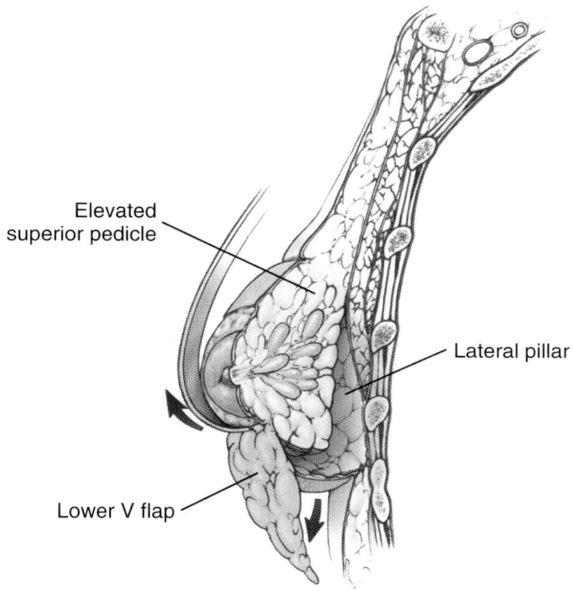

Some subcutaneous tissue is then removed medially and laterally to reduce the vertical length of the pillars of the breast to about 6 cm.

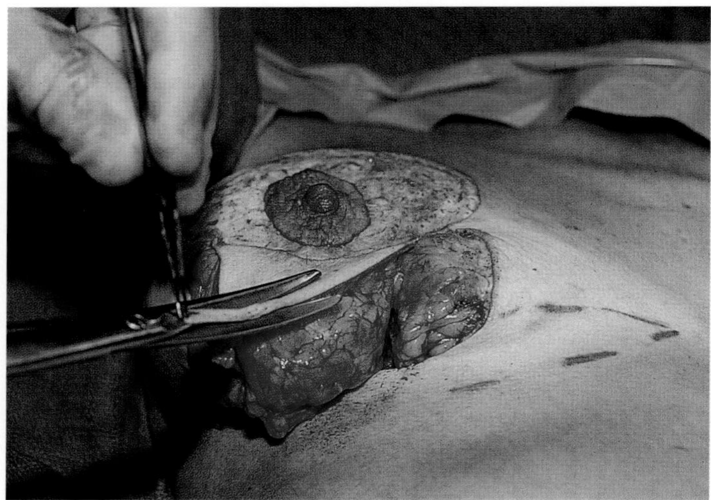

After the medial and lateral resections are completed, the skin over the breasts is deepithelialized.

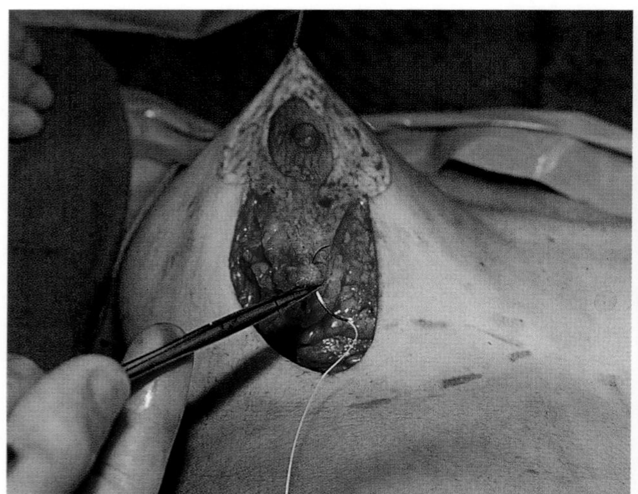

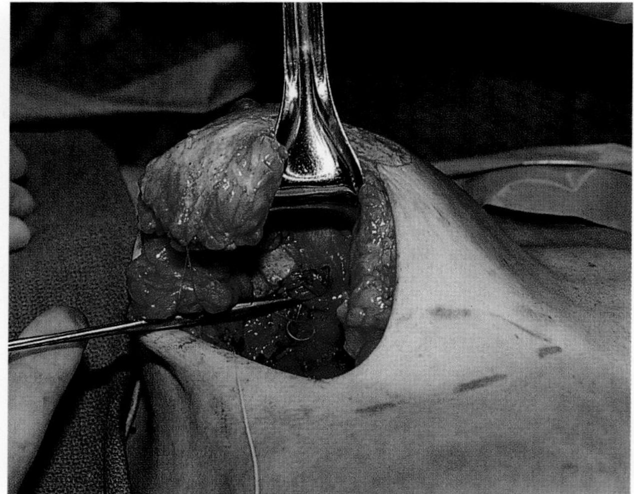

The central V is then lifted and dissected up beneath the breast area and the breast is separated centrally from its attachments to the outer pectoralis major fascia. A suture is placed at the tip of the V and sutured to the pectoral muscle fascia in the upper breast region, rotating this flap underneath the breast to provide additional upper breast fill.

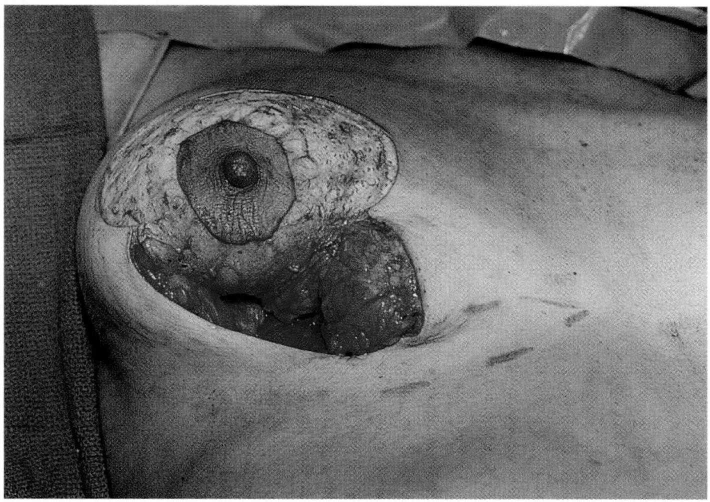

Some additional fullness is noted in the upper breast region following suture placement.

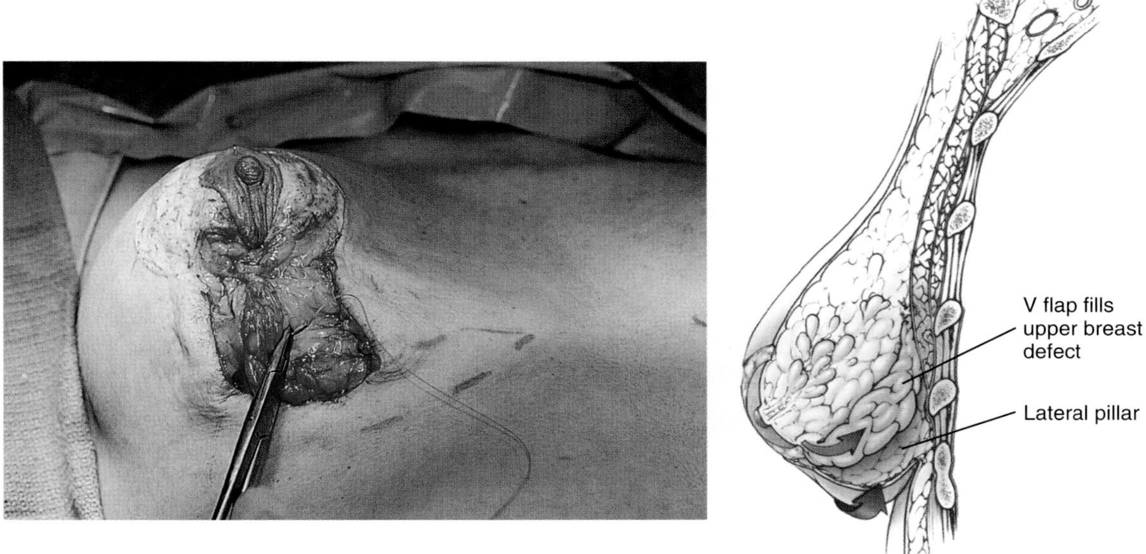

Next the pillars of the breast are closed to narrow the lower breast and to contain the rotated upper breast flap.

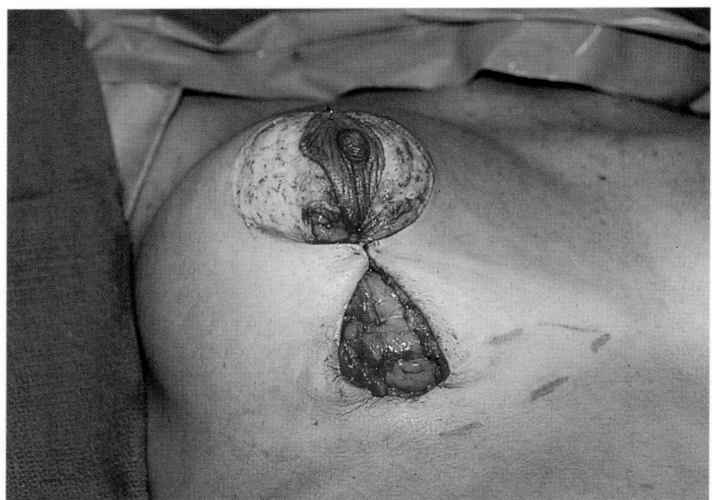

The areolar site is closed to produce the circle for the areola.

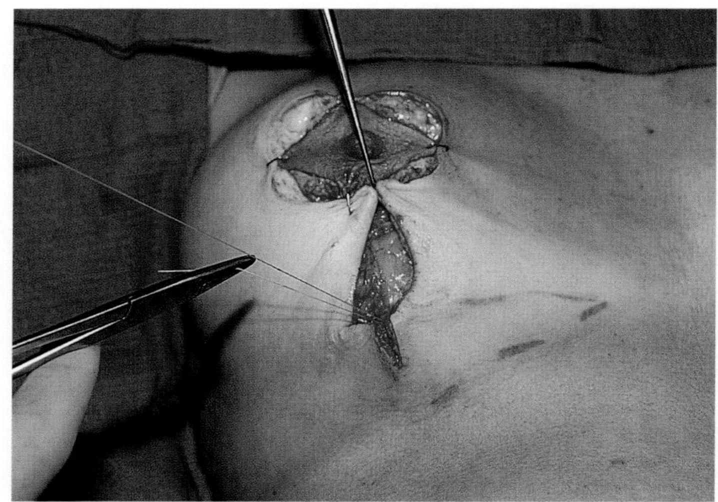

The vertical incision is closed with interrupted 3.0 absorbable sutures followed by intracuticular 3.0 clear PDS to allow shortening of the incision.

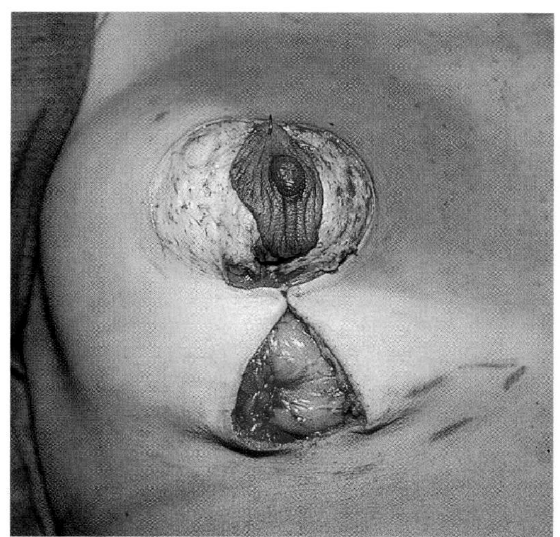

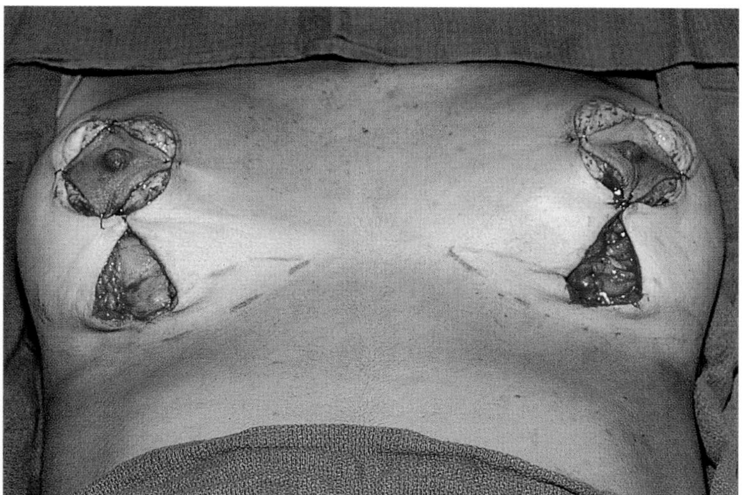

The upper portion of the breasts are shown following closure of the areolar sites. The breasts are checked for symmetry before any additional repositioning or skin adjustment is done.

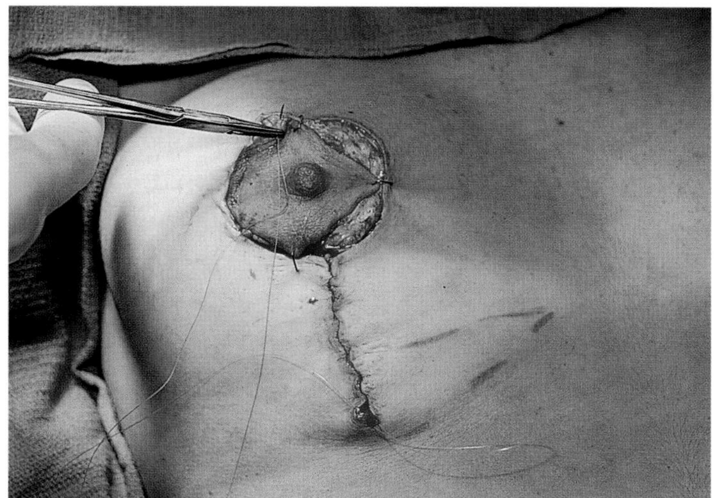

The closure is accomplished with intracuticular 3.0 absorbable sutures in the periareolar region and intracuticular 3.0 PDS below, which can be pulled tight to shorten the vertical scar.

Results

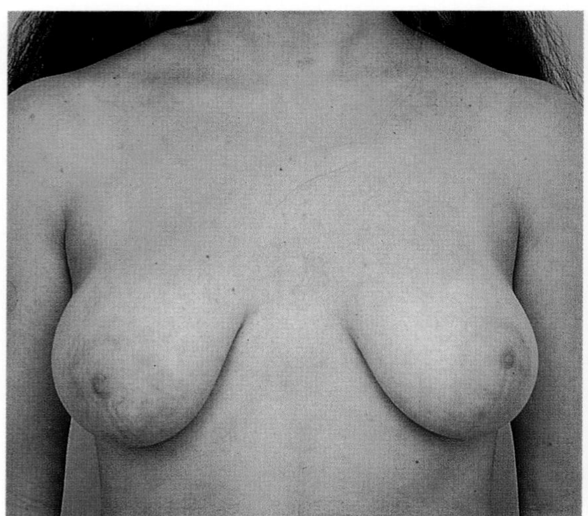

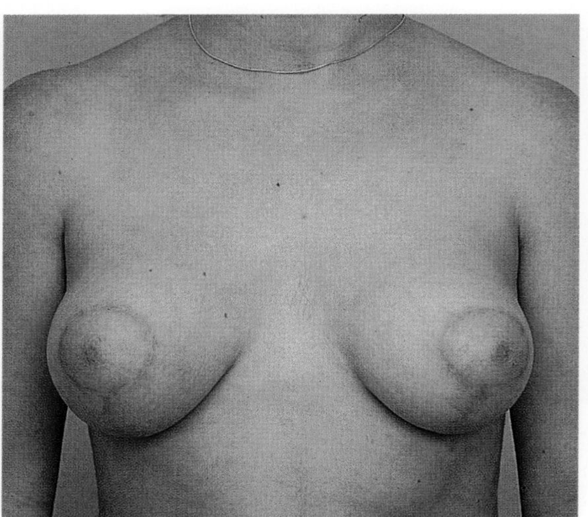

This 25-year-old woman had breast asymmetry and minor breast ptosis. She requested a mastopexy to elevate her breasts with improved upper breast fill. She was in good general health and had no dominant breast masses. She also desired some reduction of her lower breast fullness. A vertical approach was chosen in which some of the lower central breast tissue was removed, and about half of it was used as a flap that was transferred to the upper breast area and turned under to provide central breast projection and upper breast fill. Postoperatively her breasts appear more elevated, her lower breast narrower, and the overall breast contour improved. Additional upper breast fullness is minimal.

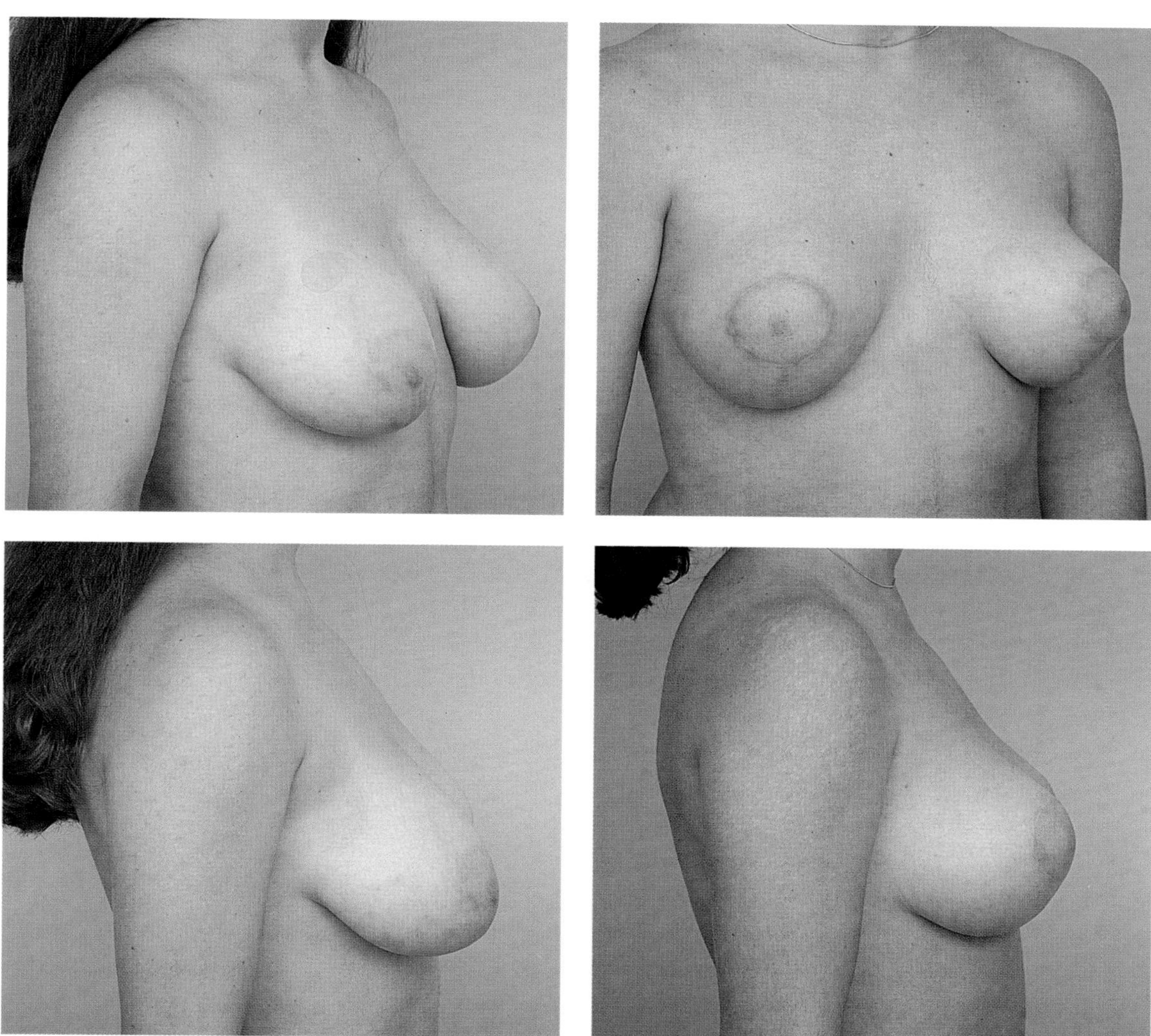

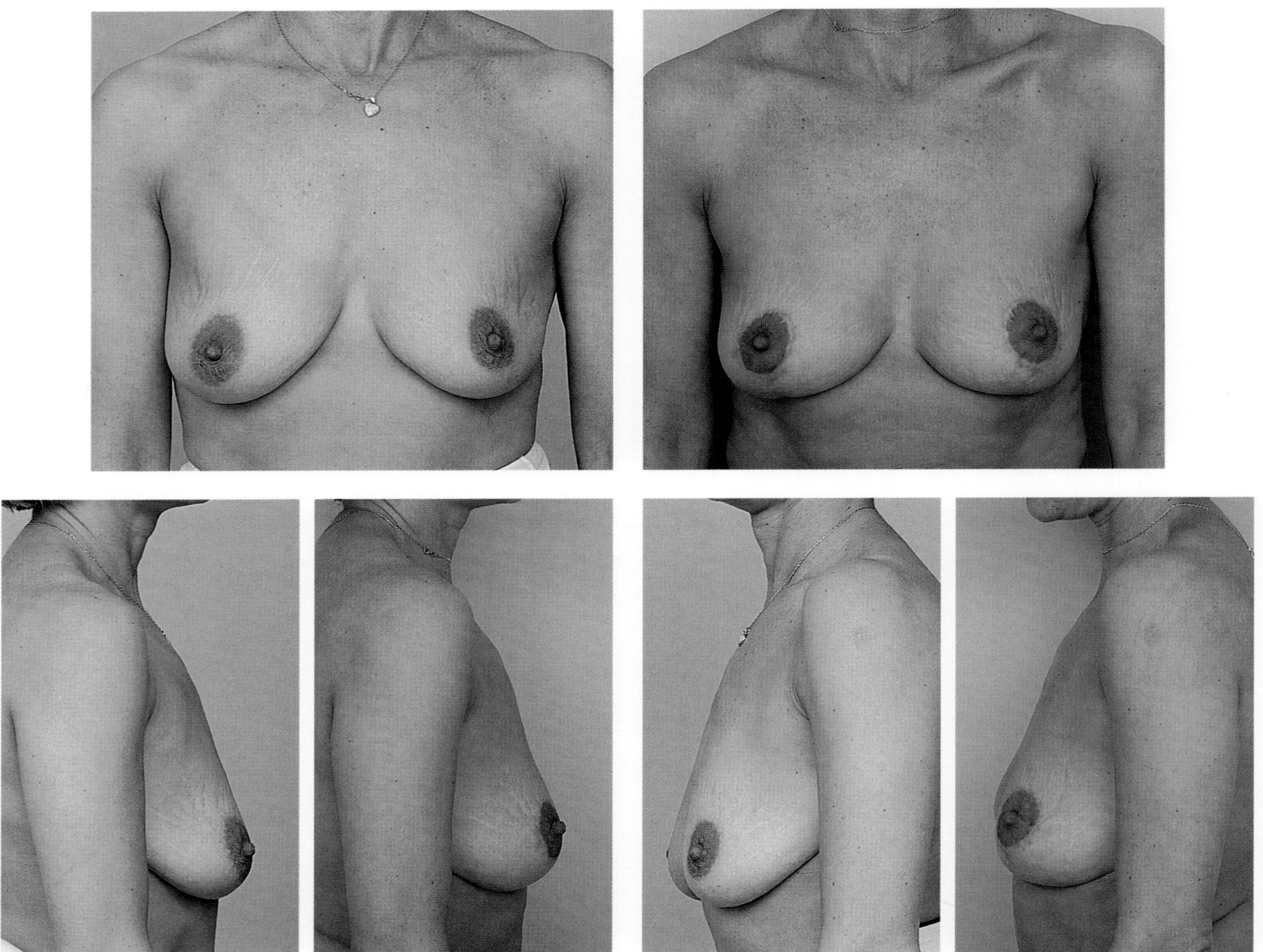

This 44-year-old woman has two children ages 20 and 24. She is very athletic and enjoys excellent health. She sought mastopexy because she disliked her sagging breasts, the low position of her nipples, and the absence of central breast fullness. She wanted her breasts to have a more youthful, uplifted appearance, but she did not want breast implants used. During preoperative discussions I explained that an operation with incisions around the areola and vertically would be necessary, but she could expect only a modest improvement. The patient was determined to proceed. She had bilateral vertical mastopexies.

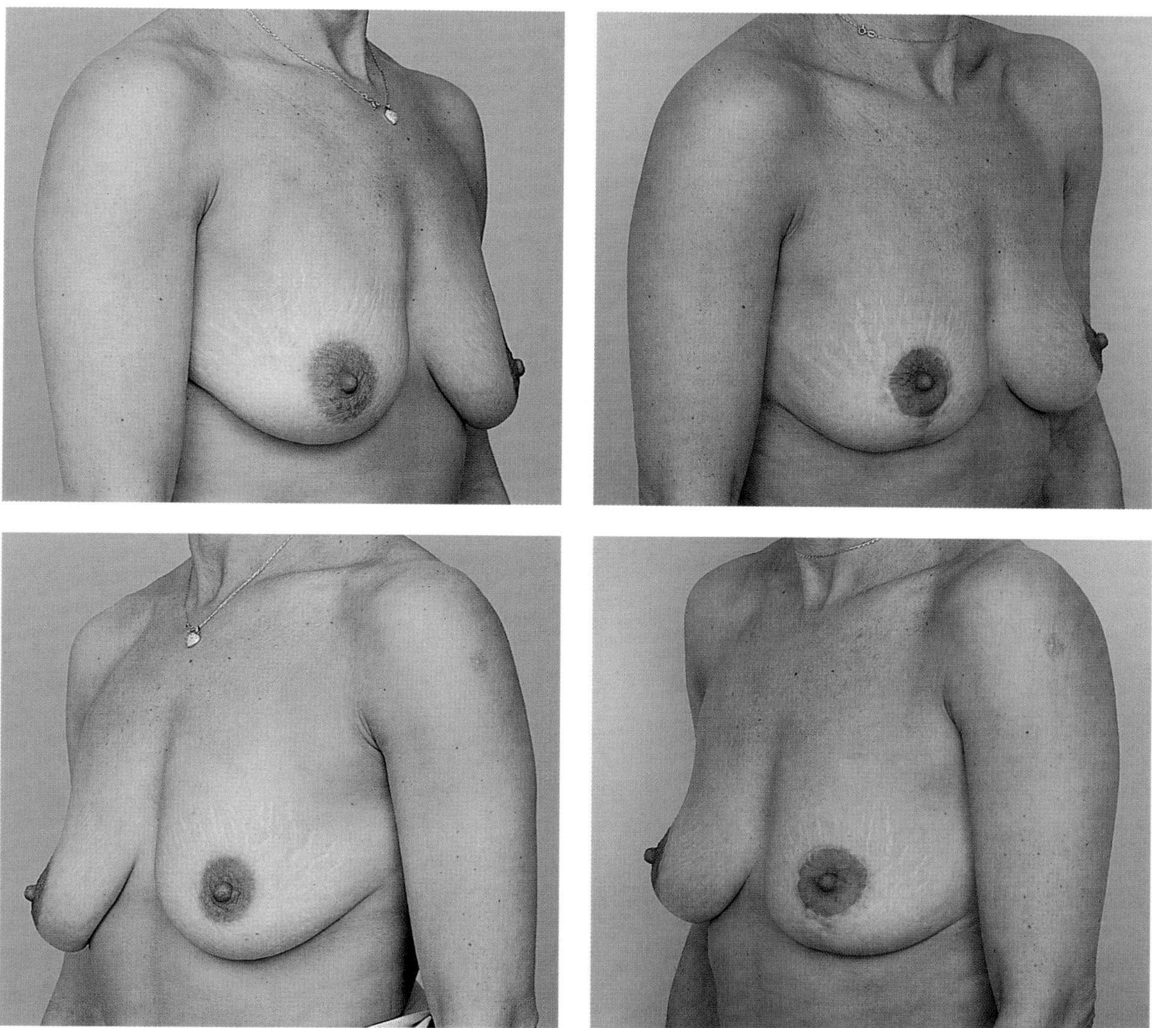

The parenchyma and tissue of the lower V were preserved and turned underneath to produce some additional central breast projection. The nipple-areolae were moved to a higher position; the closure narrowed the breast further, reducing some of the breast ptosis. Breast symmetry as well as the low position of the right areola was somewhat improved by this correction. Two years following the operation the patient is satisfied with her improvement even though the projection could use additional enhancement. We have discussed the placement of the breast implants to create further breast projection, but the patient has declined this option.

VERTICAL SCAR TECHNIQUE AND SHORT HORIZONTAL INCISION

This technique is a variation of the vertical scar technique described previously. I use this technique primarily for moderate ptosis, when the patient's areola to inframammary crease distance is longer than 7 to 8 cm. The short horizontal skin ellipse is preferable to the alternative of extending the vertical ellipse below the inframammary crease. The amount of skin excision depends on the amount of excess skin as well as skin elasticity.

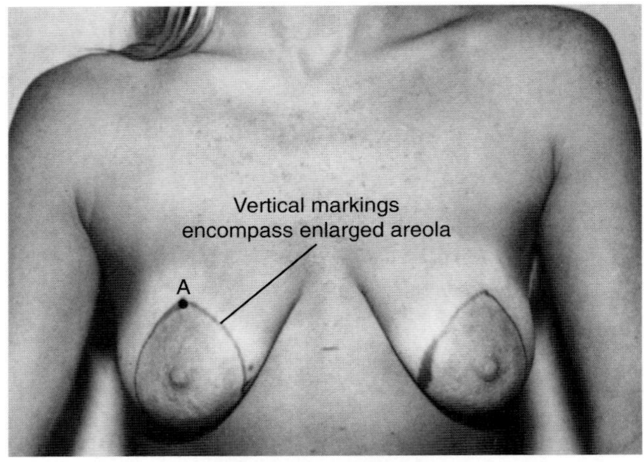

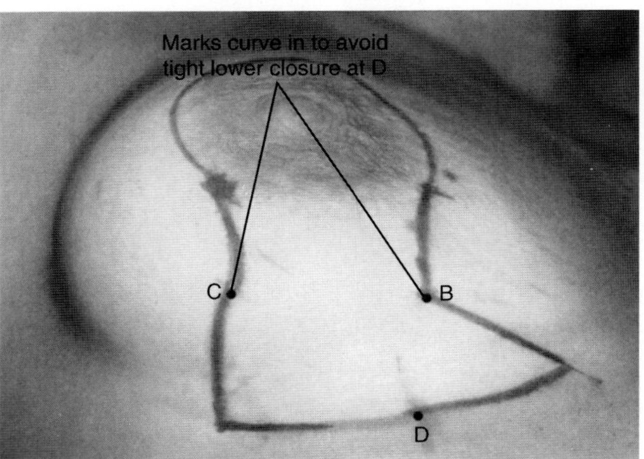

This woman experienced major breast enlargement during pregnancy and breast-feeding. After she stopped nursing, marked mammary hypoplasia developed. She was displeased with the degree of mammary involution, particularly the upper pole flatness, and the enlarged areolae. The plan included reduction of the nipple-areolar diameter, upward elevation of the nipple-areolae, a vertical as well as a short horizontal ellipse to shorten the areola to inframammary crease distance, and a subpectoral breast implant. The initial preoperative markings are shown.

Special considerations for surgical planning*

- Preoperative markings for short horizontal ellipse to reduce length of scar and prevent excess folding of skin
- Planning of vertical limb approximately 7 to 8 cm from areola to inframammary fold to ensure short vertical limb and placement of horizontal scar in inframammary fold
- Use of more traditional inverted T scar for excision of wider, lower skin ellipse to improve breast elevation

Markings and Technique

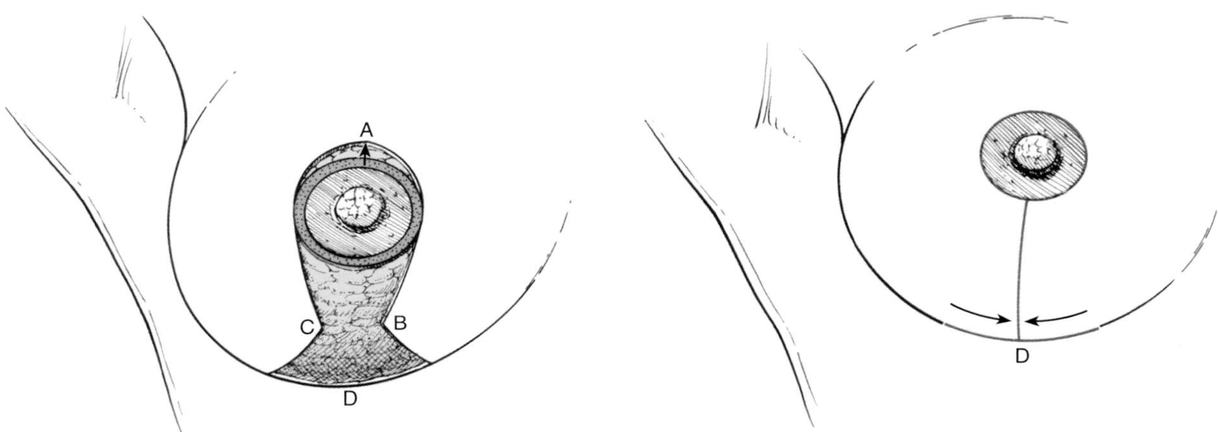

Accurate nipple placement is the first consideration, for it determines the location and extent of the vertical and horizontal ellipses. The amount of skin resection of the lower pole as well as the size and position of the implant also influences these incisions. For this reason I usually make the final determinations as to skin excision after these steps of the procedure are completed. The proposed nipple position is determined as mentioned in the preceding section. When the distance from the future lower areola margin will exceed 7 to 8 cm, then some plan for a lower short horizontal ellipse is made. Markings for the ellipse are conservative; the final skin excision is done after implant placement and parenchymal adjustment.

*Basic planning steps for vertical mastopexy procedure are listed on p. 530.

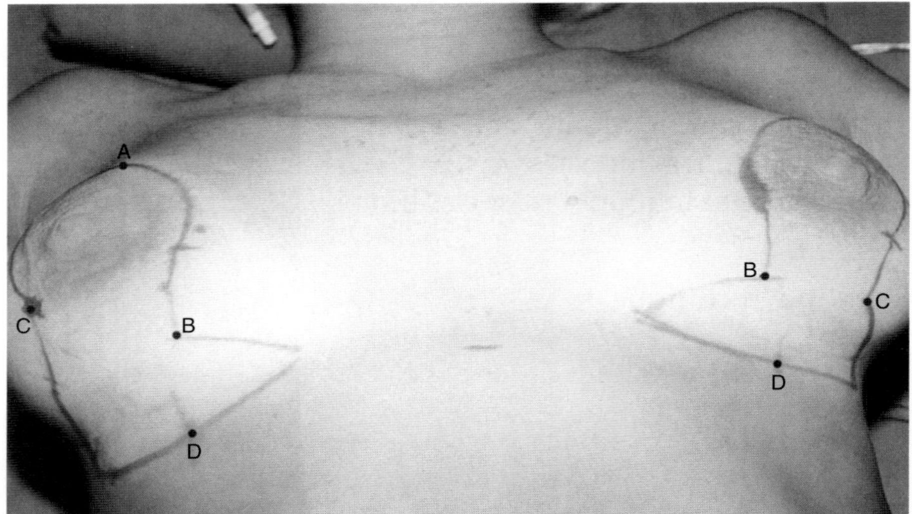

The horizontal component is reduced by excising the vertical portion first and then excising only the excess horizontal skin. Preoperative markings for the standard inverted T pattern can result in a closure that is too tight and leave long horizontal scars. Problems related to too much skin excision can be reduced by tailoring and excising the excess skin to fit the new breast mound.

The incision is made about the proposed new areolar circumference, and the skin of the vertical ellipse is excised. The dissection next proceeds around the lower pole of the breast parenchyma. A subpectoral dissection is made for placement of the implant beneath the pectoralis major muscle above and in the subglandular position below. After the 325 cc implant is placed, the margins of the skin excision are approximated and the nipple-areola moved to the new position. Then the distance is determined from the lower areola margin, and a point about 6 to 8 cm, depending on the implant diameter and breast width, is selected and marked at the inframammary fold. The skin between these two points is the amount to be removed. It is marked out as the shortest possible ellipse, excised, and closed with layered absorbable sutures.

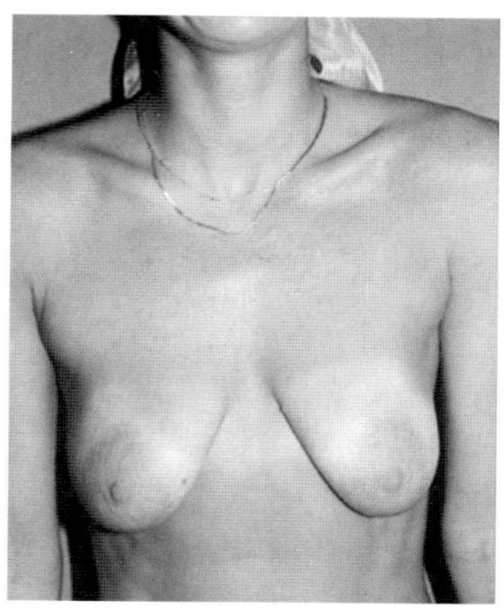
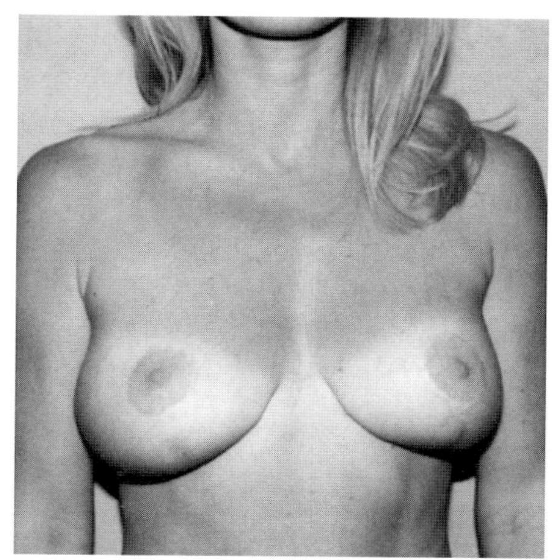
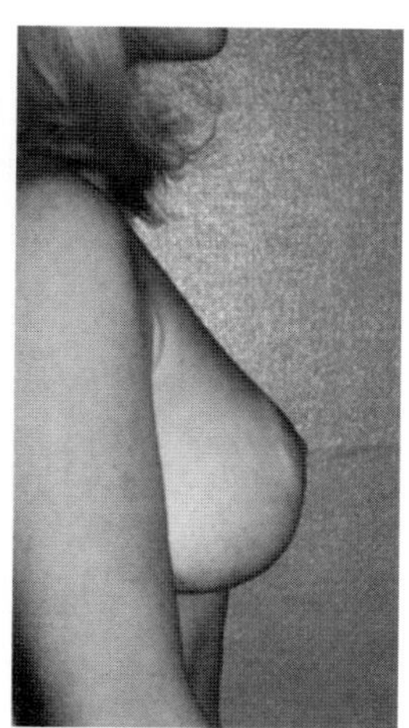

An additional 1 cm wide ellipse was excised from the vertical limb 2 years after the initial procedure. The patient remains pleased with her reshaped breast 4 years following mastopexy, although the large implants have created the appearance of some glandular ptosis.

VERTICAL AND HORIZONTAL SCAR TECHNIQUE (INVERTED T) WITH IMPLANT PLACEMENT

The vertical and horizontal scar technique is used when there is major ptosis, the lower breast area is relatively full, and the nipple-areola requires a relatively long transposition. The technique is similar to superior pedicle breast reduction except that less breast tissue is removed. Patients suitable for this approach often have an acceptable breast volume, but they exhibit marked flattening in the upper breast region and most of the breast parenchyma has ptosed below the inframammary crease.

The surgeon must determine if the patient's breast volume is satisfactory for this approach. This is done by manually elevating the breast to the position the patient desires. If she then desires upper breast fullness, a breast implant will be necessary. Simply tightening the skin over the supporting breast will not accomplish this. If the breast volume is appropriate, I resect the ptotic lower breast parenchyma below the inframammary crease and replace this volume with a breast implant to give upper breast fullness and some central breast projection.

Special considerations for surgical planning*
- Preoperative markings adjusted to accommodate 1 to 2 cm additional vertical and inferior tissue resection to prevent tight closure
- Long-term correction based on lower tissue pole resection
- Transfer of areola on superior breast parenchyma and excision of additional skin after implant placement and before final closure

Markings and Technique

Preoperative markings are similar to those for reduction mammaplasty; however, since an implant will be positioned, I do not mark as much skin for excision. I prefer to excise additional skin after the implant has been placed.

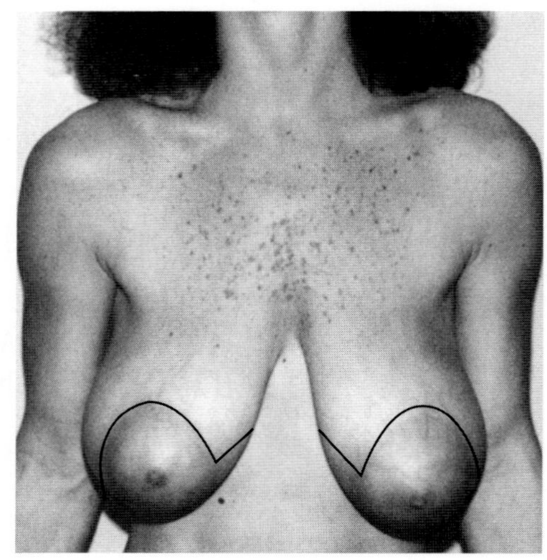

Markings are made with the patient in the sitting position. The point for the top of the areola is about 1 to 2 cm above the inframammary crease, depending on the breast volume. The central V is designed beginning at the point of the areola apex and goes around the nipple-areola to a point approximately 8 to 9 cm below the top of the areola. This is a conservative skin ellipse; additional skin can be removed at the end of the procedure. The markings are then made in the inframammary crease. By displacing the breast first laterally and then medially, lines are connected to mark the future inframammary crease. The new diameter of the nipple-areola circle is drawn, usually 38 to 42 mm. The incision is made around the nipple-areola, and the upper skin within the V markings is deepithelialized.

Next the inframammary crease incision and the future inframammary crease incisions are made. Any ptotic breast tissue below the inframammary crease is excised and the amount recorded. Dissection then goes along the depths of the breast and upward to the pectoralis major muscle, and a subpectoral pocket is created above.

* Basic planning steps for vertical mastopexy procedure are listed on p. 530.

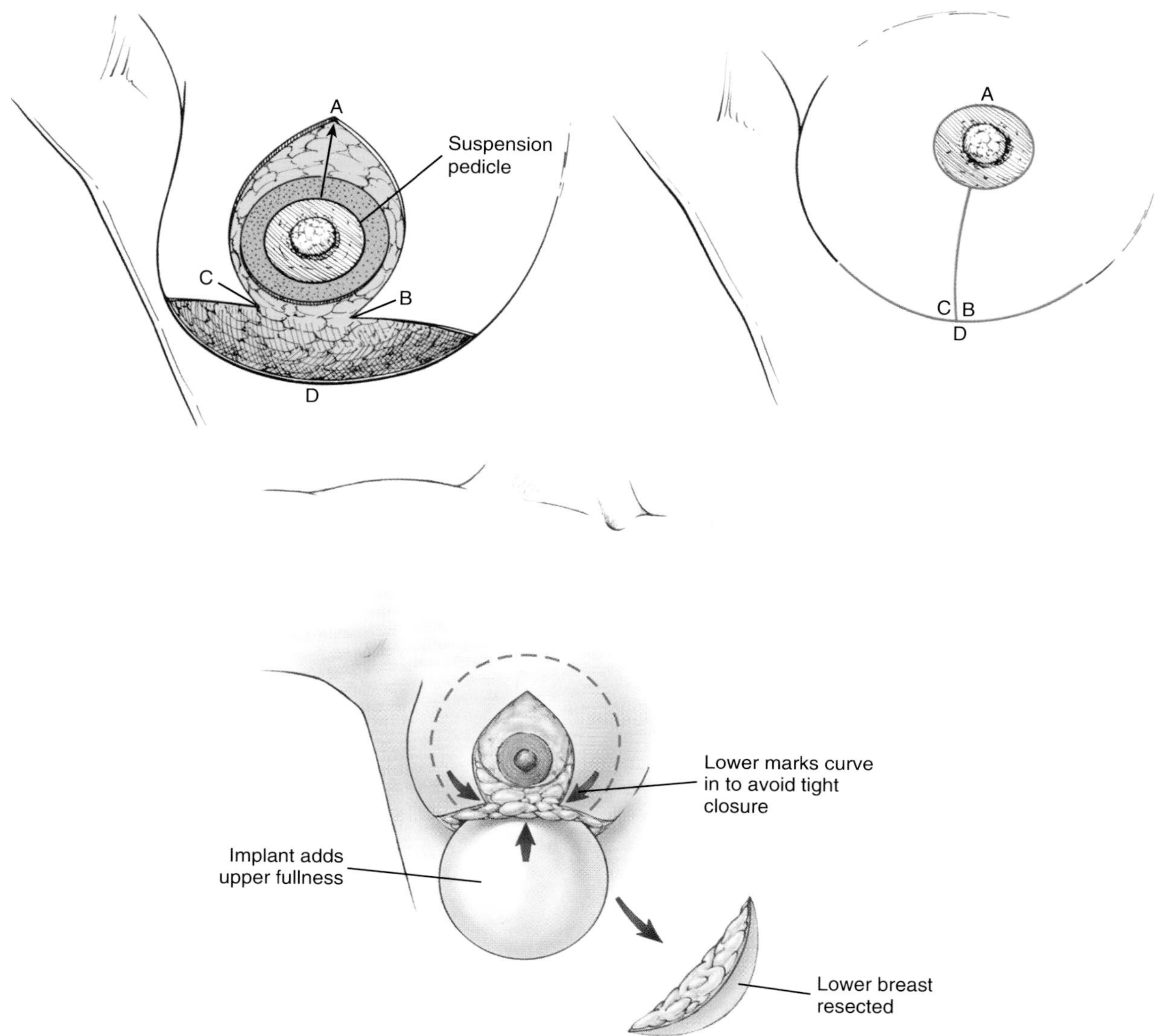

This pocket is expanded medially to accommodate the breast implant when the patient wants significant upper breast fullness. I prefer to use a smooth-surface implant. The implant is selected to give the desirable general fullness in the central breast as well as the upper breast region. Wound closure is accomplished in layers, and the lower breast parenchyma is sutured to the inframammary crease to give good nipple-areolar coverage. An incision is made around the periphery of the V to permit mobilization of the nipple-areola to its new position. The wound is then closed laterally and medially toward the center of the T. Any excess skin along the vertical limb is excised. The incision is closed from the point of the T up to about 5 to 6 cm. The nipple-areola is cut out as a circle with a few millimeters less diameter to avoid a tight areolar closure and a widened scar. The incision is then closed with layers of absorbable intracuticular sutures.

Result

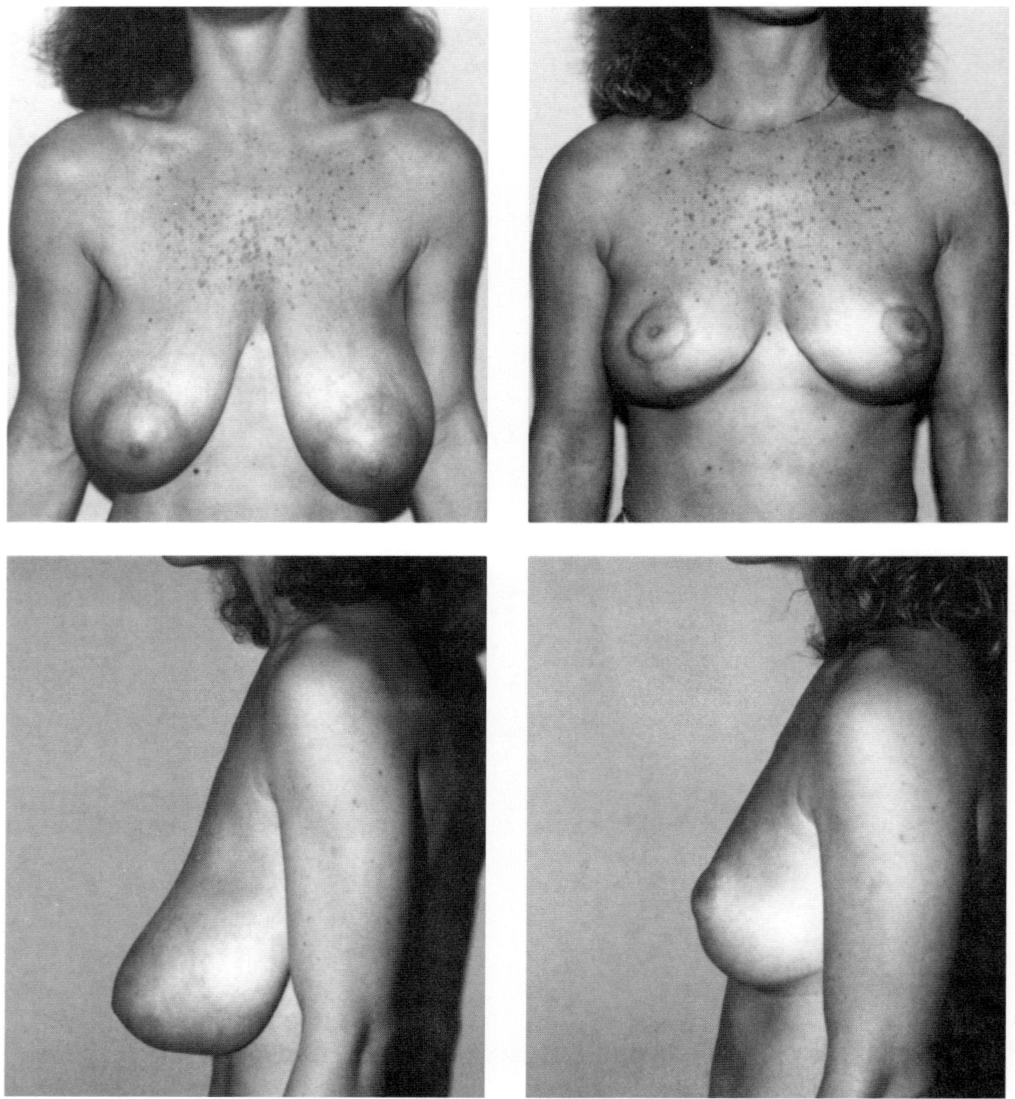

This 24-year-old patient had major ptosis. Although she felt her breasts were somewhat heavy, she was primarily focused on correcting the upper pole flattening. She requested a mastopexy with a small decrease in breast volume. The vertical and horizontal scar technique just described was used as well as a lower pole breast resection of 200 gm. A small 100 cc implant was then positioned in the subpectoral position to give some central breast fullness, and the areola was pedicled on the superior breast parenchyma. The patient is shown 6 months following the procedure. ***Resection of the lower pole tissue is the key to a more lasting correction.***

Postoperative Considerations

Steri-Strips are placed over the incisions and a gauze dressing is secured by a brassiere. I tell patients to avoid arm abduction for 2 to 3 weeks after surgery. I also alert them to signs of a developing hematoma—unilateral pain or swelling—with instructions to notify me if these occur.

Some ptosis overcorrection should be evident during the first few weeks after mastopexy. The breast is usually fuller in its upper portion, and the nipple-areola may be pointing downward. After some of the initial swelling has subsided and the breast has settled, it will fill out below. The final result will usually exhibit less upper breast fullness. When the breast settles, the scars will fade as they heal. Explaining to the patient that this is the normal healing process will make it easier for her to get through the postoperative period.

Any obvious aesthetic shortcoming—nipple-areola asymmetry, volume discrepancy, or implant malpositioning—should be discussed with the patient, a plan devised, and correction scheduled. However, it is usually wise to delay the secondary procedure for 6 to 12 months to ensure the best correction.

Problems and Complications

HEMATOMA

Although uncommon, hematoma is best prevented by careful hemostasis and by avoiding medications that affect platelet aggregation. I rarely use drains for mastopexy. A large, tight hematoma is an indication that the patient should be returned to the operating room for reopening the incisions, reestablishing hemostasis, and resuturing.

INFECTION

Infections are rare but are usually associated with loss of skin at the T incision along with underlying parenchyma. Infection is most often seen in patients with poor vascularity and microcirculation, such as cigarette smokers. Patients are asked to abstain from smoking both pre- and postoperatively for the best result and lowest rate of complications related to tissue vascularity.

NIPPLE-AREOLA NECROSIS

The techniques described here are predicated on good vascularity of the nipple-areola based on the underlying breast parenchyma. Patients with decreased microcirculation, such as heavy cigarette smokers and those with collagen vascular diseases or diabetes mellitus, may be subject to decreased vascularity with minimal breast trauma. Most of the patients I have seen who have problems with nipple-areolar survival after mastopexy have been heavy cigarette smokers with over a 40 pack-year history who continued to smoke in the perioperative period. Care, however, should be taken when considering a periareolar purse-string mastopexy and a subglandular implant. This technique cuts the central parenchyma circumferentially and necessitates wide subglandular undermining to accommodate a breast implant, which can compromise the nipple-areola.

NIPPLE AND BREAST ASYMMETRY

When there is a vertical asymmetry, it is difficult to lower the nipple-areola without leaving scars above the new nipple-areola. Sometimes the nipple-areola looks as if it is positioned too high because of glandular ptosis; this can be corrected by secondary mastopexy with implant placement. If there is an asymmetry of nipple-areolar diameter or an unacceptable nipple-areola, revisions can be made during a secondary procedure. Tissue expansion can also be used to lower the nipple-areola. In this situation the upper pole skin is expanded sufficiently to allow the nipple-areola to be lowered without an incision in the skin above it.

RECURRENT PTOSIS AND "BOTTOMING OUT" WHEN EXCESS LOWER BREAST TISSUE IS PRESERVED

The most common secondary procedure after mastopexy is to address recurrent ptosis. This condition can be anticipated when considerable lower breast tissue is preserved beneath the skin closure and can be delayed by resection of this tissue at the initial procedure. The excision of an ellipse of skin below the areola will correct this problem temporarily.

When the breast parenchyma extends below the crease and the nipple remains in the proper position, an unattractive bottoming-out deformity occurs. This glandular ptosis can be mistakenly attributed to a nipple that is positioned too high on the breast. Correct diagnosis and analysis of the problem are key to a successful revision. A second procedure is required to excise additional breast parenchyma along the lower pole of the breast and resect and recontour the skin over the reduced lower pole. The breast parenchyma protruding below the inframammary crease when the patient is standing upright is removed. (See Chapter 9 for details on reoperation.)

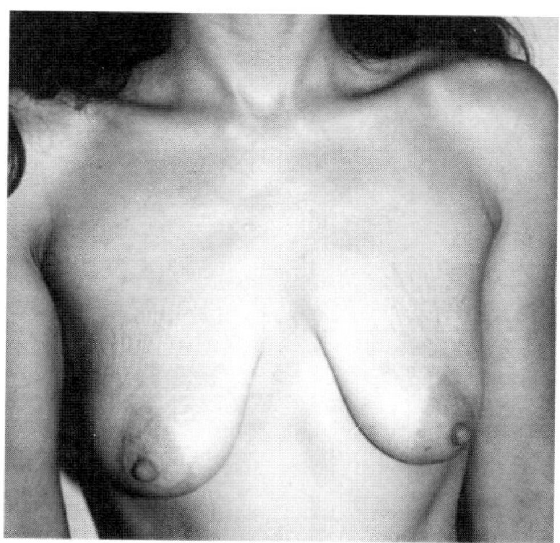

This 22-year-old woman had developmental breast ptosis. Significant additional breast ptosis occurred after the delivery of her first child. She requested mastopexy, but declined breast implants. For this reason it was necessary to excise skin both vertically and horizontally to reduce the skin envelope. Her nipple-areolae were moved up approximately 3 cm.

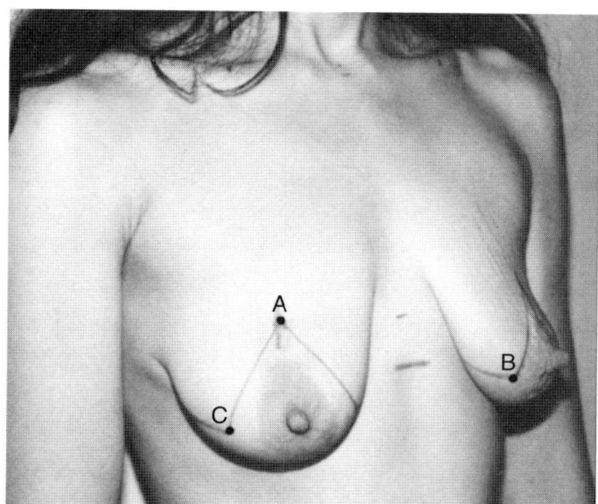

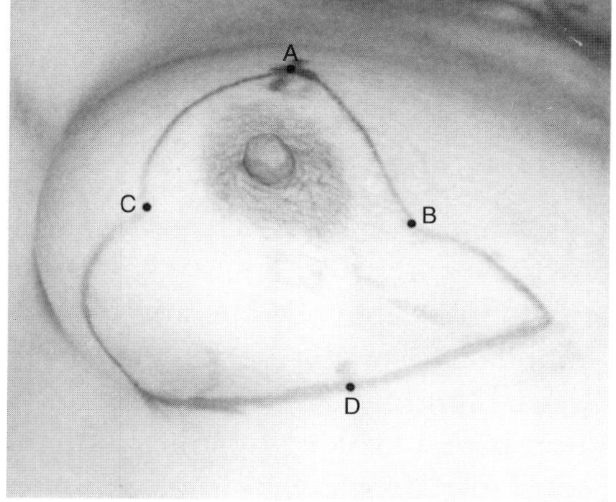

Preoperative markings are shown as well as the proposed skin excision. The top of the areola is made approximately 2 cm above the inframammary fold. This probably should have been lower, as can be seen on postoperative views of the inframammary fold. The preserved central breast tissue will contribute to additional ptosis later on. However, this procedure was done before the vertical approach was developed. Another alternative would have been to use the lower V tissue and turn it into the upper breast region, thereby leaving less lower breast tissue to develop recurrent ptosis. Today a better approach to this problem would be the vertical mastopexy.

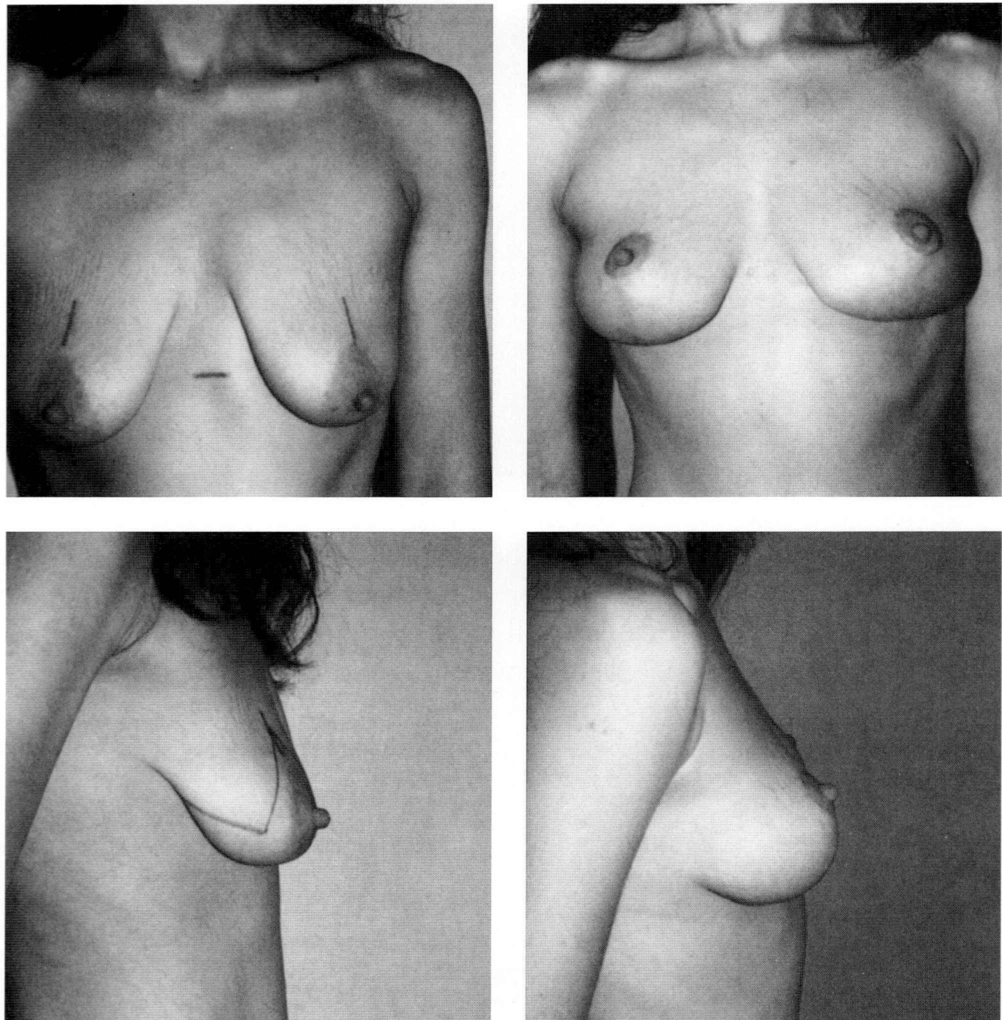

Six months after the operation early recurrence of ptosis is evident, and the nipple-areolae are too high relative to the breast parenchyma. They were placed too high and have not descended with the parenchyma. This condition is best avoided by not making the areola too high and by transferring some of the widened lower breast parenchyma to the central and upper breast region as demonstrated earlier in this chapter.

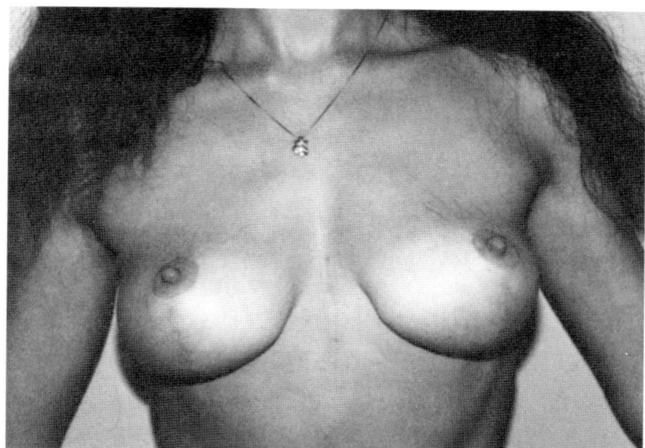

Two years later the deformity has progressed. This is a difficult condition to treat. It is best to avoid positioning the nipple too high. Improvement could be obtained with a small subpectoral implant and some resection of the lower breast skin and parenchyma. This would restore some upper breast fullness and disguise the upward nipple-areola inclination.

UPPER BREAST FLATTENING

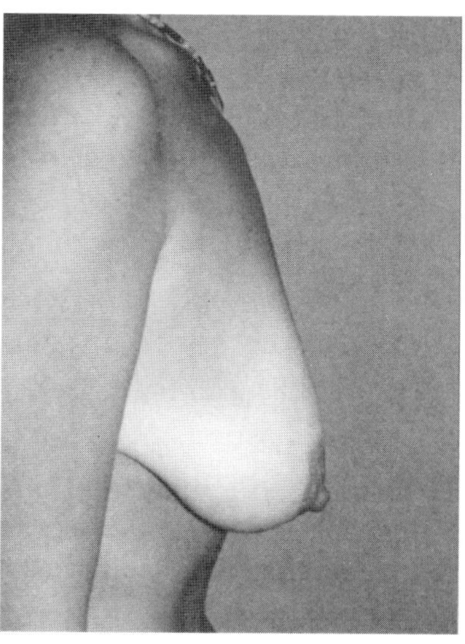

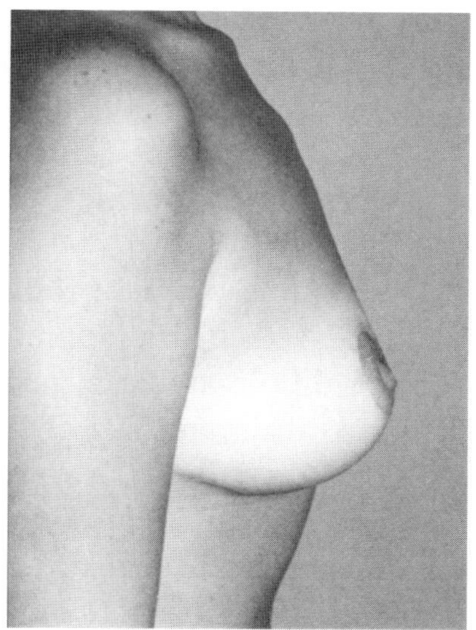

If unassisted by other procedures, mastopexy has distinct limitations. When patients want additional upper breast fullness, I recommend placement of appropriate sized smooth-surface implants in the subpectoral position. Additional contouring of breast tissue on the outer surface of the gland will achieve the appropriate breast volume.

An additional option would be to rotate some of the lower breast parenchyma to the central and upper breast region and also perform a reverse periareolar purse-string mastopexy to bring the areola down. Another option is to use a lower parenchymal flap with the vertical approach and to turn additional tissue into the upper breast region.

IMPLANT-RELATED PROBLEMS

The use of breast implants for ptosis correction introduces the gamut of possible implant-associated complications in addition to the expected sequelae of recurrent breast ptosis and scarring after a mastopexy. ***When a capsular contracture develops after a mastopexy-augmentation, the breast implant within the spherical contracture becomes elevated. An unnatural upper breast fullness develops, and glandular tissue descends over the implant and inframammary fold.*** This deformity can also occur when the breast implant is elevated by a tight closure of the T, effectively preventing the implant from descending low enough. To be effective an implant should remain in a low position behind the breast to contribute fullness in the central and upper poles.

The implant is placed under the pectoralis major muscle in the upper pole of the breast; the lower medial fibers of the pectoralis major muscle are released. In the lower portion of the breast it is positioned behind the gland but in front of the deep fascia. Its lower margin rests at the inframammary crease and is less likely to move upward. A more natural contour for mastopexy-augmentations can be achieved using this strategy, and the implant predictably retains its low profile.

To correct this double-bubble problem when it does occur, the deformity must first be analyzed. If the nipple-areolar position is low, a mastopexy or elevation of the nipple-areola is necessary. If there is ptotic breast parenchyma below the inframammary crease, then this tissue is resected. The capsular contracture must also be corrected. Thus a capsulectomy is necessary after the original implant is removed. If the breast tissue is extremely thin above, then the upper portion of the implant is placed in the subpectoral position. The lower portion of the implant is in the subglandular position so that it will assume a properly low position and not tend to ride up too high above the nipple-areola, but it will give proper upper pole contour. At times, when the inframammary fold is lowered, the lower portion of the implant is under the skin; this discrepancy of implant cover cannot be corrected without a major flap of autologous tissue.

When the patient feels that the breasts are too large after a mastopexy-augmentation, use of a smaller implant is indicated. If there is still too much projection, then a tangential reduction of the outer surface of the breast parenchyma can decrease this projection.

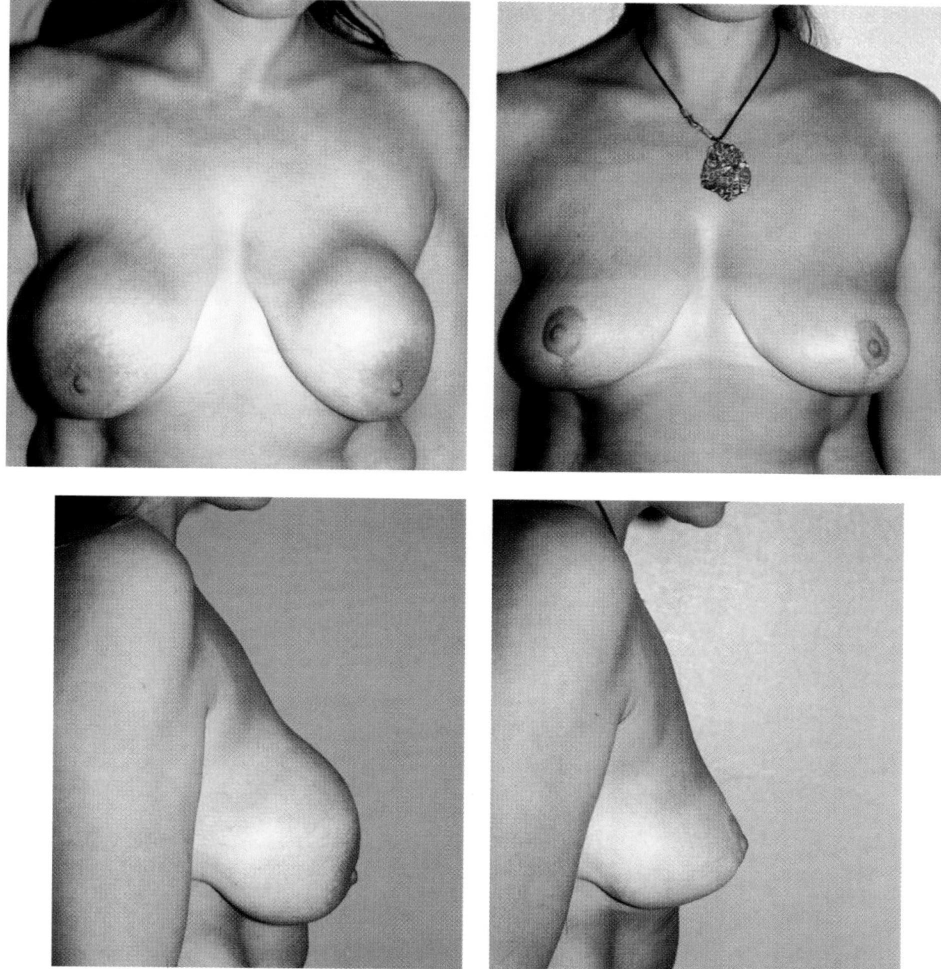

This 28-year-old patient with major ptosis had breast augmentation with implants placed in the subglandular position. Capsular contracture enhanced upper pole fullness and caused further breast parenchymal rotation over the breast implant. This problem was corrected with a vertical and horizontal ellipse and elevation of the nipple-areolae after removal of the implants. Smaller implants were repositioned in the subpectoral position above and the subglandular position below.

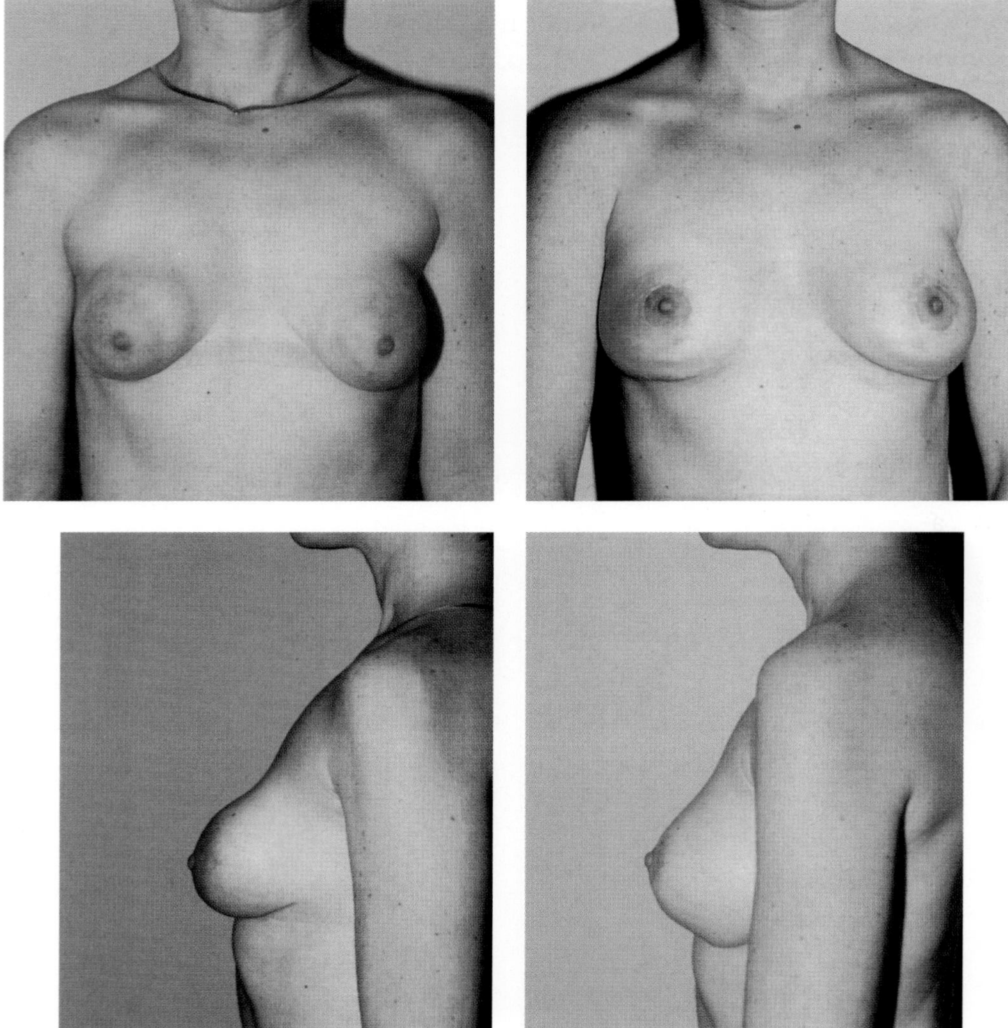

This 32-year-old woman had breast augmentation with 160 cc implants placed in the subglandular position. Her very large areolae, mild breast constriction, some asymmetry, and nipple-areolar ptosis were corrected by reducing the nipple-areolar diameter and slightly elevating the nipple-areolae. A capsulectomy was done and 220 cc implants were placed in the subglandular position. The breast parenchyma was redraped, the nipple-areolae were moved to the new position, and a short vertical closure was done to repair the previous nipple-areolar sites. A new inframammary crease was created about 2 cm below the initial crease to accommodate the larger diameter implants and reduce the appearance of a constricted breast. The patient is shown 2 years following the procedure.

SCARS

Scar revisions are sometimes necessary after mastopexy. Selection of patients who are not prone to hypertrophic scarring and avoidance of a tight closure below the nipple-areola and in a vertical position offer the best conditions for good scars after mastopexy. Cigarette smokers tend to have poor and delayed healing with widened scars. During mastopexy some pigmented tissue may need to be left below the new nipple-areola to prevent the closure from being too tight. This pigmented tissue can be excised later as a secondary procedure. I wait until additional skin laxity develops and resect it as an outpatient procedure. I prefer this strategy to placing a V flap from the inframammary area to relieve tightness.

The most objectionable scars are usually on the extremes of the horizontal incision. It is best to avoid these long horizontal scars; a breast implant inserted at the time of the mastopexy-augmentation takes up some of the skin and permits a shorter incision. Good support of the scars postoperatively with taping and compression helps to prevent healing problems. Pressure over the incisions even with a Steri-Strip can affect wound healing, improve the chances of a thinner, flatter scar, and reduce the likelihood of hypertrophic scarring.

When hypertrophic scarring develops, lidocaine-diluted triamcinolone, 10 mg/ml, can be injected serially within the hypertrophied scar. Higher concentrations of triamcinolone, 40 mg/ml, can actually cause tissue atrophy, thereby thinning the cover over the breast implant. Usually these scars are wide rather than thick; reexcision rarely improves them significantly. If the scars widen or persist, I prefer to continue the postoperative measures just described and delay reexcision for at least 1 year. (See Chapter 9 for information on scar revision.)

Long-Term Results

Mastopexy is generally a temporary procedure and long-term results usually reveal some recurrence of the problem. The use of breast implants to enhance upper breast fullness and take up some of the excess skin and lower breast parenchymal excision have been real advances in improving the permanence of mastopexy.

Mild degrees of breast ptosis can sometimes be disguised with breast augmentation, avoiding the periareolar and vertical incisions required for the traditional mastopexy procedures. By planning mastopexy incisions on a continuum, any additional breast excision or parenchymal excision can be done later. Mastopexy scars tend to improve with time, and if the mastopexy has been closed without undue tension, the scars can become very acceptable. The length of the scars, however, does not shorten significantly, and placement of a breast implant can produce a shorter scar, particularly along the inframammary crease's portion of the T.

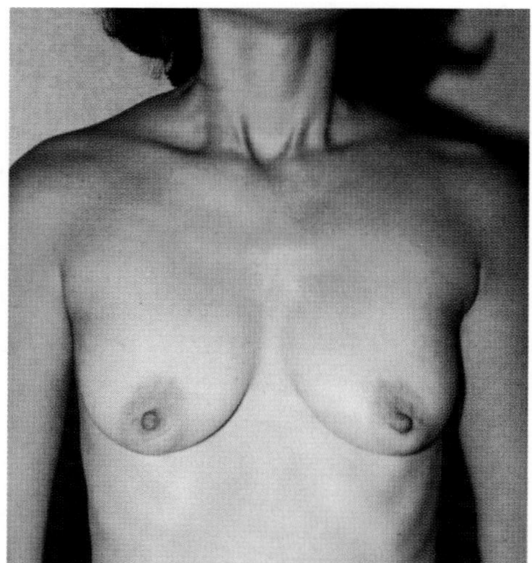

This patient had minimal mammary ptosis and flattening in the upper portion of her breasts. She requested a breast lift and upper breast fullness.

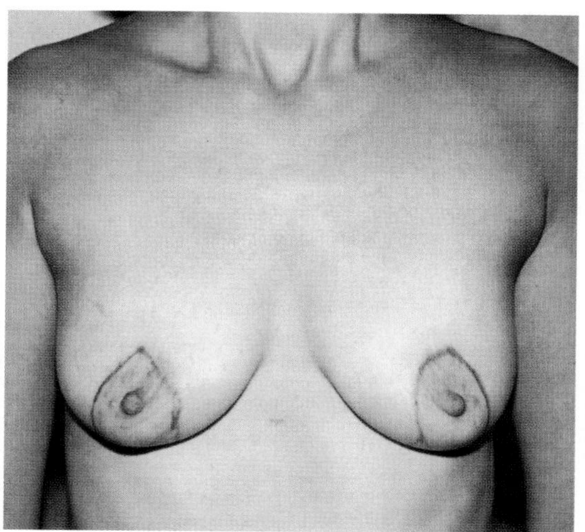

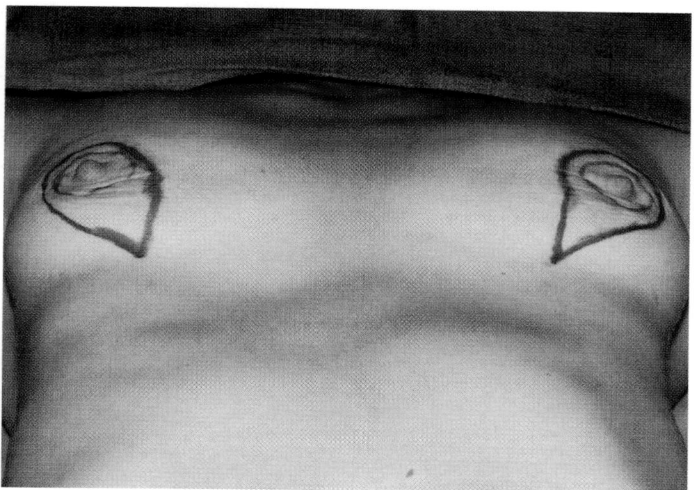

A vertical mastopexy with subpectoral breast augmentation was planned. The nipple-areolae will be elevated on the breast parenchyma. The breast augmentation will be done through the lower vertical scar.

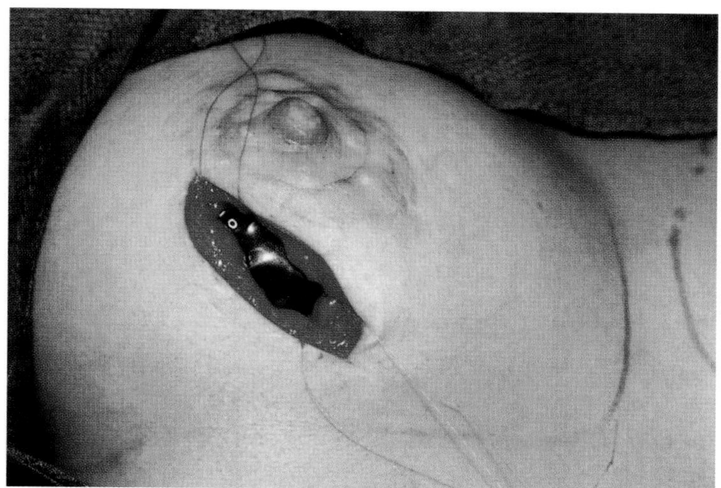

An incision is made through the parenchyma around the lower portion of the breast in the subpectoral space, and a subpectoral pocket is dissected bilaterally. The 220 cc breast implants are positioned to provide upper breast fullness. The deep portion of the wound is then closed; a 4 cm diameter nipple-areola is left, and the remainder of the skin of the ellipse is excised.

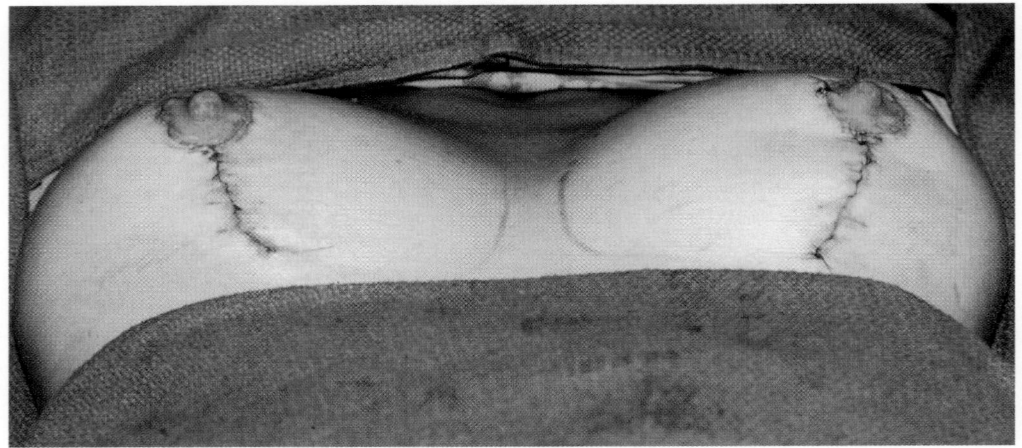

The nipple-areolae are moved to their new position. The remainder is cut out as a circle and closed vertically.

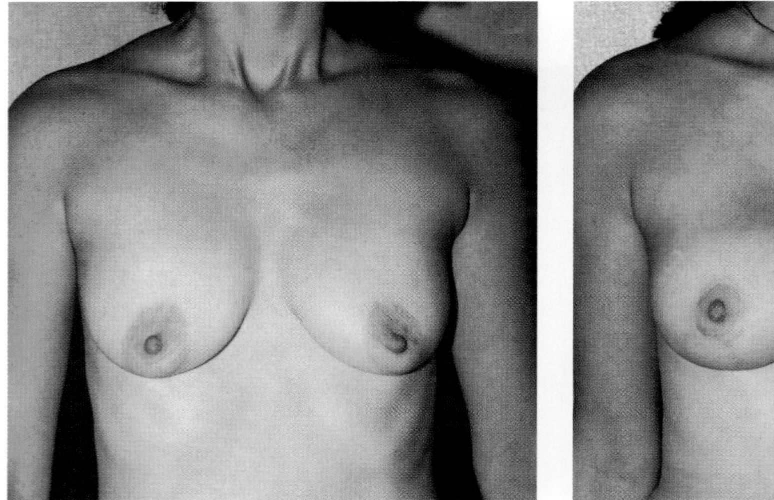

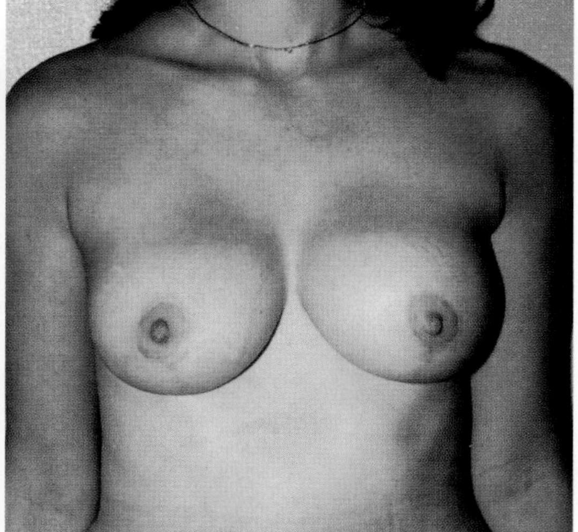

The patient is shown 1 year following the procedure. Note the elevation of the nipple-areolae, smaller diameter nipple-areolae, and additional fullness in her upper breast.

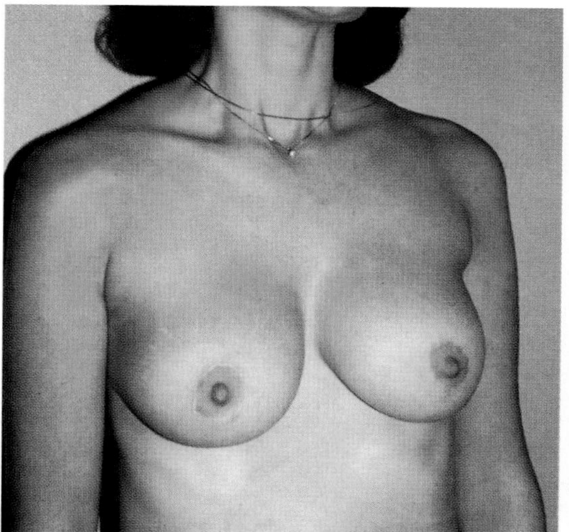

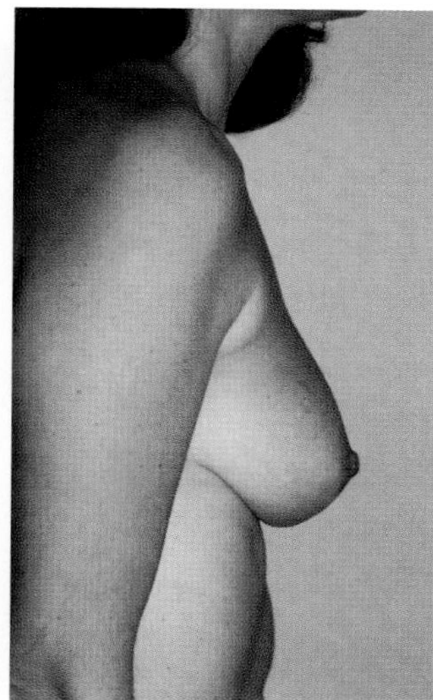

The improvement has persisted 3 years following the procedure. The scars have faded significantly and the implant continues to produce upper breast fill. Although gradual ptosis of the breast parenchyma is evident, this is a predictable sequela of the aging process and is not significant enough at this time to be bothersome to the patient.

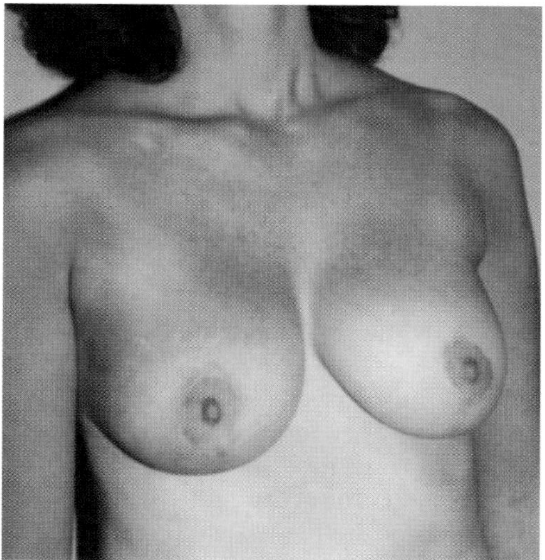

Four years after the procedure she still has enhanced upper breast fullness, although some lower breast tissue has descended below the inframammary crease, and the patient has gained approximately 10 pounds. Lower breast excision at the time of the mastopexy would possibly have delayed recurrence of some of this lower breast ptosis.

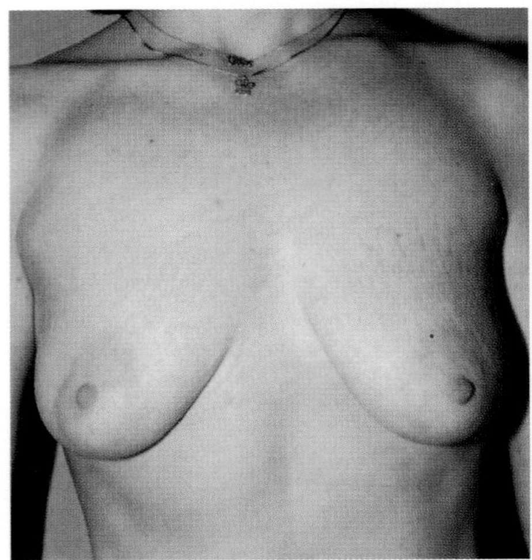 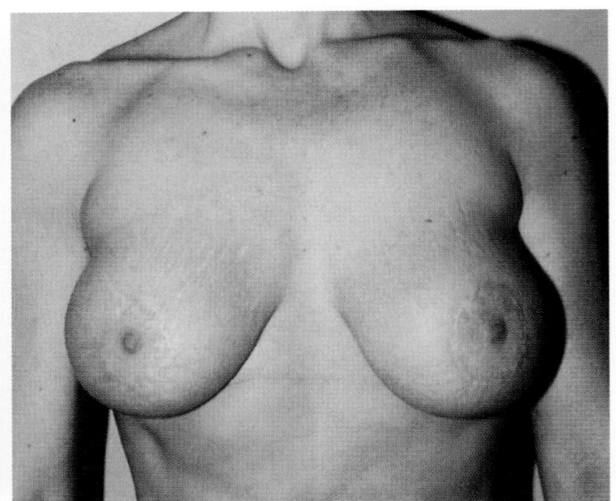

This 28-year-old woman noticed flattening in the upper pole of her breast and some ptosis. Her primary concern was upper breast flattening, and she requested some nipple-areolar elevation. Bilateral circumareolar excisions were used to tighten the central breast region; 260 cc subglandular implants were inserted through this area. She is seen 12 years later. The implants have corrected the breast flattening, but a more definitive nipple elevation would have been helpful, such as a short vertical incision would have produced. In addition some lower breast excision would reduce the breast ptosis beneath the inframammary crease over the long term.

REFERENCES

Benelli L. A new periareolar mammaplasty: The "round block" technique. Aesthetic Plast Surg 14: 93, 1990.

Brink RR. Evaluating breast parenchymal maldistribution with regard to mastopexy and augmentation mammaplasty. Plast Reconstr Surg 86:715, 1990.

Erol OO, Spira M. A mastopexy technique for mild to moderate ptosis. Plast Reconstr Surg 65:603, 1980.

Flowers RS, Smith EM Jr. "Flip-Flap" mastopexy. Aesthetic Plast Surg 22:425, 1998.

Gasperoni C, Salgarello M, Gargani G. Experience and technical refinements in the "donut" mastopexy with augmentation mammaplasty. Aesthetic Plast Surg 12:111, 1988.

Goulian D Jr. Dermal mastopexy. Plast Reconstr Surg 47:105, 1971.

Goulian D Jr, Conway H. Correction of the moderately ptotic breast: A warning. Plast Reconstr Surg 43:478, 1969.

Gruber RP, Jones HW Jr. The "donut" mastopexy: Indications and complications. Plast Reconstr Surg 65:34, 1980.

Hagerty RC. External mastopexy with imbrication following explantation. Plast Reconstr Surg 103: 976, 1999.

Kahn S, Hoffman S, Simon BE. Correction of nonhypertrophic ptosis of the breasts. Plast Reconstr Surg 41:244, 1968.

Lassus C. A 30-year experience with vertical mammaplasty. Plast Reconstr Surg 97:373, 1996.

Lejour M. Evaluation of fat in breast tissue removed by vertical mammaplasty. Plast Reconstr Surg 99:386, 1997.

Lejour M. Vertical mammaplasty and liposuction of the breast. Plast Reconstr Surg 94:100, 1994.

Lejour M. Vertical Mammaplasty and Liposuction. St. Louis: Quality Medical Publishing, 1994.

Leone MS, Franchelli S, Berrino P, Santi PL. Vertical mammaplasty: A personal approach. Aesthetic Plast Surg 21:356, 1997.

Marconi F. The dermal pursestring suture: A new technique for a short inframammary scar in reduction mammaplasty and dermal mastopexy. Ann Plast Surg 22:484, 1989.

Mladick RA. Mastopexy after explantation. Plast Reconstr Surg 103:330, 1999.

Owsley JQ Jr. Simultaneous mastopexy and augmentation for correction of the small, ptotic breast. Ann Plast Surg 2:195, 1979.

Peled IJ. Periareolar subcuticular pursestring suture. Plast Reconstr Surg 103:1094, 1999.

Rees TD, Aston SJ. The tuberous breast. Clin Plast Surg 3:339, 1976.

Regnault P Breast ptosis. Definition and treatment. Clin Plast Surg 3:193, 1976.

Regnault P. The hypoplastic and ptotic breast: A combined operation with prosthetic augmentation. Plast Reconstr Surg 37:31, 1966.

Rohrich RJ, Beran SJ, Restifo RJ, Copit SE. Aesthetic management of the breast following explantation: Evaluation and mastopexy options. Plast Reconstr Surg 101:827, 1998.

Spear SL, Kassan M, Little JW. Guidelines in concentric mastopexy. Plast Reconstr Surg 85:961, 1990.

Tapia A, Blanch A, Salvador J, Prat J, Albert I. Evolution of the vertical scar in Lejour's mastopexy technique. Aesthetic Plast Surg 20:377, 1996.

Whidden PG. The tailor-tack mastopexy. Plast Reconstr Surg 62:347, 1978.

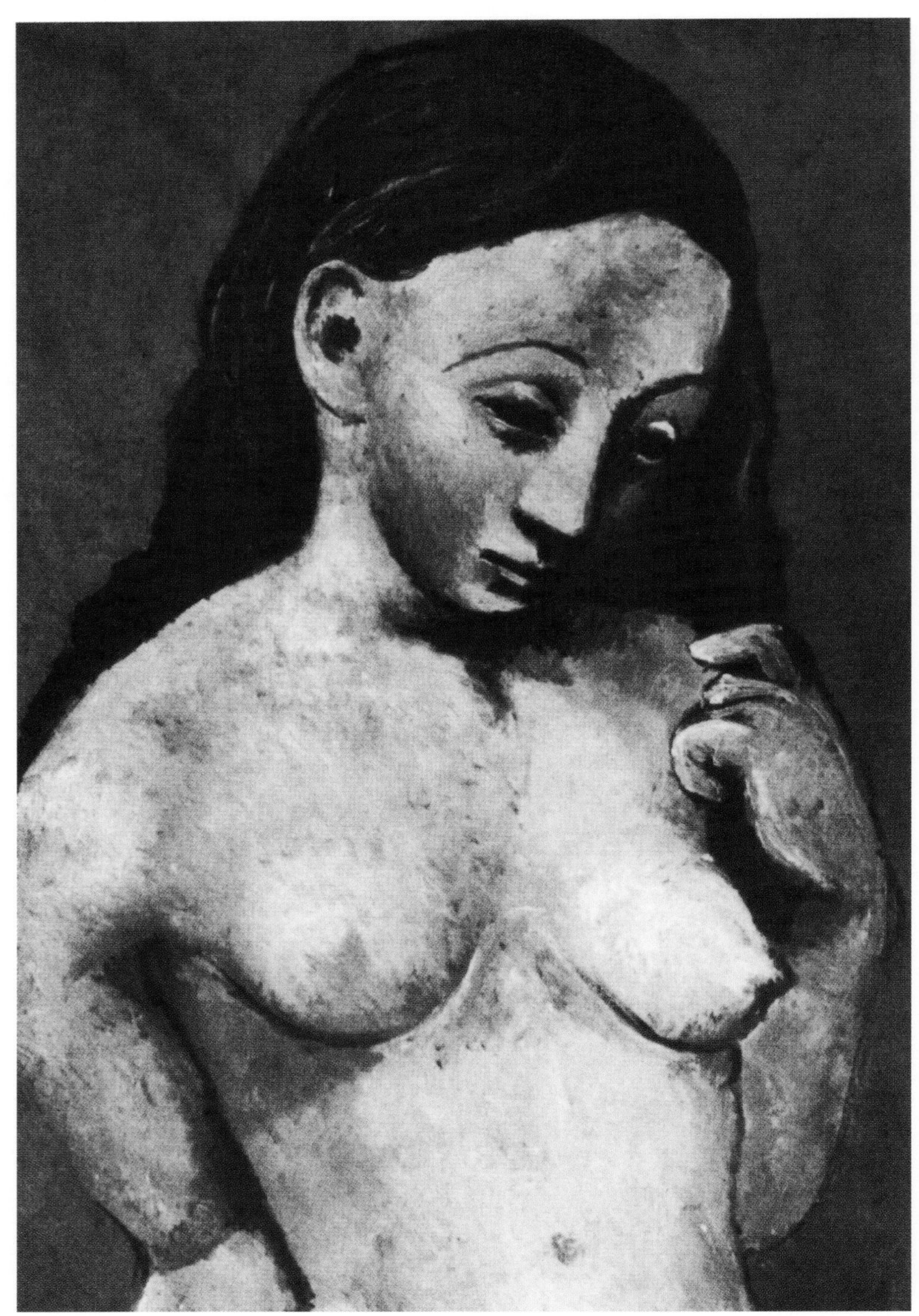

9 Aesthetic Problems

Key Topics

Axillary Breasts

Submammary Breasts

Gynecomastia

Symmastia With Breast Implants

Constricted Breasts

Nipple Problems

Chest Wall Abnormalities

Low Inframammary Fold

Breast Asymmetry

Reoperative Aesthetic Breast Surgery

Scarring After Aesthetic Breast Surgery

Observations

Some aesthetic breast problems defy categorization and simple solution. They transcend the more commonly treated aesthetic breast deformities discussed in previous chapters and require a more advanced level of decision making. Axillary and submammary breasts, gynecomastia, constricted breasts, and nipple problems pose particular challenges, as do chest wall abnormalities and breast asymmetries. Ingenuity is required when reoperation is necessary for surgical revision. Some of these patients have already had multiple operations. Implant problems may extend beyond exchanging or repositioning of implants. Long-standing complications may have left the implant envelope thinned and subject to rupture, or the tissues may be severely compromised by repeated efforts to treat capsular contracture. Patient concerns over implants, dissatisfaction with results, or persistent complications may require permanent explantation with the need for subsequent corrections or tissue replacement to prevent breast deformity. In these situations a mixing and matching of techniques are often required to produce the best aesthetic results. Augmentation may need to be converted to mastopexy-augmentation. Endoscopic techniques may be needed to minimize incisions or ultrasound-assisted liposuction to liquefy and cavitate dense parenchyma. Customized implants or implant removal may be indicated. Even reconstructive techniques may be necessary to produce the best results. The surgeon needs to be well versed with a variety of different techniques to be able to individualize treatment to solve these complex aesthetic problems.

Axillary Breasts

Breasts can develop anywhere along the embryologic breast line. One of the most common sites is the axilla. Axillary breasts are distressing to the patient; they have an unnatural upper outer breast and axillary fullness. This condition can be associated with normal, hyperplastic, or hypoplastic breasts.

To improve the appearance of axillary breasts the axillary breast tissue can be excised directly using a transverse ellipse in the axilla. If breast hypoplasia coexists, the same axillary incision can then be used to place a breast implant in the submusculofascial position. When the patient has breast hypertrophy, this axillary fullness is often accentuated. For these patients I usually reduce their breasts through an inverted T incision but use a separate axillary incision to remove redundant axillary tissue or use liposuction or ultrasound-assisted liposuction to reduce this fullness as well as any lateral fullness that is present. Care must be taken to preserve the sensory nerves, especially the intercostobrachial nerve that innervates the upper inner arm. Standard liposuction is also helpful for less severe deformities.

Patient Example

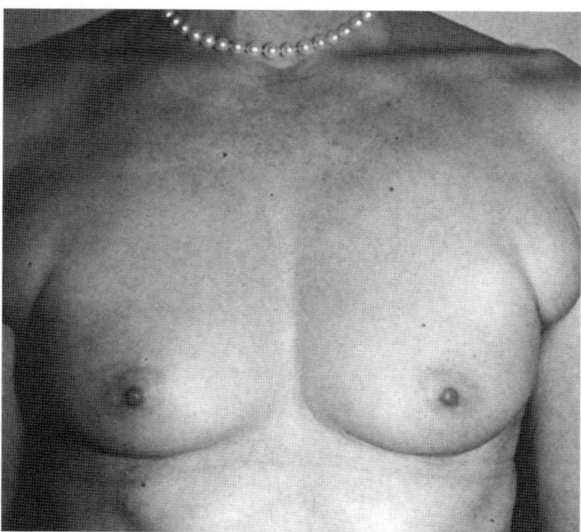

This patient was concerned about an abnormal fullness in her axillary and upper lateral chest region. On mammography this fullness was shown to be breast tissue, but there was no indication of a premalignant condition. Examination demonstrated significant axillary fullness extending from the upper outer quadrant of her breast. This condition was visible in sports clothing and produced an unattractive fullness anterior to the axilla and under the arm. A total of 150 gm of tissue was excised from the axillary region through a horizontal incision in the axilla. It is important to understand breast and axillary anatomy in this area to ensure that the intercostobrachial nerve is preserved when dissecting the axillary breast parenchyma.

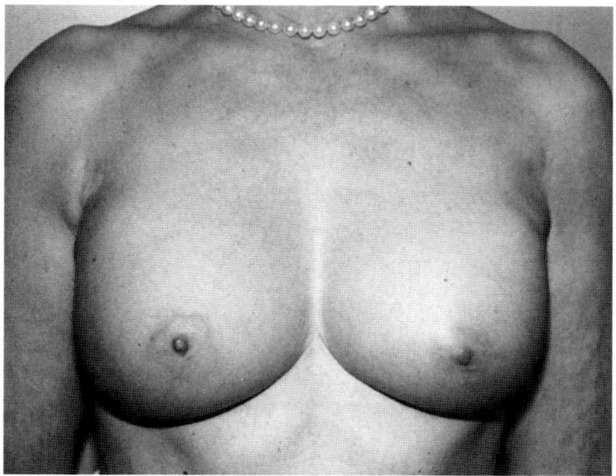

Note the results 2 years after excision of the axillary breast tissue through a transverse incision. A 300 cc subpectoral implant was positioned during the same procedure using the axillary approach.

Submammary Breasts

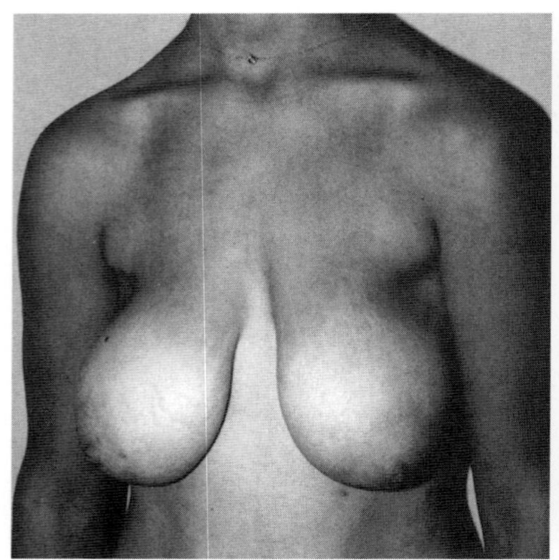

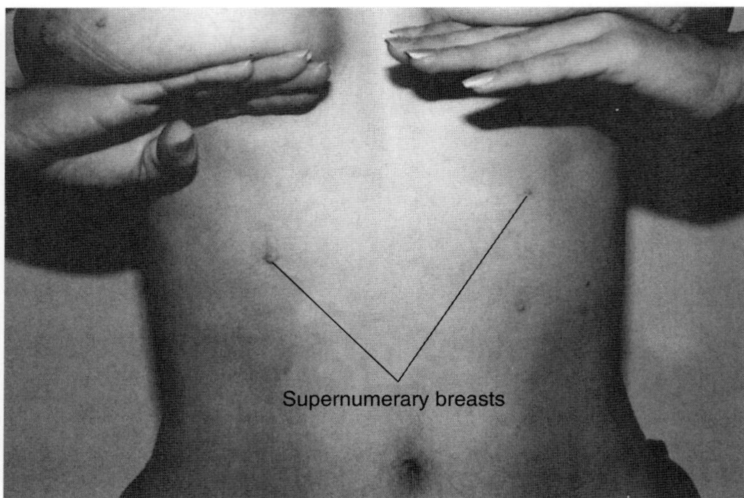

Some patients have supernumerary breasts either below the inframammary crease or in the axilla. Since these breasts can function during pregnancy or other periods of hormonal activity or may be the site for breast cancer, I recommend that they be excised when the patient has any concerns about them. They often have a remnant of nipple and areola, and I usually excise the breast tissue through this incision.

Gynecomastia

Gynecomastia is enlargement of the male breast and is a common problem. Drugs, medications, hormonal imbalances (especially the estrogen/testosterone ratio), genetic conditions, and exogenous hormones can all cause this condition.

During puberty it is normal for most boys to develop some proliferation of breast parenchyma. Ordinarily this condition is self-limited and subsides within 6 to 18 months. When gynecomastia persists, usually in both breasts or occasionally in one breast, it is often embarrassing and psychologically debilitating. Removing the excess breast parenchyma is the only effective treatment.

Gynecomastia

Physiologic	**Increased Estrogen**	**Drugs**
Puberty	Testicular tumors	Alcohol
Elderly	Estrogen	Amphetamines
Familial	Diethylstilbestrol	Chemotherapeutic agents
Idiopathic	Androgens	Cimetidine
		Digitalis
Systemic Conditions	**Decreased Testosterone**	Haldol
Obesity	Klinefelter's syndrome	Hydroxyzine
Renal failure	Chronic illness	Isoniazid
Hemodialysis	Orchiectomy	Methyldopa
Hyperthyroidism		Marijuana
Hypothyroidism		Opiates
Liver disease		Phenothiazines
Adrenal tumors		Progestins
Hermaphroditism		Reserpine
		Spironolactone
		Tricyclic antidepressants

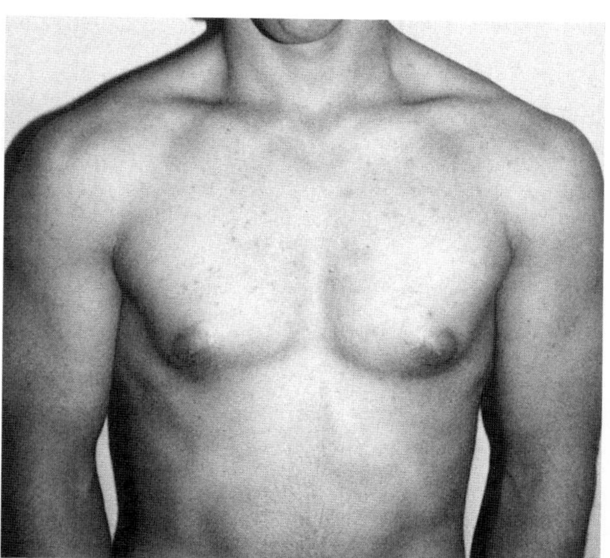

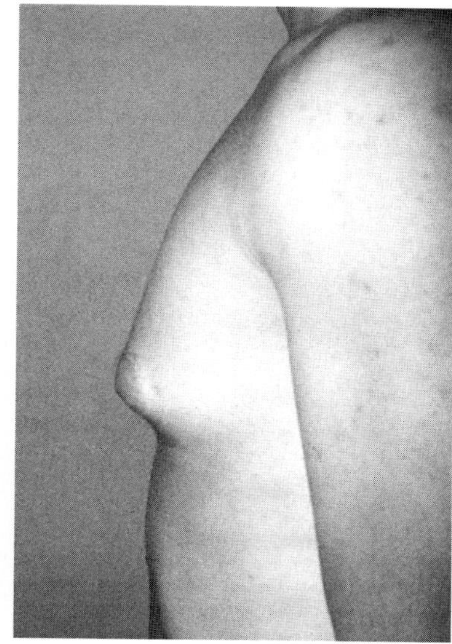

This 18-year-old man had pubertal gynecomastia. His breasts had a feminine appearance, and dense breast parenchyma was present in the subnipple region. He was psychologically troubled by this condition, which made him reticent in social situations if there was a possibility that his breasts would be revealed.

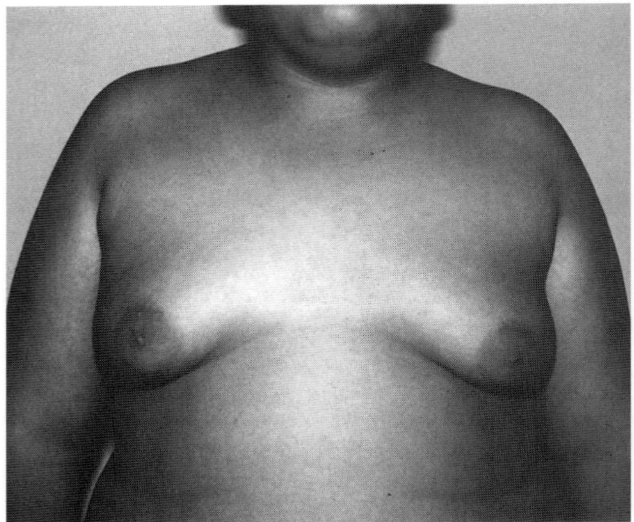
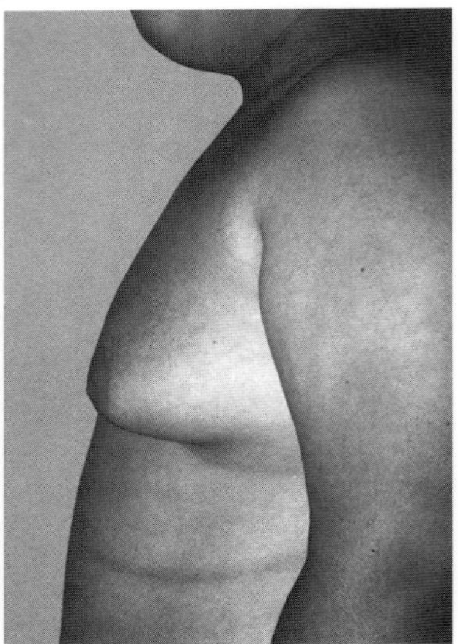

The condition can be accentuated if the patient is overweight, as is evident in this 15-year-old boy with pubertal gynecomastia and obesity. No etiology for their condition could be determined. As in women, the breast tissue contains a significant amount of fat within the parenchyma. This can add to breast volume and the appearance of larger breasts. This fat must be removed to get the best result. ***For overweight individuals the extra anterior and lateral chest fullness must also be treated in the presence of excess fat.***

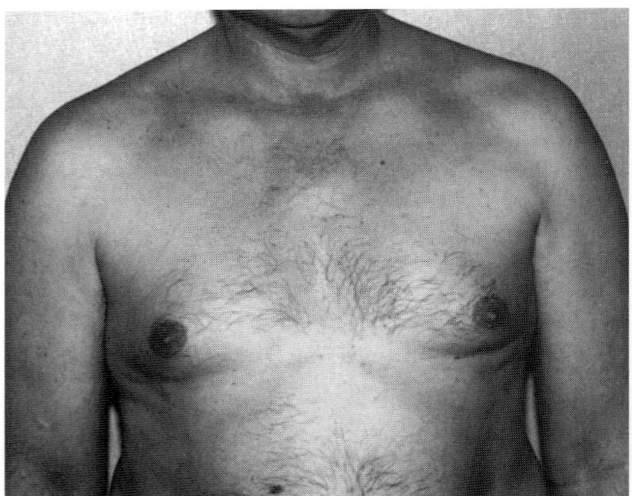
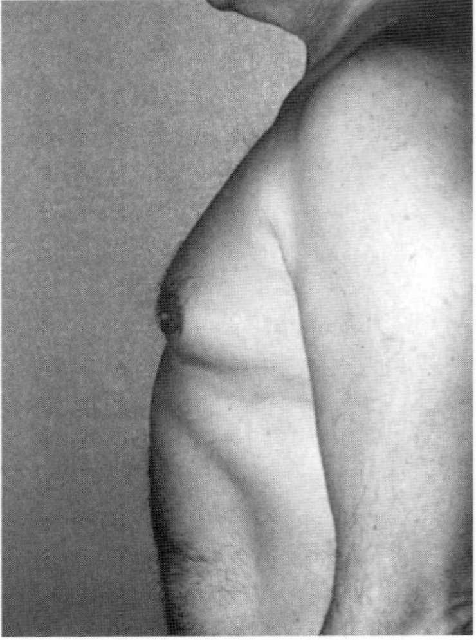

Marijuana usage is commonly linked to gynecomastia, as in this 55-year-old man who said he developed gynecomastia after frequent cannabis inhalation. Men who are taking estrogens or testosterone inhibitors because of prostate cancer or patients with liver disease who have a hormonal imbalance are also susceptible to this condition. Patients with gynecomastia usually exhibit a proliferation of fatty tissue and breast parenchyma in the chest wall area.

Men can develop gynecomastia as a result of taking anabolic steroids to enhance athletic performance or for bodybuilding. These patients usually have low body fat, but the exogenous testosterone suppresses the endogenous testosterone, permitting increased production of estrogens, which upsets the normal ratios and contributes to gynecomastia. This feminine breast appearance, which can be associated with genital atrophy, is especially distressing to these young men who are subjecting their bodies to this regimen in an attempt to achieve a more masculine physique.

Patient Evaluation

A detailed patient evaluation should be completed prior to the treatment of gynecomastia or a breast mass to determine whether the breast enlargement has a hormonal, oncologic, or idiopathic etiology. In addition, the prepubertal gynecomastia patient should be evaluated for duration of symptoms and psychological impact. Breast enlargement will resolve with expectant management in the majority of these patients.

The physical examination includes a survey to determine the treatable causes of breast enlargement. The breast itself is carefully palpated for the presence of discrete lesions as well as to assess the amount of contained fat and parenchyma and their relative proportions. The axillary space is examined for adenopathy. Further evaluation is mandatory when discrete masses indicate possible malignancy. If the breast enlargement is primarily attributable to excess adipose tissue, liposuction may be the only therapy needed.

Depending on the history and physical examination, appropriate diagnostic studies are ordered prior to treatment, particularly for individuals taking anabolic steroids. These patients should also be evaluated for liver and cardiac disease prior to correction of the gynecomastia.

TREATMENT OPTIONS

Multiple variations in operative technique have been designed to remove the excess tissue and reduce the scarring and deformity associated with mastectomy in the male subsequent to treatment for gynecomastia. Treatment approaches to gynecomastia have evolved as new techniques and technology have permitted improved tissue removal with reduced incisions.

In my experience, standard liposuction effectively reduces the bulk of breast fullness only in the overweight patient or the man who has a high percentage of fat as a component of his breast enlargement. ***If the breast enlargement is primarily attributable to excess adipose tissue, as in patients with pseudogynecomastia with large fatty deposits in the breast region but not a large volume of fibrous breast parenchyma, liposuction alone may provide adequate contour improvement, sparing the patient the breast scars from direct excision of the breast.*** Liposuction can be performed through a distant site, either the axilla or inframammary region, obviating the need for scars on the breast. In addition, the resection can be tailored laterally to provide good contour while promoting skin contraction.

Unlike the loose subcutaneous fat, the denser, hypertrophied fibrous breast parenchyma may prove resistant to removal with a blunt liposuction cannula. In this situation ultrasound-assisted liposuction or an endoscopic mastectomy technique may be a useful adjunct. Ultrasound-assisted liposuction permits cavitation and emulsification of the fibrous breast parenchyma. Standard liposuction is then used to remove excess fat and to evacuate the liquefied tissue remaining after cavitation.

When significant breast parenchyma is present and ultrasound-assisted liposuction will not completely liquefy all of the dense tissue, open mastectomy is still frequently required, often in combination with standard liposuction and ultrasound-assisted liposuction. Suctioning prior to sharp excision appears to reduce the incidence of postoperative hematoma and promotes skin contraction and a smoother contour at the resection margins. This traditional approach may be used with endoscopic visualization through axillary incisions.

The endoscopic technique makes it possible to excise this parenchymal tissue through limited, distant incisions, thereby avoiding a breast or areolar scar, which is a source of concern to most men. Excess fatty tissue is initially treated with ultrasound energy and removed with liposuction. In patients in whom a discrete mass is to be removed, an open surgical biopsy should be completed so that the tumor can be evaluated histologically and the pathologic report obtained prior to liposuction.

ULTRASOUND-ASSISTED LIPOSUCTION WITH STANDARD LIPOSUCTION

In patients who have dense breast parenchyma in addition to fatty tissue I generally perform traditional liposuction initially after infiltration of wetting solution. The remaining dense subareolar glandular tissue is then treated with ultrasound energy. The ultrasound probe is introduced via an axillary or inframammary fold incision. It is advanced slowly through the dense parenchymal tissue to allow the energy to slowly cavitate and then emulsify the breast parenchyma. The remaining fluid is evacuated using standard liposuction. A drain and compression dressing are used postoperatively. Open surgical excision, either through traditional periareolar incisions or with endoscopic assistance through the axilla, is used if standard or ultrasound-assisted liposuction does not achieve sufficient correction.

Technique

The patient is placed in the supine position with the arms abducted. A 3 to 4 mm incision is made in each axillary fold. The standard wetting solution is infiltrated into the chest wall and breast. A 5 to 6 mm blunt-tip, three-hole cannula is inserted and the anterior chest wall and breasts are suctioned.

Suctioning is performed in a radial fashion using multiple smooth strokes. The area of central fullness is treated as well as the entire chest wall. Care is taken not to oversuction the region, which can create a saucer deformity.

After the initial suctioning is completed, ultrasound-assisted liposuction is used to treat the firm mass in the subareolar region. The amplitude is increased, and the tissue is elevated manually to facilitate passage of the cannula. Approximately 10 to 15 mm of tissue, depending on the thickness of the chest wall fat, is left on the flaps and slightly more beneath the nipple-areola to avoid depression in this region.

Patient Example

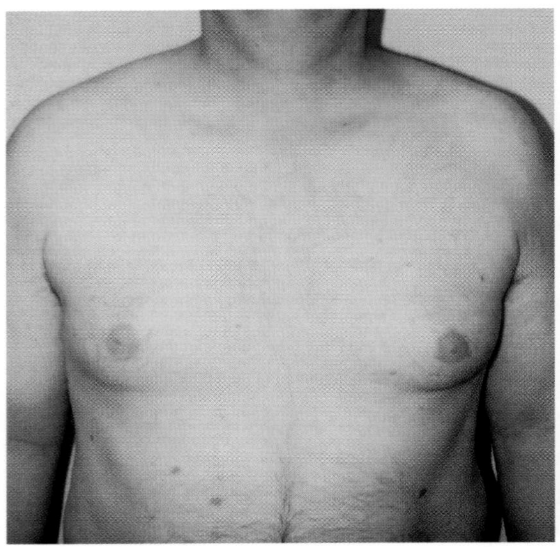

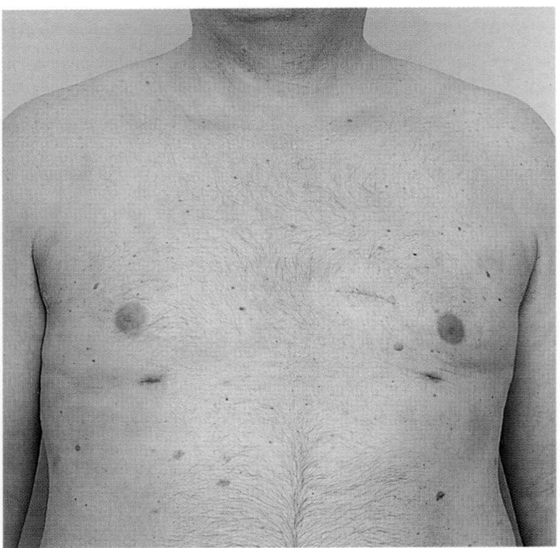

This 48-year-old man developed gynecomastia following the treatment of metastatic prostate cancer. His breasts were uncomfortably full, and their large size limited his choice of clothing and physical activity. He requested correction of the gynecomastia with minimal scars. Axillary and inframammary approaches were used. Wetting solution was infiltrated throughout the breast region. Liposuction was first used to reduce the fatty excess in the overall breast and upper and lateral chest regions. The remaining central breast parenchyma was then treated with ultrasound energy. The ultrasonic probe was effective in cavitating and emulsifying the breast parenchyma so that the excess breast tissue could be removed. He is shown 2 months after surgery. Although there is some residual postoperative edema and the inframammary access site is visible, he was delighted with the result and no longer felt embarrassed about the appearance of his breasts. The associated discomfort was also alleviated.

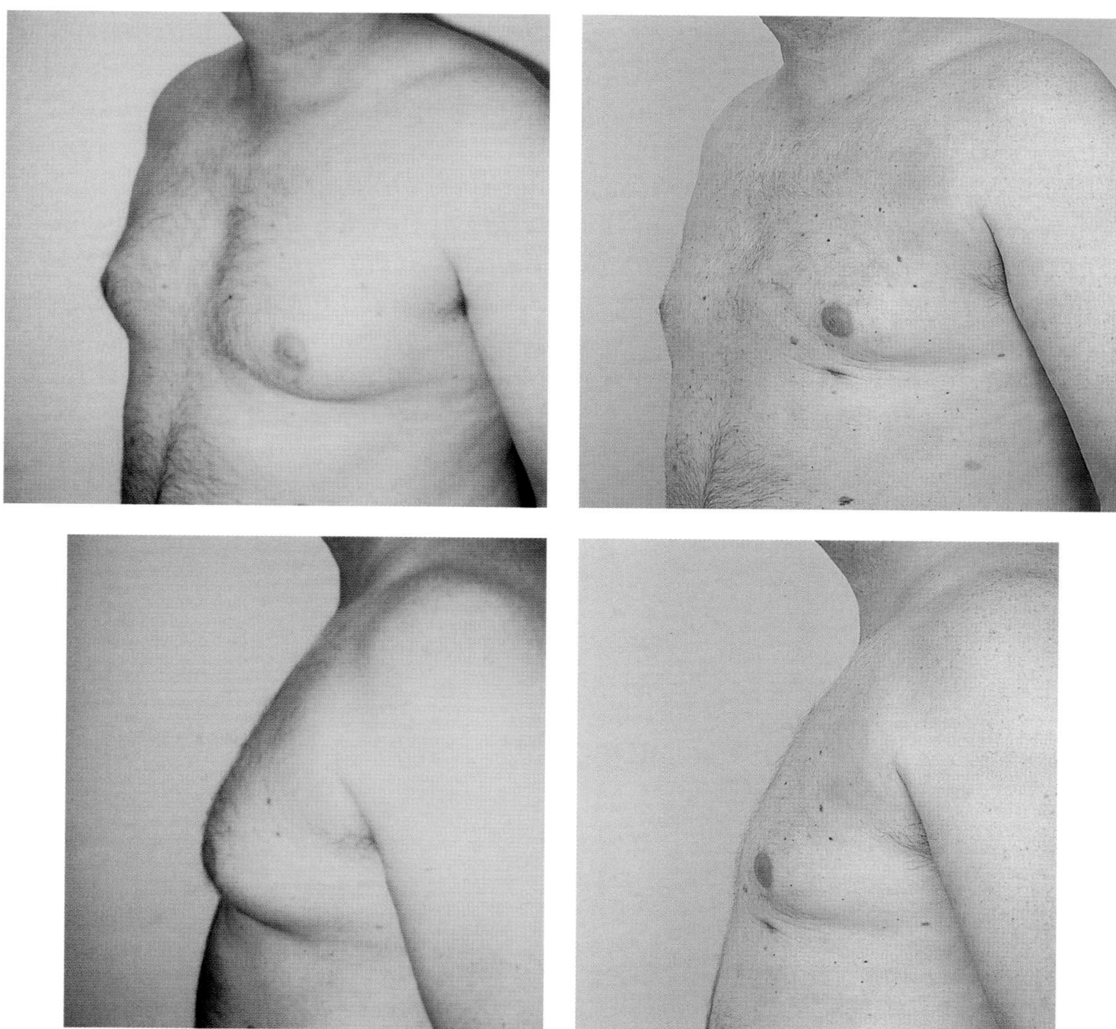

ENDOSCOPIC-ASSISTED MASTECTOMY WITH LIPOSUCTION

When an endoscopic technique is used for resection of breast parenchyma to further reduce fullness after liposuction, it is traditionally completed through a periareolar incision and combined with liposuction. The same routes can potentially be used for excision of breast masses, especially those that are benign. ***Although the intra-areolar incision usually heals with minimal visible scarring, placement of the incision away from the breast is an important consideration in the gynecomastia patient since it provides access to the parenchyma but preserves a layer of tissue between the areola and pectoralis muscle, which may help prevent areolar depression.*** The same axillary incision can be used for liposuction and endoscopic access. Finally, some patients may simply prefer an axillary to a circumareolar incision.

Operating Room Setup and Patient Positioning

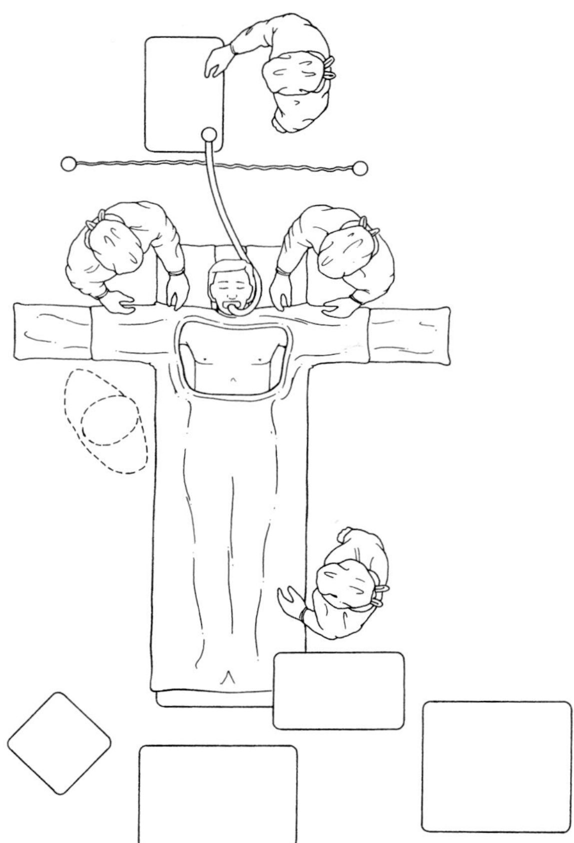

The setup for endoscopic mastectomy or endoscopic breast biopsy is the same as for endoscopic transaxillary augmentation except that space must be allocated for the liposuction machine and tubing if these are used instead of a syringe suction technique. If the patient has a unilateral deformity, the endoscopic cart may be positioned directly at the foot of the operating table (as in bilateral procedures) or on the contralateral side of the operating table. The patient is placed in a supine position with the arms extended to 90 degrees and secured.

Markings

As with other endoscopic breast procedures, the preoperative markings are made with the patient in an upright position. The extent of planned liposuction is marked and generally extends well beyond the area of breast enlargement, often to the clavicle superiorly and the costal margin inferomedially. The fullness can extend laterally and into the axilla. ***Wide suctioning maximizes skin contraction, obviating the need for skin excision mastectomy techniques in all but the most severe cases.*** If a biopsy is to be performed, the site of the mass is marked on the skin, and liposuction is delayed until the mass is proved benign. In either case an appropriate crease is chosen within the hair-bearing portion of the axilla for the access incision.

Technique

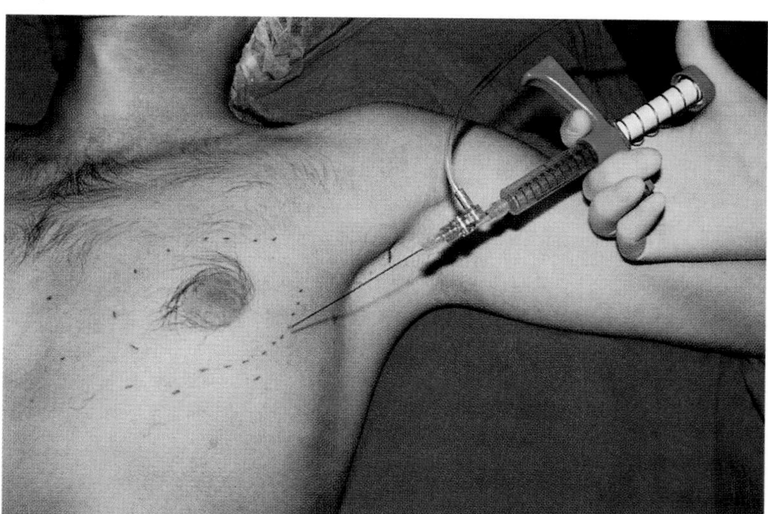

After anesthesia is induced, the breast area is infiltrated with a generous amount of wetting solution of Ringer's lactate, epinephrine, and lidocaine to promote vasoconstriction and postoperative analgesia. Several minutes are required for full vasoconstriction to take effect. During this time the final sterile skin prep is completed and the surgical drapes applied. The light and endoscopic camera cords and the liposuction tubing are secured to the drapes.

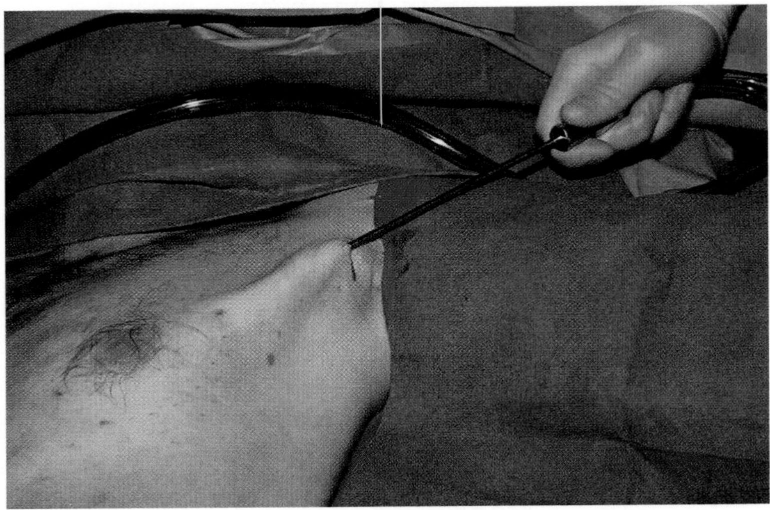

A small axillary incision is made at the site of the skin marking to expose the subcutaneous tissue of the axilla. A round-tipped, three-hole liposuction cannula approximately 5 mm in diameter is chosen. The cannula is inserted through the axillary incision, and pretunneling and suctioning are completed along the deep surface of the breast. Since in this patient the entire breast was removed except the nipple-areola complex and some underlying tissue, the actual suctioning was done at this preliminary stage. Liposuction is also used to refine the contour after the specimen is removed. When significant subcutaneous fat is contributing to the breast deformity, more aggressive suctioning is undertaken to remove all tissue necessary to produce the desired contour. ***Frequent palpation of the breast tissue will demonstrate areas of tissue thinning, guide additional areas of suctioning, and delineate the presence of a residual parenchymal bud that requires sharp resection.*** If resection of the breast bud is necessary, suction is stopped prior to removal of the desired amount of fat. This allows follow-up suctioning to smooth contour irregularities after sharp resection. Palpation will also demonstrate the mobility of the breast-skin plane, which facilitates optical cavity elevation after presuctioning.

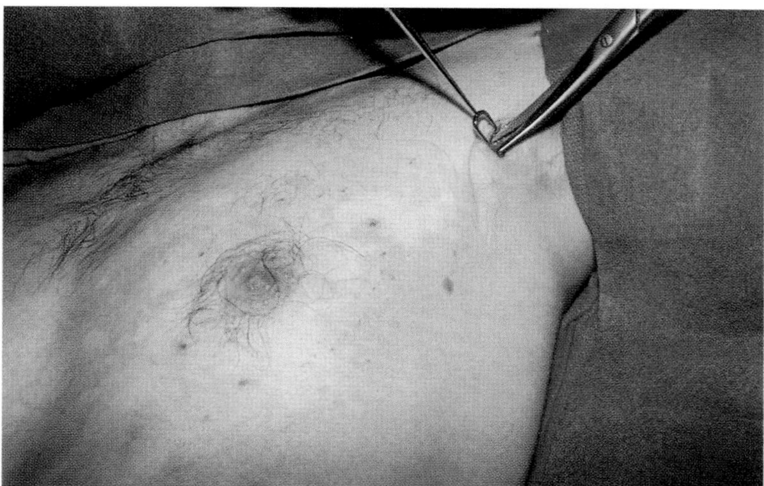

If parenchymal resection is necessary, the axillary incision is lengthened to 2.0 to 2.5 cm to provide sufficient room for the endoretractor and dissecting instruments. Spreading scissors dissection is performed superficially through the subcutaneous tissue of the axilla toward the anterior axillary line. At this line the scissor tips are guided anteriorly over the lateral border of the pectoralis major muscle, again using a spreading rather than a cutting motion. Pretunneling and/or presuctioning establishes a ready dissection plane immediately on top of the pectoral fascia in the subglandular plane. Development of the optical cavity can continue as long as the dissection in this plane can progress without resistance.

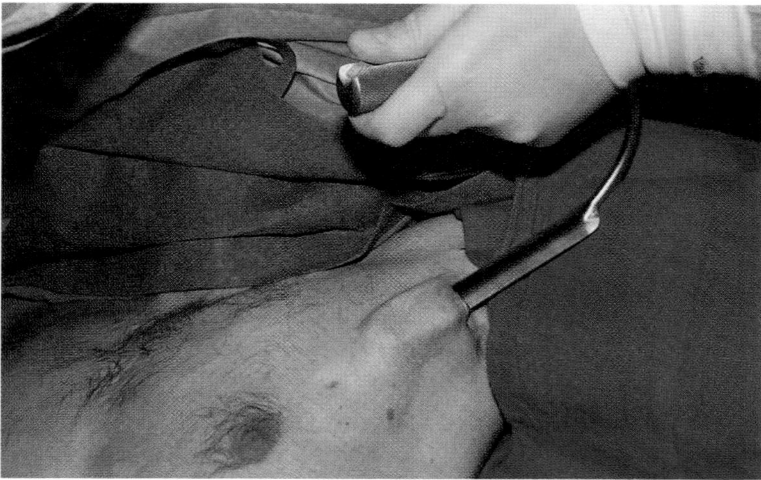

When the limits of scissors dissection are reached, the endoretractor is positioned within the subglandular prepectoral optical cavity. ***As in endoscopic augmentation mammaplasty, it is generally preferable to inset the endo-***

retractor separate from the endoscope. The endoscope may then be advanced into the sheath of the retractor with less likelihood of lens contamination. The camera is focused to provide a good view of the pocket.

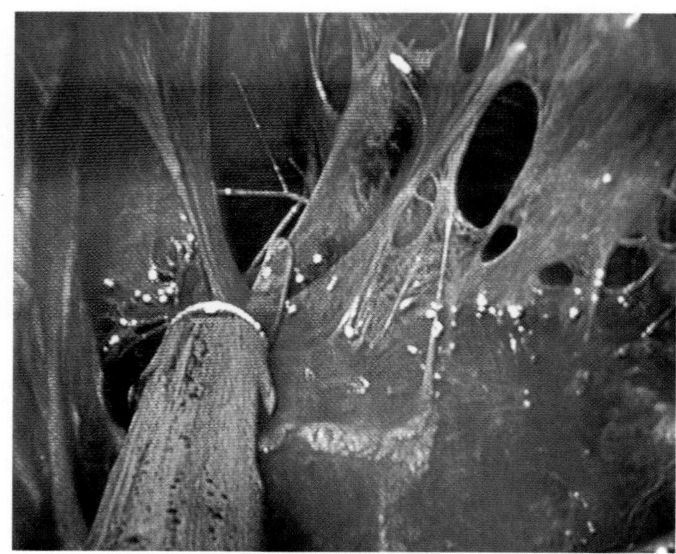

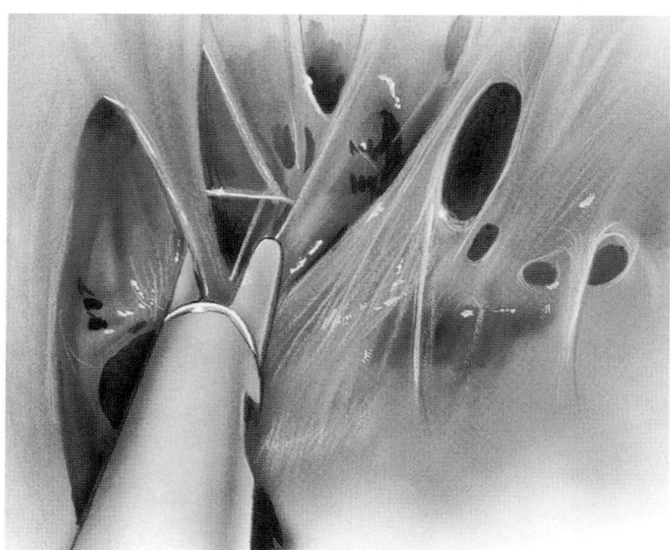

The subglandular tissues will have a honeycomb appearance subsequent to the initial suctioning, which is easily seen on the monitor. Minimal bleeding is encountered, and the surgeon can usually complete the development of the optical cavity without the need to control bleeding. Cavity development is completed using 5 mm laparoscopic scissors to lyse the "walls" of the honeycomb. This dissection can be done rapidly. ***The limits of the optical cavity must be extended past the area of desired resection to allow efficient tissue removal without instrument crowding.***

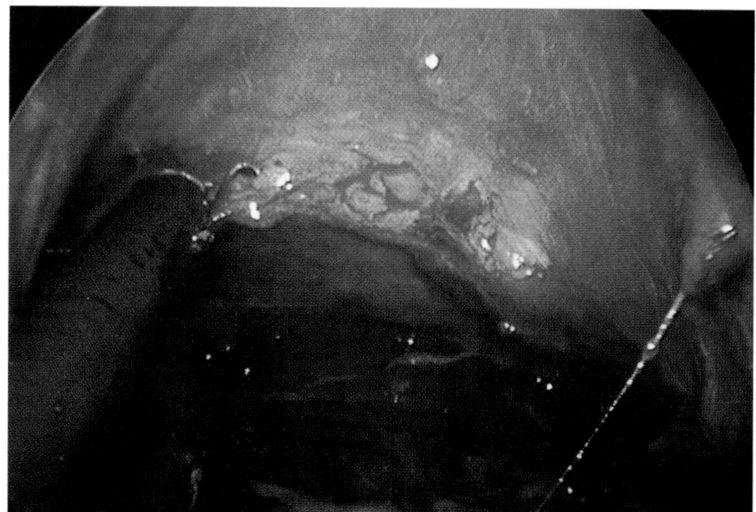

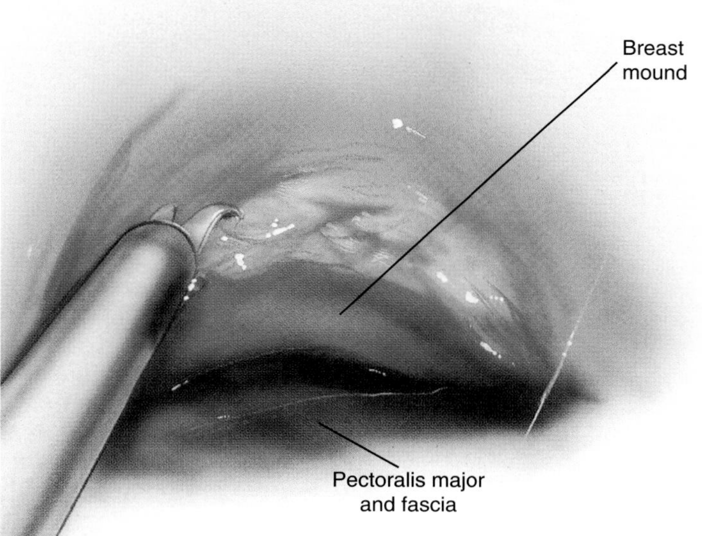

The superolateral line of dissection is then developed using the endoscissors. The dissection is kept thin on the edges and becomes thicker toward the middle, producing a discoid sample of tissue and avoiding overresection centrally. Frequent and careful palpation is necessary to guide the limit and depth of dissection to prevent a central depression postoperatively.

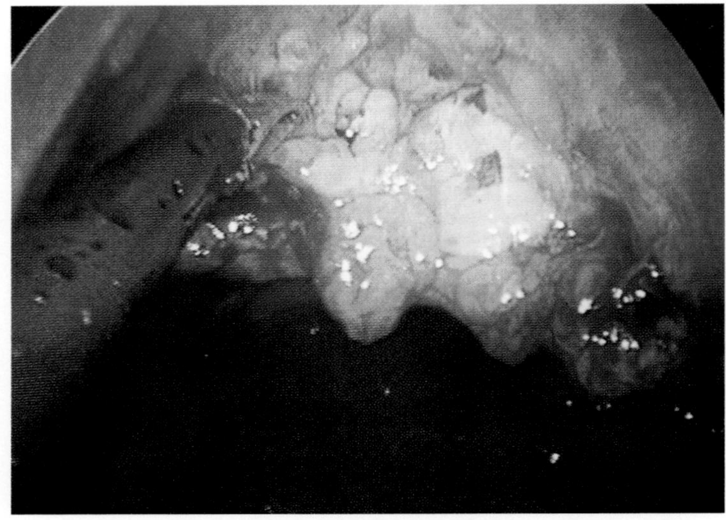

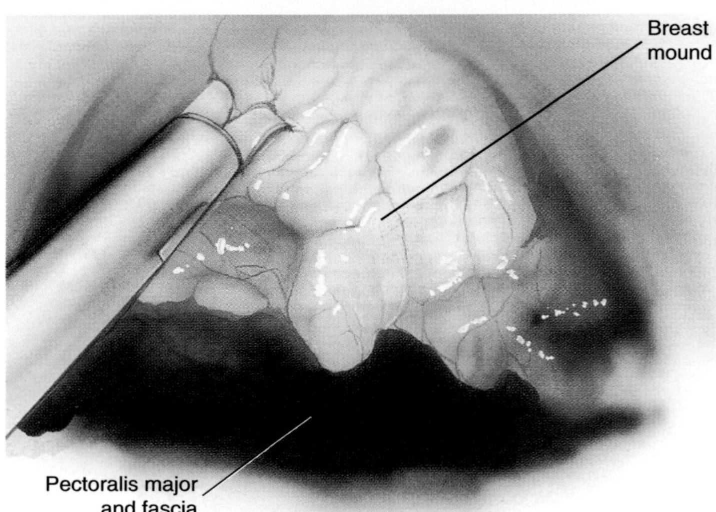

Dissection is most difficult immediately beneath the areola where the fibrous parenchymal and ductal tissues are most dense. Grasping the margins of the specimen may create enough tension to make the dissection easier; however, this does cause instrument crowding. Hemostasis is maintained by activating the monopolar cautery through the endoscopic scissors.

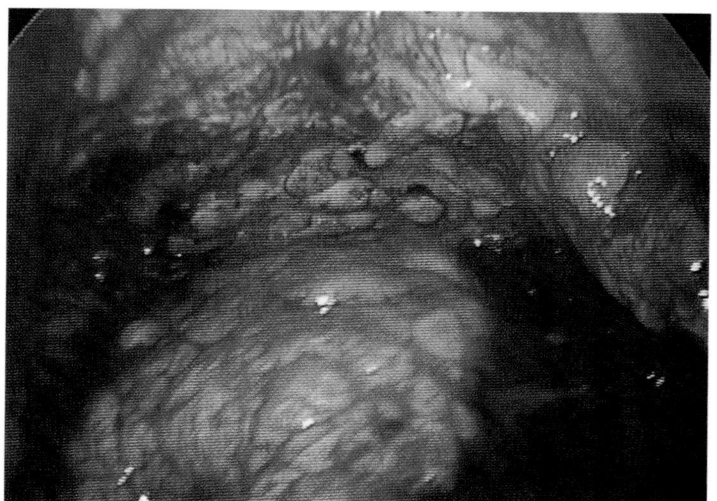

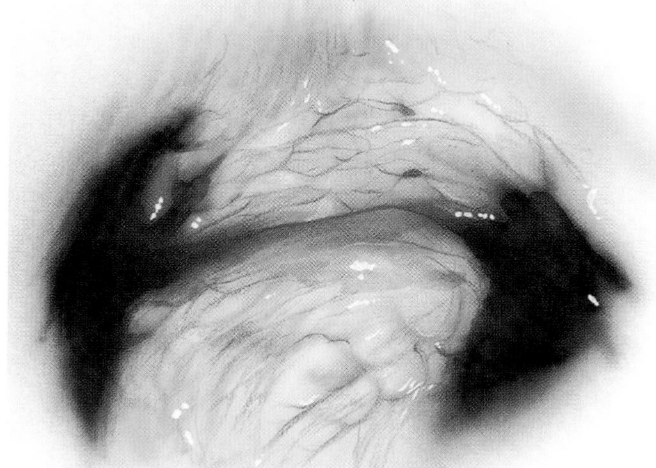

The specimen must again be thinned as the dissection proceeds past the level of the areola. Repeated palpation guides the dissection. As the inferomedial margin of the breast is divided, the specimen is freed of all its surrounding tissue and drops back against the pectoralis. The endoscissors can be used to cauterize any bleeding points.

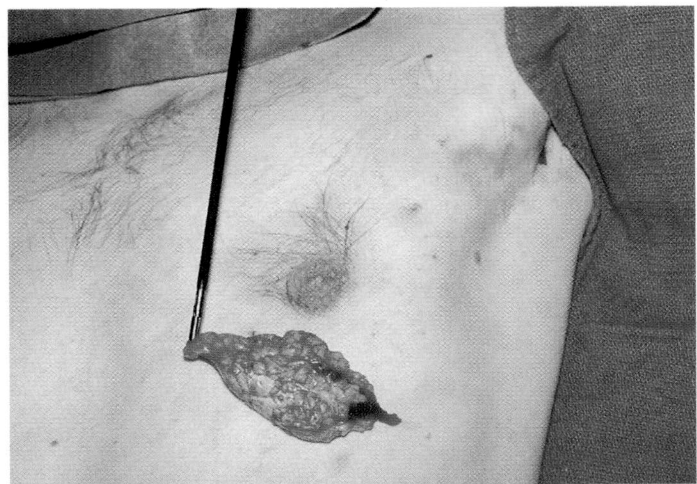

Endoscopic graspers are used to secure the specimen on its lateral surface under endoscopic guidance. The endoretractor-mounted endoscope is removed. This provides additional space for withdrawing the specimen from the optical cavity. The specimen is marked as necessary along its deep and lateral surface to give the pathologist the proper orientation. Ultrasound energy is used to remove any residual breast elements, allowing some contraction of the breast and the overlying skin. Any excess skin contracts during the healing process as the postoperative edema slowly subsides.

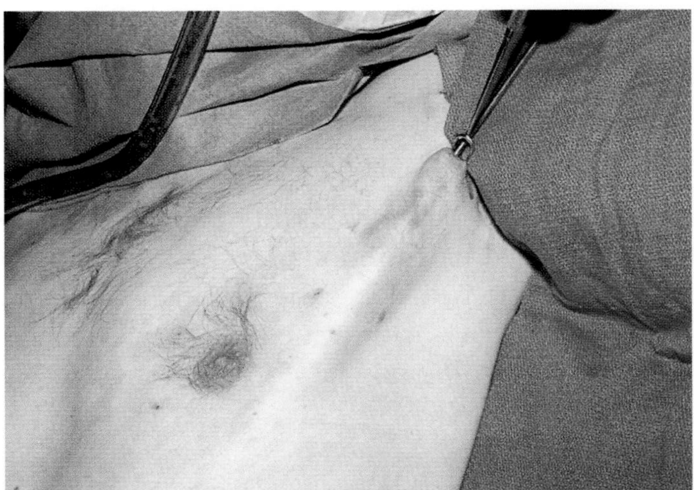

The skin and soft tissue of the breast area are carefully palpated and compared with the opposite side. The liposuction cannula is then reinserted through the axillary incision and activated to remove residual tissue and any contour irregularities to ensure a smooth contour. The optical cavity is reinspected through the endoscope, hemostasis is ensured, and a small suction drain is placed through either the access incision or a small separate axillary incision. A compression dressing is placed over the chest. The dressing and drain are generally removed 24 to 48 hours postoperatively. The patient is placed in an elastic garment to provide support while the chest skin contracts and redrapes.

Patient Example

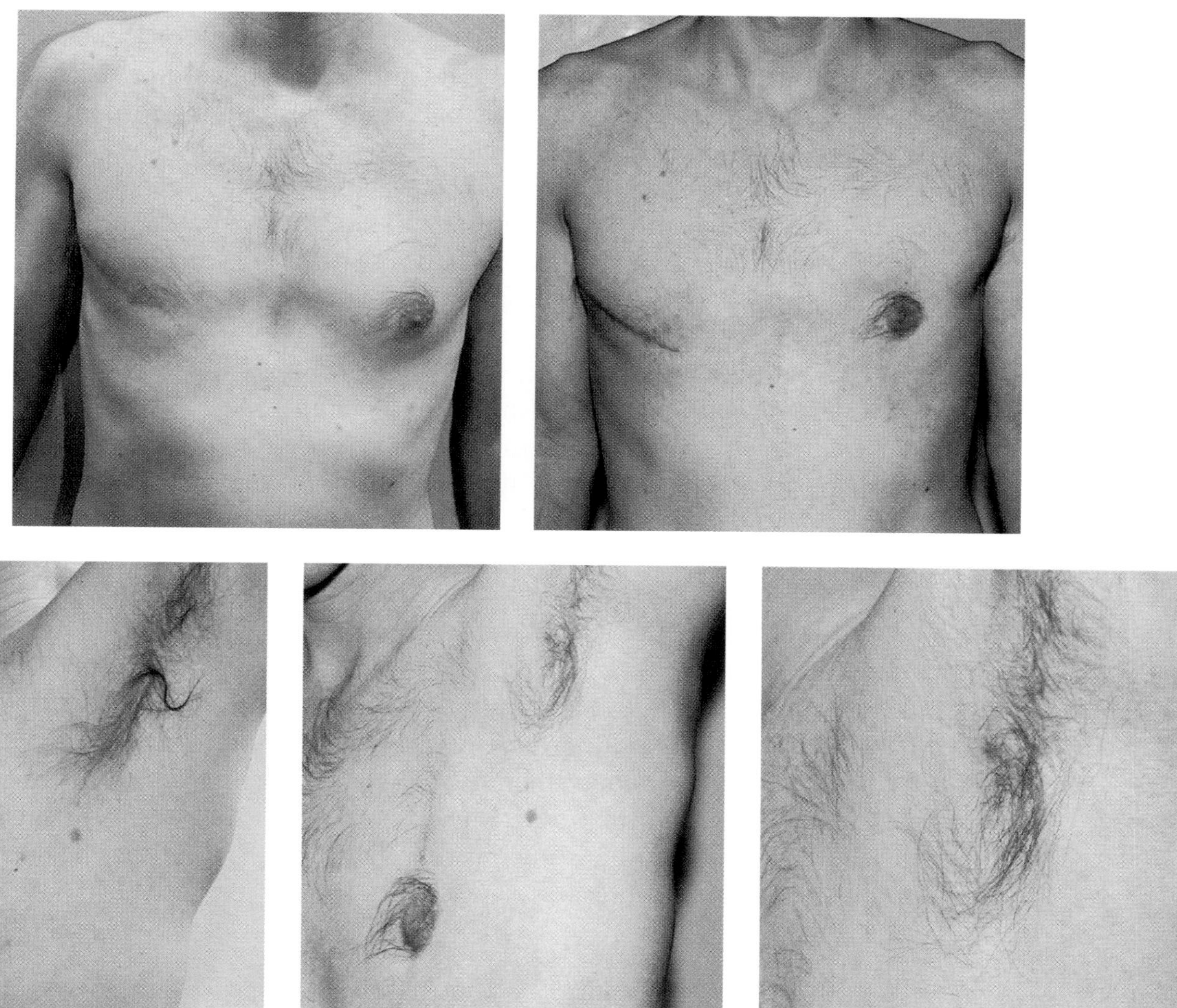

This 39-year-old patient demonstrated in the operative series had an earlier right modified radical mastectomy for infiltrating ductal carcinoma. He requested a left mastectomy because he was concerned that cancer would develop in that breast and he also wanted to improve breast symmetry. He is shown 3 months after endoscopic mastectomy on the left side. The subglandular space was pretunneled, but minimal liposuctioning was performed prior to specimen removal. Liposuctioning was deferred for final contouring. Because of this patient's history of breast carcinoma, a total mastectomy with nipple-areola preservation was performed. The resection left very little soft tissue in the chest region; simultaneous scar revision with flap thinning on the contralateral side helps minimize postoperative asymmetry and deformity. A close-up view of the axilla at early follow-up reveals that there is minimal scarring.

OPEN SURGICAL EXCISION WITH LIPOSUCTION

When open surgical excision is necessary for specific removal of the dense parenchyma in the central breast region that is not amenable to liposuction, I usually perform liposuction through a small axillary incision and then remove the subareolar and central breast tissue through a lower periareolar incision. This approach produces a minimal lower periareolar scar and permits accurate direct excision. When significant skin excess, ptosis, and fatty tissue are present, a two-stage procedure is performed to avoid major skin resection. First the bulk of the fatty tissue is removed with standard liposuction. Ultrasound-assisted liposuction is used to remove most of the residual breast elements, allowing some contraction of the breast and the overlying skin. The excess skin contracts during the healing process as the postoperative edema slowly subsides. During a second procedure 6 to 12 months later after the skin has contracted, the excess breast parenchyma is removed through a low periareolar incision or via the axilla with endoscopic assistance.

Care is taken to restore normal chest wall contour, maintaining a thin layer of subcutaneous tissue in the anterior chest wall that is consistent with the subcutaneous tissue of the upper abdominal wall. ***The goal is to create a flattened but not concave appearance, thereby avoiding the unattractive saucer deformity.*** This problem develops when too much central breast tissue is resected, particularly when all the tissue is excised between the dermis of the areola and the pectoralis major, allowing these structures to adhere to the underlying pectoralis major muscle.

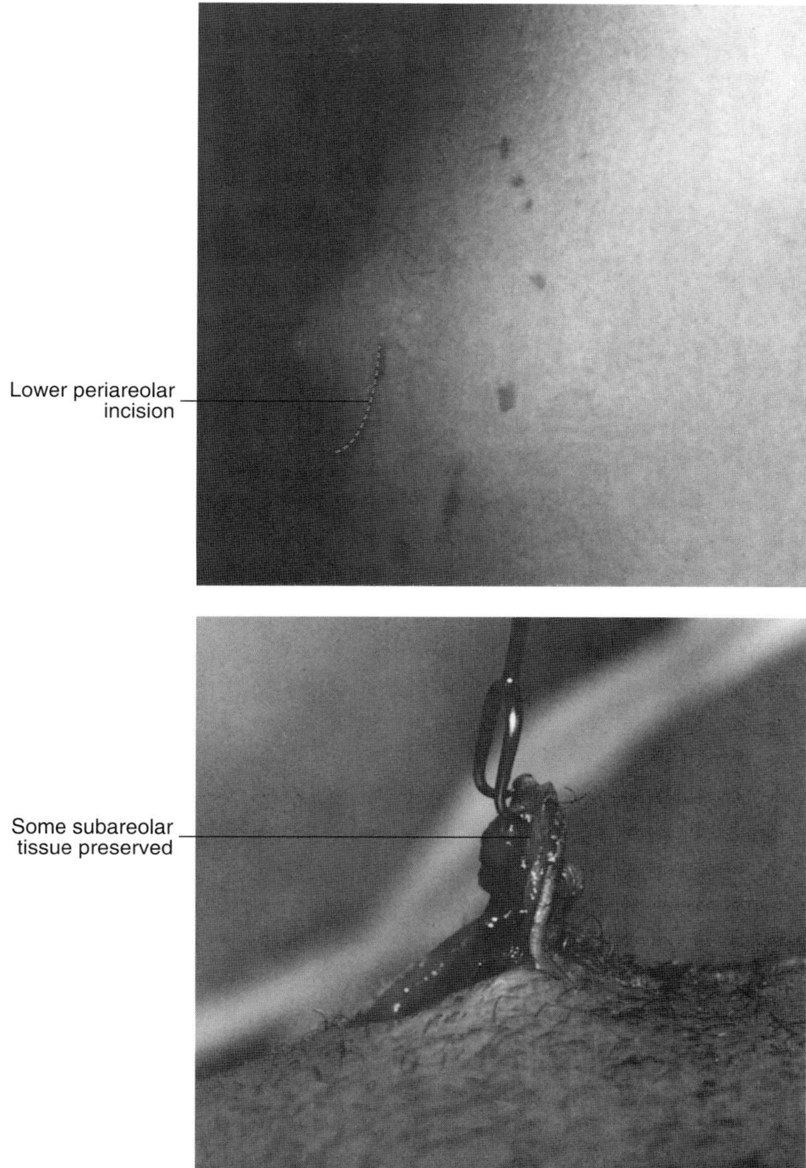

Preoperative lower periareolar markings and the extent of the breast resection are delineated. Wetting solution is infiltrated in the region before liposuction is initiated. The lower periareolar incision is made and the nipple-areola undermined, including some subareolar tissue to prevent a central depression.

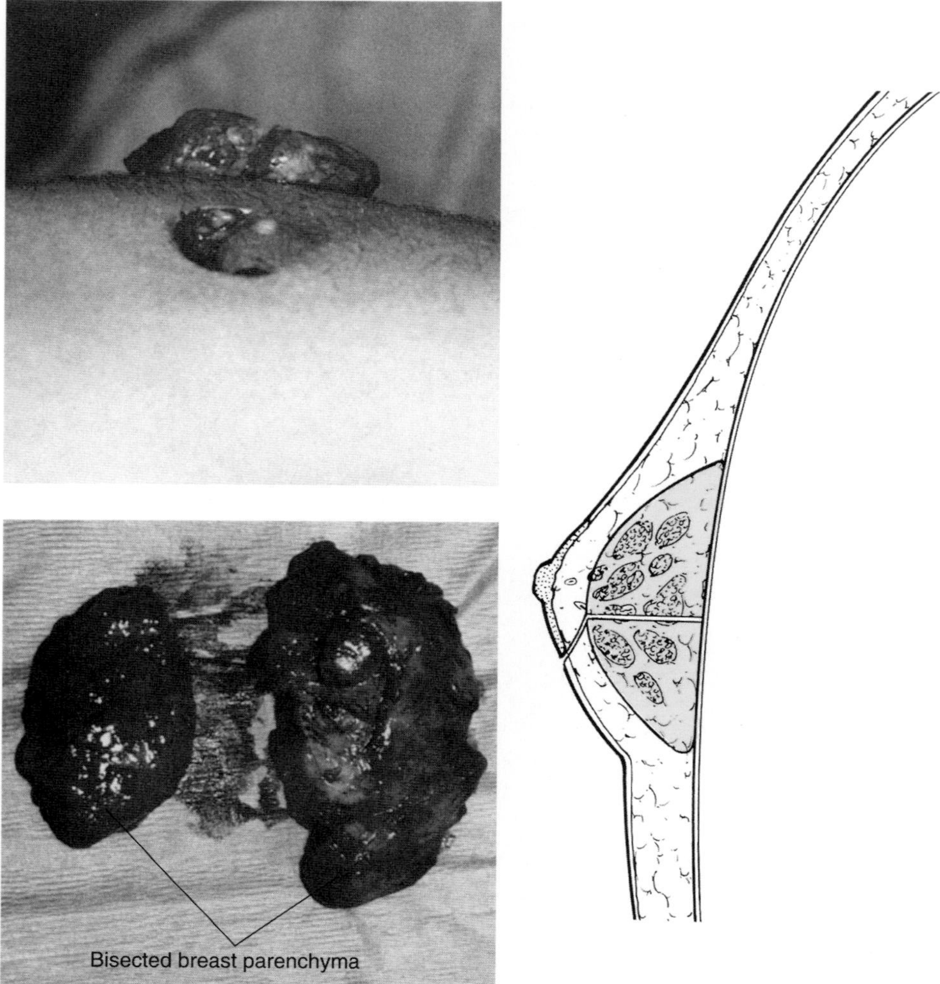

The breast is bisected transversely down to the subglandular plane, and subglandular resection lifts the breast parenchyma off the deep fascia. The breast is then removed in two segments by undermining the breast skin at the level of thickness of the cutaneous tissue of the upper abdomen. Elevating it to this level obviates a central breast depression.

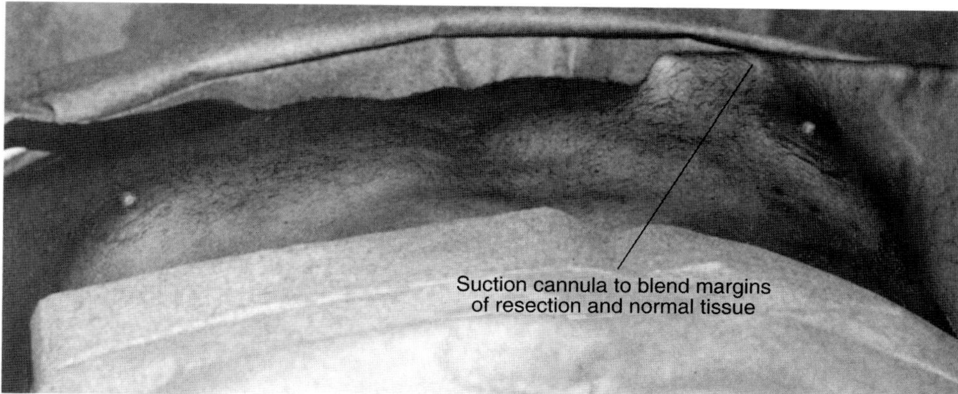

Some peripheral suctioning is done after the mastectomy to soften the junction of the breast resection and the remainder of the chest wall. Because these patients are prone to hematoma formation, special attention is directed to maintaining hemostasis. The chest wall is wrapped with an elastic bandage for a few days postoperatively, and the patient is advised to avoid strenuous activity involving the arms or upper torso for 2 weeks.

Patient Examples

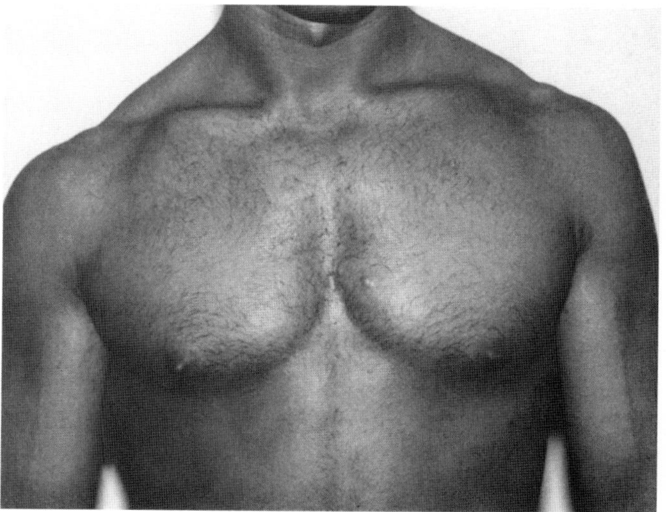

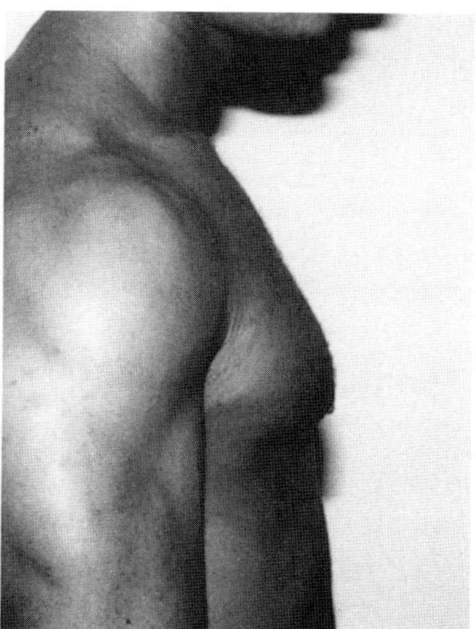

The patient is shown 6 months following periareolar subcutaneous mastectomy that removed 50 gm of tissue.

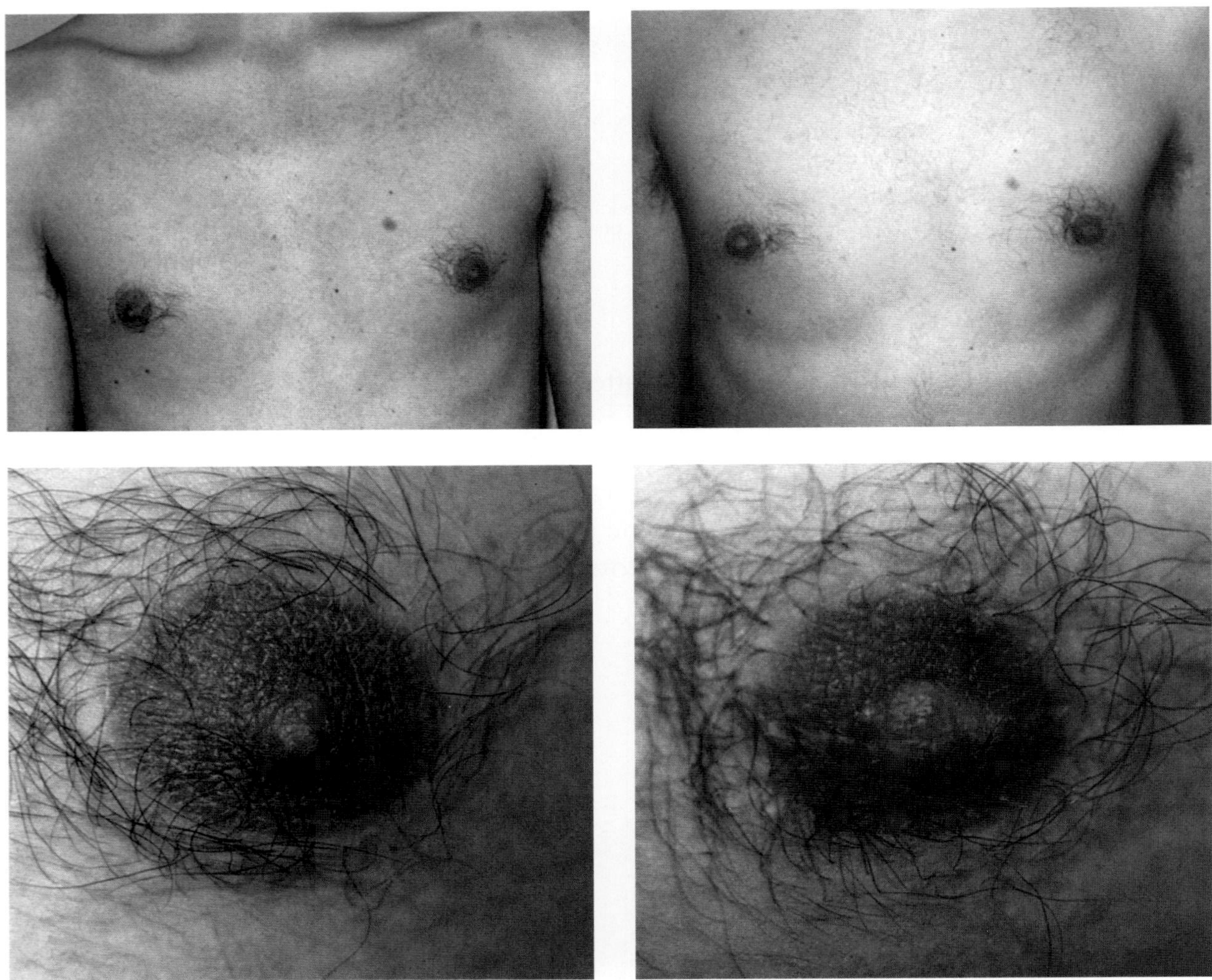

The transnipple-areolar approach is an alternate incision for subcutaneous mastectomy to treat gynecomastia. This 20-year-old patient is shown 1 year following subcutaneous mastectomy to remove 40 gm of breast tissue. The nipple-areolar scar is somewhat noticeable. For this reason I prefer a lower periareolar incision.

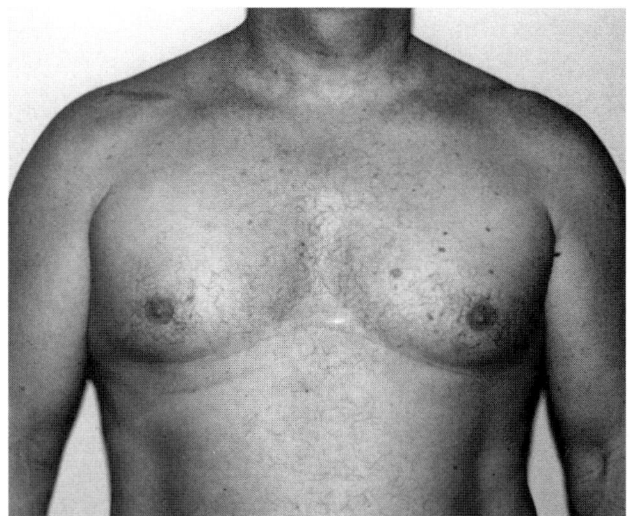

When gynecomastia is associated with breast asymmetry with some obesity and excess subcutaneous fat in the chest region, I prefer to combine standard liposuction of the anterior chest with ultrasound-assisted liposuction. The ultrasound energy cavitates the parenchyma and permits removal by aspiration.

ENDOSCOPIC BREAST MASS EXCISION

The axillary approach can be used for endoscopic breast mass excision in those patients with relatively unsuspicious breast lesions that warrant removal but who insist on limited incisions and scars. This technique is most appropriate for the young patient presenting with probable fibroadenoma, especially a lower or upper lateral lesion that might otherwise require an incision on the breast itself for removal. Certainly it is technically possible to remove a segment or quadrant of the breast and also to dissect axillary lymph nodes through a small axillary incision; however, before this approach is used for the patient with possible breast cancer, a thorough evaluation by a surgical oncologist is mandatory.

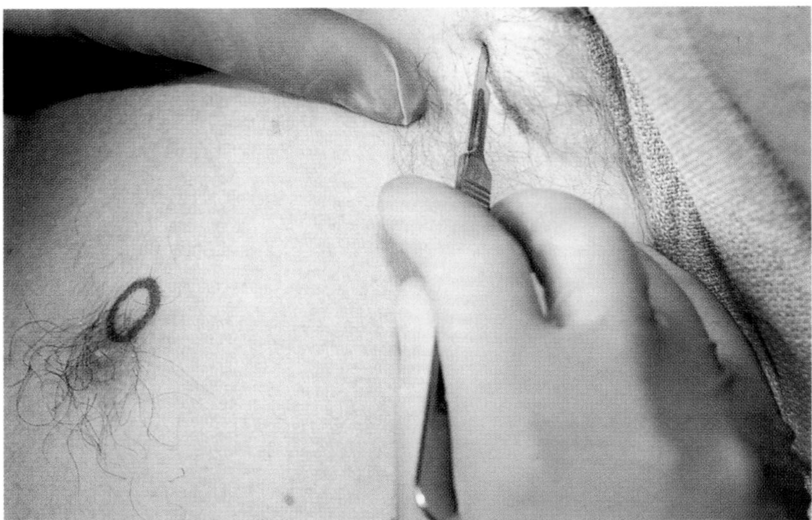

The location of the mass and the proposed access incision site are marked on the skin preoperatively. Unlike mastectomy for gynecomastia, the entire breast area is not infiltrated with local anesthetic. Rather the access incision and the superficial axillary fat to the level of the lateral pectoral border are infiltrated with a solution of 0.5% lidocaine with 1:200,000 epinephrine to minimize oozing within the access channel.

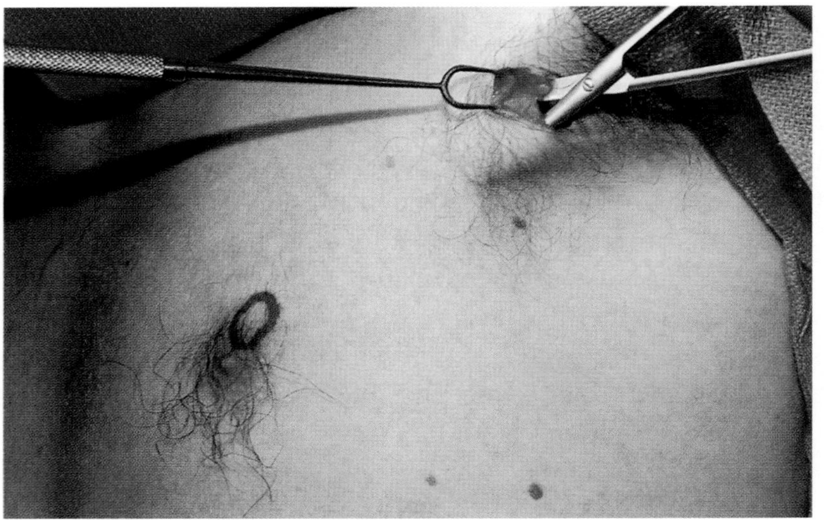

Liposuction is not performed prior to endoscopic transaxillary breast biopsy. The dissection begins with blunt spreading scissors dissection to the lateral border of the pectoralis major. Some pretunneling can reduce the bleeding.

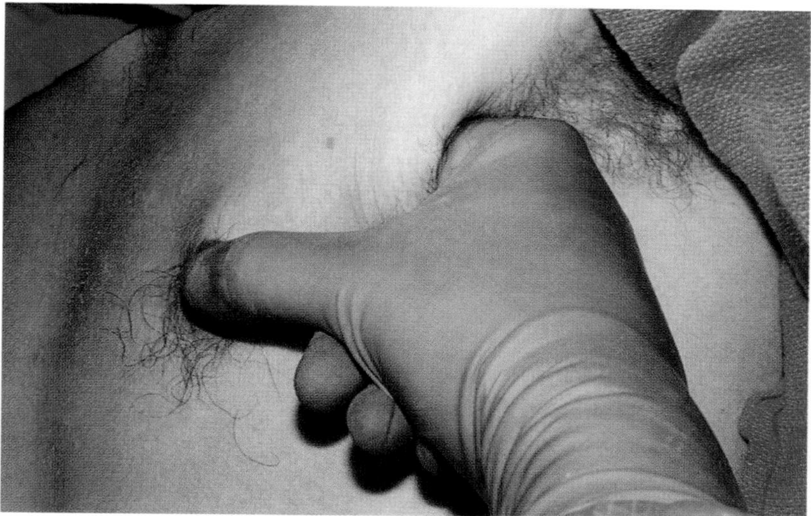

Bimanual palpation through the axillary incision and external palpation are helpful for identifying the mass. Bimanual palpation also helps determine the route of dissection and extent of intervening soft tissue that must be divided to expose the mass from the axilla.

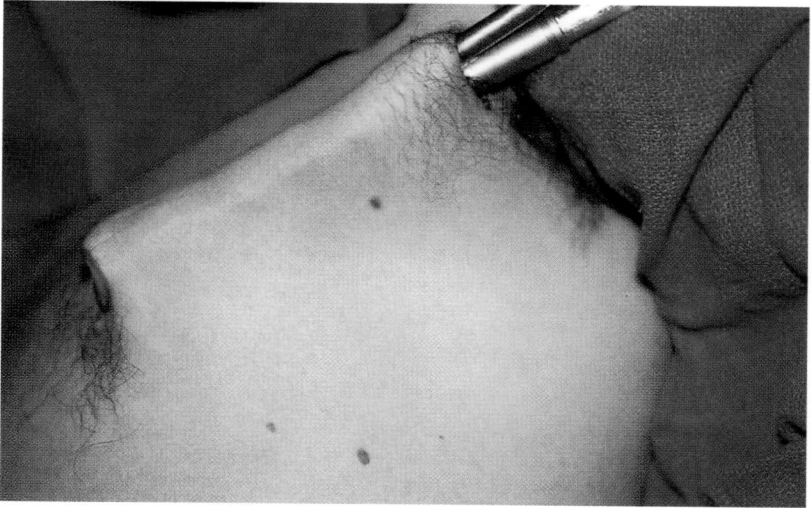

The retractor and endoscope are placed through the axillary incision and directed toward the area where the mass is located.

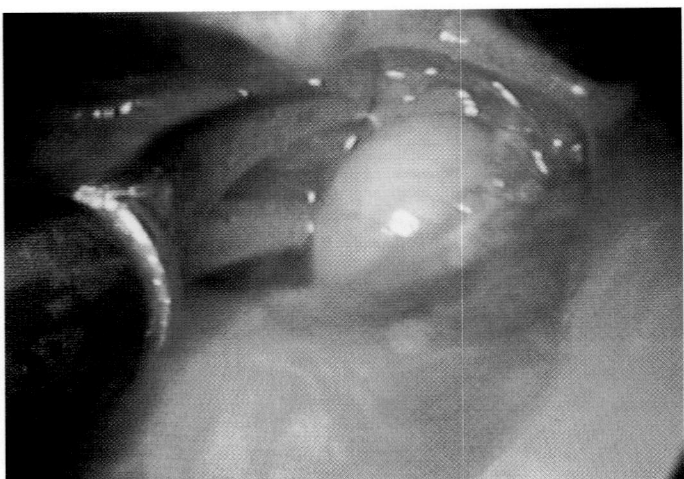 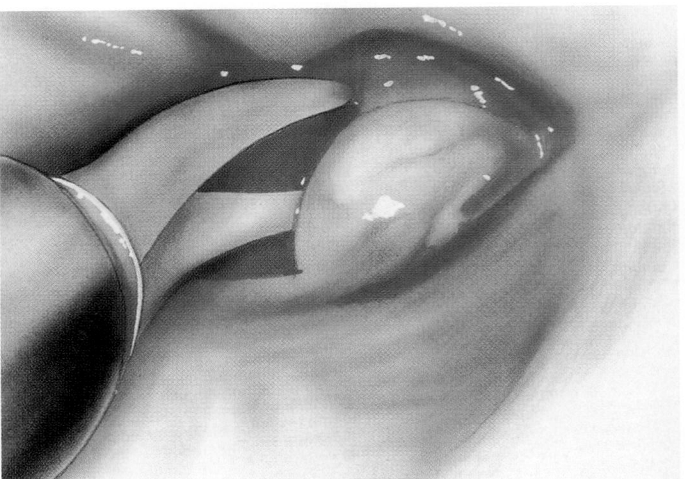

Dissection with the endoscopic Metzenbaum or hook scissors and repeated palpation will expose the mass.

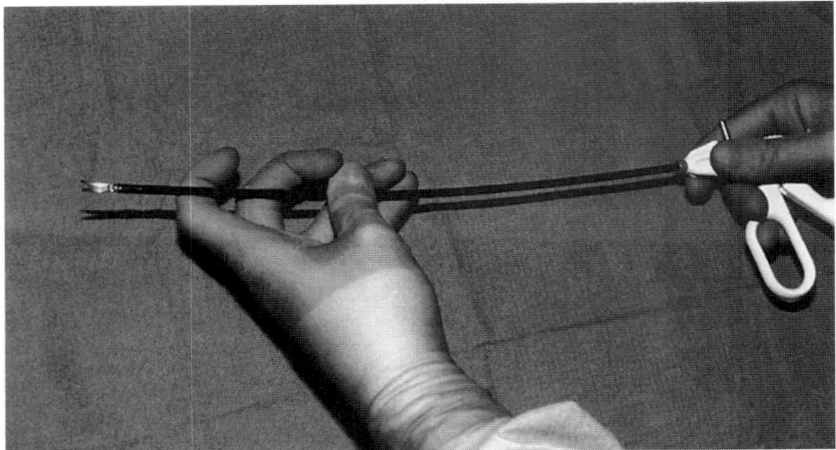

If necessary, the disposable laparoscopic scissors can be bent slightly to help navigate the curvature of the chest wall and reduce instrument crowding against the extended arm.

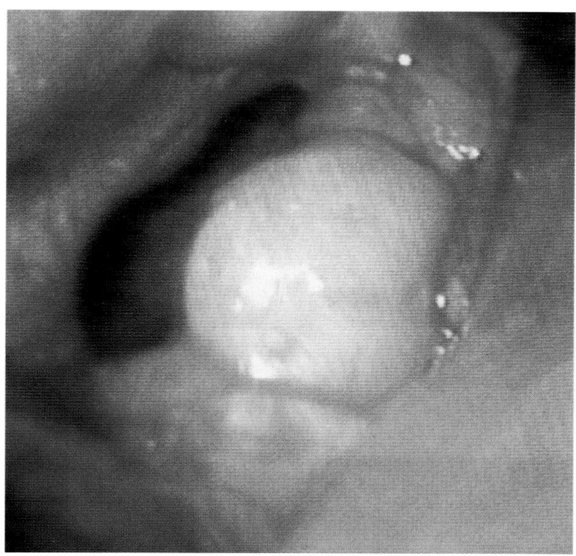

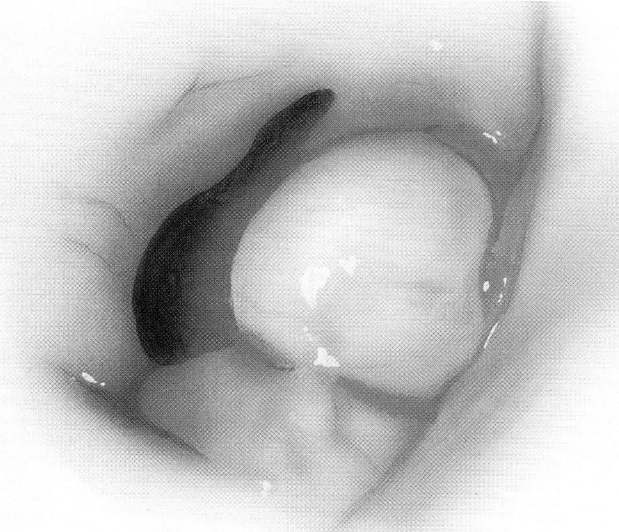

Scissors dissection is used to completely free the mass. Placement of a grasper on the mass may facilitate dissection, but instrument crowding is the trade-off when using a single access incision.

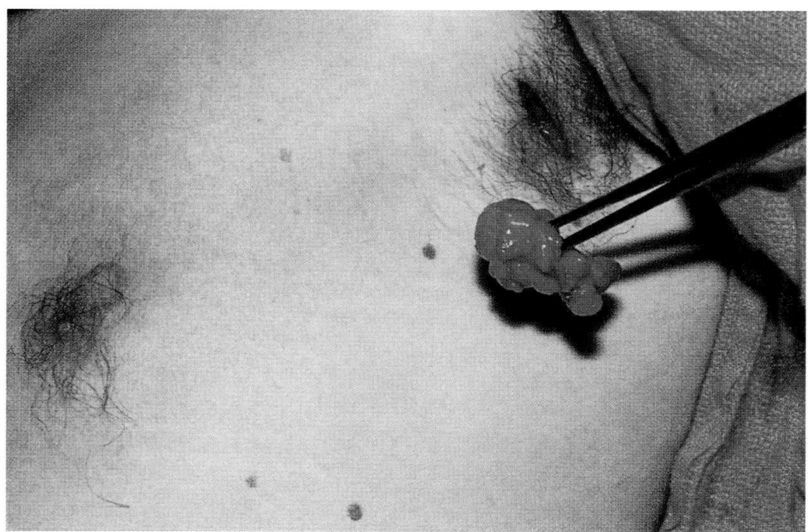

In this situation the mass was removed with a margin of surrounding soft tissue. After the optical cavity is examined for bleeding, a compression dressing is applied over the breast. Drains are not usually placed since the size of the optical cavity is smaller than that used for endoscopic-assisted mastectomy.

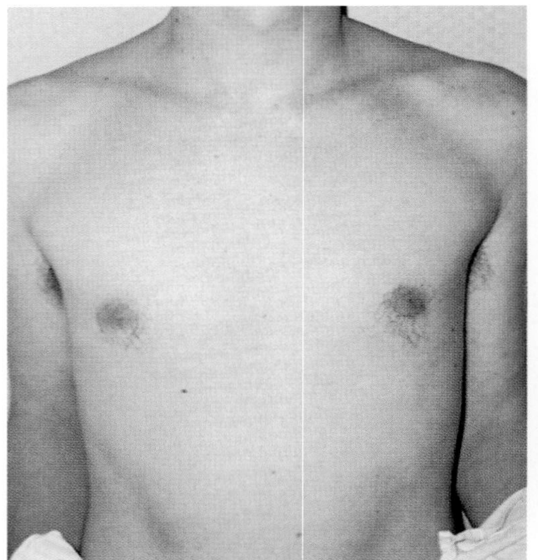

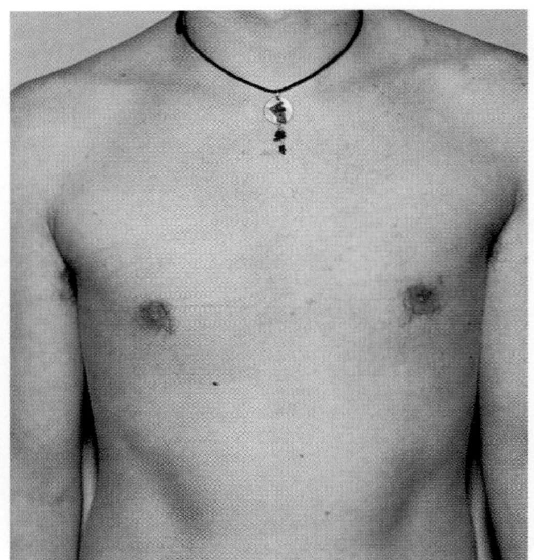

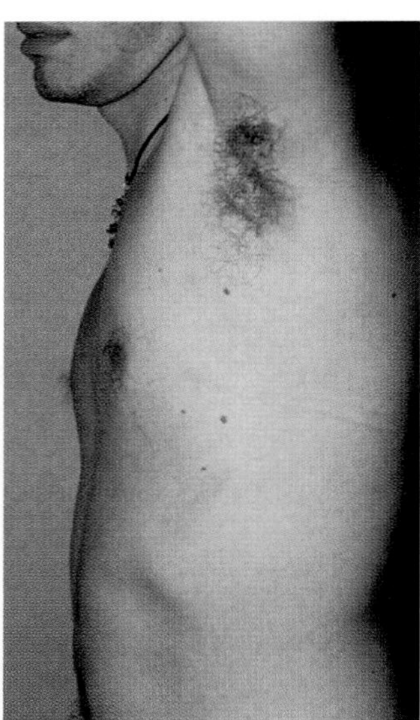

The patient in this operative sequence presented with a residual mass after open transareolar biopsy. Analysis of the pathologic specimen demonstrated only fibrous and glandular tissue. The original scar remained red for a prolonged period even though the final scar quality was excellent. The patient wanted to avoid any incisions near the breast that would leave obvious scars. He is shown 1 month after surgery. Minimal ecchymosis and edema permitted a rapid return to normal activities.

Symmastia With Breast Implants

After breast augmentation or breast reconstruction the implants (whether subglandular or submuscular) can become displaced medially, obliterating the medial juncture of the breast and sternum. This problem usually occurs when the surgeon, in attempting to meet the patient's expectations for maximum cleavage, places the implants as close together as possible. Sometimes the submuscular dissection extends across the midline after detaching the pectoralis major muscles in the upper breast region. When the implants are touching, however, the natural cleavage is lost.

Breast cleavage is restored by using textured-surface implants combined with central capsule excision and flaps developed from these medial capsules. The presternal region is resutured, and the capsules and the medial breast parenchyma are sutured to the chest wall. Although it is difficult to place sutures in the sternal periosteum and the dermis of the presternal region, this is essential for a successful outcome. Textured-surface implants are the best solution for this problem. Their outer surface inhibits motion and displacement, and following appropriate capsulectomy, the contracted pockets are dissected laterally so that the implants are not forced too far medially. I still use some medial sutures to recreate the medial margin of the pockets. I perform capsulectomies so that the textured-surface breast implants can be placed in new pockets that provide the best opportunity for the implants to adhere and remain soft. Dressings are placed centrally for a few days, and the patient wears a tube top to avoid central movement of the implants.

Constricted Breasts

The aesthetic breast surgeon should evaluate each patient's breasts for constriction. Constricted breasts are narrower than normal with a higher inframammary fold that begins more laterally than normal; they look abnormal and deformed. They usually have a tight inframammary fold and often show early changes associated with a tubular or ptotic appearance. ***The inframammary fold, an important breast landmark aesthetically and surgically, is the focal point in correcting breast constriction.*** It marks the inferior extent of the breast parenchyma and the beginning of the abdomen. Fibrous attachments extend from the dermis to the fascia at the level of the inframammary crease; breast tissue is contained above this fold. Constrictions or shortening or tightness of the inframammary fold are markedly variable and can produce unnatural and often asymmetric breasts. This is usually associated with some medial and inferior breast deficiency. A tight fold with or without breast hypertrophy often causes large breasts to fall over the fold, giving a ptotic or pseudoptotic appearance. The constriction can vary in degree from minor fold tightness, a more lateral takeoff of the inframammary folds, and a widened interbreast distance to severe tightness with tubular-shaped breasts. ***As the inframammary fold becomes tighter and higher inferiorly and the distance from the lower areola to the inframammary fold shortens, the breasts develop an increasingly constricted appearance until much of the breast is contained below an enlarged areola.*** The etiology of this developmental problem is unknown; however, inadequate development of the lower central and inferior breast tissue seems to be a major component of the problem. Deficient or missing tissue in the medial and inferior portion of the breasts does not permit the development of a normally positioned inframammary fold; the inframammary fold first moves laterally, then superiorly. This condition can be so marked that most of the breast is found centrally in the subareolar region, and little actual breast parenchyma is found beyond the confines and periphery of the areola. When the areola cannot contain the central breast tissue, this tissue protrudes centrally either as a tubular deformity or a tuberous deformity.

The underlying condition must be diagnosed and the implications of breast constriction understood prior to attempting breast surgery. Many breast asymmetries are related to unilateral or bilateral constriction. When this condition accompanies breast hypoplasia, either unilaterally or bilaterally, the surgeon must plan to modify, reposition, and extend the inframammary folds so that they are symmetric and normally positioned. Additionally, the deficiency in the lower breast region down to the new inframammary fold must be restored. The surgeon must determine the degree of breast parenchyma constriction. This condition could compromise correction with a breast implant because the tight, underdeveloped breast parenchyma and the tight, high fold restrict the anticipated fullness provided by the breast implant. When the areolar diameter is enlarged and protrudes, a periareolar and areolar excision of the excess areolar skin is sometimes necessary in addition to implant placement. When the protrusion is rather marked, it can be reduced by additional excision and areolar elevation. This tightening, however, tends to reduce the amount of central breast protrusion further and produces a more boxy, less protruding breast appearance. Breast implants can be placed through this periareolar or circumareolar incision at the time of the correction to enhance breast shape and define the lower breast pole and inframammary crease. The results produced by surgical correction of the constricted breast usually fall short of ideal. Scars are produced and some residual abnormality persists. Implants can contract and become visible through the skin. The patient must be informed of these limitations and this explanation carefully documented preoperatively.

PATIENT WITH A HIGH INFRAMAMMARY FOLD AND BREAST CONSTRICTION

To create a lower or new inframammary fold the existing fold must be detached. The skin extending up from its attachments to the dermis along the inframammary area and down to the new position must also be dissected. The breast that is constricted in the lower breast area is elevated at the time of breast augmentation, and radial incisions are made in the breast parenchyma to allow it to expand over the underlying breast implant. If the breast tissue is somewhat nodular, an obvious demarcation may be created below the breast after implants are positioned in the subglandular and subcutaneous region of the lower breast; this lower breast tissue is excised tangentially to provide a smooth juncture in this area. I prefer smooth-surface implants placed in an adequately released lower pocket. They also are more likely to produce a soft result, particularly when the implants are placed subcutaneously and subglandularly in the lower breast region.

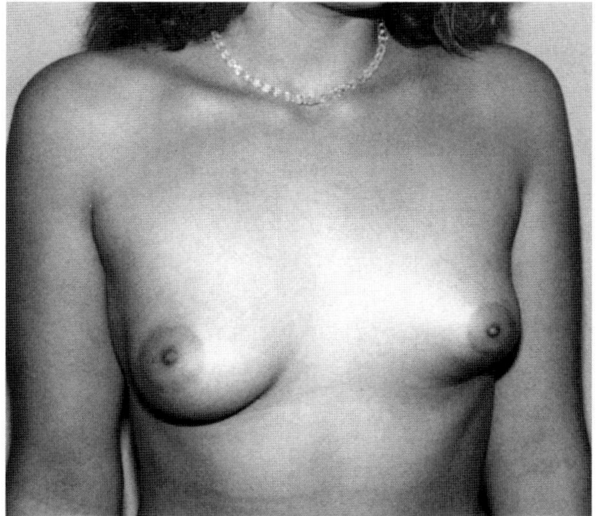

This 18-year-old patient had asymmetric breasts. Her right breast appeared essentially normal but had a lateral takeoff of the inframammary fold. The fold was about 1 cm high, and the breast ptosed over the fold. The inframammary fold began near the midline. Her left breast was constricted and had a higher inframammary crease. It demonstrated a lateral takeoff from the midline. There was some central constriction of the breasts with early signs of tubular breast deformity.

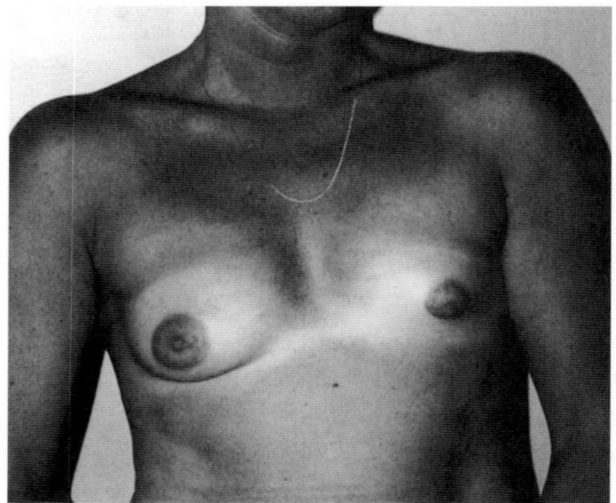

This patient had bilaterally constricted breasts with asymmetry. Her right breast, however, was not as affected as the left, demonstrating a somewhat lateral takeoff from the inframammary crease with a slightly high inframammary crease and a deficiency in the inferior and medial quadrants of the breast. Her left breast was hyperplastic with a very high and ill-defined inframammary crease; there was a suggestion of breast constriction and tubular deformity.

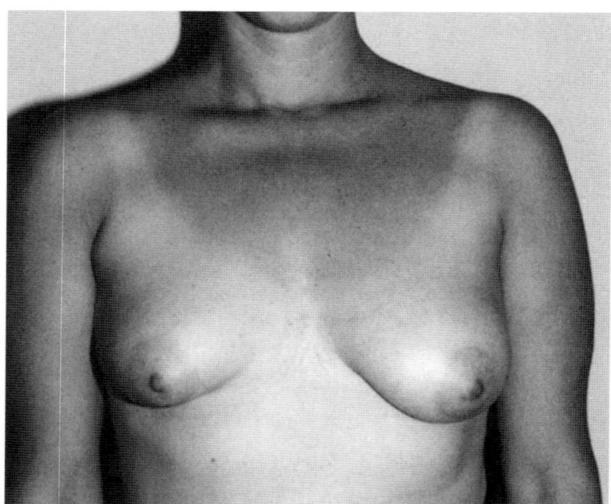

This patient had a normal left breast that exhibited mild fullness and a low nipple-areola. Her right breast had a high inframammary crease that began more laterally. There was a marked deficiency of the breast inferiorly and medially.

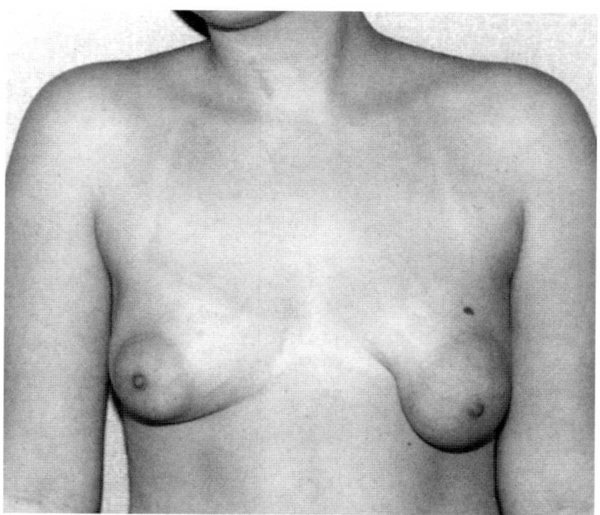

This patient demonstrated a more marked degree of this condition. Her right breast was normal, whereas the left breast had an even higher takeoff of the inframammary crease and a tubular breast deformity. Her ptotic breast rotated over the high, tight inframammary crease.

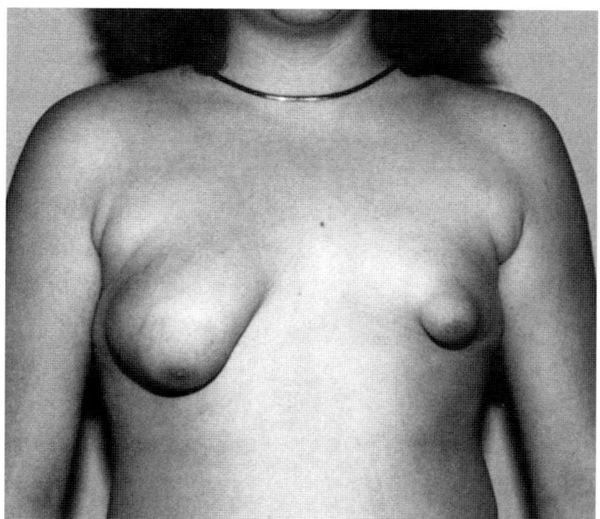

This woman had an even greater degree of breast asymmetry. The right breast had a normal volume but was constricted in its lower portions with a very high crease. The breast was underdeveloped inferiorly and medially. Her left breast had practically no inframammary crease, and most of the breast parenchyma was contained within the protruding central tubular breast deformity.

Patient Examples

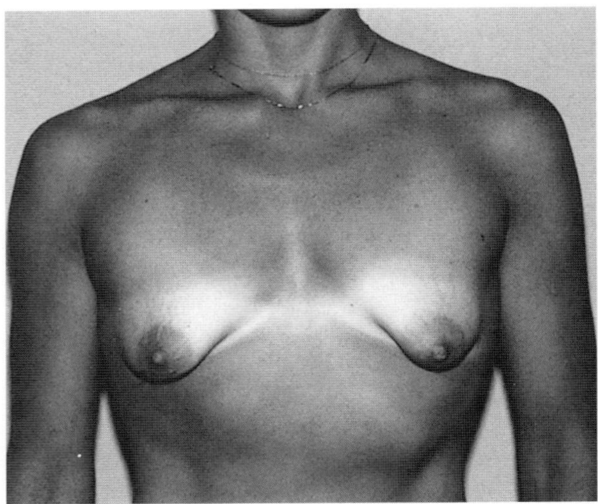
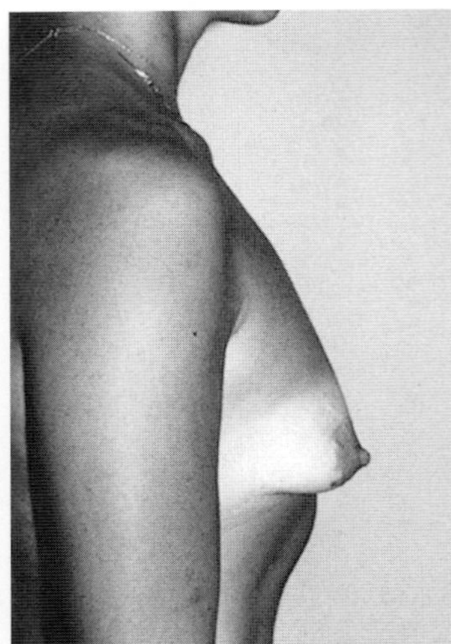

This 28-year-old mother of two children had bilaterally constricted breasts and high inframammary folds with a lateral takeoff. The intermammary breast width was greater than normal, and there was a deficiency of the breast inferiorly and inferomedially. Skin laxity had caused some ptosis of the breast parenchyma over the high, tight inframammary fold. The left nipple was 1 cm lower than the right, and there was central breast protrusion with a tubular deformity.

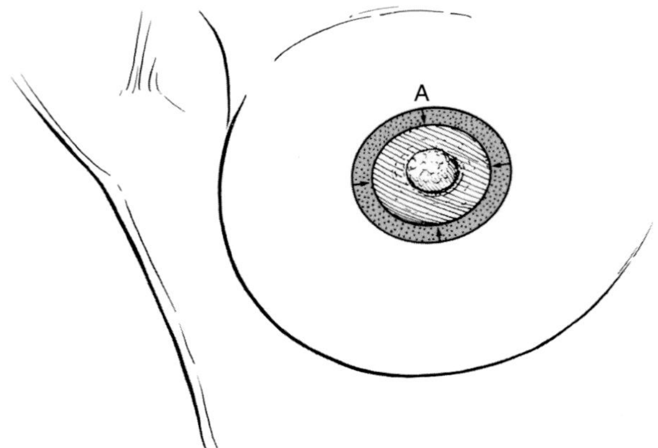

The preoperative plan was to tighten the protruding nipple-areola using a circumareolar incision. The left nipple was elevated 1 cm. A subpectoral dissection was done. The lower dissection extended beneath the gland, over the fascia, subcutaneously, and down to the level of the future inframammary crease, thereby detaching and eliminating the original inframammary crease. The inframammary crease was lowered to a normal distance of 6 cm between the inframammary crease and the lower portion of the repositioned areola. The periareolar purse-string suture tends to widen the breast and elevate the nipple-areola. ***A vertical mastopexy, particularly with a wide areola, is usually avoided in patients with constricted breasts since closure of the areola donor site further narrows the lower breast region.***

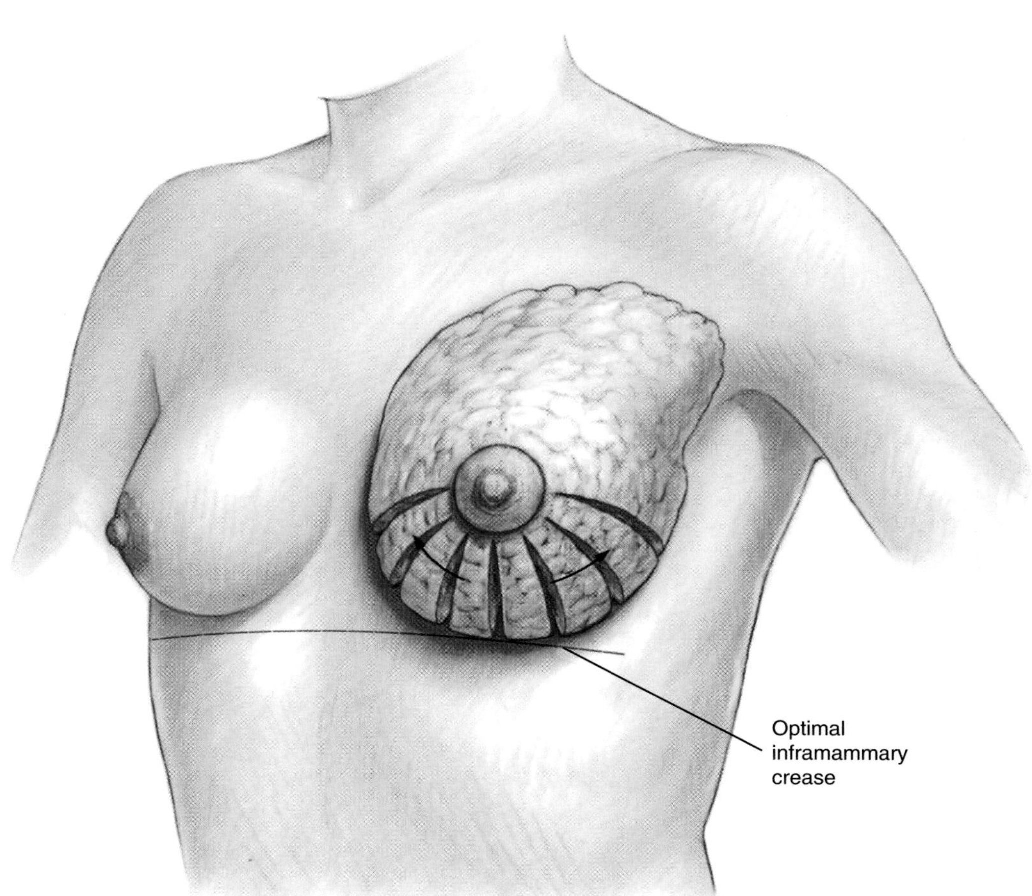

Radial incisions were made in the lower breast parenchyma to allow intraoperative expansion. Intraoperative expansion manually as well as with the expander device is helpful in releasing the lower breast to lessen the constriction and produce more lower pole fullness. Two 260 cc implants were positioned to give the best contour and symmetry.

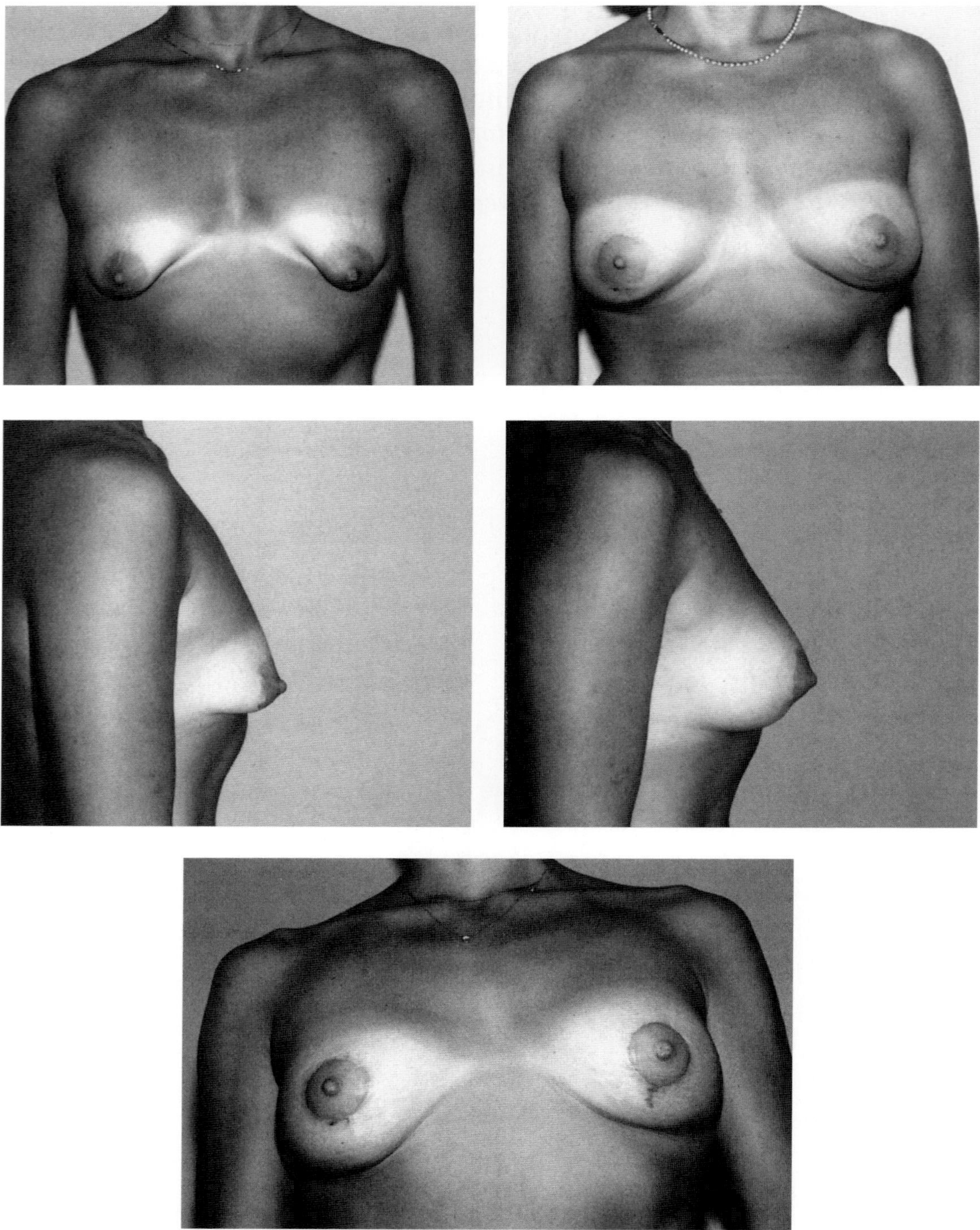

The patient is shown 15 months following the procedure with her improved contour and larger breast size. The intermammary space is still too wide, however, and additional release of the medial pectoralis major muscle would have permitted the implants to be positioned more medially.

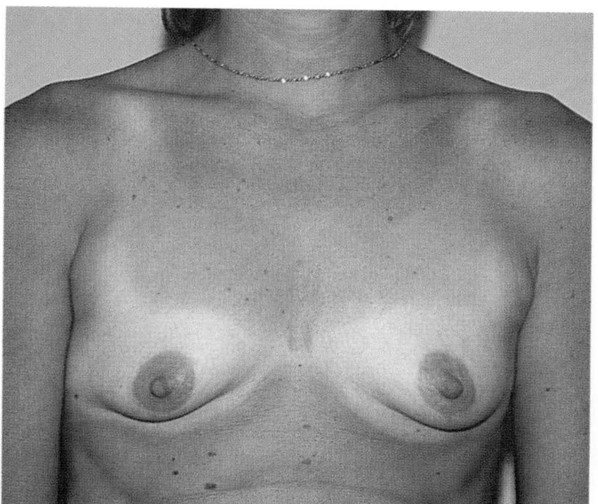

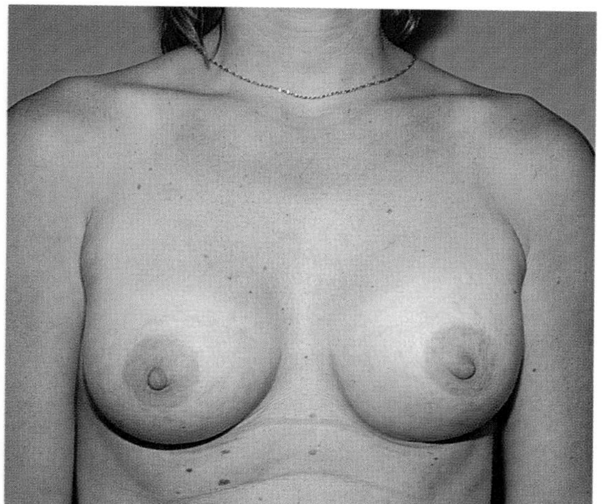

This 32-year-old woman had constricted breasts with a high inframammary fold. She felt that her breasts appeared small and droopy and wanted larger, more uplifted breasts similar in size to the way they were 5 years earlier when she was pregnant. Her health in general was good and she had no dominant breast masses and no family history of breast cancer. The preoperative plan addressed the high and constricted inframammary folds and the need to expand the lower breast parenchyma through a periareolar approach. The high inframammary fold was lowered to an appropriate position to accommodate 325 cc smooth-surface saline implants. The hemisphere of the implants was placed at the level of the nipple-areola. The pectoral muscle was released through the periareolar incision inferiorly, and smooth-surface saline implants were placed in subglandular pockets below. The patient is highly satisfied with the improvement in her breast appearance. Her breasts have remained soft and symmetric for 5 years, and there is minimal implant palpability in the lower breast region. A double-bubble deformity attributable to a difference in thickness between the breast parenchyma and the subcutaneous tissue covering the lower aspect of the breast implant has not developed, even though the patient was forewarned that this commonly occurs when constricted breasts have been augmented.

CONSTRICTED TUBULAR HYPOPLASTIC BREASTS

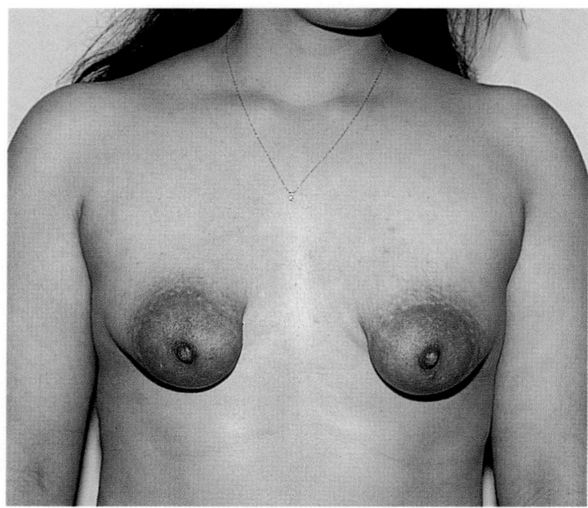

This 26-year-old woman had constricted, tubular breasts; most of the breast parenchyma was contained within her enlarged areolae. She desired larger breasts with smaller areolae. However, her breasts would be very tight and stretched if the areolae were reduced and breast implants placed. Therefore a periareolar purse-string mastopexy was planned with insertion of postoperatively adjustable implants.

Surgical plan

- Reduction of excess central breast skin with periareolar skin excision
- Elevation of nipple-areola by tightening central breast skin and moving areola upward
- Redefinition of inframammary fold
- Expansion of lower breast parenchyma
- Development of subpectoral pocket
- Placement of subpectoral saline implant to give additional breast volume
- Replacement of 325 cc adjustable implant for postoperatively adjustable implant

Markings and Technique

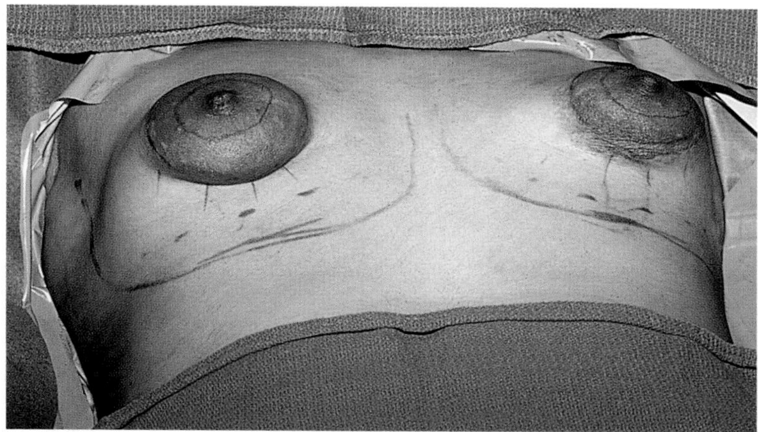

The markings for the initial incision are drawn around the areola, and a second line is marked to define the new areola. The present inframammary fold line is drawn as a dotted line, and the future inframammary fold is marked 2 cm below.

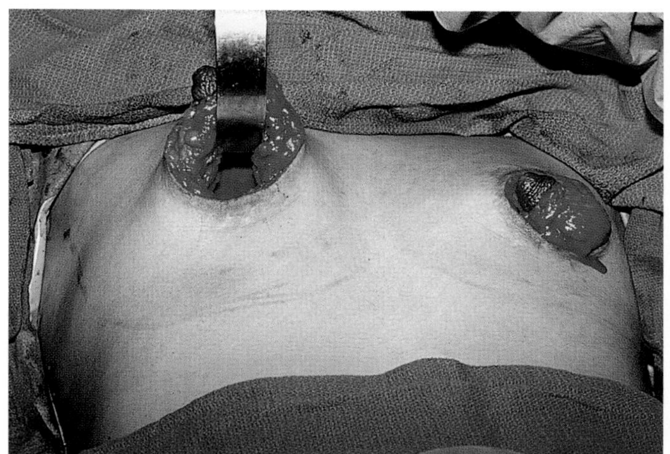

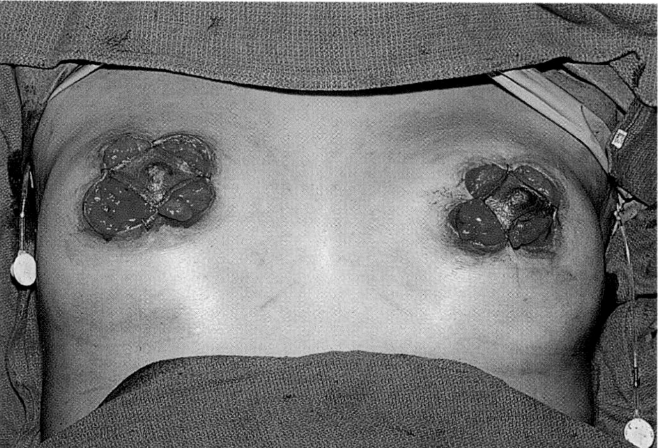

After the periareolar incision is made and the retroglandular area approached through the lower breast parenchyma, three short incisions are made in the parenchyma and intraoperative expansion begun. Next the pectoral muscle is elevated to the lower medial pectoral muscle. The implant pocket is developed subpectorally above and subglandularly below. Two 325 cc postoperatively adjustable implants are selected and positioned appropriately. Any protruding breast parenchyma is resected prior to closure with two layers of intracuticular sutures.

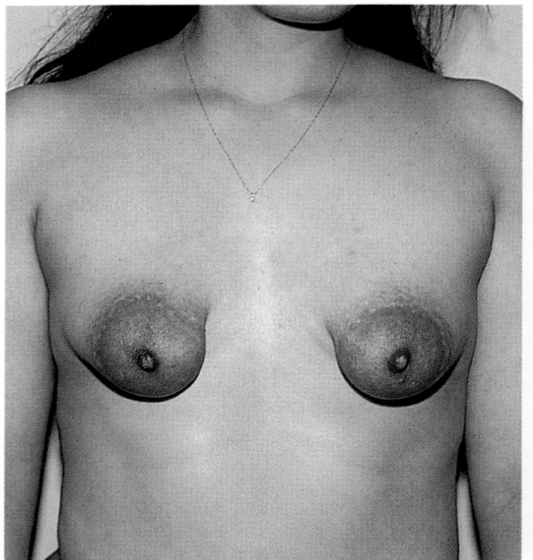

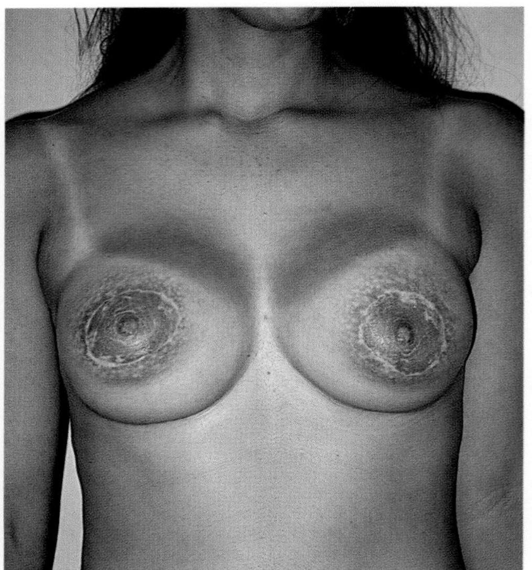

Delayed healing of the periareolar incision resulted in postoperative scarring. The intraoperative expansion produced the size breasts the patient desired. Overall the contour and shape of the breasts are good, but the scars are unattractive and would benefit from a scar revision, which the patient declined.

Patient Example

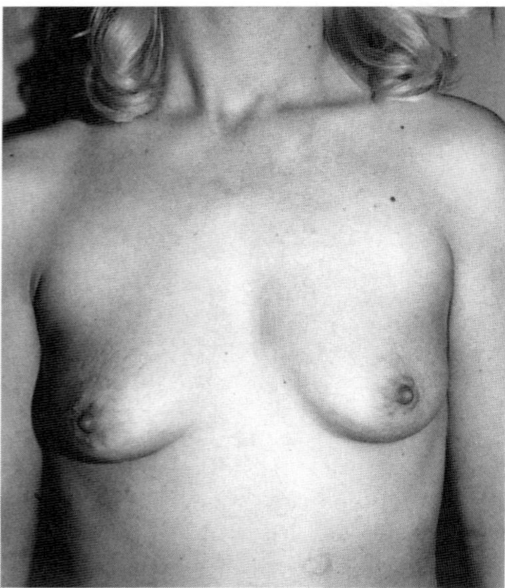

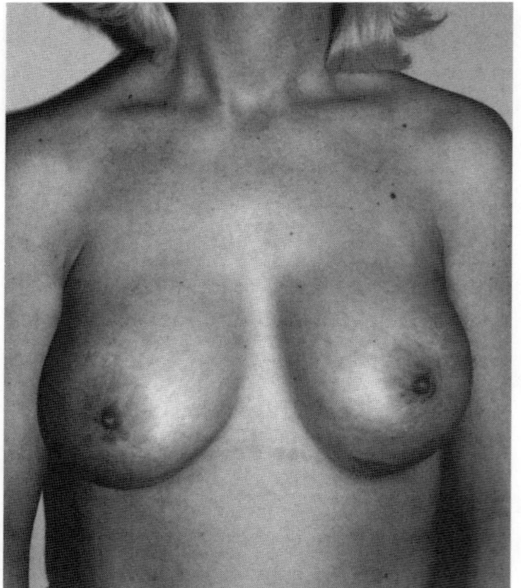

This 25-year-old patient had mammary hypoplasia and also a short 3 cm distance between her inframammary crease and areola. She requested a large breast augmentation. An inframammary approach was used and the incision placed just below her original inframammary fold. The implant was placed in a subpectoral position above and a subglandular position below. Radial incisions were made in the lower breast parenchyma to allow expansion of this area. The original inframammary crease was disrupted with sharp dissection, and the dissection was carried lower to permit repositioning of the inframammary crease. Two 320 cc implants were positioned subpectorally in the upper breast and subglandularly below. The patient is shown 4 years following the procedure.

Nipple Problems

Nipple problems are usually related to congenital absence of the nipple-areola, a rare condition; nipple-areolar asymmetries; and specific problems such as nipple discharge, nipple inversion, and nipple hypertrophy.

Congenital absence of the nipple is frequently associated with breast asymmetry and Poland's syndrome. The best approach is to correct the breast asymmetry primarily and wait to reconstruct the nipple-areola, just as is done in breast reconstruction (see Chapter 20).

NIPPLE INVERSION

Nipple inversion is usually caused by shortening of the breast ducts and fibrous tissue binding the nipple-areola to the subnipple-areola parenchyma. Breast tumor and Paget's disease of the nipple should be considered in the preoperative evaluation. The deformity can be predictably corrected by dividing the ductal and fibrous tissue within the nipple-areola and stretching it outward while healing takes place with a supporting suture that does not compromise the vascularity of the nipple-areola.

Patient Example

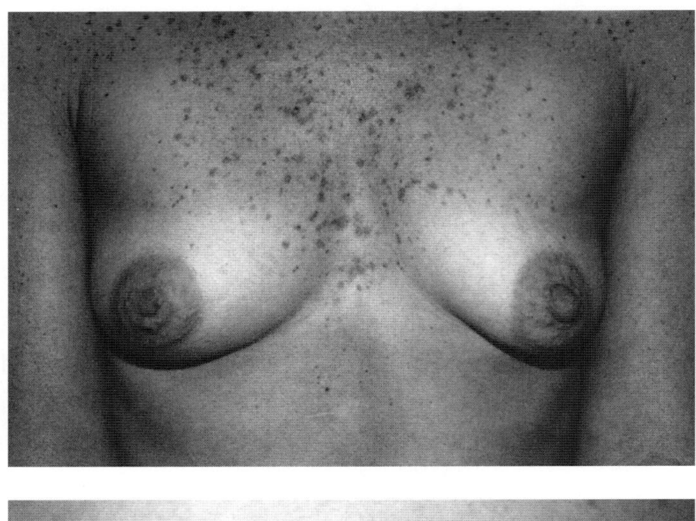

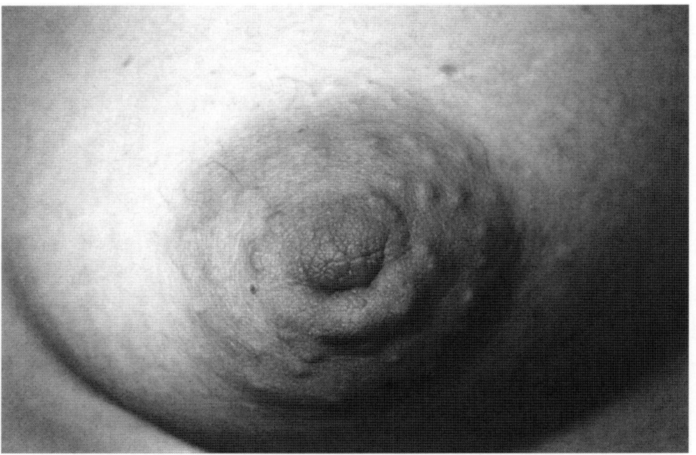

This 23-year-old woman's right nipple inversion had been evident since puberty. No underlying breast masses could be palpated, and her mammograms were negative. There was no nipple rash.

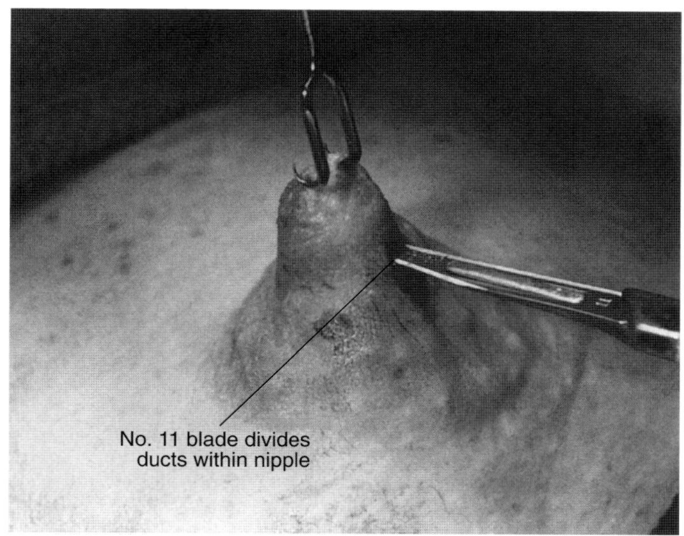

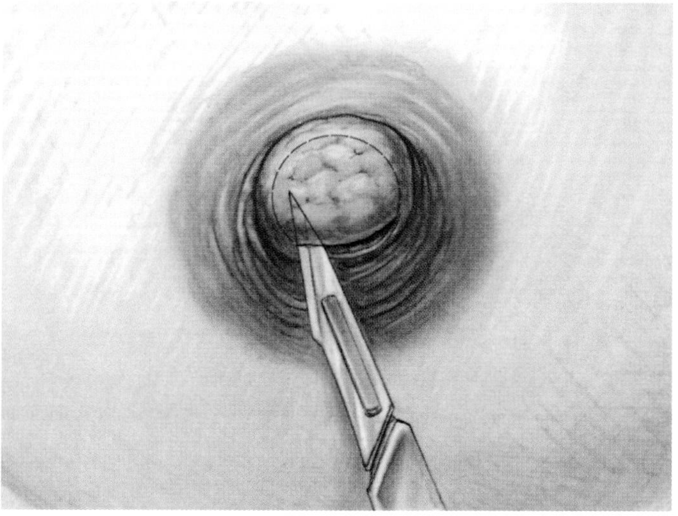

The inversion was corrected by everting the nipple with a skin hook and dividing the fibrous tissue and ducts within the nipple with a No. 11 blade. Care was taken not to damage the dermis and to preserve nipple viability; however, enough ducts must be divided to permit the nipple to remain in its corrected position without sutures. After the ducts were divided, a pair of horizontal mattress 4-0 chromic sutures were positioned at right angles through the nipple and secured so as to mildly compress the base without constricting the blood supply to the nipple.

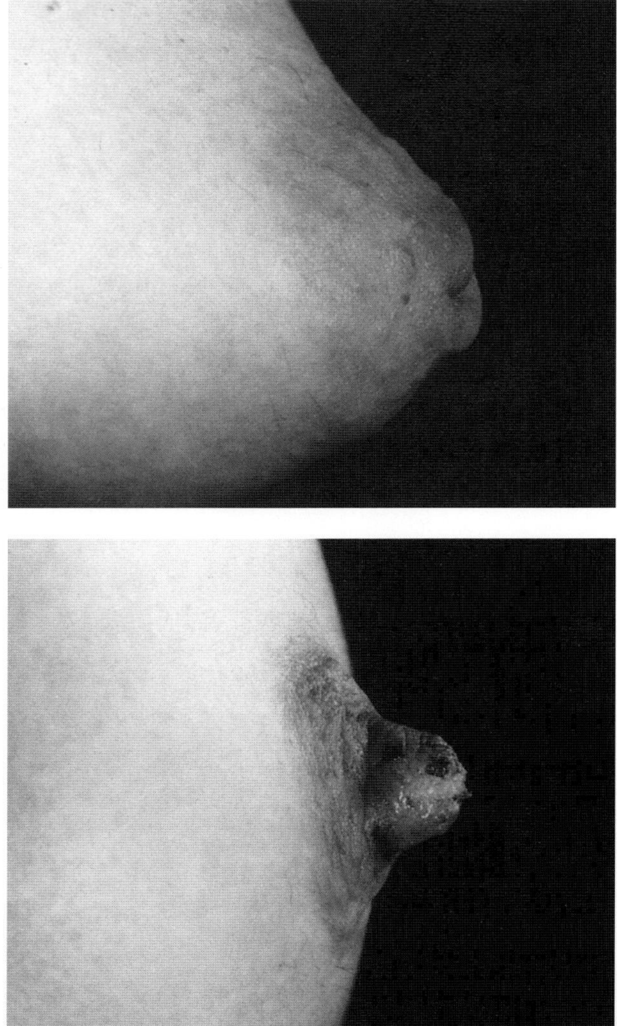

The patient, shown immediately after correction of the nipple-areola, demonstrates good long-term results.

NIPPLE HYPERTROPHY

Nipple-areolar hypertrophy can be corrected via two methods. When a patient has successfully completed lactation (commonly the case in patients with hypertrophy), a simple transection to reduce the end of the nipple is the best solution. The end is allowed to reepithelialize, and the duct openings are preserved and reconstituted during reepithelialization. When the patient wants to preserve the ability to lactate I do a sleeve resection of the nipple-areola to drop it downward and thus avoid any ductal injury.

Patient Example

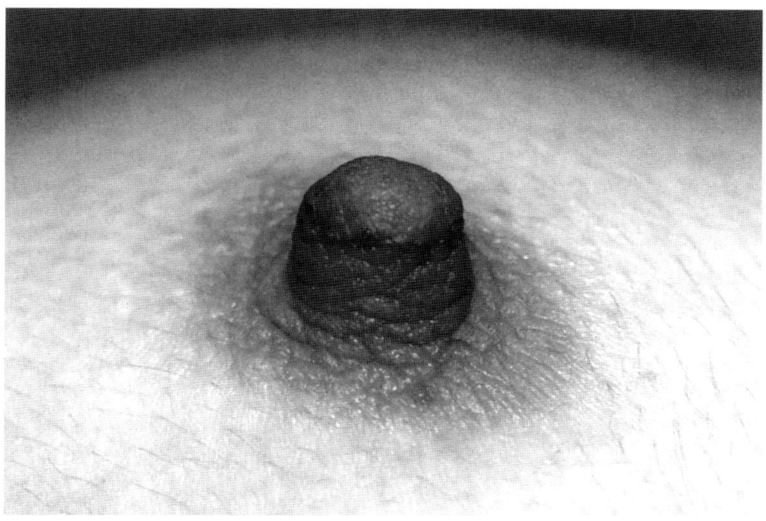

This patient had a prolapsed nipple with excessive projection. She requested that her nipple-areola be shortened. This was done by a tangential excision at the level indicated on the preoperative markings. The wound was left open and allowed to reepithelialize from the cut ends of the nipple duct. This simple technique effectively shortened the nipple to obtain the desired projection. This technique is useful for harvesting a nipple for opposite breast nipple reconstruction when the nipple has a greater projection than its diameter. Otherwise I harvest the lower half of the nipple. (This topic is discussed further in Chapter 20.)

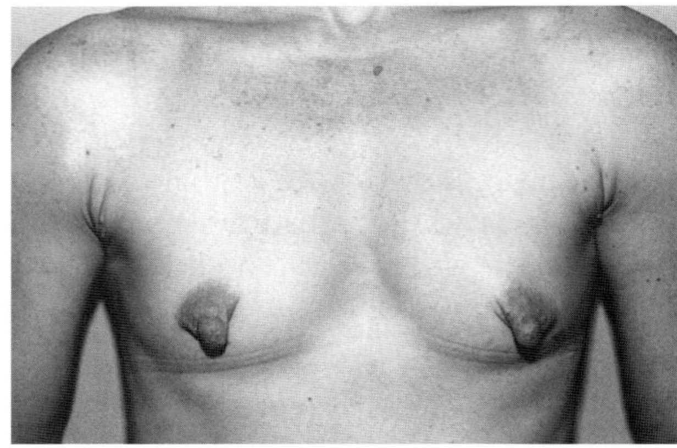

An alternate method of nipple reduction is sleeve resection, as selected for this patient who had prolapsed projecting nipples after pregnancy and breast-feeding. Since she wanted to be able to breast-feed in the future, the nipple ducts were preserved with this technique.

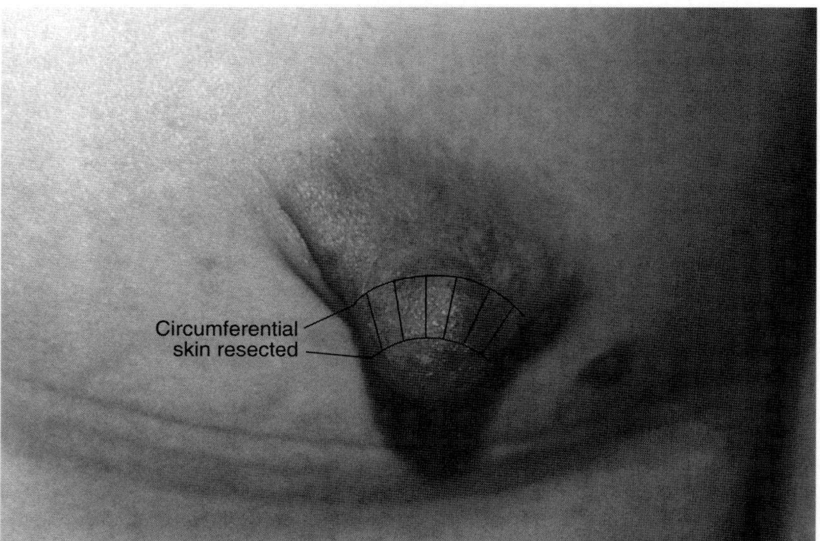

The sleeve resection extended from the base of the areola to about 2 to 3 mm proximal to its end.

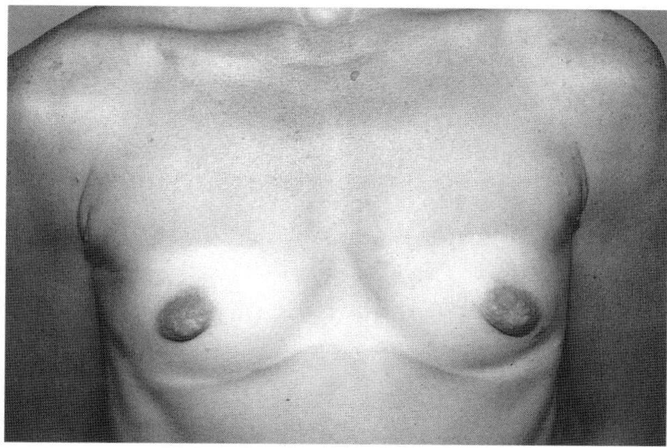

After resection the nipple was telescoped back into the breast to reduce the nipple-areolar projection. This approach effectively reduced the patient's nipple-areolar projection without disturbing the primary nipple ducts. Her breast-feeding potential was preserved.

Chest Wall Abnormalities

SPINAL CURVATURE AND SCOLIOSIS

Chest wall abnormalities such as spinal curvature and scoliosis can make one breast appear larger than the other. Patients with these problems are often seen in their late teens; they may present with a rotary deformity in which one hemithorax is more prominent than the other because the deformed thorax has pushed one breast forward and the opposite breast back. The rotation of the breast is also asymmetric; one is more compact and the other is wider and spread out over the deformed, rotated rib cage. Examination of the backs of these patients reveals the scoliosis. When observed from above, the spinal and thoracic curvature is evident. ***The key to this problem is identifying the chest wall curvature and understanding that breast augmentation requires additional projection on the side that is rotated more posteriorly.*** Infraclavicular implants are often needed to fill out the infraclavicular and upper chest wall area on the more posterior side. Correction for most of the patients usually requires augmentation.

PECTUS EXCAVATUM

Pectus excavatum is a congenital condition characterized by an abnormal concavity of the midchest. Specifically it involves an inward rotation of the sternum and the costal cartilages. The condition can exhibit subtle to marked changes. Children with severe pectus excavatum deformities often have corrective surgery at the age of 5 to 10 years by thoracic or pediatric surgeons. Correction at this time usually requires division of the costal cartilages, repositioning of the sternum, and osteotomies of the sternum to improve the contour. Patients who are seen in their teens or later usually do not demonstrate as marked a deformity, and the condition can frequently be improved with custom implants to fill out the central sternal area. Many of these patients have concomitant breast hypoplasia, accentuated by central third midchest depression. A marked deformity can also be filled with a custom-designed implant. A moulage is taken of the deformity and a custom implant is made. ***If at all possible, I try to avoid placing implants centrally to correct the pectus excavatum deformity because of the incidence of palpability and capsular contracture.***

Breast augmentation can be performed at the same time the pectus excavatum deformity is corrected. The inframammary incision for placement of the central implant can be extended medially and also be used to place the implants.

Patient Example

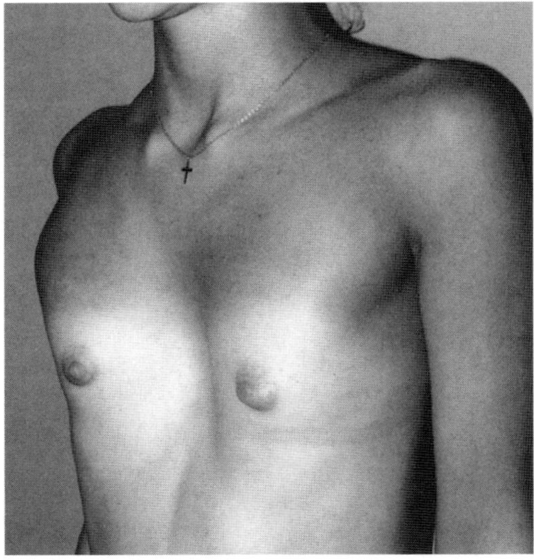

This 22-year-old patient had rather marked pectus excavatum with significant breast asymmetry. The central concavity of her chest was associated with an inward rotation of her breasts. This condition was corrected in a combined procedure performed with the thoracic surgeon. The thoracic surgeon repositioned the ribs and sternum through a bilateral inframammary incision connected with a V extension across the midline. At the same time bilateral submusculofascial breast implants were positioned to correct the breast hypoplasia.

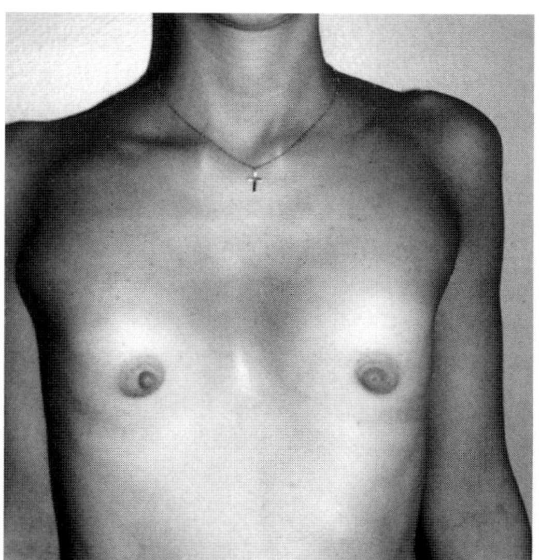

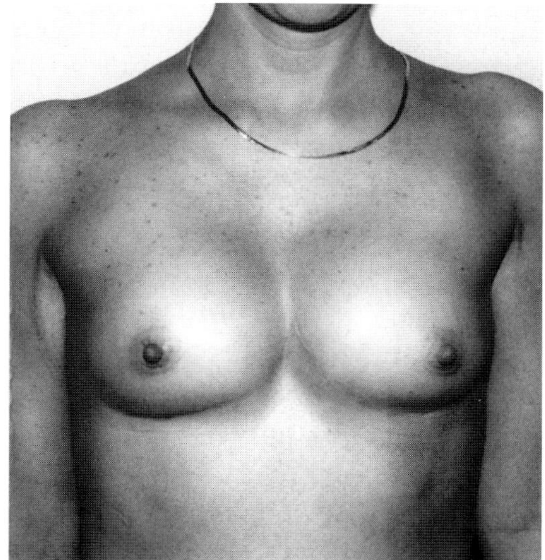

The patient is shown 6 years following this procedure. Her implants have retained their position and produced attractive cleavage. The medial positioning of the implants has filled the cavity medially and created a significantly improved, more natural contour with additional fill in the upper portion of her right breast. She also requested additional augmentation of the right breast to improve the projection on that side. The procedure was done via an inframammary incision and the implants placed in a subpectoral position. She liked the bilateral enlargement, particularly the improved fullness in the right upper chest and the projection of the right breast.

Low Inframammary Fold

A low inframammary fold in a patient with breast hypoplasia usually occurs after breast augmentation or breast reconstruction. Often this low fold is caused by an expander, a smooth-surface implant, or more rarely a textured-surface implant that has extended lower than is aesthetically acceptable. This problem can develop when the surgeon has attempted to lower the inframammary fold at the initial procedure or when an implant with a large diameter has been selected for a particularly large breast augmentation.

To elevate the inframammary fold a breast implant of the correct diameter and size must be selected and positioned properly. An implant with a textured surface is preferred in this situation because it will hold its position and not descend, particularly in the first few weeks after the correction. This implant must be placed in contact with virgin tissue; otherwise it can become displaced postoperatively.

The elevated inframammary fold must be accurately positioned and secured with sutures from the deep fascia or the deep capsule up to the dermis of the skin. I generally use an inframammary incision for this condition and remove the original implant to give the inframammary fold better definition. The implant can, however, drift downward over time. An internal capsulorrhaphy, which precludes an inframammary fold incision, is another strategy for treating this problem.

Breast Asymmetry

Most individuals exhibit some degree of breast asymmetry. Ordinarily patients with developmental breast asymmetries are seen after initial breast development. They often present at 15 or 16 years of age and can demonstrate a range of asymmetries. One normal breast may be paired with an opposite larger, smaller, or constricted breast. Both breasts may appear abnormal, either too large or too small or sizes in between. Constriction of one or both breasts, particularly asymmetric constriction, can also produce an asymmetric breast appearance. Acquired asymmetry can occur after several or multiple breast biopsies, particularly if a lumpectomy is performed. The condition is also accentuated when the breast tissue is irradiated. (Patients who have acquired asymmetries related to lumpectomy and radiation are discussed in Chapter 19.)

A proper diagnosis is necessary before correcting problems of asymmetry. The aesthetic breast surgeon must remember that a tumor can be responsible for this problem, and the breasts must be examined with this in mind. Hypoplasia, hyperplasia, and breast constriction must be identified. The patient's input is important. She should tell the aesthetic breast surgeon what she thinks about her breast size and appearance—her assessment may be very different from the surgeon's. Specific areas of asymmetry are noted, whether of the lower pole of the breast, inframammary fold, the lateral breast tissue, or central or upper breast tissue. Each of these areas must be evaluated separately prior to finalizing a plan for surgical correction. To ensure that the reconstructive procedure chosen to treat the asymmetry produces the desired symmetric appearance, certain principles merit attention:

- The breasts will behave more similarly over time when breast implants are placed behind both breasts. This is obvious when augmentation is needed on both sides.
- The symmetry will be even better if the implants are close to the same size.
- Sometimes the normal breast parenchyma of the fuller breast will need to be resected before placing implants.
- When there is a probability that the breast size may change or when the surgeon is concerned about the possibility of getting the best symmetry, particularly with asymmetric implants, the permanent expander implant with the small fill valve can be used. This expander allows the surgeon to alter implant volume to reflect breast growth or to make postoperative changes to adjust for asymmetric breast size or satisfy patient preferences.

BILATERAL BREAST HYPOPLASIA

Patients whose breasts are asymmetric and hypoplastic may also have breasts that are constricted; this condition must be identified because it may be contributing to the breast asymmetry. The position of the inframammary folds may be altered at the time the asymmetry is corrected. ***The aesthetic breast surgeon must remember that the asymmetry may be evident both in the breast diameter and projection.*** If there is no breast ptosis or marked hypoplasia, asymmetric-sized implants can be used to correct the problem. I prefer textured-surface implants for this purpose; they can be placed through the usual augmentation incisions. Using the proper-sized implants is critical. Preoperative dimensional measurements are important as is the versatility of saline implants; breast sizers are useful in determining the correct size prior to selection of the final implants. The volume of the asymmetry is estimated. In making this assessment it is important to remember that the volumes of brassiere cups are related to chest diameters. The degree of asymmetry that is noticeable is related to the size of the breasts. For instance, a 100 cc discrepancy is much more apparent in a woman with breasts that are 100 and 200 gm than it is in a woman with breasts that are 1500 and 1600 gm, respectively. Simply placing larger breast implants improves breast symmetry in a small-breasted woman who has a 100 cc difference; this discrepancy is even smaller if 300 cc implants are placed in each side or if a smaller implant is placed on the smaller side. Intraoperative expansion of the smaller breast may help to expand the skin and the submusculofascial pocket to accept a larger breast implant.

Patient Examples

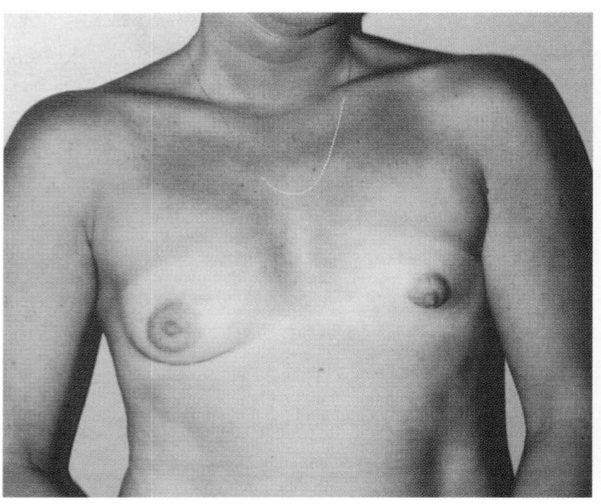

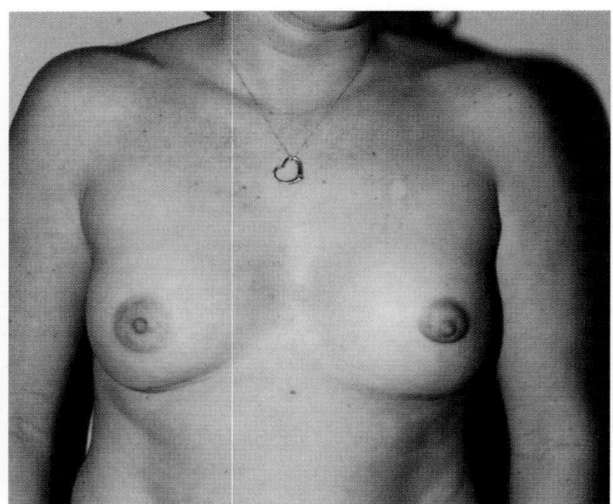

This 22-year-old patient had breast asymmetry. Her right breast was mildly hypoplastic and constricted. The left breast was more constricted and hypoplastic with some tubular deformity. Inframammary incisions were made at the site of the future inframammary crease. Subpectoral dissections were done bilaterally. On the left side, however, the skin was separated from the rudimentary inframammary crease up to the nipple-areola. Radial incisions were made in the diminutive breast parenchyma, and intraoperative manual expansion was performed to expand the lower portion of the breast. Breast implants were then positioned subpectorally above and subglandularly below. A 240 cc implant was placed on the left side and a 220 cc implant on the right.

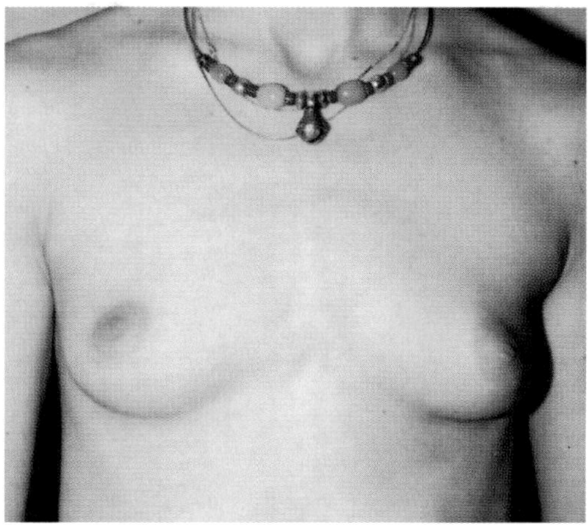

This 22-year-old woman had mammary hypoplasia with breast asymmetry. The right breast was higher than the left, and there was relative flattening in the left supra-areolar region. Asymmetry of the inframammary creases as well as the supra-areolar region was noted; the left crease was lower than the right. Subpectoral implants were positioned using a periareolar approach. The inframammary creases were dissected symmetrically and the implants positioned. With the patient in a sitting position the implant on the left was inflated further to determine the best intraoperative symmetry.

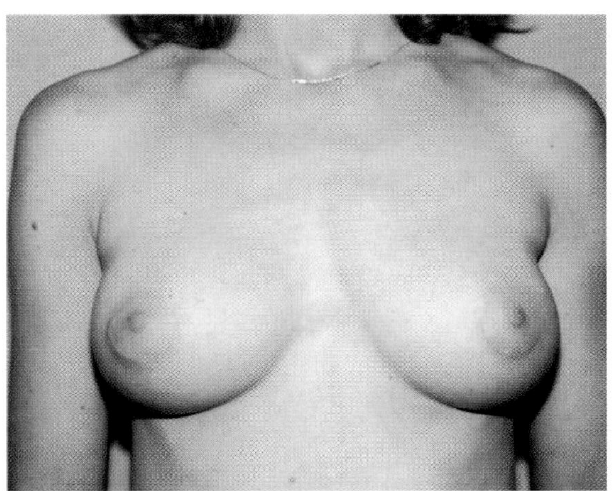

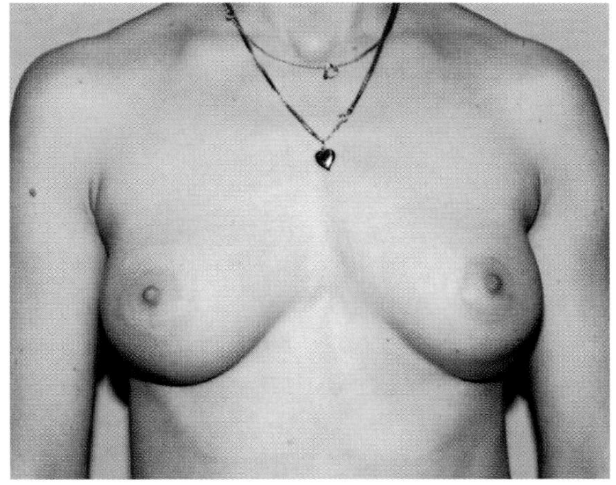

The patient is shown 1 year and 6 years after the procedure. The appearance of her correction has persisted. No significant capsular contracture has developed and there is reasonable symmetry. A double contour is observable beneath the left areola in the lower portion of the left breast, but she was alerted to this possibility preoperatively and it is not a problem for her. For some women, however, this lower breast distortion would be a source of disappointment. That is why the patient needs to be fully advised of this possibility prior to scheduling an operation.

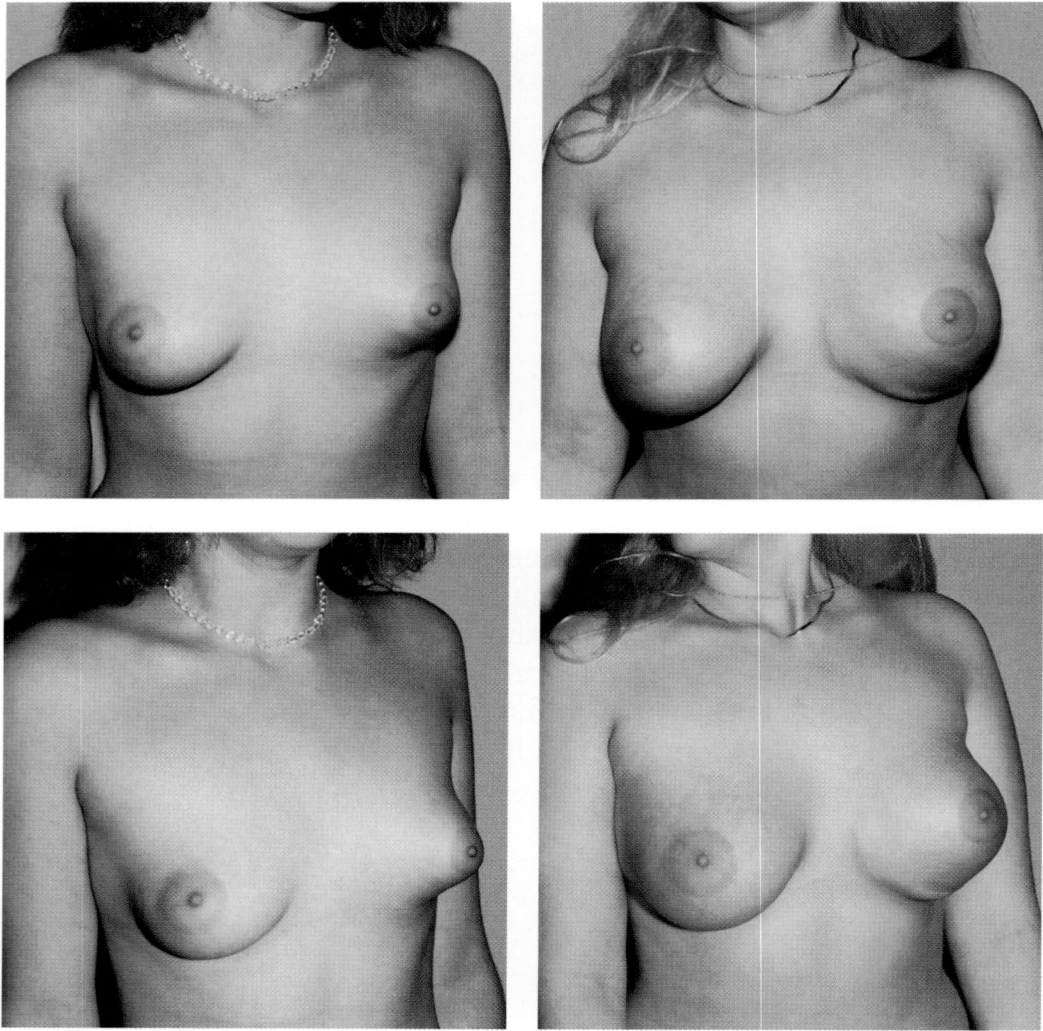

This patient had mammary hypoplasia with constriction of both breasts but more constriction of the left breast. Inframammary incisions were used for this correction. The left inframammary crease was repositioned and recreated downward by freeing up the constricted inframammary crease and radial divisions of the breast parenchyma. Implants, 260 cc on the left and 180 cc on the right, were used to obtain breast symmetry. The patient is shown 2 years following correction. She has gained approximately 20 pounds during this time.

Since her weight gain the heavier breast has assumed a lower position, and a mild capsular contracture has developed around the left implant. A capsulectomy in the lower portion of the left breast with placement of a slightly larger implant would provide some additional ptosis. Replacement of the original silicone implant with a saline implant, which is heavier, would also create somewhat more ptosis on the left side.

UNILATERAL BREAST HYPOPLASIA

When the patient has one breast that she considers normal and a smaller breast on the other side, the surgeon must ascertain whether the normal breast can be matched. The smaller breast is often constricted, and this must be considered in the surgical plan. If it is ptotic or hypertrophic, it is unlikely that symmetry can be achieved simply by placing a full implant in the opposite breast. If the opposite breast has a normal full shape with upper pole fullness, then placement of an implant in the hypoplastic breast may provide symmetry. If there is any ptosis or unusual fullness in the lower pole of the breast that the patient considers normal, I use the size of the normal breast as the model for correction but resect some of its ptotic lower breast tissue so that breast implants can be positioned bilaterally and the distances from the lower areola border to the inframammary crease can be controlled.

If a decision is made to place an implant in only one breast, the patient should know that her breasts will not behave the same over time and that future alterations may be necessary. The breast without the implant will respond differently than the breast with the implant to weight fluctuation, hormones, pregnancy, lactation, and menopause. All these influences can affect the opposite breast more than the implanted breast. For this reason I prefer to maintain similar amounts of breast skin and parenchyma and to use comparably sized implants that are more likely to act similarly over time.

BILATERAL ASYMMETRIC BREAST HYPERTROPHY

Breast asymmetry frequently accompanies breast hypertrophy. The patient's breasts are carefully checked to determine the extent of asymmetry and areas of excess tissue. For patients with this problem, plans are made to remove the excess tissue from these areas so that the tissue that is left is symmetrically positioned and of similar size. It is helpful to mark estimates of the larger and smaller breast volumes on the breasts and to estimate preoperatively the amount of tissue to be excised. During the procedure the amount of the excised breast tissue is recorded and can be compared to the preoperative estimate of breast reduction. The excess breast tissue is usually found in the lower and outer poles of the breasts. These patients also demonstrate a general increase in breast projection. The superior and superior medial techniques are effective for resecting this lower and lateral breast tissue (see Chapter 7).

Patient Examples

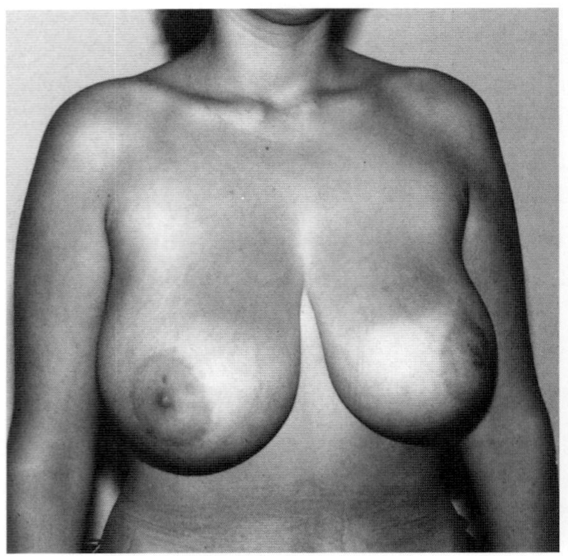

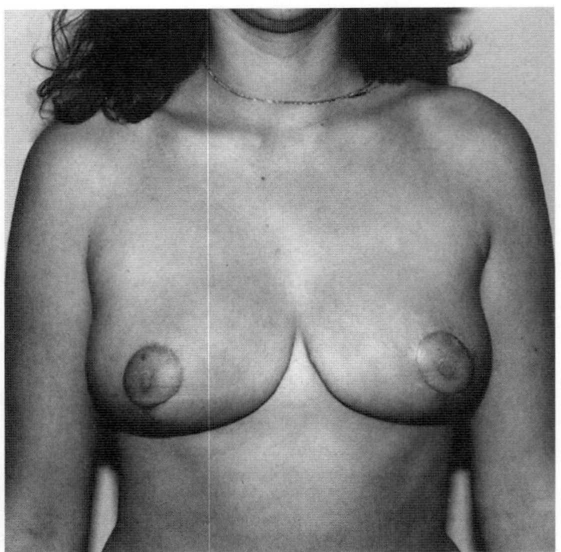

This patient had bilateral mammary hyperplasia with the right breast larger than the left. The superior medial pedicle technique was used for breast reduction. A total of 500 gm was removed from the left side and 650 from the right. When correcting asymmetric breast hypertrophy I have found it helpful to estimate the grams of asymmetry preoperatively. The preoperative markings for the nipple-areola of the heavier breast will usually be lower. If the positions of the nipple-areola are marked at the identical level, after the breast tissue is resected, the larger breast will recoil more and will become higher than the smaller side. To accommodate this condition I mark the nipple-areolar position with the breast lifted upward. The patient is shown 4 months following the procedure. Her breasts have been effectively reduced and exhibit improved breast symmetry.

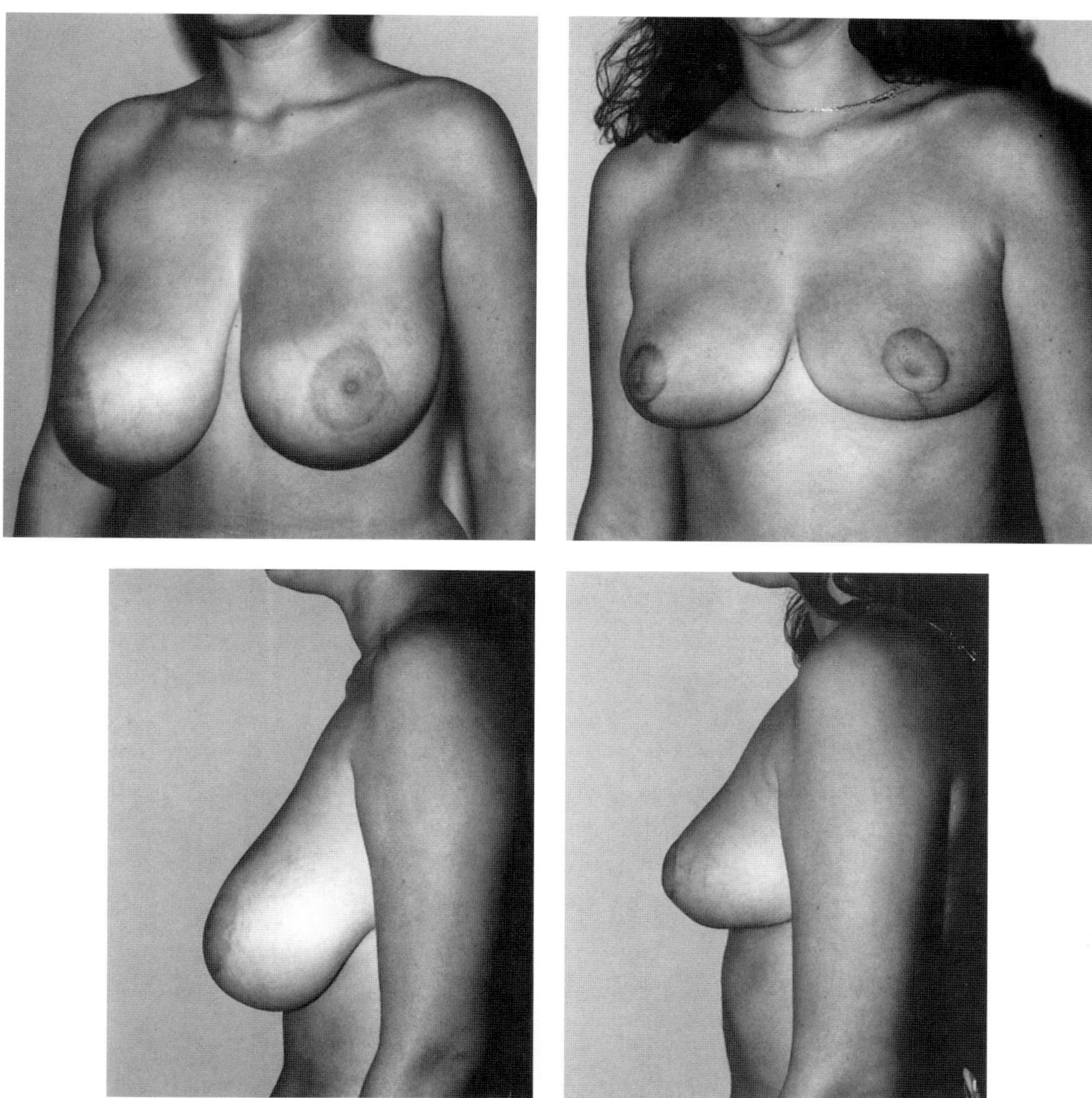

UNILATERAL BREAST HYPERTROPHY AND UNILATERAL BREAST HYPOPLASIA

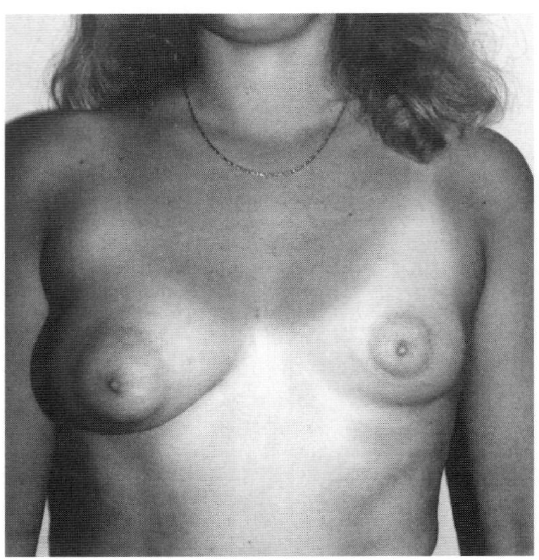

When one breast is too large and the other breast is too small, neither is usually pleasing to the patient and both require some alteration. Because a breast implant will be necessary for the breast that is too small, I recommend that the patient consider having the larger breast reduced to permit placement of bilateral breast implants. This approach affords the best opportunity for maintaining long-term symmetry. The plan for this patient called for a vertical reduction mammaplasty on the right breast and a breast augmentation via the inframammary approach on the left.

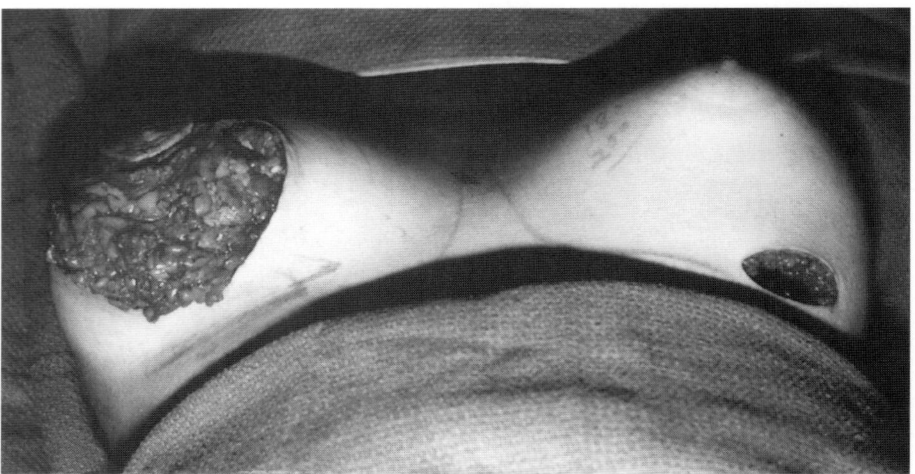

After the inframammary augmentation with the implant placed in the subpectoral position above and the subglandular position below, a submusculofascial resection was done on the right side and a 120 cc implant positioned.

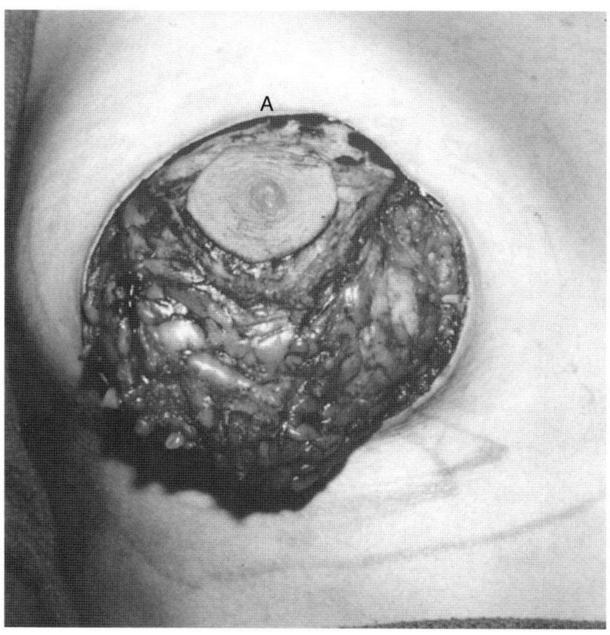

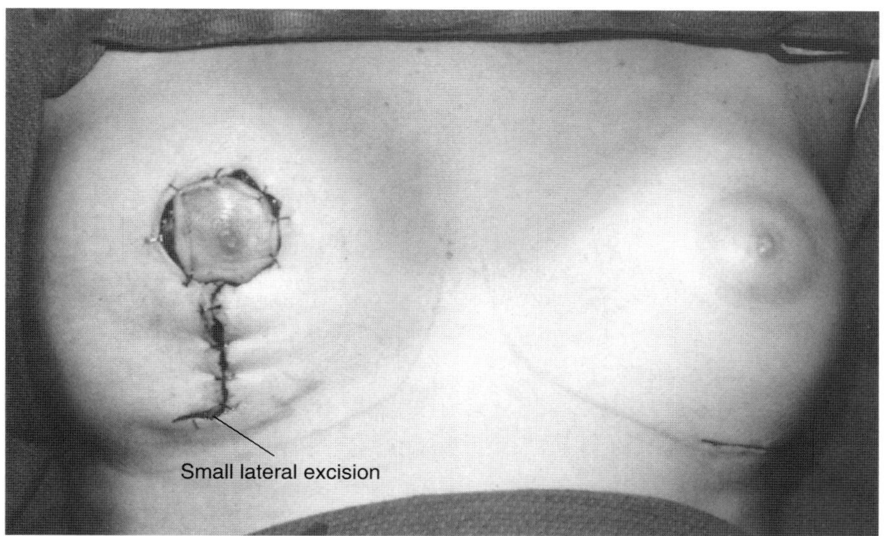

The breast was then reduced to a volume to match the opposite left breast to produce relatively symmetric breasts.

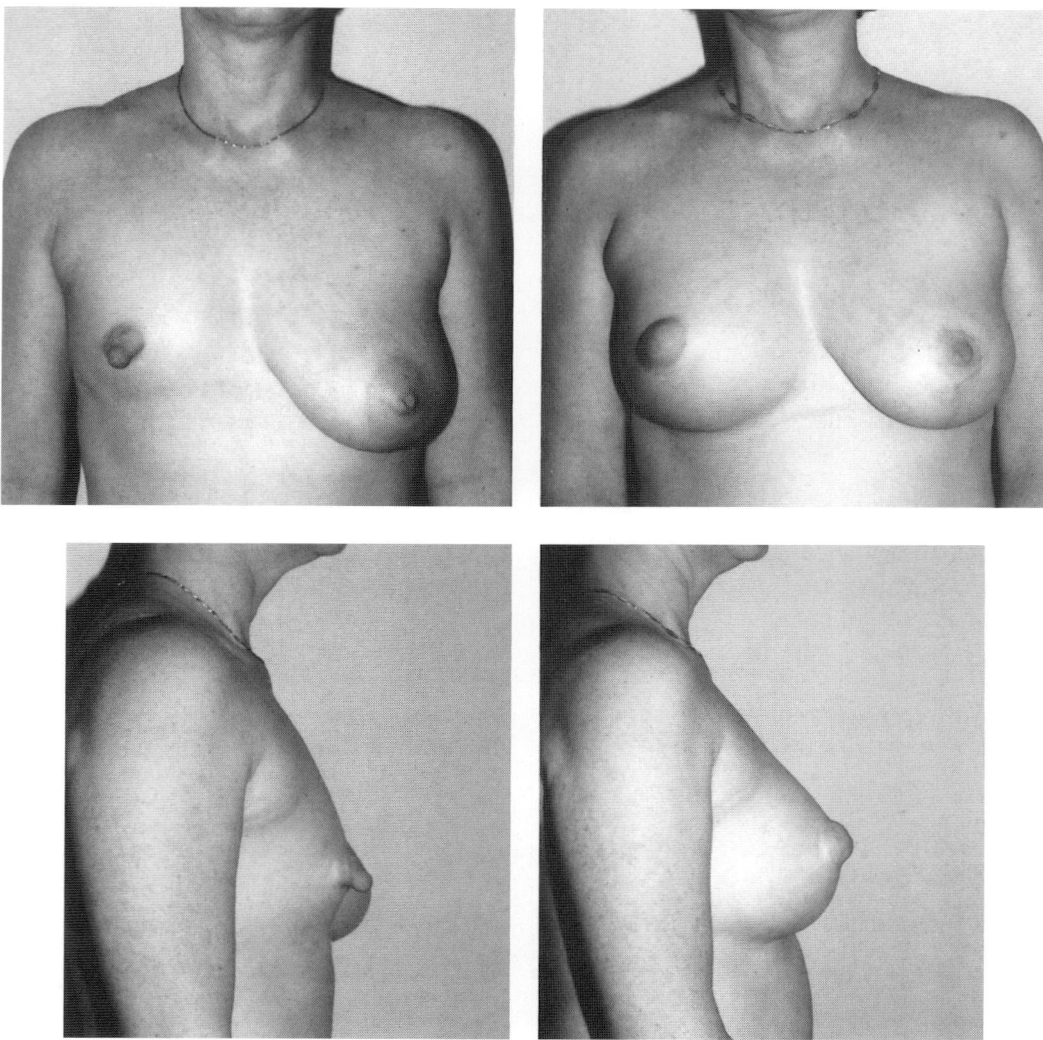

This woman had marked breast asymmetry with right mammary hypoplasia and left mammary hyperplasia. She requested a right breast augmentation and a left breast reduction. Breast augmentation was performed via the inframammary approach using a textured-surface implant. With the patient in a sitting position a reduction mammaplasty was done using the superior pedicle technique. The left breast was reduced and elevated to match the right breast as closely as possible. One year later the left breast shows signs of early ptosis. Better symmetry may be achieved with a small breast implant and additional lower left breast resection.

UNILATERAL BREAST HYPERPLASIA AND UNILATERAL HYPOPLASIA WITH CONSTRICTION

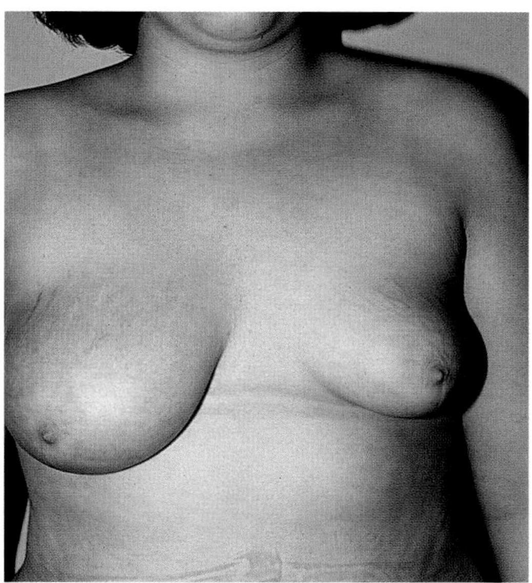

This young woman had major breast asymmetry and wanted her breasts to be more balanced and uplifted. Her right breast was ptotic and hyperplastic and her left breast was constricted with a laterally positioned areola. She liked the size of her right breast but disliked the droopy appearance. The surgical plan called for a right mastopexy and placement of a subpectoral breast implant to correct the left breast constriction. The periareolar approach was planned for the left side to move the areola to a more central, elevated position.

Surgical plan

- Augmentation of left breast and elevation and medial repositioning of left nipple-areola
- Right vertical mastopexy with elevation of right nipple-areola and narrowing of right breast
- Placement of breast implant in left subpectoral position for symmetry
- Left periareolar mastopexy to move nipple-areola superiorly and medially and to avoid narrowing constricted lower left breast
- Periareolar approach to left subpectoral space
- Expansion of lower breast parenchyma
- Placement of saline implant
- Right vertical mastopexy with movement of right nipple-areola to position to match left side and increase diameter
- Resection of lower breast parenchyma and closure of vertical mastopexy incision

Markings and Technique

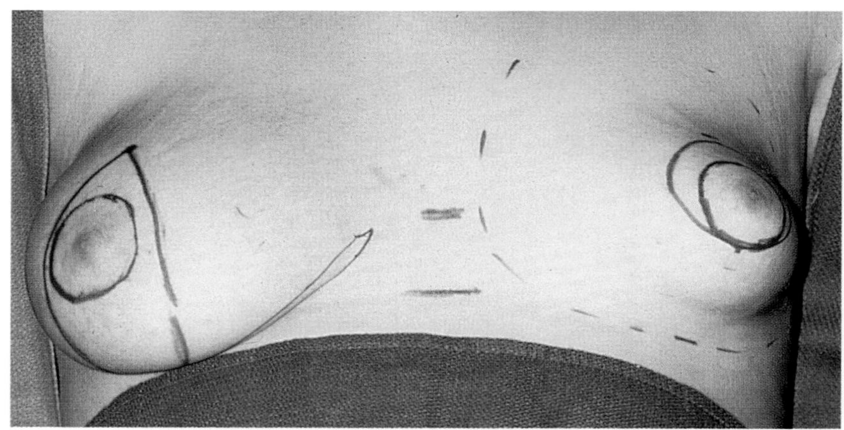

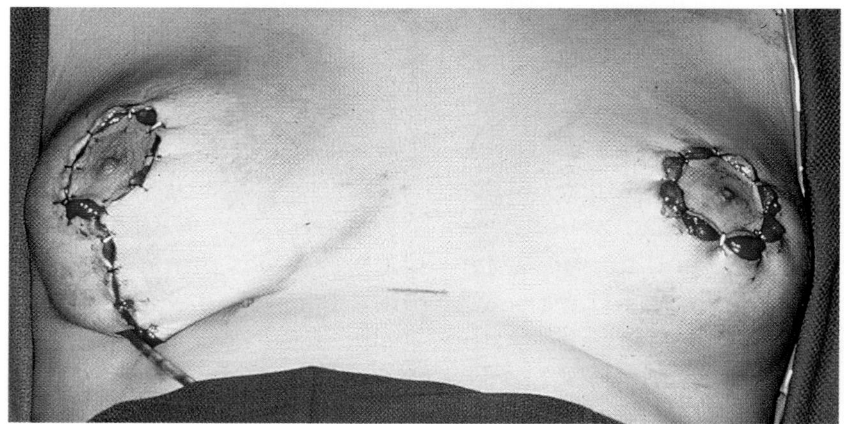

A vertical mastopexy is done on the right side, removing approximately 40 gm of parenchyma from the lower breast area to reduce the possibility of ptosis recurrence. The markings for the periareolar purse-string mastopexy are drawn on the left side to show how the final closure will move the areola in. The subpectoral pocket is created through this periareolar approach with release of the pectoral muscle medially and inferiorly. The initial intraoperative closure is shown after placement of the subpectoral 280 cc implant. Intracuticular sutures are used for the final closure.

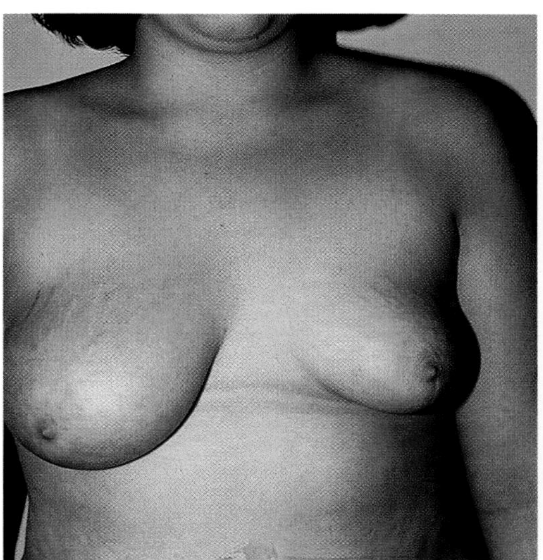
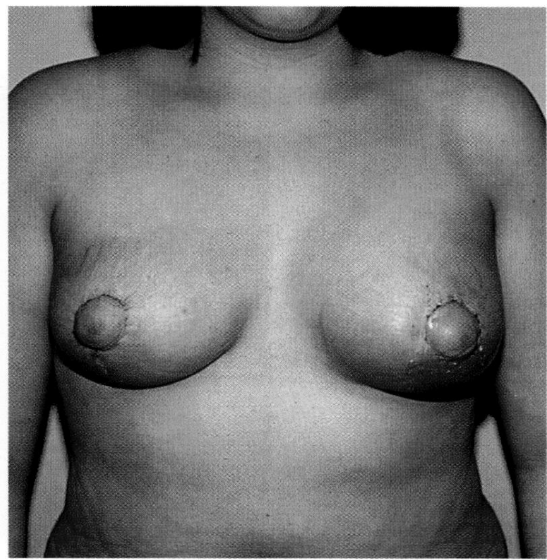

Postoperatively the appearance of the right breast is much improved. The ptosis has been slightly overcorrected to counter later recurrence, particularly since the left side will probably elevate somewhat with time. If she gains weight, she will have a larger breast on the right than on the left. She was alerted to this possibility in advance.

UNILATERAL OR BILATERAL PTOSIS WITH OTHER ASYMMETRIES

Patients who present with ptosis and asymmetry usually require breast recontouring and resection of lower breast tissue to preserve similar amounts of breast parenchyma to drape over the implants. The implants are then placed in the submusculofascial position above and in the subglandular position below. During resection it is important to shave the breast tangentially so that there is a good parenchymal cover over the implant. The same amount of skin and breast parenchyma should be preserved. I try to be very conservative in the markings for this condition and use the tailor-tack approach to mastopexy so that no extra skin is removed and no tight areas are left to cause postoperative dehiscence.

I use textured-surface implants in the upper subpectoral position for most mastopexy-augmentation patients when there is good cover to ensure that the implants are positioned low enough and will not move upward in the postoperative period. If the lower cover is thin, I use smooth-surface implants to avoid rippling and palpability. A complete lower and medial pectoralis major muscle release is necessary to ensure properly positioned implants.

Patient Examples

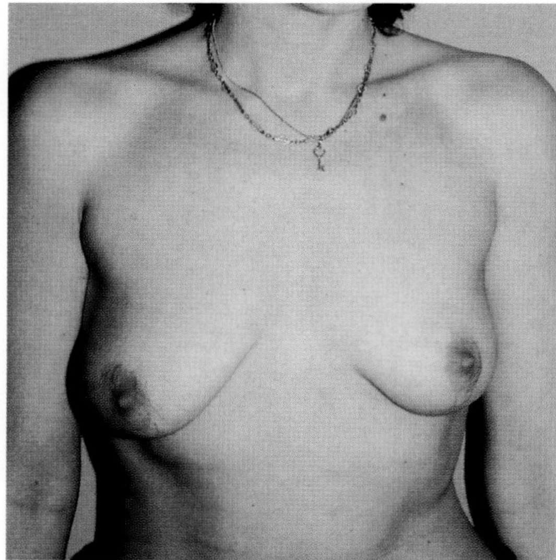

This young woman was always bothered by her asymmetric breasts. Her right breast was mildly ptotic, whereas her left breast exhibited signs of glandular ptosis with some constriction. She requested improved symmetry with larger breasts. Bilateral short horizontal incisions were planned. The procedure was done before I began using the vertical approach, which would be my preference if I were to operate on this patient today.

Surgical plan

- Bilateral correction of breast ptosis with upward mobilization of right nipple-areola and tightening of lower breast skin
- Subpectoral positioning of smooth-surface implants to give appropriate symmetry
- Inflation of implants for best volume adjustment
- Closure of mastopexy incisions

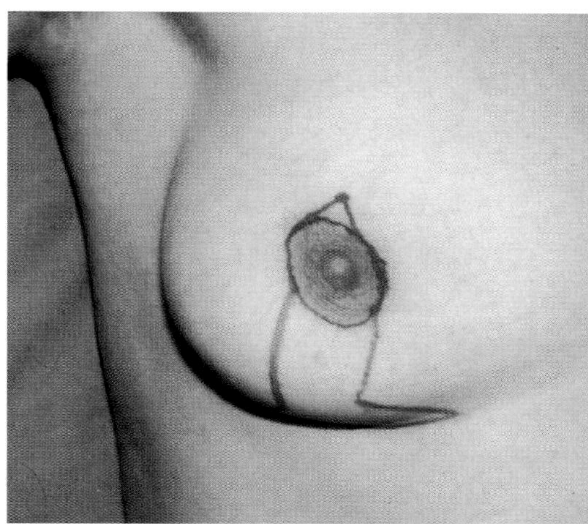

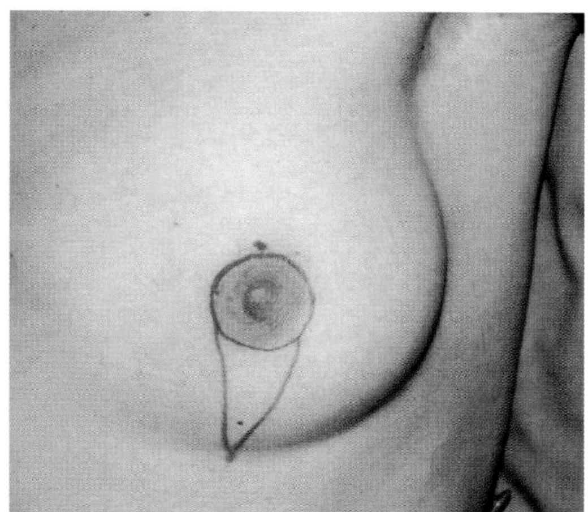

The patient was marked preoperatively for bilateral nipple-areolar elevation with a vertical incision on the left side and a vertical and short horizontal incision on the right side to more precisely define the areola-inframammary crease distance. Augmentation mammaplasty with the implant placed in the subpectoral position was planned.

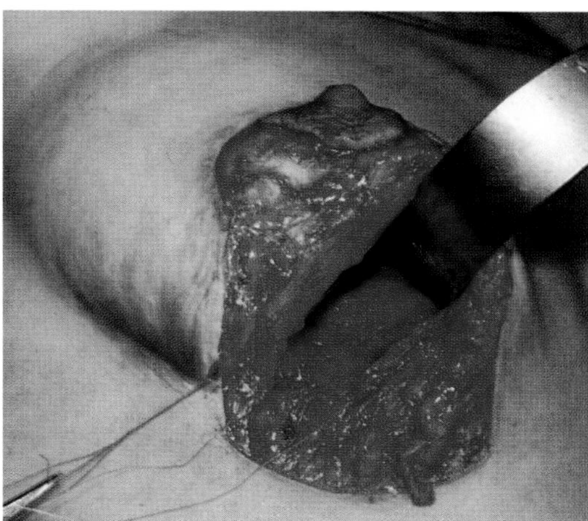

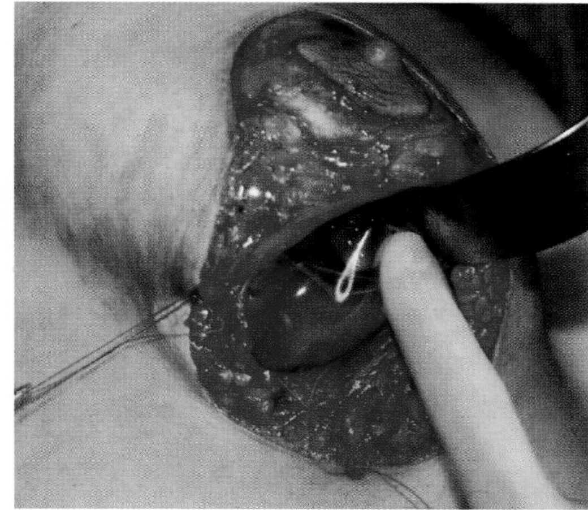

The submuscular dissection was completed, the implant positioned, and the incisions closed. The implant size was adjusted by additional inflation of the left implant.

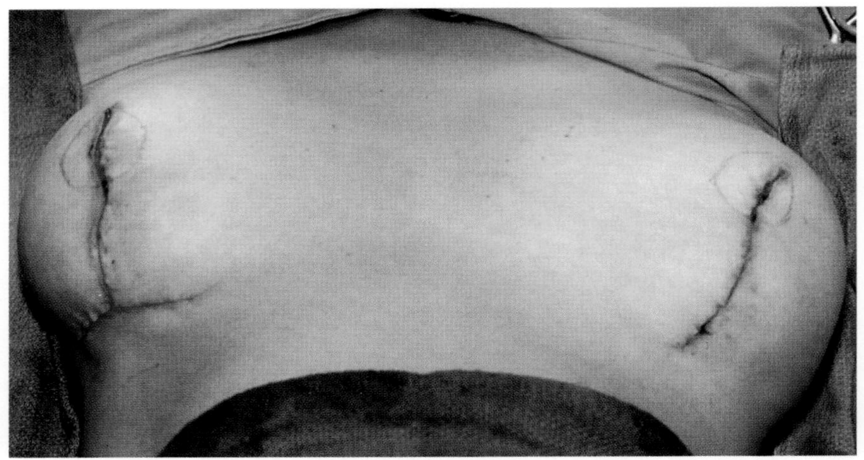

The nipple-areolar position was determined with the patient in the sitting position, and the nipple-areolae were brought out through the circular incisions. The nipple-areolae were based on the breast parenchyma.

Results

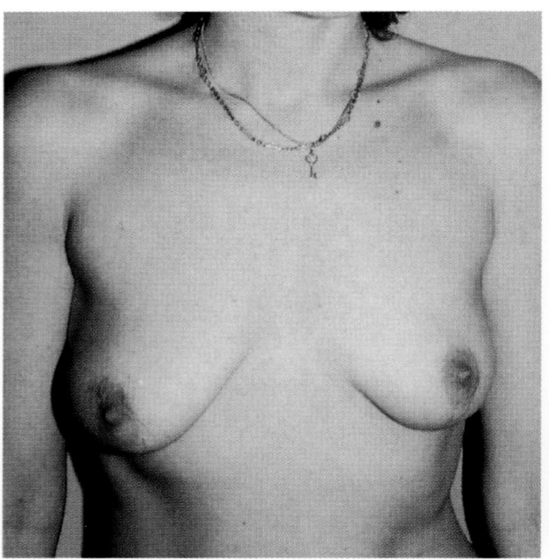

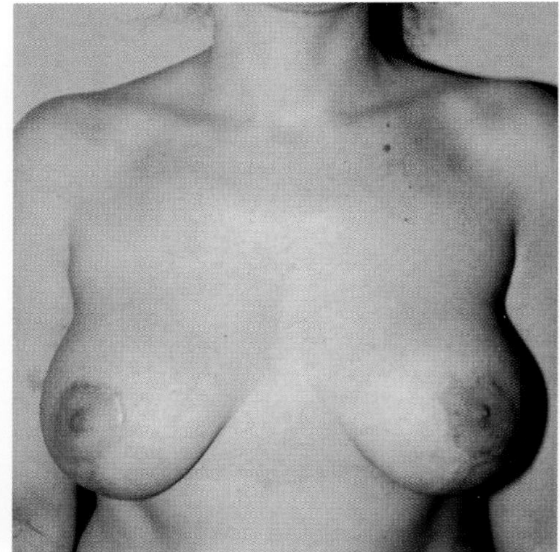

The patient is shown 6 months following the operation. She likes the improvement in her breast contour and size. Some widening of the breast scars has occurred, but healing is acceptable at this point in her recovery.

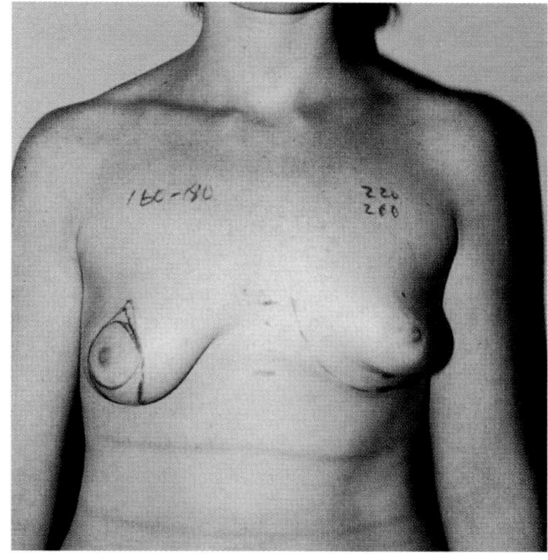

This 21-year-old patient had breast asymmetry. Both breasts were constricted, but the right breast was larger than the left. The right breast was ptotic over a high, constricted inframammary crease. Early ptosis and a tubular deformity of the left breast were noted. The plan called for a right vertical mastopexy and augmentation with a 180 cc implant and left inframammary subpectoral augmentation with a 260 cc implant. Some breast parenchyma must be removed from the right breast to correct the breast asymmetry. The future inframammary crease markings were drawn on the left side. Plans to lower the inframammary crease to this point called for radial incisions in the lower breast parenchyma.

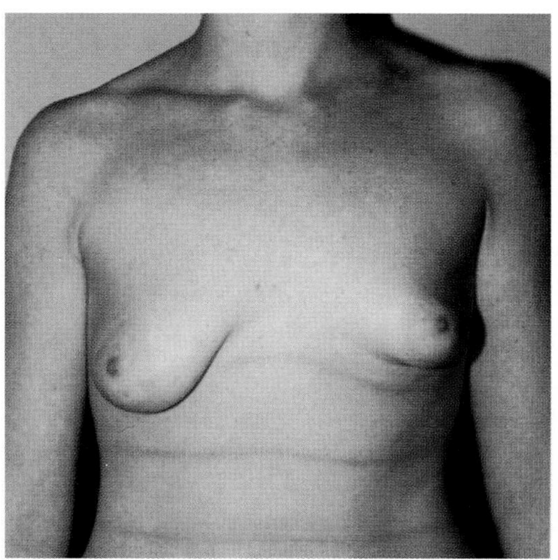

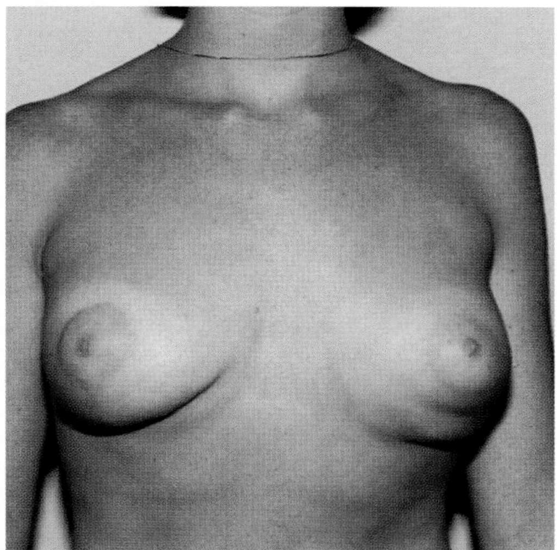

The patient is shown 1 year following the procedure. Although breast volume and symmetry are good, there is an irregular bulge in the lower portion of her left breast. Further release of the constricted lower breast parenchyma and intraoperative expansion may have improved the postoperative result. She demonstrates the double-bubble appearance, which is a common sequela following placement of implants in the extremely constricted and tubular breast.

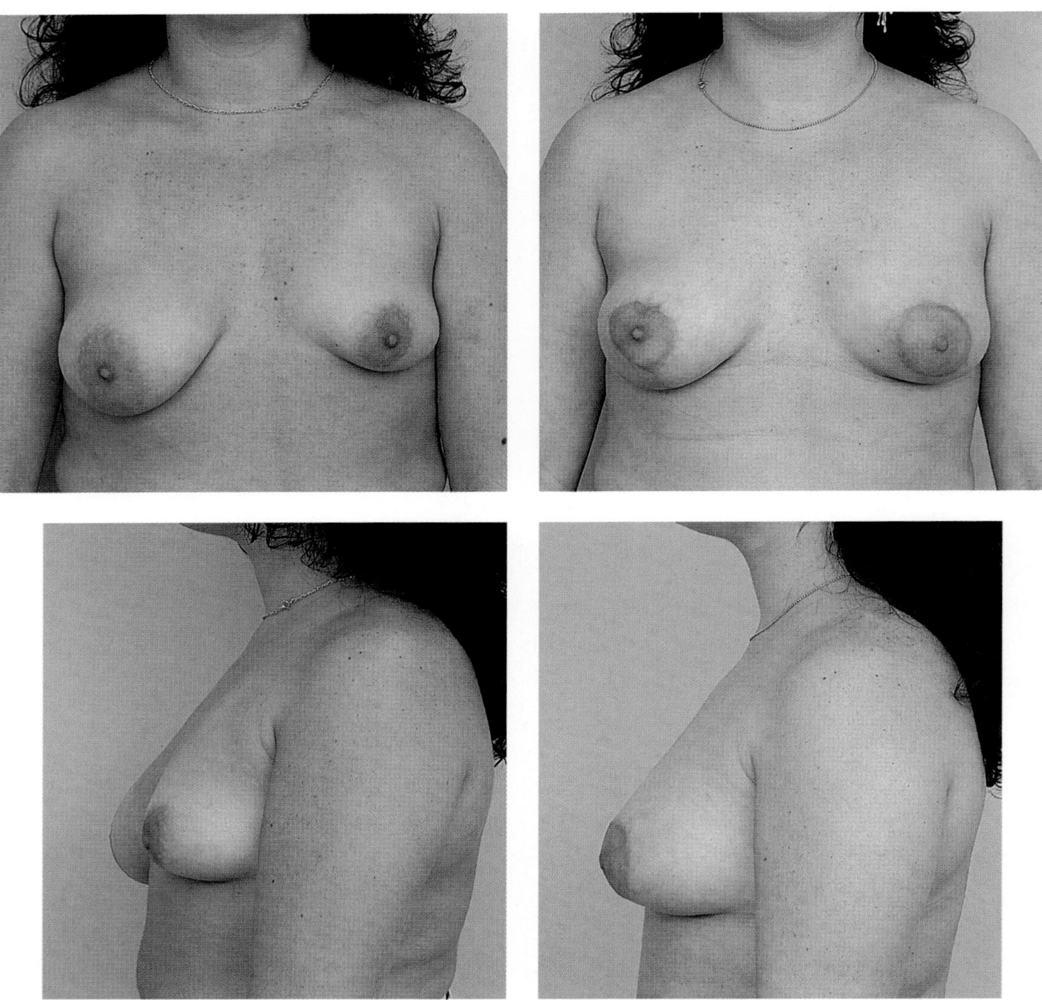

This 25-year-old woman had moderate ptosis of the right breast with a constricted left breast and requested correction of breast asymmetry. The surgical plan called for a right vertical mastopexy and a left periareolar purse-string elevation with expansion of the constricted breast and placement of a saline implant. Her general health was good and she had no family history of breast cancer. The right vertical mastopexy required removal of some central breast parenchyma with some rotation of central breast parenchyma to the upper breast region. The left subpectoral space was approached using the periareolar approach. The medial and inferior pectoral muscles were released. A 240 cc saline implant was selected to provide symmetry with the opposite breast and was placed in the subpectoral position above and the subglandular position below. The inframammary fold was lowered on the left side to obtain symmetry with the other breast; the lower breast parenchyma was released radially to expand and widen the lower breast. The periareolar approach elevates the areola and also widens the lower breast, as can be seen by comparing the patient's preoperative and postoperative photographs.

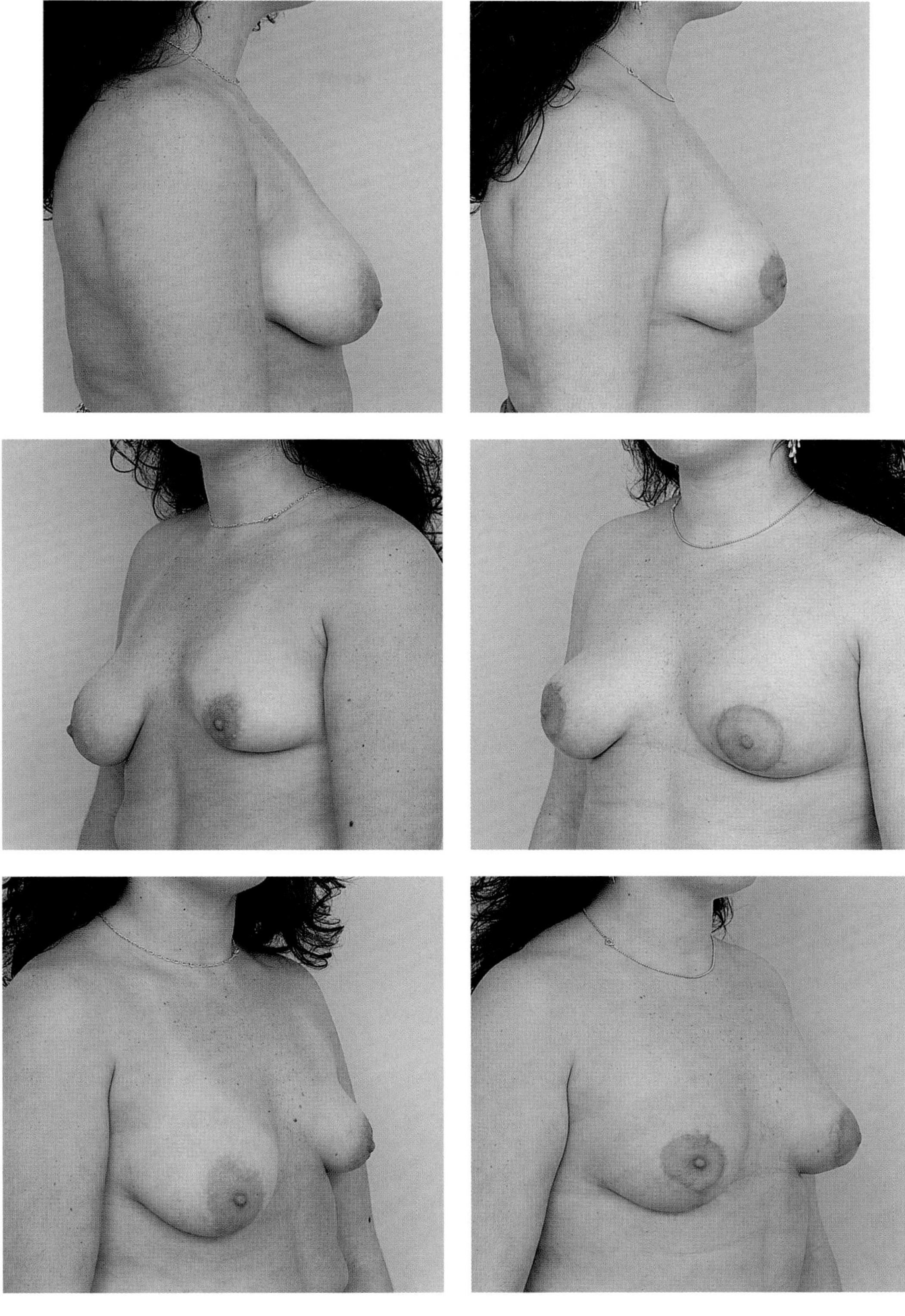

Reoperative Aesthetic Breast Surgery

AUGMENTATION MAMMAPLASTY

Reoperation following augmentation mammaplasty is usually performed to correct aesthetic problems related to capsular contracture, asymmetries, and patient dissatisfaction with breast size. The asymmetries can be related to volume, ptosis, or nipple-areolar position (see Chapter 6).

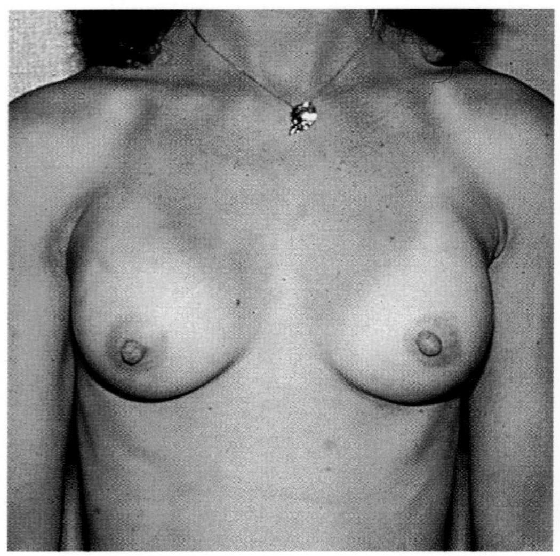

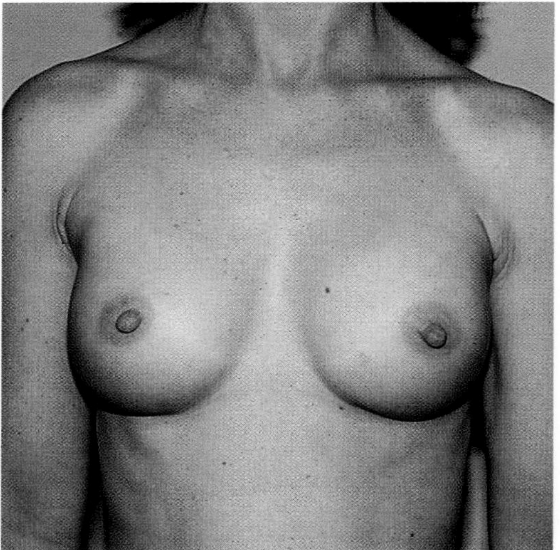

Ten years before this photograph was taken, this 38-year-old woman had breast augmentation with implants placed using the axillary subglandular approach. She had never been happy with her breast contour after the initial augmentation but became deeply dissatisfied after bilateral capsular contracture developed. She now felt that her implants were too high and too firm, a common problem with standard axillary breast augmentation techniques before the endoscope afforded better control and visualization for more accurate implant placement. Correction was planned through an inframammary approach. Capsulectomies were done inferiorly and laterally, and new subglandular pockets were created at the level of the proposed inframammary fold. The original 280 cc implants were removed and replaced with 340 cc smooth-surface saline implants. Her breasts have remained soft and the contour is much improved.

REDUCTION MAMMAPLASTY

Problems requiring reoperation after reduction mammaplasty include asymmetries, healing problems, overreduction, and underreduction. Inadequate breast reduction is the most frequent patient complaint; a secondary reduction is usually done as an outpatient procedure through the previous breast reduction incisions. If the initial reduction mammaplasty was performed by another surgeon, it is important to know what type of reduction procedure was performed, particularly how the nipple-areola was moved to its new position. The surgeon should discuss this with the patient; the initial operative note is also helpful. I have witnessed major problems with nipple-areola necrosis when the blood supply was divided at a secondary breast reduction, especially when appropriate consideration was not given to the initial pedicle and its blood supply. The patient is advised of the possibility of nipple-areola necrosis after transfer of the nipple-areola as a free graft.

Patient Example

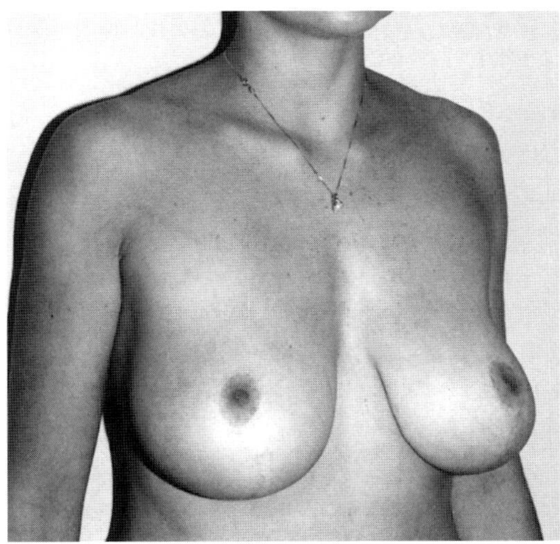

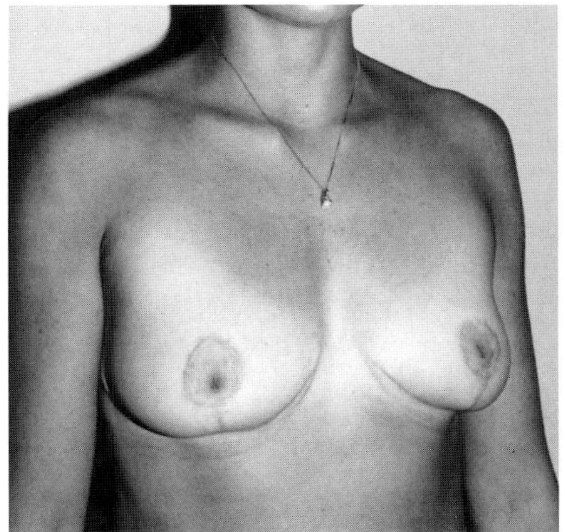

This 26-year-old woman had a breast reduction 6 years before her consultation. She said she had been a 34DD and was now a 34D. She was unhappy with the amount of reduction, feeling that her breasts were still too large. She requested a significant secondary reduction and correction of ptosis. Because the nipple-areolar position was nearly correct, the nipple-areolae were moved only a short distance based on the underlying parenchyma. A superior pedicle technique was used to reduce the lower portions of the breast and the width of the breast. The patient is shown 1 year following secondary breast reduction. She is pleased with the improvement and hopes that the scars will fade with time.

MASTOPEXY

Reoperative aesthetic problems usually involve ptosis recurrence. When a dermal mastopexy is performed initially and ptosis recurs, it is frequently associated with decreased upper pole fullness as well as ptosis of the breast parenchyma below the inframammary fold. When not used initially, I generally suggest placing breast implants at the secondary procedure. The ptotic breast parenchyma is resected, and textured-surface implants are placed in the submusculofascial position above and subglandularly below to reconstitute upper pole fullness. The resection eliminates the tissue that will ptose in the future. ***In the mastopexy patient it is not advisable to rely on the elasticity of the skin to support the breast if it failed to do so initially.*** When the closure of the T is too tight, especially when the patient is a cigarette smoker, separation and delayed healing of the T in the periareolar region are likely; this also requires reoperation.

MASTOPEXY-AUGMENTATION

Problems after mastopexy-augmentation can be caused by capsular contracture resulting in upward displacement of the breast implant. If a smooth-surface implant was used initially and the breast has ptosed over a capsular contracture, the implant becomes elevated; correction involves removing the implant and performing a capsulectomy or submuscular repositioning of the implant and substituting a textured-surface implant for the smooth-surface implant.

Patient Example

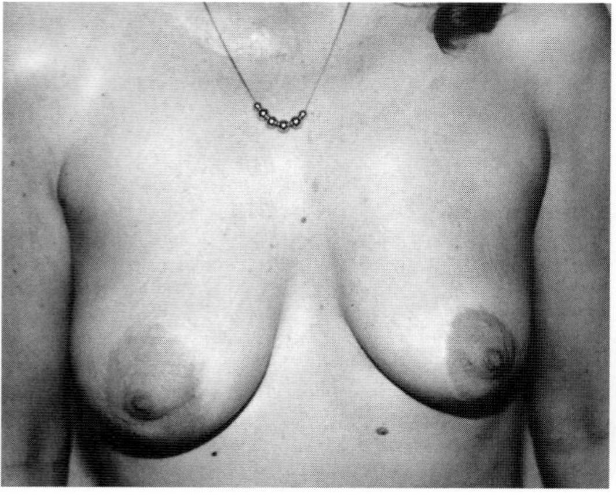

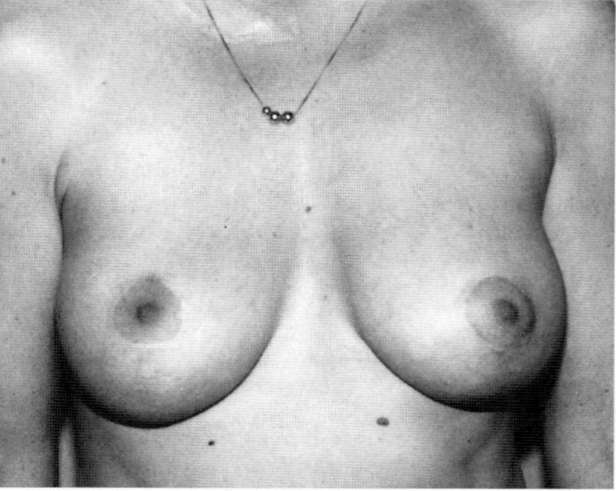

This woman exhibited breast asymmetry after unilateral mastopexy of her left breast. A secondary bilateral mastopexy was performed with placement of subpectoral implants. Additional breast tissue was removed from the lower portion of the right breast so that identically sized implants could be positioned bilaterally to provide future symmetry. The patient is shown 1 year following the procedure. Symmetry is improved and the breasts have remained soft. Generally long-term symmetry is enhanced when the same volume of breast parenchyma is retained and the same size breast implants are used. However, the development of capsular contracture or weight gain or loss will likely produce additional asymmetry.

Scarring After Aesthetic Breast Surgery

The patient who develops hypertrophic scarring after aesthetic breast surgery is predisposed to healing problems. With time, the hypertrophic scarring often settles down. Other strategies for obtaining finer scars include:

1. Injection of triamcinolone, 10 mg/ml, intralesionally
2. Postoperative pressure applied to the scars either with a foam pad inside a brassiere or with Steri-Strips
3. Long-term support of the wound with Steri-Strips after the initial sutures have been removed
4. Silicone sheeting to reduce scar hypertrophy

Hypertrophic scars are best avoided by not operating on the patient who has demonstrated a predisposition to keloids or hypertrophic scarring. Elimination of tension at the time of closure of the breast, using a short-scar technique, and keeping the scars central and below the nipple-areola also minimize the possibility of hypertrophic scar formation. This is particularly important after breast reductions. ***When tight medial and lateral closures are used to shape the breasts, I have noted that widened and hypertrophic scars can develop.*** Now that breast reductions are done so that there is minimal tightness laterally and the scars are shortened laterally and medially this has become less of a problem.

If the hypertrophy persists and the scars remain unattractive after a suitable postoperative period, I consider a scar revision. With this procedure the scar is excised, leaving possibly 0.5 mm of scar tissue along the margin of the wound. The skin flaps are undermined and freed up for about 1 cm so that when they are advanced together there is some eversion of a deeper dermal suture. An intracuticular pull-out permanent suture such as Prolene is used for the final closure. The sutures are left in place for several weeks. Following suture removal, prolonged support is maintained with Steri-Strips for 2 to 3 months or even longer until signs of wound activity as demonstrated by hyperemia are no longer evident.

REFERENCES

Abramo AC, Viola CJ. Liposuction through an axillary incision for treatment of gynecomastia. Aesthetic Plast Surg 13:85, 1989.

Balch CR. A transaxillary incision for gynecomastia. Plast Reconstr Surg 61:13, 1978.

Baroudi R, Lewis JR. The augmentation-reduction mammaplasty. Clin Plast Surg 3:301, 1976.

Beer GM, Kompatscher P, Hergan K. Diagnosis of breast tumors after breast reduction. Aesthetic Plast Surg 20:391, 1996.

Behrman RE, Vaughan VC, eds. Nelson's Textbook of Pediatrics, 12th ed. Philadelphia: WB Saunders, 1983.

Berrino P, Galli A, Rainero ML, Santi P. Unilateral reduction mammaplasty: Sculpturing the breast from the undersurface. Plast Reconstr Surg 82:88, 1988.

Bi DJ. Inverted nipple: A method of correction. Plast Reconstr Surg 87:1147, 1991.

Bostwick J III, Eaves FF III, Nahai F. Endoscopic Plastic Surgery. St. Louis: Quality Medical Publishing, 1995.

Broadbent TR, Woolf RM. Unsatisfactory results in augmentation mammoplasty: Chest and breast asymmetry. Aesthetic Plast Surg 2:251, 1978.

Carlson HE. Gynecomastia. N Engl J Med 303:795, 1980.

Corso PF. Plastic surgery of unilateral hypoplastic breast. Plast Reconstr Surg 50:134, 1972.

Courtiss EH. Suction lipectomy: A retrospective analysis of 100 patients. Plast Reconstr Surg 73: 780, 1984.

Crestinu JM. Correcting the inverted nipple. Plast Reconstr Surg 89:1181, 1992.

Eade GG. The radial incision for gynecomastia excisions. Plast Reconstr Surg 54:495, 1974.

Eaves FF III, Bostwick J III, Nahai F, Murray DR, Styblo TM, Carlson GW. Endoscopic techniques in aesthetic breast surgery. Augmentation, mastectomy, biopsy, capsulotomy, capsulorrhaphy, reduction, mastopexy, and reconstructive techniques. Clin Plast Surg 22:683, 1995.

Elliott RA, Hoehn JG. Asymmetrical breasts. In Georgiade NG, ed. Reconstructive Breast Surgery. St. Louis: CV Mosby, 1976.

Elliott RA, Hoehn JG, Greminger RF. Correction of asymmetrical breasts. Plast Reconstr Surg 56: 260, 1975.

El-Sharkawy AG. A method for correction of congenitally inverted nipple with preservation of the ducts. Plast Reconstr Surg 95:1111, 1995.

Fee TE, Caffee HH. Predictors of postoperative aesthetics following explantation of the augmented breast. Ann Plast Surg 38:217, 1997.

Ferreira LM, Neto MS, Okamoto RH, Andrews J de M. Surgical correction of nipple hypertrophy. Plast Reconstr Surg 95:753, 1995.

Gliosci A, Presutti F. Asymmetry of the breast: Some uncommon cases. Aesthetic Plast Surg 18:399, 1994.

Gruber RP, Jones HW Jr. The "donut" mastopexy: Indications and complications. Plast Reconstr Surg 65:34, 1980.

Hauben DJ, Mahler D. A simple method for correction of the inverted nipple. Plast Reconstr Surg 71:556, 1983.

Hueston J. Unilateral agenesis and hypoplasia: Difficulties and suggestions. In Goldwyn RM, ed. Plastic and Reconstructive Surgery of the Breast. Boston: Little, Brown, 1975.

Juri J. Mammary asymmetry: A brief classification. Aesthetic Plast Surg 13:47, 1989.

Kaye BL. Axillary breasts: An aesthetic deformity of the trunk. Clin Plast Surg 2:397, 1975.

Kaye BL. Axillary breasts. Plast Reconstr Surg 53:61, 1974.

Letterman G, Schurter M. Gynecomastia. In Courtiss EH, ed. Male Aesthetic Surgery. St. Louis: CV Mosby, 1982.

Letterman G, Schurter M. History of the surgical correction of mammary asymmetry. In Owsley JQ, Peterson RA, eds. Symposium in Aesthetic Surgery of the Breast. St. Louis: CV Mosby, 1978.

Lewis CM. Lipoplasty: Treatment for gynecomastia. Aesthetic Plast Surg 9:287, 1985.

Maclaren NK. Gynecomastia. In Gellis SS, Kagan BM, eds. Current Pediatric Therapy 11. Philadelphia: WB Saunders, 1984.

Marks F. The hazards of using the inferior pedicle technique for reduction in a patient with a previous submammary augmentation. Plast Reconstr Surg 98:751, 1996.

Mladick RA. Gynecomastia. Clin Plast Surg 18:815, 1991.

Murphy TP, Ehrlichman RJ, Seckel BR. Nipple placement in simple mastectomy with free nipple grafting for severe gynecomastia. Plast Reconstr Surg 94:818, 1994.

Netscher DT, Sharma S, Thornby J, Peltier M, Lyos A, Fater M, Mosharrafa A. Aesthetic outcome of breast implant removal in 85 consecutive patients. Plast Reconstr Surg 100:206, 1997.

Pitanguy I. Transareolar incision for gynecomastia. Plast Reconstr Surg 38:414, 1966.

Perras C. Asymmetry of the breast and the thoracic cage. Aesthetic Plast Surg 4:117, 1980.

Radlauer CB, Bowers DG. Treatment of severe breast asymmetry. Plast Reconstr Surg 47:347, 1971.

Rees TD. Mammary asymmetry. Clin Plast Surg 2:371, 1975.

Rees TD, Aston SJ. The tuberous breast. Clin Plast Surg 3:339, 1976.

Rees TD, Dupuis CC. Unilateral mammary hypoplasia. Plast Reconstr Surg 41:307, 1968.

Regnault P. Ptosis, asymmetry, tubular breast, and congenital anomalies. In Owsley JQ, Peterson RA, eds. Symposium on Aesthetic Surgery of the Breast. St. Louis: CV Mosby, 1978.

Regnault P. Nipple hypertrophy. Clin Plast Surg 2:391, 1975.

Reyes RJ, Zicchi S, Hamed H, Chaudhary MA, Fentiman IS. Surgical correction of gynaecomastia in bodybuilders. Br J Clin Pract 49:177, 1995.

Rintala AE, Nordstrom RE. Treatment of severe developmental asymmetry of the female breast. Scand J Plast Reconstr Surg Hand Surg 23:231, 1989.

Rohrich RJ, Beran SJ, Kenkel JM. Ultrasound-Assisted Liposuction. St. Louis: Quality Medical Publishing, 1998.

Rosenberg GJ. Gynecomastia. Suction lipectomy as a contemporary solution. Plast Reconstr Surg 80:379, 1987.

Shulman Y, Westreich M. Treatment of mild breast asymmetry. Plast Reconstr Surg 67:31, 1981.

Simon BE, Hoffman S, Kahn S. Treatment of asymmetry of the breasts. A report of 30 cases of developmental origin. Clin Plast Surg 2:375, 1975.

Simon BE, Hoffman S, Kahn S. Classification and surgical correction of gynecomastia. Plast Reconstr Surg 51:48, 1973.

Smith GA. Hazard of inferior pedicle breast reduction concurrent with explantation of old subglandular implants. Plast Reconstr Surg 97:254, 1996.

Slavin SA, Goldwyn RM. Silicone gel implant explantation: Reasons, results, and admonitions. Plast Reconstr Surg 95:63, 1995.

Smoot EC III. Eccentric skin resection and purse-string closure for skin reduction with mastectomy for gynecomastia. Ann Plast Surg 41:378, 1998.

Spence RJ, Feldman JJ, Ryan JJ. Symmastia: The problem of medial confluence of the breasts. Plast Reconstr Surg 73:261, 1984.

Teimourian B, Adham MN. Surgical correction of the tuberous breast. Ann Plast Surg 10:190, 1983.

Teimourian B, Perlman R. Surgery for gynecomastia. Aesthetic Plast Surg 7:155, 1983.

Teimourian B, Adham MN. Simple technique for correction of inverted nipple. Plast Reconstr Surg 65:504, 1980.

Thomas WO III, Harper LL, Wong SW, Michalski JP, Harris CN, Moore JT, Rodning CB. Explantation of silicone breast implants. Ann Surg 63:421, 1997.

Vandenbussche F. Asymmetries of the breast: A classification system. Aesthetic Plast Surg 8:27, 1984.

Von Heimburg D, Exner K, Kruft S, Lemperle G. The tuberous breast deformity: Classification and treatment. Br J Plast Surg 49:339, 1996.

Williams G, Hoffman S. Mammoplasty for tubular breasts. Aesthetic Plast Surg 5:51, 1981.

Williams JE. Complete breast absence. Plast Reconstr Surg 49:253, 1972.

Index

C

D

E

Q

R

S

U

V

W